PERINATAL PROGRAMMING

Early Life Determinants of Adult Health & Disease

Edited by

DEBORAH M HODGSON PhD
Director of the Laboratory of Neuroimmunology
School of Behavioural Sciences
University of Newcastle
Callaghan
NSW
Australia

CHRISTOPHER L COE PhD
WB Cannon Professor of BioPsychology
Department of Psychology
Director of the Harlow Center for Biological Psychology
University of Wisconsin
Madison, WI
USA

Foreword by
DAVID BARKER FRS
MRC Epidemiology Resource Centre
Southampton General Hospital
Southampton
UK

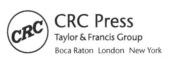

CRC Press
Taylor & Francis Group
Boca Raton London New York

CRC Press is an imprint of the
Taylor & Francis Group, an **informa** business

CRC Press
Taylor & Francis Group
6000 Broken Sound Parkway NW, Suite 300
Boca Raton, FL 33487-2742

First issued in paperback 2019

© 2006 by Taylor & Francis Group, LLC
CRC Press is an imprint of Taylor & Francis Group, an Informa business

No claim to original U.S. Government works

ISBN-13: 978-1-84214-294-3 (hbk)
ISBN-13: 978-0-367-39144-7 (pbk)

A CIP record for this book is available from the British Library.

Typeset by J&L Composition, Filey, North Yorkshire

Visit the Taylor & Francis Web site at
http://www.taylorandfrancis.com

and the CRC Press Web site at
http://www.crcpress.com

Contents

SECTION I PRENATAL DETERMINANTS OF FETAL GROWTH, BIRTH OUTCOMES AND LATER DISEASE RISK

SECTION II PRENATAL PROGRAMMING OF THE NEUROENDOCRINE SYSTEM – LINKS TO TYPE 2 DIABETES, OBESITY, AND CARDIOVASCULAR DISEASE

Contributors

Elie D Al-Chaer PhD JD
Section of Critical Care Medicine
University of Arkansas for Medical Sciences
Arkansas Children's Hospital
Little Rock, AR, USA

Kanwaljeet Singh Anand MBBS Dphil
Associate Professor of Pediatrics
Anesthesia and Anatomy
University of Arkansas for Medical Sciences
Arkansas Children's Hospital
Little Rock, AR, USA

David Barker FRS
MRC Epidemiology Resource Centre
Southampton General Hospital
Southampton, UK

Sheri A Berenbaum PhD
Department of Psychology
The Pennsylvania State University
Pennsylvania, PA, USA

Adnan T Bhutta MD FAAP
Critical Care Medicine
Department of Pediatrics
University of Arkansas for Medical Sciences
Arkansas Children's Hospital
Little Rock, AR, USA

Frank H Bloomfield BSc MB ChB MRCP FRACP PhD
Liggins Institute
Faculty of Medicine and Health Sciences
University of Auckland
Auckland, New Zealand

Wim JA Boersma PhD
Animal Sciences Group
Wageningen University and Research Centre
AB, Lelystad, The Netherlands

Laura Rosa Brunet PhD
Centre for Infectious Diseases and International
Health
Windeyer Institute of Medical Sciences
Royal Free and University College Medical School
London, UK

Irina P Butkevich PhD
IP Pavlov Institute of Physiology RAS
Laboratory of Ontogeny of Nervous System
Nab Makarova
St Petersburg, Russia

John RG Challis DSc FRSC
Departments of Physiology and Obstetrics &
Gynaecology
University of Toronto
Toronto, ON, Canada

Francesco Chiappelli PhD
Associate Professor of Oral Biology & Medicine
School of Dentistry
University of California, Los Angeles, CA, USA

Vicki L Clifton PhD
Mothers and Babies Research Centre
Hunter Medical Research Institute
University of Newcastle
Callaghan, NSW, Australia

Christopher L Coe PhD
WB Cannon Professor of BioPsychology
Department of Psychology
Faculty of Medicine
Harlow Primate Laboratory
University of Wisconsin
Madison, WI, USA

Miles J De Blasio BSc
Department of Physiology
University of Adelaide
Adelaide, SA, Australia

Johanna de Groot PhD
Animal Sciences Group
Wageningen University and Research Centre
AB, Lelystad, The Netherlands

Josie Diorio BSc
Developmental Neuroendocrinology Laboratory
Douglas Hospital Research Centre
Departments of Psychiatry, and Neurology and
Neurosurgery
McGill University
Montréal, QC, Canada

Nancy A Dreschel DVM
Department of Dairy and Animal Science
College of Agricultural Sciences
The Pennsylvania State University
Pennsylvania, PA, USA

Jaime A Duffield BSc
School of Molecular and Biomedical Science
University of Adelaide
Adelaide, SA, Australia

Janet Dunstan BAppSc PGDip PhD
School of Paediatrics and Child Health
Department of Paediatrics
University of Western Australia
Perth, WA, Australia

Marie Dziadek BSc DPhil
School of Biological Sciences
Molecular Genetics and Development Group
Mammalian Development Laboratory
University of Auckland
Auckland, New Zealand

Ilona S Federenko PhD
Assistant Professor
Department of Psychology and Social Behaviour
University of California, Irvine
Irvine, CA, USA

Kathryn L Gatford PhD
Department of Obstetrics and Gynaecology
University of Adelaide
Adelaide, SA, Australia

Warwick B Giles MB BS FRACOG PhD DDU CMFM
Mothers and Babies Research Centre
Hunter Medical Research Institute
University of Newcastle
Callaghan, NSW, Australia

Vivette Glover MA PhD DSc
Professor of Perinal Psychobiology
IRDB, Imperial College London
London, UK

Douglas A Granger PhD
Behavioral Endocrinology Laboratory
Department of Biobehavioral Health
Pennsylvania State University
Pennsylvania, PA, USA

Richard W Hall MD
Department of Pediatrics
University of Arkansas for Medical Sciences
Little Rock, AR, USA

Jane E Harding MB ChB Dphil FRACP FRSNZ
Professor of Neonatology
Liggins Institute
Faculty of Medical and Health Sciences
University of Auckland
Auckland, New Zealand

Ian Hellstrom BSc MSc
Douglas Hospital Research Centre
Research in Molecular and Cellular Neuroscience
Montréal, QC, Canada

Deborah M Hodgson PhD
School of Behavioural Sciences
University of Newcastle
Callaghan, NSW, Australia

Dane M Horton BSc
Department of Obstetrics and Gynaecology
University of Adelaide
Adelaide, SA, Australia

Ludmila I Khozhai PhD
IP Pavlov Institute of Physiology RAS
Laboratory of Ontogeny of Nervous System
Nab Makarova
St Petersburg, Russia

Karen L Kind PhD
Department of Obstetrics and Gynaecology
University of Adelaide
Adelaide, SA, Australia

Sietse Jan Koopmans PhD
Animal Sciences Group
Wageningen University and Research Centre
AB, Lelystad, The Netherlands

Gabriele R Lubach PhD
Assistant Scientist
Harlow Center for Biological Psychology
University of Wisconsin
Madiston, WI, USA

Patrick McGown PhD
McGill Program for the Study of Behavior, Genes and
Environment
Department of Pharmacology
McGill University
Montréal, QC, Canada

I Caroline McMillen DPhil MB BChir
Faculty of Medicine
Chair in Physiology
University Research Centre for the Physiology of
Early Development
University of Adelaide, SA, Australia

Roberta Martinelli PhD
Centre for Infectious Diseases and International
Health
Windeyer Institute of Medical Sciences
Royal Free and University College Medical School
London, UK

Stephen G Matthews BSc PhD
Department of Physiology
Faculty of Medicine
University of Toronto
Medical Sciences Building
Toronto, ON, Canada

Michael J Meaney PhD
Departments of Psychiatry, and Neurology and
Neurosurgery
Douglas Hospital Research Centre
McGill University
Montréal, QC, Canada

Viktor A Mikhailenko PhD
IP Pavlov Institute of Physiology RAS
Laboratory of Ontogeny of Nervous System
Nab Makarova
St Petersburg, Russia

Beverly S Muhlhausler BSc
School of Molecular and Biomedical Science
University of Adelaide
Adelaide, SA, Australia

Vanessa E Murphy PhD
Mothers and Babies Research Centre
Hunter Medical Research Institute
University of Newcastle
Callaghan, NSW, Australia

John P Newnham FRANZCOG MD
School of Women's and Infant's Health
The University of Western Australia
and
The Women and Infants Research Foundation
King Edward Memorial Hospital
Perth, WA, Australia

Theo Niewold PhD
Faculty of Bioscience Engineering
Catholic University of Leuven
Heverlee, Belgium

Moffat J Nyirenda MRCP PhD
Lecturer in Medicine
Endocrinology Unit
University of Edinburgh
School of Medicine
Western General Hospital
Edinburgh, UK

Thomas G O'Connor PhD
Department of Psychiatry
University of Rochester Medical Center
Rochester, NY, USA

Mark H Oliver BSc MSc PhD
Liggins Institute
Faculty of Medicine and Health Sciences
University of Auckland
Auckland, New Zealand

Vladimir A Otellin PhD
Professor of Neuromorphology
The Chief of Laboratory of Ontogeny of Nervous
System
IP Pavlov Institute of Physiology RAS
Laboratory of Ontogeny of Nervous System
Nab Makarova
St Petersburg, Russia

Julie A Owens PhD
Department of Physiology
University of Adelaide
Adelaide, SA, Australia

Juha Pekkanen MD
Head of the unit of Environmental Epidemiology,
National Public Health Institute
Kuopio, Finland

David IW Phillips MA PhD FRCP
University of Southampton
Medical Research Council
Southampton, UK

Susan L Prescott MBBS BMedSci FRACP PhD
Associate Professor in Paediatrics
Consultant Immunologist and Allergiest
School of Paediatrics and Child Health
Department of Paediatrics
University of Western Australia
and
Princess Margaret Hospital
Perth, WA, Australia

Sami T Remes MD MPH
Pediatric Allergist
National Public Health Institute
Kuopio, Finland

Jeffrey S Robinson BSc MB BCh BAO FRCOG
FRANZCOG
Department of Obstetrics and Gynaecology
University of Adelaide
Adelaide, SA, Australia

Graham AW Rook BA MB Bchir MD
Professor of Medical Microbiology
Centre for Infectious Diseases and International
Health
Windeyer Institute of Medical Sciences
Royal Free and University College Medical School
London, UK

Cynthia R Rovnaghi MS
University of Arkansas for Medical Sciences
Arkansas Children's Hospital
Little Rock, AR, USA

Teun Schuurman PhD
Animal Sciences Group
Wageningen University and Research Centre
AB, Lelystad, The Netherlands

Jonathan R Seckl FRCPE FmedSci FRSE
Moncrieff-Arnott Professor of Molecular Medicine
Endocrinology Unit
Centre for Cardiovascular Science
Queen's Medical Research Institute
Edinburgh, UK

Deborah M Sloboda PhD
School of Women's and Infant's Health
The University of Western Australia
and
The Women and Infants Research Foundation
King Edward Memorial Hospital
Perth, WA, Australia

Roger Smith MB BS FRACP PhD
Faculty of Medicine
Mothers and Babies Research Centre
University of Newcastle
Callaghan, NSW, Australia

Norbert Stockhofe DVM Vetpath
Animal Sciences Group
Wageningen University and Research Centre
AB, Lelystad, The Netherlands

Moshe Szyf PhD
McGill Program for the Study of Behavior, Genes and
Environment
Department of Pharmacology
McGill University
Montréal, QC, Canada

Anna N Taylor PhD
Department of Neurobiology
UCLA School of Medicine
Los Angeles, CA, USA

Susan H Tritt MD PhD FACOG
Department of Neurobiology
UCLA School of Medicine
Los Angeles, CA, USA

Tette van der Lende PhD
Animal Sciences Group
Wageningen University and Research Centre
AB, Lelystad, The Netherlands

Franz Josef van der Staay PhD
Animal Sciences Group
Wageningen University and Research Centre
AB, Lelystad, The Netherlands

Pathik D Wadhwa MD PhD
Behavioral Perinatology Research Program
Departments of Psychiatry & Human Behavior and
Obstetrics and Gynecology
University of California, Irvine
College of Medicine
Gillespie Neuroscience Research Facility (GNRF)
Irvine, CA, USA

Ian CG Weaver BSc MSc
McGill Program for the Study of Behavior, Genes and
Environment
Department of Pharmacology
McGill University
Montréal, QC, Canada

Marta Weinstock BPharm MSc PhD
Department of Pharmacology
School of Pharmacy
Hebrew University Medical Centre, Ein Kerem
Jerusalem, Israel

Tao Wu BSc
McGill Program for the Study of Behavior, Genes and
Environment
Department of Pharmacology
McGill University
Montréal, QC, Canada

Raz Yirmiya PhD
Department of Psychology
The Hebrew University of Jerusalem
Mount Scopus, Jerusalem, Israel

Dedication

This book is dedicated to all of our parents, who provided the formative and nurturing experiences that ensured the success of our own academic and personal trajectories.

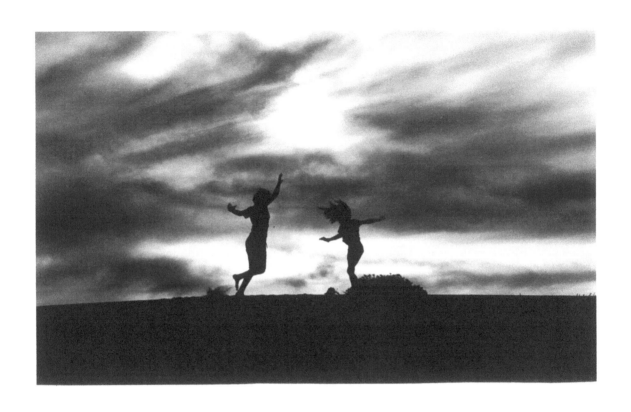

'Facts which at first seem improbable will, even on scant explanation, drop the cloak which has hidden them and stand forth in naked and simple beauty' Galileo

Foreword

The hypothesis that common chronic diseases are initiated through developmental processes in utero arose from geographical studies published twenty years ago. The evidence was circumstantial and the mechanisms unknown. The publication of this book shows that the developmental origins of chronic disease now has a rapidly expanding scientific basis, built on studies in humans and animals.

The new developmental model for chronic disease postulates not only that initiating events, such as restriction of the functional capacity of an organ, occur during early development but that an individual's vulnerability to the environment in later life is acquired at that time. A number of obstacles have had to be overcome in order to create this developmental perspective for the commonest causes of premature death and disability, which include coronary heart disease, stroke, hypertension, type 2 diabetes and osteoporosis. It was initially argued that the associations between these diseases and low birthweight were the result of confounding variables. Specifically the argument was that people whose growth was impaired in utero because of an adverse environment continue to be exposed to adversity after and it is this that produces the effects attributed to low birthweight. There is now strong evidence against this.

A consistent feature of the associations with birthweight is that disease rates fall progressively across the entire range of weight so that people who weighed 7 pounds at birth are at lower risk than those who weighed 6 pounds, and those who weighed 9 pounds are at lower risk than those who weighed 8 pounds. This implies that what were regarded as normal variations in the delivery of nutrients to the human fetus have profound implications for health in later life, a concept that has proved difficult for some clinicians, whose attention is necessarily focussed on people with pathologically low birthweight. There are similar graded associations between disease and weight at one year of age.

There is an emerging consensus that the nutrient supply to the baby, rather than other influences such as hypoxia, is the major influence that shapes its organs and systems. An obstacle to acceptance of this has been that fetal nutrition is sometimes equated with maternal nutrition. Because western women appear adequately nourished, the argument runs, western babies must also be adequately nourished. Such a view does not take into account the long and vulnerable fetal supply line, which includes the placenta, through which nutrients are transferred to the baby; nor does it acknowledge the sometimes competing demands of mother and baby. Because, in western communities, supplementation of the diets of pregnant women has relatively small effects on birthweight, the view has formed that fetal development is little influenced by normal variations in maternal diet. This neglects growing evidence from experimental studies and assisted reproductive technology that periconceptional nutrition establishes the trajectory of fetal growth and thereby sets the demand for nutrients in mid-late gestation. The view also takes no account of the balance of nutrients in the mother's diet, which is now known to be important.

Another obstacle that has had to be overcome is that some of the associations between birthweight and intermediary markers of disease, including blood pressure, are small. This contrasts, however, with the large effects of birthweight on clinical cardiovascular disease, including hypertension. It suggests that lesions accompanying poor fetal growth which lead to hypertension have a small influence on blood pressure because counter-regulatory mechanisms are able to maintain normal blood pressure levels for many years after birth. Ultimately these mechanisms fail to maintain homeostasis and clinical hypertension develops.

These obstacles can now be set aside and the stage is set for rapid progress towards the main goals of research into the developmental origins of disease. These goals are the primary prevention of chronic adult disease, the identification of childhood markers of disease and an understanding of the biological processes that link early development and later health. Disease prevention will depend on improvements in fetal, infant and early childhood nutrition. As a marker of disease risk, low birthweight is convenient but crude. The war-time famine in Holland produced lifelong insulin resistance in babies who were in utero at the time with little alteration in birthweight. Nevertheless the combination of small body size at birth and during infancy followed by rapid weight gain in childhood is a powerful marker of risk.

This book describes a wonderful and diverse array of biological processes that occur during development and affect later health. The book moves beyond established areas such as the developmental effects on insulin resistance, renal function and body composition. It describes effects on endocrine axes, on pain, behaviour, emotion, reproduction, well-being. It reviews the 'hygiene hypothesis', a phrase first used to explore the developmental origins of appendicitis but now used to explore the origins of asthma. The theme of this book is that the environment of the mother, baby and young child is critical. Some systems of the body have to be evoked by environmental experience during development: vision is a well-known example. Environmental and epigenetic influences on gene expression during development determine lifelong biological variations between one individual and another. Even small changes in nutrition, or other aspects of the environment at critical periods of development can lead to profound and lasting changes in the body's homeostasis. Well-being reflects the body's ability to maintain constancy in its internal environment in the face of challenges. Homeostatic systems that develop in an undernourished baby, or in one stressed in other ways, may be less able to withstand the challenges of rapid nutritional excess, childhood weight gain or poor living conditions in postnatal life. A child unloved, stressed or deprived may be less able to accommodate the emotional ups and downs of life.

Models of disease causation based on the unidirectional effects of genes have largely failed. There are many reasons for protecting early human development and increasing our understanding of it. This book strengthens the case.

David Barker
University of Southampton, UK
Oregon Health and Science University, USA

Preface

The concept of prenatal programming formulated initially from the effects of malnutrition and undernutrition on the developing infant has now been extended to many other domains. The fundamental concept that there can be a recalibration of the regulatory set points in the baby also seems to apply to many physiological processes beyond just later glucoregulation and the cardiovascular system in the adult. In particular, the development of the neuroendocrine system in the baby appears to be especially sensitive to extrinsic events that impinged upon the mother. These findings concur with the well-established view that there is a critical period during fetal life when many physiological systems become 'organized', and that the nature of that organizational influence then has extensive ramifications throughout the lifespan.

This conclusion that the fetal stage is a malleable one, during which the environment already begins to shape the individual, is a logical extension of the large body of research demonstrating that young infants are very responsive to early experiences during rearing. Developmental studies have clearly shown that many aspects of the brain, endocrine, and immune systems are not fully mature at birth, and depend upon environmental stimuli to shape and guide normal maturation. In a very real sense, each can be thought of as a 'learning system', responsive to the environmental context, which affords a critical degree of plasticity that optimizes flexibility and adaptation.

This books brings together many different perspectives supporting and extending the idea of 'fetal programming', and highlights the importance of the prenatal environment. It is now clear that the trajectory toward health or illness is started *in utero*. There are many important social and medical implications of this realization. For example, it appears that there can be long-lasting and inter-generational effects of gestating babies under adverse societal and economic conditions, which requires us to think more compassionately about the welfare of others, especially in the developing world. We are just beginning to understand the full significance of these prenatal influences on brain development and learning ability, and the ramifications for the competence of the immune system to fight off pathogens and prevent disease.

A relationship between early life events and long-term health outcomes was already postulated over 30 years ago. Professor David Barker and colleagues from Southampton demonstrated that children of lower birth weight were at increased risk for high blood pressure, cardiovascular disease, and type 2 diabetes. These provocative findings led to a large corpus of subsequent research, which focused on the role of undernutrition in determining fetal outcomes. The first two chapters of our book discuss the important role played by maternal, placental, and fetal processes that regulate growth *in utero*. Maternal nutrition and the balance of nutrients, *even at the moment of conception*, all appear to be significant predictors of fetal growth and birth outcomes. However, there has been a shift away from the unidimensional idea that birth phenotype alone is the exclusive, causal factor increasing disease risk in adulthood. Dr P. Wadhwa in Chapter 3 emphasizes the point that whilst availability of energy is a major determinant of development, a second equally important determinant is the repeated demands placed on the developing organism as it adapts to psychological and physiological threats to homeostasis, often described as stress. Numerous associations between prenatal stress, fetal development and adverse birth outcomes have been elucidated with an obvious connection to the hypothalamic-pituitary-adrenal (HPA) axis as a putative mechanism underlying poor fetal outcomes.

The HPA axis is one of the physiological systems most widely studied in this area of research because of its links to stress, and the likelihood that the adrenal hormones may be involved in mediating many of the maternally induced effects on the fetus. Drs Nyirenda and Seckl introduce the concept of neuroendocrine programming in Chapter 4 and discuss the potential role of overexposure of the fetus to glucocorticoids as a mechanism that may account for the association between maternal stress and low birth weight. Glucocorticoids play a critical role in growth, organ and tissue maturation and neural development. In general, it is only when there is excessive exposure that it has been proposed that there would be the potential for disturbances in programming. Excess exposure to glucocosteroids can be a consequence of repeated or chronic stress exposure, and even more commonly they occur in the context of medical interventions involving the use of antenatal corticosteroid agonists like dexamethasone and betamethasone to rapidly mature the lungs and prevent intraventricular hemorrhage in preterm infants. Because glucocorticoids can affect so many systems, including cardiovascular function, glucose metabolism, and behavior, it is reasonable to suspect that this pathway mediates many programming effects via the placental transfer of maternal cortisol into the fetal compartment. Some intellectual tension does however exist in the field right now because the fetus appears able to protect itself from excess cortisol by the placental enzyme 11β-hydroxysteroid dehydrogenase type 2 (11β-HSD2), which converts bioactive cortisol into inactive cortisone. Perturbations to the placental 11β-HSD barriers may account for some of the programming effects, but just how this occurs and if it is more common at certain stages of pregnancy remains to be addressed. The presence of this placental enzyme would also suggest that there are additional mediators.

The multifactorial underpinnings of programming are described further in the next three chapters in Section II. Drs Mathews and Phillips in Chapter 5 point out that while there is a large body of evidence focused on the HPA axis, other endocrine axes including the hypothalamic-pituitary-thyroid and the hypothalamic-pituitary-gonadal axes can also be permanently affected by environmental manipulations early in life. Chapters 6 and 7 detail the impact of the intrauterine environment on the development of the pancreas, documenting the lasting effects of malnutrition and antenatal corticoid exposure. Intrauterine growth restriction is consistently associated with impaired insulin sensitivity in animal models. Subsequently these perturbations may explain the association with the increased risk of developing type 2 diabetes in later life. In Chapter 6, Dr McMillen and co-workers suggest that the nutrient environment before and after birth predicts patterns of postnatal growth and the predisposition towards obesity in later life. They discuss how the *preconception* profile of the mother's nutrition is also a predictor of adult obesity in offspring. Epidemiological studies of the children born after the Dutch famine during World War II have emphasized the importance of specific windows of sensitivity for inducing permanent changes to hormonal programming. Exposure to famine during early gestation did not affect birth size, but instead correlated with obesity in adulthood. Exposure to famine during mid- and late gestation was more likely to result in low birth weight and insulin resistance. Multiple mechanisms underlie these effects. Dr McMillen discusses the programming impact of prenatal nutrition on the deposition pattern of fat cells, the programming of appetite in the brain, and regulation of hunger and weight by the adipokine, leptin. Leptin, the adipocyte-derived hormone encoded by genes related to obesity, is an important regulator of energy balance through effects on food intake and thermogenesis. The causal relationships between nutritional history and obesity are still unclear, but multiple processes have already been identified, including a stimulatory effect of estradiol on leptin production and the inhibitory effect of glucocorticoids on leptin responsiveness. This work has broader ramifications because it highlights the concept of amplification, suggesting that maternal body composition and the level of maternal nutrition may contribute in an additive fashion to programming the infant. The possibility of these intergenerational effects is very important now in light of the global trend toward obesity and its known association with type 2 diabetes. Further progress on these questions will require the combined effort of human research and creative use of animal models. The final chapter in this section by De Groot and co-workers discusses the use and need for developing additional animal models for programming research. Past research has relied heavily on the use of rodent models given the advantages of ready availability, reduced genetic variability and lower cost. But there is also much to be learned from agricultural and other domesticated animals, and farmers have often intuitively incorporated ideas and procedures into their husbandry that reveal an awareness of programming and early rearing effects. This last chapter advocates for greater use of bovine and porcine models, and describes the many lessons that have already been learned about growth and biology from studies of developing piglets.

Section III of our book illustrates the expansion beyond the traditional emphasis on neuroendocrine programming and focuses on a rapidly evolving interest in the impact of the fetal and maternal environment on the development of the immune system. Important work by Drs Coe and Lubach in primates demonstrates that both the psychological and hormonal state of the mother can have lasting effects on the offspring's immune system. Even relatively benign and acute disturbances during pregnancy can produce results that persist for 2–3 years postpartum. Also raised is the issue of variation in vulnerability; when is the critical period of exposure and what is the minimal perturbation required to produce illness in later life? Moreover, some effects on the offspring may not become evident unless they are exposed to additional stressors later in life. Pathology is then a consequence of the additive or cumulative effects as emphasized in stress-diathesis models of disease. These physiological challenges could also be the result of exposure to environmental toxins or teratogens. Alcohol exposure *in utero*, for instance, has been associated with changes in immune and endocrine responses, which appear to reflect an aspect of re-programming. Alcohol is well known to activate the HPA axis in animals, and Dr Taylor and colleagues in Chapter 13 report that fetal exposure to moderate levels of alcohol alters later HPA activity, and humoral and cellular aspects of immunity. Fetal alcohol exposure was also associated with an impaired fever response when the young rats were exposed to bacterial antigens. The fever response is an important component of the acute phase response to infection coordinated, in part, by the release of proinflammatory cytokines that serve to enhance the response of the host to infection. This effect of prenatal alcohol on immunological outcomes appears to be mediated by maternal glucocorticoids, but some of the later effects in the offspring suggest the involvement of changes in both central (prostaglandins) and peripheral (sympathetic) neurochemical signalling. Beyond highlighting concerns about alcohol consumption during pregnancy, this chapter more broadly raises the question about whether the effects of teratogens in general should be considered under the rubric of disruptions in the developmental program.

Other basic and clinical research on the immune system concurs with these data showing that the maternal and fetal environments shape the immunophenotype of the infant. The findings may have particular relevance to allergies and asthma, and help to explain the growing incidence of these two conditions in industrialized countries. In many countries asthma will impact between 6 and 25% of developing children, and some of the explanation may be attributable to prenatal events and the influence of the early rearing environment during the first year of life. During the early 1990s, a provocative idea was proposed: the 'hygiene hypothesis', suggesting that a decreased exposure to certain infectious agents during infancy and early childhood might provide one explanation for the rise in allergies. In particular, the reduction in exposure to parasites and the move from rural to urban environments seemed to coincide with the rise in asthma. While many studies have provided support for the 'hygiene hypothesis', the evidence remains inconclusive, and some viral infections, especially upper respiratory ones, will increase the risk for asthma. Chapters 11 and 12 discuss the complexity of the determinants of asthma by demonstrating that the predisposition extends far beyond simple childhood environmental exposures to allergens, and also includes genetic predisposition, fetal growth, premature birth, and interactions between the immature host's biology and the environment. The last chapter in this section extends beyond the 'hygiene hypothesis' to a more encompassing theory, attempting to explain the general increase in atopic, autoimmune, and inflammatory bowel disease. Rook and colleagues speculate that a lack of exposure to microbes in our neonatal environment has led to a failure in the development of immunoregulatory mechanisms, specifically acting on a type of lymphocyte known as the T regulatory cell (Treg). One of the functions of this Treg cell is to modulate and prevent over-reactions of the immune system, and thus it could be implicated in diseases where excessive inflammatory or immune responses are integral to the pathophysiology. This review offers a provocative evolutionary perspective, which highlights the fact that multicellular organisms came into being while other life forms were already here. Thus, the immune system might have always had to be prepared to respond to parasite loads and bacterial infections of the gastrointestinal tract and other exposed body surfaces. With cleaner environmental conditions, the need for such a response has been reduced and, possibly has been inappropriately diverted toward more benign antigens in the environment.

This is an aspect of anticipatory immune programming that could be referred to as 'preparedness' – that is, over the course of evolution, the genetic program was selected toward preparing us for the most likely environment and thus appears to anticipate some of the needs in the postnatal environs. Rook et al. argue that the preparedness could even include the emergence of symbiotic relationships with commensal microbiota. The evolution of multicellular organisms involved the creation of a type of inter-specific social contract with bacteria. The importance of this relationship is most dramatically conveyed by the fact that we are comprised of 10^{13} cells, while serving as the substrate for 10^{14} bacteria within our gut and on our skin. Indeed, digestion and life would not be possible without this mutually beneficial collaboration, which must certainly be anticipated by the developmental program. Clearly, while improved hygiene and the advent of vaccines and antibiotics represent some of the greatest medical and social achievements of the last century for reducing infant mortality, we still have a lot more to learn about the implications of reduced infection for the development of immunity and later health in adulthood.

Further broadening the scope of the 'fetal origins' perspective is the work reviewed in Sections IV and V of the book. Drs Anand and Butkevich detail important clinical research on pain illustrating the plasticity of the neonatal brain with regard to the development of the processing of pain and the emergence of pain inhibitory systems, both of which appear susceptible to programming. Rather than desensitizing to pain, it appears that early exposure of premature human infants and neonates to painful stimuli results in exaggerated responses to pain in childhood. These observations have significant clinical ramifications because preterm babies are often exposed to many painful procedures, often performed without analgesics, in some cases reaching 400 before the baby leaves the Neonatal Intensive Care Unit. Basic science studies in animal models have further supported the conclusion that pain and inflammation in newborns alters the development of sensory pathways and will induce both central and peripheral sensitization. Dr Butkevich and co-workers show that these effects may be mediated by changes in sensory processing as well as by changes in important neurotransmitters, such as in the serotonergic pathways. The prenatal programming of nociception is a relatively new area, but one with profound importance for understanding the etiology of seemingly inexplicable chronic pain disorders of adulthood, such as fibromyalgia. Although the most straightforward change is in the subsequent response to pain, there is also a growing body of literature indicating that exposure to pain and stressors early in life alters other behavioral processes in adulthood. Neonatally stressed animals show decreased exploratory behavior in novel environments, an increased preference for alcohol, greater anxiety, a lower threshold for the emergence of learned helplessness reactions, and increased loss of hippocampal neurons associated with an earlier onset of cognitive defects. In human studies, exposure to repeated pain as a neonate has been associated with lower cognitive scores in infancy and a three-fold increase in the risk of being diagnosed with attention deficit hyperactivity disorder (ADHD). Some of these long-term changes have been attributed to altered plasticity in the neonatal hypothalamus, but the range of effects suggests that there are influences on limbic and cortical regions as well. Section V continues this discussion of the role of early life events in the programming of behavior.

Dr Weinstock in Chapter 18 extends the conclusions discussed in previous chapters on the role of stress and activation of the HPA axis in programming behavior. Her extensive research on prenatal stress in rodents has demonstrated the increased emotionality and attentional and memory deficits of pups disturbed *in utero*. Prenatal stress was associated with offspring that exhibited increased anxiety behavior in many tests such as the elevated plus maze and the open-field. Offspring of dams stressed during pregnancy exhibited impaired cognitive performance in learning tests including the Y-maze, T-maze, radial arm maze, and in passive avoidance conditioning. As suggested for other types of outcome measures, it appears that exposure to high levels of corticosterone may result in deleterious actions on areas such as the dorsal and ventral hippocampus, causing reduced synaptic density and neurogenesis. In addition, in Chapter 20, Dr Granger reveals yet another pathway by which early life events could program adult brain functioning and behavior: via activation of the immune system. Cytokines are integrally involved in immune-to-brain communication. Early life exposure to stimuli that markedly activate this immune-brain pathway, such as exposure to endotoxins and septic shock, has the potential to produce neural damage and dysfunction. It may be that there are also immune-related actions at a more subtle programming level, which can continue to modulate perceptual, arousal and cognitive processes.

The contributory influence of other hormones and intrinsic processes is considered in Chapters 18 and 19. In particular, these chapters bring up the important issue of gender differences in vulnerability and discuss the important programming role of androgen in driving the female form toward a more masculine one. Dr

Glover provides an extensive review of the effects of pregnancy stressors in humans, and highlights the possibility that testosterone may be involved in the genesis of higher numbers of behavioral disorders in male children. Dr Berenbaum covers the topic of androgen's actions more specifically in her extensive review of the effects of exposure to prenatal androgen in several clinical conditions in girls. Prenatal androgens are not only involved in sexual differentiation of physical appearance, they also mediate the emergence of sexual dimorphism in behavior. In rodents, females administered high doses of androgens in the newborn period show behavior more typical of males; conversely males that are castrated or given anti-androgens show behavior more typical of females. Similar behavioral effects of androgenic hormones are also found in non-human primates, with genetic females exhibiting a masculinization of sexual behavior, rough-and-tumble play, and aggressiveness. While the picture is a little less clear in humans, there seems to be a similar androgenic effect on gender-typical preferences and perhaps also some influences on sexual orientation. The prenatal effects of testosterone provide convincing evidence for the potentially powerful and long-reaching effects of *in utero* conditions. These findings are certainly important for providing more insight into how best to help patients who experienced these atypical fetal exposures that differed from the normal programming hormone milieu.

The final section of our book is comprised of two chapters that take us into the future of programming research. Dr Dziadek offers a comprehensive and scholarly discussion of the role played by genes in fetal programming and the implications for health and disease. In addition, the traditional view that genes control behavioral expression in a unidirectional manner is contrasted with the newly emerging perspective emphasizing bidirectional influences: environmental or epigenetic influences on gene transcription. Epigenetic influences may even be passed on through effects on cell division and how gene regulation occurs into adulthood. Indeed, epigenetic modifications may reflect a long history of environmental exposure, which may have many health implications. The final chapter is by Dr Meaney and colleagues, whose research demonstrates the potential of this new avenue of research for documenting how environmental influences can 'get under the skin' and become biologically embedded. The discovery that maternal licking and grooming behavior can alter so many brain processes in rodent pups, and literally change the expression of the genetic program is one of the most dramatic illustrations of the influence of 'early experience'. The

detail and the resolution of the mechanisms that have been elucidated by Dr Meaney and co-workers in their efforts to understand these maternal influences set a very high standard for the whole field. These two chapters reveal an important future emphasis for research on fetal programming, both at the theoretical and mechanistic levels, raising many new and significant questions to be addressed.

For instance, how does one begin to characterize the nature and most important aspects of gene and environment interactions during development? When do such interactions result in sustained programming of gene expression and function? What magnitude of environmental perturbation is required to drive this type of epigenetic modification? Finally, one is compelled to ask, from an evolutionary standpoint, how do we discern when prenatal influences are adaptive or will result in later pathological consequences? Clearly some but not all aspects of programming serve to maximize the survival potential of offspring by more efficiently matching the individual to the extant environmental conditions.

Hopefully, in bringing together this diverse literature on many types of fetal programming, our book will raise awareness about the multifactorial nature of programming and the profound influence that the early environment has on development. The fetal and maternal environment, not surprisingly, plays a critical role in determining how we respond to stress or pain, behave as adults, parent our own children, age and ultimately succumb to certain illnesses, perhaps even setting the clock for our longevity. Beyond the consequences for our children, the new discoveries have many implications for animal husbandry, especially with domesticated farm animals. If growth processes that will be sustained postpartum and the path toward health really start in fetal life, then it also raises many questions about the optimal living conditions for the gravid female animal, which have both economic and ethical ramifications. At a basic science level, these studies also point to an important source of the individual variation commonly seen in behavioral and physiological systems across populations of animals and humans. Not all of these individual differences are attributable to the genes, but rather to how the genetic program becomes manifest in the growing baby within the womb. In many ways it seems similar to a statement recently written to describe how the context in which an individual cell grows can result in a marked divergence in its differentiation: 'The difference between radically different destinies often reflects disarmingly small variations in timing or circumstance'.[1] There is even some evidence that the emergent phenotype could be sustained over time, changing the progeny that will be produced in the next generation. These are provocative ideas that could alter our traditional views about the inheritance of traits. They also argue for much more societal concern about the well-being of mothers and for ensuring the optimal prenatal conditions for developing babies. Better policies to improve developmental health are perhaps the most important agenda item for governments across the industrialized and developing world.

DMH and CLC

---

[1] Shaywitz DA, Melton DA. The molecular biology of the cell. Cell 2005; 120: 729–33.

Acknowledgments

There are many individuals to thank for the 'birth' of this book. Firstly, our publishers Taylor & Francis, whose support was paramount. Thank you to Nick Dunton for supporting our idea in the first instance and to Kelly Cornish for her hard work in preparing and editing each manuscript and for keeping us on task and ensuring that all of the pieces came together in a timely manner. We would also like to thank Dr Stuart Marlin and the Women and Infants Research Foundation of Western Australia for permission to use their photographs in our book. Of course, there is no way that this book would have been possible without the contributions from all of our authors. It is their work that provided the richness, depth, and breadth of the material for this book. Contributions came from Australia, Canada, Finland, Israel, The Netherlands, New Zealand, Russia, the United Kingdom and United States. Bringing together individuals from such different backgrounds to present a united message clearly indicates how science can represent the best of the collective human endeavour, where international affiliations and borders present no boundaries or obstacles to scientific creativity and sharing. We thank them for their hard work and willingness to see and enable the vision we had.

Deborah M Hodgson and Christopher L Coe

Section I – Prenatal determinants of fetal growth, birth outcomes and later disease risk

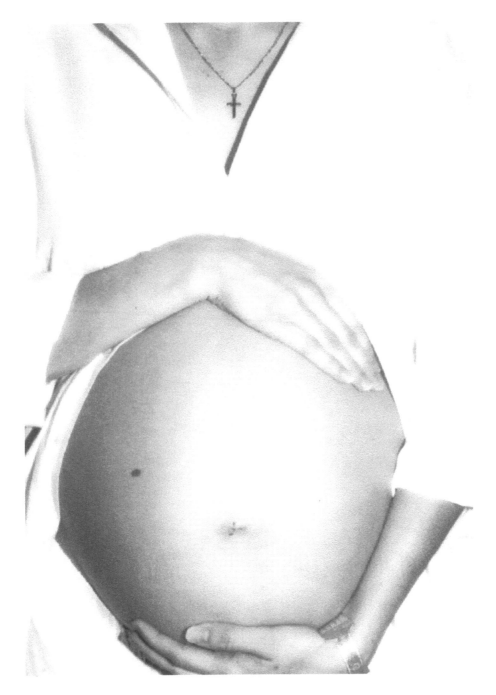

'And when our baby stirs and struggles to be born it compels humility: what we began is now its own' Margaret Mead

1

The role of the mother, placenta, and fetus in the control of fetal growth during human pregnancy

Vanessa E Murphy, Roger Smith, Warwick B Giles, and Vicki L Clifton

INTRODUCTION

The environment in which the fetus develops is critical for its long-term survival and health. Currently, there is interest in the developmental origins of adult disease and the ways in which altered nutrition affects the fetus both in the short and long term. Central to progress in this area is an understanding of the determinants of fetal growth. This chapter describes maternal, placental, and fetal processes that regulate human growth *in utero*.

The mother plays an essential role in supplying nutrients and oxygen to the fetus via the placenta. The placenta is the site of nutrient exchange between mother and fetus. Increased uteroplacental blood flow and adequate trophoblast invasion in early pregnancy are required for growth of the uterus, placenta, and fetus. The placenta secretes hormones into both the mother and fetus, which influence maternal metabolism to mobilize nutrients and directly regulate fetal and placental development. Placental metabolism of maternal glucocorticoids by 11β-hydroxysteroid dehydrogenase type 2 (11β-HSD2) protects the fetus from the growth-inhibiting effects of glucocorticoid exposure. Expression of insulin-like growth factors and their receptors along with 11β-HSD2 in fetal tissues allows local control of growth by the fetus. Understanding the regulation of fetal growth will provide insights relevant to the long-term programming of the fetus.

NORMAL FETAL GROWTH

Size at birth for all mammals is a function of the rate of maternal investment and length of gestation. At the beginning of intrauterine life, embryogenesis occurs and the basic body structure is created. During this period, cell number increases maximally up to 16 weeks gestation.[1] At this stage, growth as assessed by ultrasound is essentially linear. At the completion of embryogenesis, the embryo is formed and becomes a fetus. Fetal growth involves an increase in cell number, but from 16 to 32 weeks there is also an increase in cell size, which becomes more pronounced after 32 weeks.[1] Fetal growth is also essentially linear, although the rate of increase is greater than observed during embryogenesis. The growth of the fetus is critically dependent on the size of the mother both in terms of her height and her weight. Fetal sex is a modifier of growth with males growing faster than females.

LOW BIRTH WEIGHT

Low birth weight is defined by the World Health Organization as birth weight less than 2500 g.[2] Small for gestational age (SGA) refers to neonates less than the 10th percentile for gestational age in relation to a reference population.[1]

Low birth weight independent of prematurity is a significant contributor to neonatal morbidity and mortality[1] and represents a large health-care cost, both in economic and social terms. The risk of postnatal death in term infants weighing 2000–2499 g has been estimated to be increased two-fold compared to infants weighing 2500–2999 g and increased four-fold compared to infants weighing 3000–3499 g.[3] Low birth weight has been shown to be associated with an increased risk of mortality up to 15 years of age, which is mostly accounted for by higher infant mortality rates, and with increased morbidity including birth asphyxia, meconium aspiration, persistent fetal circulation, hypoglycemia, hypothermia, and hypocalcemia, and therefore represents a significant public health issue.[1]

INTRAUTERINE GROWTH RESTRICTION (IUGR)

Fetal growth restriction refers to fetal growth that is below that of the genetic potential of the particular fetus. Intrauterine growth restriction may be symmetrical (type I) or asymmetrical (type II). Symmetrical growth restriction, where the entire body is proportionally small, accounts for 25% of IUGR cases and often results from an alteration in growth in early gestation, during the period of cellular hyperplasia, and may be the result of genetic anomalies, severe malnutrition, or maternal smoking.[1] Asymmetrical fetal growth was first recognized by Gruenwald in 1963, who found that growth-restricted infants had a higher brain weight and lower thymus weight than premature infants of the same size.[4] Such asymmetric growth restriction may occur during the periods of cellular hypertrophy later in gestation and is often the result of uteroplacental insufficiency secondary to other maternal complications.[1] In asymmetric growth restriction, there is sparing of the brain and other vital organs such as the heart, with other parts of the body such as the liver and muscle reduced in size.[1]

Fetal growth can be assessed in several ways, with common measurements including crown–heel length, head circumference, weight–height ratio, skin fold thickness and ponderal index. The ponderal index (birth weight (g)/[birth length (cm)]^3 × 100), which is unaffected by race or infant sex, is used to assess the thinness or obesity of the neonate, with symmetrically small neonates having a normal ponderal index and those with asymmetric growth restriction having a reduced ponderal index due to a normal length and low weight.[1]

DEVELOPMENTAL ORIGINS OF ADULT DISEASE

Recent interest in the developmental or fetal origins of adult disease (Barker hypothesis), has revealed that low birth weight or small size at birth is a predictor for the development of and/or death from diseases in adult life, including diabetes, cardiovascular disease, atherosclerosis, hypertension, stroke, and coronary heart disease.[5] This concept, which proposes that events *in utero* can determine long-term outcomes into adulthood, is known as fetal programming. It is thought that glucocorticoids may play a major role in programming. Adaptation of the fetus to its environment *in utero* is believed to lead to changes in body structure, physiology, and metabolism which persist into extrauterine life.

Barker's initial studies examined the geographical relationship in England and Wales between current death rates from heart disease or stroke and prior infant or maternal mortality rates.[6] The geographical distribution of death rates from stroke was more closely correlated with past maternal mortality than with any other cause of death, suggesting that the health of mothers may be linked to the risk of disease in their offspring.[6]

In 1989, Barker et al. published results of follow-up studies of almost 10,000 children at age 10, born in 1970 and over 3000 adults at 36 years of age, born in 1946.[7] They found an inverse relationship between birth weight and systolic blood pressure, which was stronger in the 36-year-old adults and independent of current weight. In the children, increased systolic blood pressure was not related to gestational age and therefore was associated only with a reduction in fetal growth aside from prematurity.[7] The relationship between higher systolic blood pressure and low birth weight has been found to be consistent in children aged 0–10 years, and adults at 36 years, 46–54 years and 59–71 years, but to become more pronounced with age.[8]

Blood pressure in adult life is also linked to placental size and particularly the ratio of fetal to placental weight. In 449 men and women born in Lancashire, England between 1935 and 1943, systolic and diastolic blood pressures were strongly related to both placental weight and birth weight independent of gestational age, current alcohol consumption, and current body mass index (BMI), with the highest blood pressures in those with a low birth weight but high placental weight.[9] Within each social class, the relationships between blood pressure and placental and birth weights were similar.[9] Placental weight was inversely correlated with length to head circumference ratio, suggesting the possibility that changes in the fetal circulation, such as diversion of blood flow to the brain at the expense of other parts of the body, may permanently alter arterial structure and blood vessel development.[9]

Barker et al. also studied the Hertfordshire and Lancashire cohorts with regard to the development of syndrome X, or the combination of noninsulin-dependent diabetes mellitus, hypertension, and hyperlipidemia.[10] In Lancashire, men and women at age 50 with syndrome X had lower birth weights as well as a small head circumference and low ponderal index at birth. The proportion of subjects with syndrome X was lower with increasing birth weight in the Hertfordshire and Lancashire cohorts.[10] The association between fetal growth and diabetes may be related to alterations in the development of the fetal pancreas and a reduction in insulin-secreting capacity.[10]

It is becoming increasingly clear that the effect of small size at birth on adult diseases is compounded by rapid rates of childhood growth.[5] It is suggested that developmental plasticity allows an appropriate phenotype for the current environment (in utero); however, when nutrition improves after birth, compensatory growth occurs. The combination of these events results in physical and physiological changes that contribute to the increased risk of developing metabolic and cardiovascular diseases later in life.[5]

Maternal diet during pregnancy may have an adverse effect on fetal growth and consequences for adult blood pressure. Several studies have demonstrated that a particularly high or low protein diet during pregnancy has adverse effects on blood pressure in offspring.[11] Maternal undernutrition has been examined in women who were pregnant at the time of the Dutch famine in 1944 and 1945, where babies exposed during mid- or late gestation were found to have reduced birth weights compared to babies born before the famine or conceived after the famine.[12,13] Follow-up studies of the offspring indicate that at approximately 50 years of age, the highest rates of impaired glucose tolerance and type 2 diabetes were seen in those exposed to maternal famine in late gestation.[12] In addition, offspring exposed to maternal famine during early gestation had a higher prevalence of coronary heart disease, respiratory disease, hypertension, diabetes, and cancer and a poorer perception of their own health at 50 years of age, which is a predictor of mortality.[13]

Alterations in susceptibility to disease in childhood and adulthood in relation to fetal growth may be related to impaired development in utero or in infancy, or to increased susceptibility to postnatal disease. Therefore, an understanding of the mechanisms which cause low birth weight is important for the development of future interventions, which may give small infants a better chance of a healthy life, both in their immediate future and in the long term. The mother, placenta, and fetus are all integral components in the regulation of fetal growth during human pregnancy.

THE ROLE OF THE MOTHER IN FETAL GROWTH REGULATION

The mother supplies oxygen and essential nutrients to the fetus via the placental blood supply. Maternal genes have a specific influence over fetal growth, and maternal size (particularly height which represents genetic potential for growth and uterine capacity), is a major determinant of fetal size.[14] Many maternal factors influence fetal growth, including height and weight, race and parity, age, energy intake, and gestational weight gain.[1] The genome of the mother is a determinant of her response to the fetus and specifically her response to the nutrient-mobilizing hormones released by the fetus.

Nutrient supply

The mother is the supplier of nutrients to the fetus, and maternal diet and caloric intake have an essential role to play.[2] The placenta has a dual role in releasing hormones into the maternal circulation, which may modify maternal appetite, and the mobilization of nutrients. The placenta also has an essential role in transferring these nutrients to the fetus. Adequate caloric intake is critical during all of pregnancy and an increase is necessary during the second and third trimesters when most fetal and placental growth occurs.[15] Additional protein intake is specifically required for growth of maternal, placental, and fetal tissues.[15]

Nutrient availability in maternal blood is clearly an important regulator of fetal growth and supplementation of calories or vitamins to undernourished women increases birth weight. In Nepal, pregnant women supplemented with folic acid, iron, and vitamin A had an increased mean birth weight of 37 g and a 16% reduction in the rate of low birth weight compared to control subjects given vitamin A alone.[16] The effect of multiple micronutrient supplementation (folic acid, zinc, iron, vitamin A, and 10 other micronutrients) was not found to be of additional benefit compared to folic acid and iron. This study suggested that iron deficiency may be an important cause of reduced fetal growth.

During the Dutch famine in 1944 and 1945, pregnant women were undernourished due to compulsory food rationing, which was as low as 400–800 calories per day at the height of the famine.[12] Maternal weight gain and fetal growth were significantly reduced when the exposure to famine occurred during the second or third trimester.[12] In the 1960s, Scottish women in Motherwell were advised to increase their red meat intake and decrease consumption of carbohydrates during pregnancy in an attempt to avoid pre-eclampsia.[11] As pregnancy progressed, women doubled their meat consumption, while carbohydrate consumption fell by one third. As a consequence, these women had reduced weight gain during pregnancy compared to women in other parts of Scotland and their babies were of reduced birth weight.[11]

Maternal smoking

Cigarette smoking is associated with reduced birth weight, with early reports suggesting a doubling of the rate of low birth weight in smokers compared to non-smokers and an increase in low birth weight with increasing number of cigarettes smoked.[17] The entire birth weight distribution curve is shifted to the left, such that maternal smoking affects the entire range of birth weights. Infants born to smoking mothers are approximately 150–200 g lighter than infants of non-smokers, representing one of the largest preventable effects on birth weight.[17] Neonates born to smoking mothers are usually symmetrically growth restricted, having reduced weight, head circumference, and abdominal circumference.[1] Higher levels of carbon monoxide in maternal blood – which cross the placenta to the fetus, leading to fetal tissue hypoxemia – along with the vasoconstrictive effects of nicotine, are thought to contribute to these changes in fetal growth.[17] Smoking may reduce fetal growth by altering uteroplacental blood flow, as Lehtovirta and Forss demonstrated a reduced placental blood flow at the time of smoking a cigarette, which then returned to normal within 15 minutes.[18]

Sexton et al. conducted a randomized clinical trial to investigate whether a reduction in maternal smoking would improve fetal growth.[19] Women in the intervention group received health information and counselling and 43% stopped smoking by late pregnancy, as compared to only 20% in the control (no intervention) group. The significant reduction in the number of cigarettes smoked per day corresponded to a decrease in salivary thiocyanate levels, a biochemical marker of smoking, and was associated with a significant increase in birth weight (by 92 g) and birth length (by 0.6 cm) compared to the control group, confirming that smoking cessation overcomes some of the reduced fetal growth seen in smokers.[19]

Maternal oxygenation

Maternal arterial oxygenation and high altitude residence also have an effect on third trimester fetal growth. Babies born at high altitude are of lower birth weight than their low altitude counterparts regardless of socioeconomic status[20] and the effect of altitude on birth weight is independent of existing risk factors, such as maternal smoking, pregnancy-induced hypertension (PIH) and nulliparity.[21] The mean difference in birth weight between high altitude (2744–3350 m) and lower altitude (915–1524 m) in Colorado was 241 g, a difference which could not be explained only by a reduction in gestational age.[21] The entire birth weight distribution is shifted to the left, so that a greater proportion of births fall below 2500 g, indicating that altitude affects all births and not just an 'at risk' subgroup.

Decreased arterial oxygen content as a result of high altitude exposure may also lower uterine blood flow, which could contribute to reduced nutrient transport to the fetus. Uterine blood flow is altered at high altitude with less flow from the common iliac reaching the uterine artery.[22] Although uterine artery flow velocity increased, the uterine artery diameter was smaller, resulting in lower volumetric flow in late pregnancy.[22] Uterine blood flow velocity was found to be correlated with birth weight at 1600 m.[22] In 2001, Moore et al. reported that despite lower arterial O_2 content in Tibetan compared to Han Chinese residents at high altitude (3658 m), the Tibetan women had a higher uterine artery blood flow velocity and a greater distribution of blood flow to the uterine artery, which contributed to their babies being of higher birth weight than those of the Han Chinese women.[23] Women who develop pre-eclampsia at high altitude have less blood flow distributed to the uterine artery than normotensive women.[22] These studies suggest that there are physiological adaptations to residence at high altitude, which increase blood flow to the feto-placental unit, and these are beneficial for fetal growth.

Maternal inflammatory diseases

The presence of a maternal inflammatory disease may contribute to reduced fetal growth. Our group has an interest in the effect of maternal asthma on fetal growth.[24–26] Previous epidemiological evidence has linked maternal asthma with an increased risk of low birth weight, with some suggesting that poorly controlled asthma or acute asthma may be a particular risk. We found that mild asthma was associated with reduced birth weight of female neonates, and that the use of anti-inflammatory inhaled steroid medication was protective against these changes in fetal growth.[26] We observed no alterations in fetal growth as measured by ultrasound at 18 and 30 weeks gestation, suggesting a late gestation decline in growth, which may have been mediated by a reduction in placental 11β-hydroxysteroid dehydrogenase type 2 (11β-HSD2) activity.[25,26] We speculate that inflammatory factors may be involved in the regulation of placental 11β-HSD2 activity in this context.[25,26] In addition, there may be a role for reduced placental blood flow in altering fetal growth in women with moderate and severe asthma.[24]

Several other inflammatory diseases are also associated with reduced fetal growth, including rheumatoid arthritis, systemic lupus erythematosus, inflammatory bowel disease, and periodontal disease.[27] Bowden et al. found that women with active inflammatory arthritis during pregnancy had smaller babies at birth compared with healthy control women or women whose disease was in remission.[27] These data indicate that active inflammation during pregnancy may contribute to a reduction in fetal growth.

Many other maternal factors including having preeclampsia, PIH, anemia, or infections such as rubella or malaria, excess alcohol consumption or using drugs such as cocaine may alter fetal growth via changes in placental function.[1]

THE ROLE OF THE PLACENTA IN FETAL GROWTH REGULATION

The placenta is the site where nutrients and waste products are exchanged between mother and fetus. Morphometric studies have shown that the placental villous surface area for exchange is approximately 11 m^2 at term.[28] This surface area is decreased in cases of fetal growth restriction as is the mid-pregnancy or term placental volume.[28] Placental weight is an important predictor of fetal weight, with SGA neonates having significantly reduced placental weights and placental weight to birth weight ratios than appropriately grown neonates of the same birth weight, suggesting that adequate placental growth is required for adequate fetal growth. Several aspects of placental function are critical for human fetal growth. They include adequate trophoblast invasion, an increase in uteroplacental blood flow during gestation, transport of nutrients such as glucose and amino acids from mother to fetus and the production and transfer of growth-regulating hormones. In addition, the placenta plays an important role in limiting the transfer of the maternal hormone cortisol, which may have a negative effect on the growth of the fetus. The placenta also modifies the maternal environment by releasing hormones and metabolites into the maternal circulation.

Trophoblast invasion and uteroplacental blood flow

One week after fertilization, the blastocyst enters the uterus. The blastocyst contains the inner cell mass, which will develop into the fetus, and an outer layer of trophoblast, which will become the placenta. The trophoblast layer implants into the uterus, by releasing proteolytic enzymes which digest cells of the endometrium allowing subsequent penetration by the trophoblast. Adequate trophoblast invasion is required to sustain fetal growth. When the blastocyst adheres to the uterus, the fetal trophoblast cells differentiate into villous or extravillous cells.[29] The extravillous cytotrophoblasts migrate and invade the maternal uterine epithelium, a process which is essential for increased uteroplacental blood flow as pregnancy progresses.[29] In this process, maternal uterine spiral arteries are transformed into larger, low resistance vessels, capable of transporting the increased maternal blood to the placenta. Part of the modification and remodelling of spiral arteries involves a replacement of the muscular and elastic walls of the arteries with a fibrinoid layer embedded with trophoblast cells, allowing low pressure intervillous flow.[30] The absence of trophoblast-induced changes in decidual or myometrial segments of spiral arteries is a feature of some pregnancies complicated by fetal growth restriction.

Growth of the uterus, placenta, and fetus requires an increase in uterine blood flow during pregnancy in order to meet metabolic demand.[30] During pregnancy, total blood volume and cardiac output increase by approximately 40% and the total uteroplacental blood flow represents 25% of cardiac output.[30] Palmer et al. found that the diameter of the uterine artery had increased two-fold by 21 weeks gestation, and further increased between 30 and 36 weeks gestation.[31] In addition, flow velocity of the uterine artery increased throughout gestation and was eight times greater by 36 weeks compared to nonpregnant values.[31] In addition to increased uterine blood flow during pregnancy, the development of new blood vessels also occurs in the uterus, possibly promoted by human chorionic gonadotropin (hCG) and insulin-like growth factor (IGF)-II.[32] In IUGR, there is a decrease in number and surface area of terminal villi, representing a malfunction of vascularization in these pregnancies.[32]

Umbilical vein blood flow can be measured by Doppler ultrasound techniques[33] and has been shown to be decreased in IUGR fetuses in relation to fetal size, representing reduced perfusion of the fetal tissues. In a study of 70 human fetuses, Barbera et al. found a strong correlation between absolute umbilical vein flow and fetal head and abdominal circumferences, with an increase in umbilical vein diameter and mean velocity throughout pregnancy.[34] They also found an exponential increase in flow from 97.3 ml/min at mid-gestation to 529.1 ml/min in late gestation, but no corresponding increase in flow per kg of fetal weight, suggesting that increasing flow is matching the increase in fetal size in late gestation.[34] These studies suggest the importance of uteroplacental blood flow in maintaining appropriate fetal growth through the supply of oxygen and nutrients.

Nutrient transport

Glucose, amino acids, and lipids are some of the most important nutrients that are transported from mother to fetus via the placenta. These nutrients may be delivered by passive diffusion; however, concentrations of many amino acids are higher in fetal than maternal plasma, indicating the existence of active transport mechanisms across the placenta. Amino acid transporters within the fetal (basal) and maternal (microvillous) facing syncytiotrophoblast plasma membranes actively transport numerous amino acids across the placenta.[35] System A, found mostly on the microvillous membrane, is sodium-dependent and transports neutral amino acids such as alanine, proline, glycine, and serine.[35] Neutral amino acids may also be transported by system ASC, found mostly on the basal membrane, while system L is sodium independent, transporting phenylalanine and branched chain amino acids.[35] Systems y^+ and y^+L transport cationic amino acids such as arginine across the microvillous and basal membranes, respectively.[35] Amino acids may also be metabolized and processed by the placenta.

In SGA fetuses there are alterations in amino acid transport by the placenta and uptake by the fetus. Jansson et al. found that *in vitro* uptake of lysine in the basal membrane and leucine in both the basal and microvillous membranes was decreased in placentae from IUGR pregnancies, suggesting reduced activity of amino acid transporters.[36] Economides et al. found that fetal concentrations of many amino acids including branched chain, basic and essential amino acids that cannot be produced by the fetus, were reduced in SGA fetuses.[37] Moreover, the ratio of nonessential to essential amino acids was greater with increasing fetal hypoxemia, assessed by umbilical vein PO_2.[37] In IUGR, the activity of system A in the microvillous membrane is reduced, while the expression and activity of glucose transporters in the syncytiotrophoblast is not changed.[38]

Glucose transport from mother to fetus is related to the concentration gradient and is carried out by transporters found on the maternal and fetal sides of the trophoblast.[39] Nicolini et al. found that while maternal glucose concentrations were similar between normal and growth-restricted pregnancies, the fetal glucose concentration was significantly reduced in the growth-restricted group,[40] possibly reflecting reduced supply and transfer of glucose across the placenta. The glucose transporter, GLUT1, is found in abundance in the microvillous membrane of the syncytiotrophoblast at levels three times higher than the basal membrane. In a perfusion study of preterm IUGR placentae, it was found that baseline glucose consumption was two-fold higher in IUGR, suggesting that placental consumption of glucose may contribute to alterations in maternal–fetal concentration differences in glucose.[41] However, this study also demonstrated no change in glucose transfer to the fetal side of the placenta,[41] confirming previous studies showing no alteration in glucose transporter expression or activity in IUGR placentae. Another study found that in IUGR, the maternal–fetal glucose concentration gradient was increased in relation to clinical severity, possibly representing an adaptation to maintain glucose uptake across the placenta.[39]

Fatty acids, which are essential components of plasma membranes and used for energy, are also transported to the fetus across the placenta.[42] In the third trimester, fatty acids are required for changes in fetal tissue composition, particularly in the brain and adipose tissue. The n-3 and n-6 fatty acid structures can be acquired only from the maternal diet and placental transfer.[42] Free fatty acids may be transferred across the placenta via passive diffusion, due to the concentration gradient between mother and fetus, and there are fatty acid binding proteins and fatty acid transfer proteins in the microvillous and basal membranes.[42] The essential fatty acid, linoleic acid was found to be significantly higher in IUGR placentae compared with those from appropriately grown fetuses, which may have implications for fetal brain development. However, there is no clear evidence for reduced fatty acid concentrations or placental transport in fetal growth restriction.[42]

Placental production of growth factors and growth-regulating hormones

Insulin-like growth factors (IGFs)

The IGF axis is of major importance in both fetal and placental growth. Insulin-like growth factors I and II (IGF-I and IGF-II) are polypeptides with sequences similar to that of insulin, which have mitogenic properties, inducing somatic cell growth and proliferation. They may also have the ability to influence the transport of glucose and amino acids across the placenta. Alterations in the IGF axis are associated with fetal growth restriction in both animal models and humans.

Knockout and transgenic mice studies have demonstrated that IGF-I and IGF-II are required for optimal fetal and placental growth.[43–46] Null mutations in the gene encoding IGF-I result in mice that are 60% smaller than their wild-type littermates without altering placental size.[44,45] Inactivation of the IGF-II gene also results in a 60% reduction in fetal weight[43] with reduced placental growth also evident from embryonic day 13.5.[43,44] When both IGF-I and IGF-II were knocked out, birth weight was further reduced to 30% of normal size.[45] Knocking out the IGF-I receptor either alone, or in combination with IGF-I or IGF-II, resulted in postnatal death due to respiratory failure and a 50% reduction in fetal size.[45] Recent work has demonstrated that selective mutation of the placental promoter of the IGF-II gene (P0 in mice) results in a proportionate reduction in size of all parts of the placenta by embryonic day 12 and in fetal size by day 16, despite the fact that this transcript comprises only 10% of all placental IGF-II mRNA.[46] The reduced placental growth was as great as when all IGF-II was absent, suggesting that the P0 transcript is essential for determining the action of IGF-II on the placenta.[46] This study also showed that mice carrying the mutation had reduced placental passive transport but increased active transport of amino acids, possibly reflecting a compensatory mechanism to increase fetal growth.[46]

The type 1 IGF receptor is similar in structure to the insulin receptor, being a transmembrane heterotetrameric $(\alpha_2\beta_2)$ glycoprotein with disulfide links and an intracellular tyrosine kinase domain. It is able to bind both IGF-I and IGF-II through an extracellular α subunit; however, its affinity for IGF-I is 15–20 times greater than for IGF-II.[47] The type 2 IGF receptor is a single-chain polypeptide which has a high affinity for IGF-II, but does not bind IGF-I or insulin.[45] Recent studies in humans have indicated that a mutation in the IGF type 1 receptor gene, which results in reduced functioning of the receptor, is associated with poor prenatal and postnatal growth.[48]

IGF-I and IGF-II circulate in pregnant women at higher levels than in nonpregnant women and concentrations increase even further by the third trimester, suggesting that these hormones may have a role in fetal growth regulation in addition to their well-characterized effects on postnatal growth. Fetal serum concentrations of IGF-I, IGF-II, and IGFBP-3 increase significantly with advancing gestation, with the greatest rise in IGF-I.[49] Maternal IGF-I levels are regulated by growth hormone and, during pregnancy, the placenta secretes a placental variant of growth hormone which drives maternal IGF-I secretion.[50]

The actions of IGF-I and IGF-II are regulated by one of six insulin-like growth factor-binding proteins (IGFBP-1–6). IGFBP-2, 4, 5 and 6 are present in low concentrations in plasma.[51] IGFBP-3 complexes with IGF-I or II and an acid-labile subunit acting as a reservoir for IGFs in the circulation[51] and increases in maternal plasma during pregnancy. IGFBP-1 is dynamically regulated in human plasma and its levels can vary more than 10-fold in response to changes in insulin.[51] IGFBP-1 binds IGF-I and II with greater affinity than either of the IGF receptors, and thus prevents the IGFs from exerting their mitogenic actions.[51]

During pregnancy, IGFBP-1 is the major regulator of IGF-I action, since it is the main product of the decidua, the main IGFBP in the amniotic fluid and a major binder of IGFs in fetal plasma.[52] IGFBP-1 can exist in one of several phosphorylated forms. Jones et al. first described the existence of up to five phosphorylated forms, in addition to a nonphosphorylated form of IGFBP-1, finding that amniotic fluid and fetal serum contained large amounts of the nonphosphorylated form, while decidual cells contained only the phosphorylated forms.[53] This group also showed that the mix of phosphorylated forms of IGFBP-1 had six-fold higher affinity for IGF-I than the nonphosphorylated form.[53] Subsequently, Westwood et al. demonstrated the importance of post-translational phosphorylation of IGFBP-1 in pregnancy by showing that plasma from nonpregnant adults contained only the highly phosphorylated species, while pregnant plasma also contained a nonphosphorylated and three less phosphorylated variants, with concentrations at least double those of nonpregnant individuals and higher in multi-fetal pregnancies.[52] The highly phosphorylated isoform has the highest affinity for IGF-I, which is greater than that of the IGF type 1 receptor, resulting in an inhibition of IGF activity, while the nonphosphorylated form has a similar affinity for IGF-I as its receptor.[52] Dephosphorylation of IGFBP-1 may represent a mechanism by which IGF-I is released and its bioactivity increased during pregnancy. Proteolysis of IGFBPs may be an additional mechanism for altering the bioavailability of IGFs during pregnancy.

The human placenta produces IGF-I and IGF-II, which may act as local growth regulators. The mRNA abundance of IGF-II is greater than that of IGF-I in the placenta at all gestational ages.[54] IGF-II is found throughout the chorionic villi, chorionic plate, basal plate, and fetal membranes, while all IGFBPs are found in the decidua, with IGFBP-1 in greatest abundance.[54] IGFBP-1 produced by the maternal decidua may be involved in cell to cell communication, with IGF-II produced by fetal trophoblast cells, due to the close spatial positioning of the two mRNAs.[54] The autocrine or paracrine actions of IGF-II and IGFBP-1 may be especially important during implantation and trophoblast invasion. In the syncytiotrophoblast, type 1 IGF receptors are found mainly on the microvillous membrane, facing the maternal side. IGFBP-3 has been localized to both the microvillous and basal membranes, and IGFBP-1 is predominantly found on the basal surface, facing the fetal side.[55]

The role of the IGF axis in fetal growth has been studied in monozygotic twin pregnancies where the twins are genetically identical and share a common uterine environment. Twin to twin transfusion syndrome (TTTS) accounts for a high incidence of perinatal mortality in monochorionic twins and causes the growth of one twin to be compromised as it donates blood to the other.[56] Fetal serum IGF-I concentrations are thought to be determined primarily by genetic influences, while IGF-II and IGFBP-1 concentrations are determined by both maternal environment and genetic factors. Bajoria et al. found that donor twins with TTTS had significantly lower levels of IGF-II and significantly higher levels of IGFBP-1, particularly the inhibitory phosphorylated isoform, than their recipient twin.[56] In addition, there was a positive correlation between birth weight and IGF-II and a negative correlation with IGFBP-1.[56] Given that the IGF-I levels in cord blood were similar and are thought to be genetically determined, altered placental production or placental regulation was proposed to contribute to changes in IGF-II and IGFBP-1 in growth-restricted twins. Inadequate placental dephosphorylation of IGFBP-1 may lead to alterations in the mitogenic activity of IGF-I and of placental nutrient transfer stimulated by IGF-I.[56]

Alterations in the IGF axis are also observed in dichorionic twins and in singletons of low birth weight. There is a positive relationship between cord blood IGF-I and birth weight in normal term singleton infants,[57,58] and some have also found a relationship between cord blood IGF-I and other parameters of size such as birth length, crown–rump length, ponderal index or placental weight.[57] The relationship between IGF-II and birth weight is not clear, with some groups finding a positive correlation in term singletons[59] and others finding no significant correlation.[57]

The relationship between cord blood IGFBPs and fetal growth has also been examined. IGFBP-3 correlates positively with birth weight,[57] while IGFBP-1 is inversely correlated with birth weight in term and preterm infants.[60] Iwashita et al. also observed an increase in phosphorylated isoforms of IGFBP-1 and a reduced proportion of nonphosphorylated to total IGFBP-1 in SGA fetuses, suggesting that the bioactivity of IGFBP-1 is increased in cases of poor fetal growth.[61]

Many studies have described some relationship between cord blood IGFs or IGFBPs and birth weight, but whether there is any relationship between fetal growth and maternal concentrations of these factors is more controversial. Boyne et al. found a positive correlation between maternal IGF-I concentration and birth weight and a negative correlation between maternal IGFBP-1 and birth weight at 35 weeks gestation, but not earlier in gestation.[62] Reduced maternal IGF-I,[63] IGF-II[63] and elevated IGFBP-1 in cases of fetal growth restriction have been described. However, other studies could not demonstrate any association between maternal IGF-I or IGFBP-1, measured at any stage of pregnancy, with neonatal birth weight or the development of IUGR and no correlation between maternal IGFBP-3 and fetal growth was reported.[64] Despite this finding, it is likely that the IGF axis has a crucial role to play in modulating normal fetal growth during human pregnancy, with IGF-I and IGFBP-1 implicated in fetal growth, and IGF-II possibly having an important role in placental growth.

Placental metabolism of glucocorticoids

Glucocorticoids are essential for the development and maturation of fetal organs before birth. Late pregnancy in humans and in many animal species is characterized by a rise in fetal cortisol levels, which parallels the increased maturation of fetal organs. Studies in sheep demonstrated that infusion of adrenocorticotropic hormone (ACTH), cortisol or dexamethasone into the preterm fetus resulted in delivery of lambs within 4–7 days.[65] These animals had accelerated adrenal growth and maturation of the lungs comparable to term lambs, suggesting an effect of glucocorticoids on fetal lung development.[65] Glucocorticoids also contribute to maturation of other organs including the thymus, gastrointestinal tract, liver, and kidney.

In humans, betamethasone administration to women at risk of preterm delivery has confirmed the effectiveness of glucocorticoids in maturing the fetal lungs, because it lowers the incidence of neonatal respiratory distress syndrome (RDS) and its associated mortality.[66] Today, antenatal glucocorticoids are commonly given to women in preterm labor to mature the fetal lungs and successfully reduce the risk of neonatal morbidity and mortality. Recent research interest, however, has focused on the potentially harmful effects of these treatments on the fetus and particularly on fetal growth.

Glucocorticoids may have adverse effects on the fetus. Antenatal dexamethasone treatment has been associated with a reduction in birth weight, by as much as 161 g in infants delivered between 30 and 32 weeks.[67] In addition, multiple doses of antenatal glucocorticoids have been linked to reduced fetal growth when compared to single doses. French et al. found that repeated courses of betamethasone were associated with a 9% reduction in birth weight and a 4% reduction in head circumference in preterm infants born prior to 33 weeks gestation.[68] However, recent evidence from randomized controlled trials suggests that there is no additional decrease in fetal growth when repeated courses of antenatal steroids are used as compared to single doses.[69] Therefore, glucocorticoids may have a beneficial effect on fetal organ maturation before birth, but also have the potential to reduce fetal growth.

Placental 11β-hydroxysteroid dehydrogenase (11β-HSD)

Maternal cortisol concentrations are 5–10 times higher than fetal cortisol concentrations.[70] This difference is maintained by the presence of the placental enzyme, 11β-hydroxysteroid dehydrogenase type 2 (11β-HSD2), which controls the passage of cortisol from mother to fetus. Two isoforms of 11β-HSD have been cloned and characterized in humans which interconvert glucocorticoids with their 11-keto metabolites (Figure 1.1). The type 1 enzyme (11β-HSD1) is NADP(H)-dependent, catalyzes the bidirectional interconversion of cortisol and cortisone, but acts primarily as an oxoreductase, converting cortisone to the active cortisol. This action is due to its higher affinity for cortisone (K_m in the nanomolar range) compared to cortisol (K_m in the micromolar range). The type 2 enzyme (11β-HSD2) is a high affinity, NAD-dependent, unidirectional enzyme, catalyzing only the dehydrogenase reaction, converting cortisol to the inactive cortisone.

The main function of the type 1 11β-HSD isozyme is to increase the availability of glucocorticoids for the glucocorticoid receptor (GR), allowing pre-receptor control of local glucocorticoid action. 11β-HSD1 is also found in gestational tissues; predominantly the decidua and chorion, as well as the endothelium of placental villous tissue, where it modulates the effect of cortisol on other placental pathways including prostaglandin biosynthesis and metabolism.[71]

The type 2 11β-HSD isozyme is found in specific tissues, such as the kidney and the placenta.[72] Its presence in mineralocorticoid target tissues, especially the kidney, is necessary to protect the mineralocorticoid receptor (MR) from occupation by cortisol. In the placenta the main function of 11β-HSD2 is to protect the fetus from the potentially harmful effects of endogenous maternal glucocorticoids. Synthetic glucocorticoids, such as dexamethasone and betamethasone, are not thought to be extensively metabolized by placental 11β-HSD2, possibly due to protection from their 9-halogen group.[73]

Placental 11β-HSD2 and fetal growth

Reductions in 11β-HSD2 activity have been associated with reduced human fetal growth. Shams et al. demonstrated that there was a significant reduction in enzyme activity in placenta from pregnancies complicated by IUGR compared to normally grown term deliveries and appropriately grown preterm deliveries.[74] In asthmatic pregnancies, reduced birth weight in females was specifically associated with reduced placental 11β-HSD2 activity, but not protein or mRNA.[25,26] In small preterm infants (22–32 weeks gestation), a positive correlation between relative birth weight (expressed in standard deviation units compared to population standards) and placental 11β-HSD2 total activity and activity rate was observed.[75] In addition, lower birth weight was associated with reduced umbilical cord vein cortisone, also suggesting

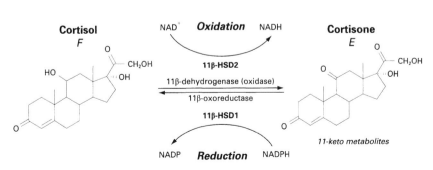

Figure 1.1 Interconversion of cortisol and cortisone by 11β-HSD. 11β-HSD2 catalyzes the oxidation of cortisol to its inactive 11-keto derivative, cortisone, with the use of NAD as a cofactor. 11β-HSD1 catalyzes the reduction of cortisone to cortisol with NADPH as a cofactor.

a reduction in transplacental cortisol to cortisone conversion in association with reduced fetal growth.[75]

One of the clinical features of patients suffering from the apparent mineralocorticoid excess syndrome (AME), which results from mutations of the 11β-HSD2 gene, is moderate IUGR.[76] Stewart et al. studied 11β-HSD2 activity in placenta obtained from a 28-week twin stillbirth in a family with two other children with AME.[76] Placental 11β-HSD2 activity was approximately 15% of that in five gestational age-matched controls and immunohistochemical staining for 11β-HSD2 was virtually absent in the AME placenta.[76] Both the siblings with AME and the placenta were shown to have a point mutation in exon V of the 11β-HSD2 gene.[76] These studies suggest that reduced 11β-HSD2 activity may be related to reduced fetal growth and possibly fetal death.

Regulation of placental 11β-HSD2

Placental 11β-HSD2 is clearly an important modulator of fetal glucocorticoid exposure and it is regulated by many hormones and factors associated with pregnancy, including estradiol, progesterone and prostaglandins, while studies in other tissues and cell lines have revealed regulation of this enzyme by inflammatory cytokines.

Glucocorticoids have an important role to play during fetal development, promoting maturation of organs required for extrauterine survival. An important pre-receptor mechanism exists to control the actions of glucocorticoids during pregnancy in the form of placental and fetal 11β-HSD2. Alterations in the activity of the placental 11β-HSD2 barrier, which result in an increase in maternal glucocorticoids crossing to the fetus, can have a deleterious effect on fetal growth and postnatal development.

THE ROLE OF THE FETUS IN GROWTH REGULATION

The fetus itself plays a role in its own growth regulation. The fetal tissues express IGFs and 11β-HSD2, allowing the fetus to adjust local levels of growth factors and glucocorticoids, thereby modulating cellular growth and differentiation in an autocrine or paracrine manner.

The mid-gestation human fetus (16–19 weeks) contains 11β-HSD2 mRNA and activity in the kidney, lung, gonad, liver, adrenal, and colon, while 11β-HSD1 mRNA has not been found in any fetal tissues at mid-gestation.[77] The presence of placental 11β-HSD2, high levels of 11β-HSD2 activity in fetal tissues, and the absence of 11β-HSD1 in the fetus all

contribute to a predominance of cortisone over cortisol in the fetal circulation. The presence of 11β-HSD2 enzyme in the fetal tissues may serve to locally regulate the positive and negative effects of glucocorticoids on the fetus.

Receptors for IGFs have also been identified in the human fetus from as early as the first trimester,[78] which allow IGF-I and IGF-II to exert growth-promoting effects on fetal cells. IGF-I and IGF-II have mitogenic actions in cultures of fetal fibroblasts, adrenal cells, and myoblasts.[79] IGF-I itself has been localized to many human fetal tissues, with high expression in the lung and intestine.[79] In addition, IGF-II has been found in the fetal kidney, liver, adrenal, and muscle and may be present in larger quantities than IGF-I.[79] IGFBP-1 has been localized to most fetal tissues including liver, lung, muscle, kidney, pancreas, adrenal, and intestine.[80] IGFBP mRNA expression studies suggest that IGFBP-1 is predominantly found in the fetal liver, while the other IGFBPs are located in most tissues of the fetus.[80] IGFs may be complexed to IGFBP-1 on the surface of fetal cells, as the pattern of immunostaining for fetal IGFs and IGFBP-1 was found to be similar in most sites.[80] The presence of IGF-I and IGF-II mRNA and protein in most fetal tissues suggests a local role for them in modulating growth.

Fetal sex is known to affect fetal growth, with male fetuses on average being larger than female fetuses.[81] This difference may not be evident until after 30 weeks, but increases as gestation progresses, with some studies reporting a 150–200 g weight difference by 38 weeks.[81] Males had a greater variation in birth weight distribution, with an increased tendency for higher birth weights.[14] Despite the difference in birth weight between male and female infants, the survival rate is greater for females than males.[14]

There are fetal sex differences in the IGF axis. IGF-II concentrations in umbilical cord serum from male neonates were significantly higher than those from female neonates[82] and cord plasma IGF-I was higher in female neonates than males.[83] A recent study of 987 healthy singletons found that IGF-I and IGFBP-3 concentrations in cord blood were higher in females than males.[84] In this study, there was no difference in IGF-II between male and female neonates, while growth hormone (GH) concentrations were higher in males than females.[84] Given that males are larger at birth and both IGF-I and IGFBP-3 correlate with birth size, these findings are counterintuitive, but do suggest that there are sexually dimorphic patterns of fetal growth regulation.

One possible mechanism by which the male fetus becomes larger than the female fetus was recently proposed by Tamimi et al., who studied maternal dietary intake during the second trimester of pregnancy.[85] They suggested that the fetus may be able to modulate its mother's nutritional input, since women pregnant with a male fetus had a higher energy intake compared with women pregnant with a female fetus.[85] After adjustment for confounding factors, this effect was related to an extra 796 kJ per day, which comprised 8% higher protein, 9.2% higher carbohydrates, and over 10% higher lipid intakes in women gestating with a male fetus as compared to those with a female fetus.[85]

Other studies have demonstrated that maternal smoking or caffeine consumption have different effects on the growth of male and female fetuses. Vik et al. studied second and third trimester caffeine consumption of mothers with SGA infants and mothers with normally grown infants.[86] They found that the risk of having an SGA infant was increased in women who consumed high levels of caffeine at 33 weeks gestation. However, when data were analyzed based on fetal sex, only the male fetus was at risk of being born small in association with high maternal caffeine intake.[86] Spinillo et al. examined a variety of risk factors for fetal growth restriction and found that overall, IUGR was more frequent in female fetuses, and that females were more sensitive to hypertension-induced growth restriction.[87] On the other hand, males were more affected by low maternal pre-pregnancy weight or BMI and maternal smoking.[87] Zaren et al. made serial ultrasound measurements throughout pregnancy and showed a significant decrease in biparietal diameter (BPD) from 18 weeks gestation with heavy maternal smoking in male fetuses, but no significant difference in BPD in female fetuses.[88] However, mean abdominal diameter in female fetuses of heavy smokers was significantly decreased from 25 weeks, while no decrease was observed in males until 33 weeks gestation.[88] All aspects of male neonatal size were reduced in the presence of maternal smoking, and while females had reduced birth weight and length, there was no significant difference in their head circumference, skin fold thickness or femur length compared to female neonates from non-smoking mothers.[88] These studies suggest that the regulation of fetal growth may be different for male and female fetuses.

Placental 11β-HSD2 may also differ depending on the sex of the fetus, thus possibly contributing to different fetal growth regulation in males and females. Placental 11β-HSD2 activity is greater when the fetus is female than when the fetus is male.[26] This difference may contribute to altered sensitivities to the effects of glucocorticoids in males and females. It is possible that many factors responsible for fetal growth regulation during human pregnancy are altered in a sex-specific manner. This could contribute to increased susceptibility to low birth weight in the male fetus, as observed with maternal smoking and caffeine intake, or to an increased likelihood of low birth weight in the female fetus, as observed with hypertension-associated IUGR.[87]

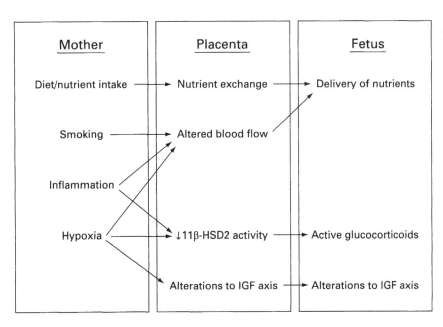

Figure 1.2 Interactions between the mother and placenta and fetus in the control of human fetal growth.

SUMMARY

- The mother, placenta, and fetus interact during pregnancy to modulate and regulate fetal growth (Figure 1.2).
- Maternal nutrients are essential for growth and development of the fetus, and transport of these nutrients occurs via the placental blood supply.
- The placenta is also important in the production and transport of growth-promoting hormones, which affect growth of the fetus, maternal nutrient levels, and growth of the placenta itself.
- Disturbances in fetal growth regulation can result in adverse outcomes for the neonate, and these adverse outcomes may persist into adult life. It is important, therefore, to understand the regulation of fetal growth, and particularly the role of mother, placenta, and fetus in complicated pregnancies. A better outcome for the fetus may be achieved, which may have health benefits into adulthood.

ACKNOWLEDGMENTS

Sources of funding were as follows. National Health and Medical Research Council (ID 252438), Hunter Medical Research Institute, NSW Health. Vanessa Murphy was the recipient of a National Health and Medical Research Council (NHMRC) Dora Lush (Biomedical) Postgraduate Scholarship and a Hunter Medical Research Institute/Port Waratah Coal Services Postdoctoral Fellowship. Dr Vicki Clifton was the recipient of the Arthur Wilson Memorial Scholarship from the Royal Australian College of Obstetricians and Gynaecologists and NHMRC Career Development Grant (ID 300786).

REFERENCES

1. Brar HS, Rutherford SE. Classification of intrauterine growth retardation. Semin Perinatol 1988; 12: 2–10.
2. Public health aspects of low birth weight: Third report of the expert committee on maternal and child health. WHO Tech Rep Ser 1961; 217: 3–16.
3. Ashworth A. Effects of intrauterine growth retardation on mortality and morbidity in infants and young children. Eur J Clin Nutr 1998; 52 (Suppl 1): S34–S41; discussion S41–S42.
4. Gruenwald P. Chronic fetal distress and placental insufficiency. Biol Neonate 1963; 33: 215–65.
5. Barker DJ, Eriksson JG, Forsen T, Osmond C. Fetal origins of adult disease: strength of effects and biological basis. Int J Epidemiol 2002; 31: 1235–9.
6. Barker DJ, Osmond C. Death rates from stroke in England and Wales predicted from past maternal mortality. BMJ (Clin Res Ed) 1987; 295: 83–6.
7. Barker DJ, Osmond C, Golding J, Kuh D, Wadsworth ME. Growth in utero, blood pressure in childhood and adult life, and mortality from cardiovascular disease. BMJ 1989; 298: 564–7.
8. Law CM, de Swiet M, Osmond C et al. Initiation of hypertension in utero and its amplification throughout life. BMJ 1993; 306: 24–7.
9. Barker DJ, Bull AR, Osmond C, Simmonds SJ. Fetal and placental size and risk of hypertension in adult life. BMJ 1990; 301: 259–62.
10. Barker DJ, Hales CN, Fall CH et al. Type 2 (non-insulin-dependent) diabetes mellitus, hypertension and hyperlipidaemia (syndrome X): relation to reduced fetal growth. Diabetologia 1993; 36: 62–7.
11. Shiell AW, Campbell-Brown M, Haselden S et al. High-meat, low-carbohydrate diet in pregnancy: relation to adult blood pressure in the offspring. Hypertension 2001; 38: 1282–8.
12. Ravelli AC, van der Meulen JH, Michels RP et al. Glucose tolerance in adults after prenatal exposure to famine. Lancet 1998; 351: 173–7.
13. Roseboom TJ, Van Der Meulen JH, Ravelli AC et al. Perceived health of adults after prenatal exposure to the Dutch famine. Paediatr Perinat Epidemiol 2003; 17: 391–7.
14. Cogswell ME, Yip R. The influence of fetal and maternal factors on the distribution of birthweight. Semin Perinatol 1995; 19: 222–40.
15. Picciano MF. Pregnancy and lactation: physiological adjustments, nutritional requirements and the role of dietary supplements. J Nutr 2003; 133: 1997S–2002S.
16. Christian P, Khatry SK, Katz J et al. Effects of alternative maternal micronutrient supplements on low birth weight in rural Nepal: double blind randomised community trial. BMJ 2003; 326: 571.
17. de Haas JH. Parental smoking. Its effects on fetus and child health. Eur J Obstet Gynecol Reprod Biol 1975; 5: 283–96.
18. Lehtovirta P, Forss M. The acute effect of smoking on intervillous blood flow of the placenta. Br J Obstet Gynaecol 1978; 85: 729–31.
19. Sexton M, Hebel JR. A clinical trial of change in maternal smoking and its effect on birth weight. JAMA 1984; 251: 911–15.
20. Giussani DA, Phillips PS, Anstee S, Barker DJ. Effects of altitude versus economic status on birth weight and body shape at birth. Pediatr Res 2001; 49: 490–4.
21. Jensen GM, Moore LG. The effect of high altitude and other risk factors on birthweight: independent or interactive effects? Am J Public Health 1997; 87: 1003–7.
22. Zamudio S, Palmer SK, Droma T et al. Effect of altitude on uterine artery blood flow during normal pregnancy. J Appl Physiol 1995; 79(1): 7–14.
23. Moore LG, Zamudio S, Zhuang J, Sun S, Droma T. Oxygen transport in Tibetan women during pregnancy at 3,658 m. Am J Phys Anthropol 2001; 114: 42–53.
24. Clifton VL, Giles WB, Smith R et al. Alterations of placental vascular function in asthmatic pregnancies. Am J Respir Crit Care Med 2001; 164: 546–53.
25. Murphy VE, Zakar T, Smith R et al. Reduced 11beta-hydroxysteroid dehydrogenase type 2 activity is associated with decreased birth weight centile in pregnancies complicated by asthma. J Clin Endocrinol Metab 2002; 87: 1660–8.
26. Murphy VE, Gibson PG, Giles WB et al. Maternal asthma is associated with reduced female fetal growth. Am J Respir Crit Care Med 2003; 168: 1317–23.

27. Bowden AP, Barrett JH, Fallow W, Silman AJ. Women with inflammatory polyarthritis have babies of lower birth weight. J Rheumatol 2001; 28: 355–9.
28. Aherne W. Morphometry. In: The Placenta and its Maternal Supply Line (Gruenwald P, ed). Baltimore: University Park Press, 1975: 80–97.
29. Rockwell LC, Vargas E, Moore LG. Human physiological adaptation to pregnancy: inter- and intraspecific perspectives. Am J Hum Biol 2003; 15: 330–41.
30. Kliman HJ. Uteroplacental blood flow. The story of decidualization, menstruation, and trophoblast invasion. Am J Pathol 2000; 157: 1759–68.
31. Palmer SK, Zamudio S, Coffin C et al. Quantitative estimation of human uterine artery blood flow and pelvic blood flow redistribution in pregnancy. Obstet Gynecol 1992; 80: 1000–6.
32. Zygmunt M, Herr F, Munstedt K, Lang U, Liang OD. Angiogenesis and vasculogenesis in pregnancy. Eur J Obstet Gynecol Reprod Biol 2003; 110 (Suppl 1): S10–S18.
33. Giles WB, Lingman G, Marsal K, Trudinger BJ. Fetal volume blood flow and umbilical artery flow velocity waveform analysis: a comparison. Br J Obstet Gynaecol 1986; 93: 461–5.
34. Barbera A, Galan HL, Ferrazzi E et al. Relationship of umbilical vein blood flow to growth parameters in the human fetus. Am J Obstet Gynecol 1999; 181: 174–9.
35. Cetin I. Placental transport of amino acids in normal and growth-restricted pregnancies. Eur J Obstet Gynecol Reprod Biol 2003; 110 (Suppl 1): S50–S54.
36. Jansson T, Scholtbach V, Powell TL. Placental transport of leucine and lysine is reduced in intrauterine growth restriction. Pediatr Res 1998; 44: 532–7.
37. Economides DL, Nicolaides KH, Gahl WA, Bernardini I, Evans MI. Plasma amino acids in appropriate- and small-for-gestational-age fetuses. Am J Obstet Gynecol 1989; 161: 1219–27.
38. Jansson T. Amino acid transporters in the human placenta. Pediatr Res 2001; 49: 141–7.
39. Marconi AM, Paolini C, Buscaglia M et al. The impact of gestational age and fetal growth on the maternal-fetal glucose concentration difference. Obstet Gynecol 1996; 87: 937–42.
40. Nicolini U, Hubinont C, Santolaya J et al. Maternal-fetal glucose gradient in normal pregnancies and in pregnancies complicated by alloimmunization and fetal growth retardation. Am J Obstet Gynecol 1989; 161: 924–7.
41. Challis DE, Pfarrer CD, Ritchie JW, Koren G, Adamson SL. Glucose metabolism is elevated and vascular resistance and maternofetal transfer is normal in perfused placental cotyledons from severely growth-restricted fetuses. Pediatr Res 2000; 47: 309–15.
42. Haggarty P. Placental regulation of fatty acid delivery and its effect on fetal growth – a review. Placenta 2002; 23 (Suppl A): S28–S38.
43. DeChiara TM, Efstratiadis A, Robertson EJ. A growth-deficiency phenotype in heterozygous mice carrying an insulin-like growth factor II gene disrupted by targeting. Nature 1990; 345: 78–80.
44. Baker J, Liu JP, Robertson EJ, Efstratiadis A. Role of insulin-like growth factors in embryonic and postnatal growth. Cell 1993; 75: 73–82.
45. Liu JP, Baker J, Perkins AS, Robertson EJ, Efstratiadis A. Mice carrying null mutations of the genes encoding insulin-like growth factor I (Igf-1) and type 1 IGF receptor (Igf1r). Cell 1993; 75: 59–72.
46. Constancia M, Hemberger M, Hughes J et al. Placental-specific IGF-II is a major modulator of placental and fetal growth. Nature 2002; 417: 945–8.

47. Germain-Lee EL, Janicot M, Lammers R, Ullrich A, Casella SJ. Expression of a type I insulin-like growth factor receptor with low affinity for insulin-like growth factor II. Biochem J 1992; 281 (Pt 2): 413–17.
48. Abuzzahab MJ, Schneider A, Goddard A et al. IGF-I receptor mutations resulting in intrauterine and postnatal growth retardation. N Engl J Med 2003; 349: 2211–22.
49. Bang P, Westgren M, Schwander J et al. Ontogeny of insulin-like growth factor-binding protein-1, -2, and -3: quantitative measurements by radioimmunoassay in human fetal serum. Pediatr Res 1994; 36: 528–36.
50. Chellakooty M, Vangsgaard K, Larsen T et al. A longitudinal study of intrauterine growth and the placental growth hormone (GH)-insulin-like growth factor I axis in maternal circulation: association between placental GH and fetal growth. J Clin Endocrinol Metab 2004; 89: 384–91.
51. Lee PD, Conover CA, Powell DR. Regulation and function of insulin-like growth factor-binding protein-1. Proc Soc Exp Biol Med 1993; 204: 4–29.
52. Westwood M. Role of insulin-like growth factor binding protein 1 in human pregnancy. Rev Reprod 1999; 4: 160–7.
53. Jones JI, D'Ercole AJ, Camacho-Hubner C, Clemmons DR. Phosphorylation of insulin-like growth factor (IGF)-binding protein 1 in cell culture and in vivo: effects on affinity for IGF-I. Proc Natl Acad Sci USA 1991; 88: 7481–5.
54. Han VK, Bassett N, Walton J, Challis JR. The expression of insulin-like growth factor (IGF) and IGF-binding protein (IGFBP) genes in the human placenta and membranes: evidence for IGF-IGFBP interactions at the feto-maternal interface. J Clin Endocrinol Metab 1996; 81: 2680–93.
55. Fang J, Furesz TC, Smith CH, Fant ME. IGF binding protein-1 (IGFBP-1) is preferentially associated with the fetal-facing basal surface of the syncytiotrophoblast in the human placenta. Growth Horm IGF Res 1999; 9: 438–44.
56. Bajoria R, Gibson MJ, Ward S et al. Placental regulation of insulin-like growth factor axis in monochorionic twins with chronic twin-twin transfusion syndrome. J Clin Endocrinol Metab 2001; 86: 3150–6.
57. Fant M, Salafia C, Baxter RC et al. Circulating levels of IGFs and IGF binding proteins in human cord serum: relationships to intrauterine growth. Regul Pept 1993; 48: 29–39.
58. Ong K, Kratzsch J, Kiess W et al. Size at birth and cord blood levels of insulin, insulin-like growth factor I (IGF-I), IGF-II, IGF-binding protein-1 (IGFBP-1), IGFBP-3, and the soluble IGF-II/mannose-6-phosphate receptor in term human infants. The ALSPAC Study Team. Avon Longitudinal Study of Pregnancy and Childhood. J Clin Endocrinol Metab 2000; 85: 4266–9.
59. Bennett A, Wilson DM, Liu F et al. Levels of insulin-like growth factors I and II in human cord blood. J Clin Endocrinol Metab 1983; 57: 609–12.
60. Wang HS, Lee CL, Chard T. Levels of insulin-like growth factor-I and insulin-like growth factor-binding protein-1 in pregnancy with preterm delivery. Br J Obstet Gynaecol 1993; 100: 472–5.
61. Iwashita M, Sakai K, Kudo Y, Takeda Y. Phosphoisoforms of insulin-like growth factor binding protein-1 in appropriate-for-gestational-age and small-for-gestational-age fetuses. Growth Horm IGF Res 1998; 8: 487–93.
62. Boyne MS, Thame M, Bennett FI et al. The relationship among circulating insulin-like growth factor (IGF)-I, IGF-binding proteins-1 and -2, and birth anthropometry: a prospective study. J Clin Endocrinol Metab 2003; 88: 1687–91.
63. McIntyre HD, Serek R, Crane DI et al. Placental growth hormone (GH), GH-binding protein, and insulin-like

growth factor axis in normal, growth-retarded, and diabetic pregnancies: correlations with fetal growth. J Clin Endocrinol Metab 2000; 85: 1143–50.

64. Orbak Z, Darcan S, Coker M, Goksen D. Maternal and fetal serum insulin-like growth factor-I (IGF-I), IGF binding protein-3 (IGFBP-3), leptin levels and early postnatal growth in infants born asymmetrically small for gestational age. J Pediatr Endocrinol Metab 2001; 14: 1119–27.

65. Liggins GC. Premature parturition after infusion of corti-cotrophin or cortisol into foetal lambs. J Endocrinol 1968; 42: 323–9.

66. Liggins GC, Howie RN. A controlled trial of antepartum glucocorticoid treatment for prevention of the respiratory distress syndrome in premature infants. Pediatrics 1972; 50: 515–25.

67. Bloom SL, Sheffield JS, McIntire DD, Leveno KJ. Antenatal dexamethasone and decreased birth weight. Obstet Gynecol 2001; 97: 485–90.

68. French NP, Hagan R, Evans SF, Godfrey M, Newnham JP. Repeated antenatal corticosteroids: size at birth and subse-quent development. Am J Obstet Gynecol 1999; 180 (1 Pt 1): 114–21.

69. Lee MJ, Davies J, Guinn D et al. Single versus weekly courses of antenatal corticosteroids in preterm premature rupture of membranes. Obstet Gynecol 2004; 103: 274–81.

70. Gitau R, Cameron A, Fisk NM, Glover V. Fetal exposure to maternal cortisol. Lancet 1998; 352: 707–8.

71. Challis JRG, Matthews SG, Gibb W, Lye SJ. Endocrine and paracrine regulation of birth at term and preterm. Endocr Rev 2000; 21: 514–50.

72. Krozowski Z, Maguire JA, Stein-Oakley AN et al. Immuno-histochemical localization of the 11 beta-hydroxysteroid dehydrogenase type II enzyme in human kidney and placenta. J Clin Endocrinol Metab 1995; 80: 2203–9.

73. Walker BR, Connacher AA, Webb DJ, Edwards CR. Glucocorticoids and blood pressure: a role for the corti-sol/cortisone shuttle in the control of vascular tone in man. Clin Sci (Colch) 1992; 83: 171–8.

74. Shams M, Kilby MD, Somerset DA et al. 11Beta-hydroxy-steroid dehydrogenase type 2 in human pregnancy and reduced expression in intrauterine growth restriction. Hum Reprod 1998; 13: 799–804.

75. Kajantie E, Dunkel L, Turpeinen U et al. Placental 11beta-hydroxysteroid dehydrogenase-2 and fetal cortisol/cortisone shuttle in small preterm infants. J Clin Endocrinol Metab 2003; 88: 493–500.

76. Stewart PM, Krozowski ZS, Gupta A et al. Hypertension in the syndrome of apparent mineralocorticoid excess due to mutation of the 11 beta-hydroxysteroid dehydrogenase type 2 gene. Lancet 1996; 347: 88–91.

77. Stewart PM, Whorwood CB, Mason JI. Type 2 11 beta-hydroxysteroid dehydrogenase in foetal and adult life. J Steroid Biochem Mol Biol 1995; 55: 465–71.

78. Shifren JL, Osathanondh R, Yeh J. Human fetal ovaries and uteri: developmental expression of genes encoding the insulin, insulin-like growth factor I, and insulin-like growth factor II receptors. Fertil Steril 1993; 59: 1036–40.

79. Han VK, Hill DJ, Strain AJ et al. Identification of somatomedin/insulin-like growth factor immunoreactive cells in the human fetus. Pediatr Res 1987; 22: 245–9.

80. Hill DJ, Clemmons DR, Wilson S et al. Immunological dis-tribution of one form of insulin-like growth factor (IGF)-binding protein and IGF peptides in human fetal tissues. J Mol Endocrinol 1989; 2: 31–8.

81. Thomas P, Peabody J, Turnier V, Clark RH. A new look at intrauterine growth and the impact of race, altitude, and gender. Pediatrics 2000; 106: E21.

82. Gluckman PD, Johnson-Barrett JJ, Butler JH, Edgar BW, Gunn TR. Studies of insulin-like growth factor-I and -II by specific radioligand assays in umbilical cord blood. Clin Endocrinol (Oxf) 1983; 19: 405–13.

83. Vatten LJ, Nilsen ST, Odegard RA, Romundstad PR, Austgulen R. Insulin-like growth factor I and leptin in umbilical cord plasma and infant birth size at term. Pediatrics 2002; 109: 1131–5.

84. Geary MP, Pringle PJ, Rodeck CH, Kingdom JC, Hindmarsh PC. Sexual dimorphism in the growth hormone and insulin-like growth factor axis at birth. J Clin Endocrinol Metab 2003; 88: 3708–14.

85. Tamimi RM, Lagiou P, Mucci LA et al. Average energy intake among pregnant women carrying a boy compared with a girl. BMJ 2003; 326: 1245–6.

86. Vik T, Bakketeig LS, Trygg KU, Lund-Larsen K, Jacobsen G. High caffeine consumption in the third trimester of preg-nancy: gender-specific effects on fetal growth. Paediatr Perinat Epidemiol 2003; 17: 324–31.

87. Spinillo A, Capuzzo E, Nicola S et al. Interaction between fetal gender and risk factors for fetal growth retardation. Am J Obstet Gynecol 1994; 171: 1273–7.

88. Zaren B, Lindmark G, Bakketeig L. Maternal smoking affects fetal growth more in the male fetus. Paediatr Perinat Epidemiol 2000; 14: 118–26.

2

Maternal nutrition and later disease risk

Jane E Harding, Frank H Bloomfield, and Mark H Oliver

INTRODUCTION

Maternal nutrition before and during pregnancy can alter fetal growth, size at birth, and later disease risk. The causal pathways that link these factors remain uncertain, but it is now clear that changes in maternal nutrition may alter outcome for the offspring without affecting size at birth. There is both human and animal evidence that fetal outcomes can be influenced not only by the overall level of maternal nutrition, but also by timing of any changes in nutrition, the balance of macronutrients, and a number of specific micronutrients. Potential mechanisms which underlie these effects are beginning to be described. Determining the optimal nutrition for women before and during pregnancy and lactation must become a research priority to optimize lifelong health of their offspring.

EPIDEMIOLOGY

A potential link between adult cardiovascular disease risk and adverse events in early life was first postulated about 30 years ago.[1] However, the strength and consistency of this link have only been established in recent years. David Barker and colleagues from Southampton were the first to conduct retrospective cohort studies that clearly demonstrated in humans the link between low birth weight and subsequent disease risk. In initial historical cohort studies from the UK, it was clearly shown that those who were of lower birth weight had an increased risk of high blood pressure,[2] cardiovascular disease,[3] noninsulin-dependent diabetes[4] and dyslipidemias.[5,6] These studies have since been replicated elsewhere in the world and in other prospective studies.

There are a number of striking aspects of these epidemiological studies. First, the effect is found across the range of normal birth weights, rather than only amongst the very low birth weight infants. Second, the effect on blood pressure is much weaker than the effect on disease, e.g. hypertension or cardiovascular disease. Although there has been debate about the size of the effect,[7] in most studies the blood pressure increases approximately 2 mmHg for every kilogram decrease in birth weight.[8] However, the risk of hypertensive disease changes much more markedly across the birth weight range,[9] suggesting that the pathophysiology might be more strongly related to size at birth than are some of the known physiological predictors of disease in adulthood.

Although initially greeted with considerable skepticism, these findings have now been widely accepted and much attention has focused on the possible underlying mechanisms. It has proved surprisingly easy to produce long-term changes in such outcomes as blood pressure and glucose tolerance in experimental animals, but the precise mechanisms underlying the observations in human populations remain to be elucidated.

CAUSES OF SMALL BABIES

In human populations there are large numbers of pathologies and pathophysiologies that give rise to small babies. However, in broad terms these can be thought to comprise four main groups (Table 2.1). Those that are 'intrinsic' to the fetus are not usually considered susceptible to nutritional influences, although there are exceptions such as folate supplementation for prevention of neural tube defects. However, it is the group that are apparently 'extrinsic' to the fetus, caused by limited fetal nutrition, that are the focus of this chapter.

It is readily demonstrable in animal studies that limited maternal nutrition leads to small size at birth. In sheep, fetal growth slows within 3 days in response to maternal undernutrition in late gestation, and resumes

Table 2.1 Main causes of small size at birth in human populations

Cause	Examples
Intrinsic to the fetus	
Chromosomal and genetic defects	Trisomy 18
	Leprechaun syndrome (mutation in the insulin receptor)
Toxins	Alcohol
	Smoking
Infections	Rubella
	Toxoplasma
Extrinsic to the fetus	
Fetal nutritional limitation	Maternal hypertension
	Placental infarction
	Placental vascular disease

promptly upon maternal refeeding (Figure 2.1). However, the major regulator of fetal growth is fetal nutrition rather than maternal nutrition. This is because nutrients must reach the fetus along a complex supply line, including not only maternal nutrition, but also the supply of those nutrients across the placenta to the fetus (Figure 2.2). Any interference with fetal nutrition by limitations at any point along the supply line can lead to impaired fetal growth. The latter processes mean that maternal nutrition is only indirectly related to fetal nutrition under some circumstances. Nevertheless, there is growing evidence in both animal and human populations that maternal nutrition can alter both size at birth and later disease risk.

ROLE OF MATERNAL NUTRITION

Global undernutrition

Chronic global undernutrition in human populations is associated with reduced average size at birth. However, direct causal relationships are difficult to

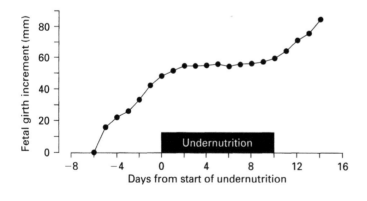

Figure 2.1 Effect of maternal undernutrition on fetal growth in sheep. Fetal growth in late gestation slows within 3 days of the onset of 10 days of maternal undernutrition, and resumes upon maternal refeeding.

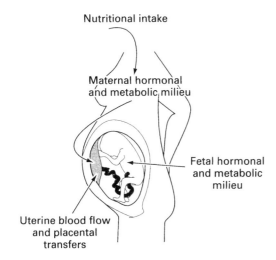

Nutritional intake

Maternal hormonal and metabolic milieu

Fetal hormonal and metabolic milieu

Uterine blood flow and placental transfers

Figure 2.2 The fetal supply line. Nutrients reach the fetus via a series of steps in the mother, uterus, and placenta, so that changes in maternal diet may or may not result in changes in fetal nutrition. Conversely, fetal nutrition may be limited by the fetal supply line, even when maternal diet is adequate.

ascribe in chronically undernourished populations where maternal size, infectious disease burden, and micronutrient deficiencies are also likely to play an important part. Animal studies in rats and guinea pigs have clearly demonstrated that global maternal undernutrition during most of pregnancy results in offspring that are small at birth. This reduced birth size is associated with long-term changes in glucose tolerance, adiposity, and cardiovascular function in the offspring after birth.[10–14]

The timing of maternal undernutrition may also be important. The best human data come from the Dutch Hunger Winter, where a 5-month period of severe famine in a previously well-nourished population provided some information about the effects of maternal undernutrition at different times of pregnancy on size at birth and health of the offspring.[15] Women who experienced famine only in late gestation had babies who were on average smaller at birth and as adults had a higher incidence of glucose intolerance.[16] Women exposed to famine in early or mid-gestation had offspring that were on average of normal size at birth.[17] Despite this, these offspring had an increased risk of cardiovascular disease, dyslipidemia, and of themselves giving birth to smaller babies.[17–19] These data strongly suggest that exposure to undernutrition in early gestation in humans can result in altered disease risk in adulthood with little or no change in size at birth.

In general, animal studies have been more helpful in clarifying the role of undernutrition of different timing in determining later disease risk. In rats, exposure to undernutrition in late gestation resulted in altered pancreatic function of the offspring;[20] a finding remarkably similar to those from the Dutch famine studies. Similarly, exposure to chronic maternal undernutrition in the first part of pregnancy in sheep resulted in offspring with altered maturation of the hypothalamic-pituitary-adrenal (HPA) axis[21] and regulation of blood pressure.[22,23] All of these changes were without effect on size at birth. In sheep exposed to either 10 or 20 days of undernutrition in late gestation, only offspring from ewes exposed for the longer duration were significantly smaller than controls at birth, consistent with previous findings that 10 days of undernutrition causes a temporary slowing of fetal growth which recovers upon refeeding, whereas 20 days causes an irreversible alteration in fetal growth trajectory.[24] However, in adult life, offspring that had been exposed to undernutrition for 10, but not for 20, days *in utero* had altered HPA axis function.[25]

It is important to note, therefore, that although the human epidemiology is based on measures of size at birth, this is because size at birth is a readily measurable variable, whereas fetal growth is not. It appears that at least some of the causal pathways linking maternal nutrition to disease risk in the offspring do not necessarily involve changes in size at birth, although they may involve altered fetal growth.[26] When a change in size at birth is also present, this difference may not necessarily be the mediator, but rather a surrogate marker of the factors that caused both adult disease and altered size at birth (Figure 2.3). Furthermore, sheep studies demonstrate that a relatively mild nutritional insult early in pregnancy, at a stage when the nutritional requirements of the developing conceptus are so small that nutritional supply would not be likely to be directly compromised, have effects late in gestation on maturation of the HPA axis[27,28] and the timing of birth.[29] These findings indicate that there must be some communication between the mother and her developing conceptus predicting later nutrient supply (Figure 2.3).[30] Once again, fetal weight in late gestation and birth weight of offspring were not altered in these studies, although fetal growth trajectory was different,[31,32] suggesting that this was set very early in pregnancy. The epidemiological findings from the women exposed to famine in the first trimester in the Dutch Hunger Winter (see above) are also consistent with such a mechanism.

Balance of macronutrients

One reason that maternal nutrition had been thought to have relatively little effect on size at birth in humans is the observation that maternal nutritional supplements in chronically undernourished populations produce only a very small improvement in mean birth weight, although they produce a greater improvement in the incidence of low birth weight.[33] Nevertheless, it appears that the balance of macronutrients, and specifically the balance of protein and carbohydrate in the supplements, does have some influence on size at birth. Studies in which women were given a calorie supplement that was of low protein density (low proportion of the calories as protein) tended to have babies of larger birth weight than unsupplemented controls, whereas women receiving a high protein density supplement tended to have smaller babies than those not supplemented.[33,34] These data suggest that the balance of protein and carbohydrate has an important influence on size at birth.

There are increasing data from epidemiological studies to support this view. Southampton women were found to be more likely to have larger babies if they had a low carbohydrate intake in early pregnancy accompanied by a high meat protein intake in late pregnancy.[35] In contrast, a prospective study in Adelaide suggested that the percentage of energy intake derived from protein in early pregnancy was positively associated with birth weight, and that the similar measure for carbohydrate in both early and late pregnancy was negatively associated with ponderal index at birth.[36] In a recent prospective study from New Zealand, women whose babies were born small-for-gestational age (SGA) were found to have a lower consumption of fish, carbohydrate-rich foods, and fresh vegetables than were those with a normal birth weight baby.[37] Smaller size at birth was also associated in an Indian study with a lower maternal intake of fruit and green leafy vegetables during pregnancy.[38] In a retrospective cohort study from Aberdeen, in which women were asked to eat 0.45 kg of red meat per day and to avoid carbohydrate-rich foods, blood pressure was lowest in the 27–30-year-old offspring of women who had consumed larger amounts of both protein and carbohydrate, and blood pressure was higher in those whose mothers' diets during pregnancy showed an imbalance between carbohydrate and protein intake.[39] Cortisol concentrations also increased with each daily portion of red meat or fish, but decreased with each portion of green leafy vegetables.[40] Similarly, in survivors of the Dutch famine, adult blood pressure was found to be more closely related to the protein density of the maternal diet than to size at birth or timing of the maternal famine exposure.[41]

A low protein diet during pregnancy has been widely used experimentally to induce reduced birth size and later disease risk. In rats, protein restriction throughout pregnancy and lactation leads to reduced birth weight, decreased nephron number, increased systolic blood pressure and insulin resistance in the offspring.[10,11,42]

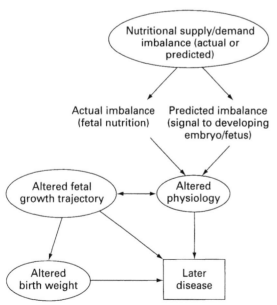

Figure 2.3 Possible causal pathways between fetal nutrition and adult disease. Altered fetal nutrition may lead directly to the physiological changes that result in adult disease susceptibility, and may or may not also lead to changes in fetal growth and size at birth.

Overnutrition in animals has also been demonstrated to result in altered physiology in the offspring. Global overnutrition in rat dams, induced by impairing hypothalamic satiety control, results in hyperglycemia and glucose intolerance in the offspring.[43] Rat dams fed a high fat diet in pregnancy have offspring with impaired glucose homeostasis,[44] altered endothelial function, lower basal heart rates, and hypertension as adults.[45] Interestingly, if the offspring are also fed a high fat diet after birth, the endothelial dysfunction, but not the hypertension, is prevented.[46] During gestation, the high fat-fed dams had a lower total food intake. As the feed is hypercaloric, their total energy intake was isocaloric compared with controls. This finding suggests that the effect may not be simply overnutrition with fat, but that there may also be an element of nutritional imbalance, perhaps with inadequate intake of other components of the diet.

The baby born to a diabetic mother may also have experienced fetal overnutrition. These babies are exposed to high glucose and fatty acid concentrations *in utero*, and have larger birth weights, but with minimal increase in other measurements of body size, with most of the increase in weight due to fat deposition. There is now good evidence that these babies are also at increased risk of glucose intolerance and type 2 diabetes mellitus in later life.[47,48]

Micronutrients

The role of micronutrients in fetal growth is more difficult to discern in human populations. This challenge is because many micronutrients are often simultaneously limited in the diet, and data must come from the randomized trials of micronutrient supplements, often in otherwise undernourished populations. These studies have provided some limited findings on the effects of some micronutrients. Higher calcium intake during pregnancy has been associated with lower blood pressure in the offspring, at least in early childhood.[49] One long-term follow-up study of a randomized trial suggested that the effect of maternal calcium supplements on the blood pressure of the offspring was still apparent when the children were 7 years old.[50] However, there was no effect on birth weight in either study.

Maternal anemia is commonly associated with reduced size at birth[51] and sometimes with a larger placenta.[52] This combination of a small baby with a proportionately large placenta has been associated in epidemiological studies with higher blood pressure in adulthood.[53] However, randomized trials of iron supplementation have generally shown no benefit in terms of increased birth weight.[54] Similarly, the addition of a multiple micronutrient supplement in one large randomized trial had no additional effect on birth weight over that of iron supplements alone.[55]

Nevertheless, it is clear that some specific nutrients, and particularly some amino acids, may have important effects on long-term outcomes even without an effect on size at birth. Glycine is a conditionally essential amino acid in pregnancy, and many women become marginally glycine-deficient during pregnancy, even in apparently well-nourished populations.[56] Glycine is essential for fetal and placental growth, because it is required for the production of many essential compounds, such as heme, creatine, collagen, and nucleic acids. Rats fed a low protein diet have offspring who develop hypertension in postnatal life. Supplementing maternal diet with glycine but not with alanine or urea prevents hypertension and endothelial dysfunction in the offspring without changing size at birth.[57,58] Glycine metabolism is also perturbed in late gestation fetal sheep after maternal undernutrition in early gestation.[59]

Similarly, taurine is a semi-essential amino acid that is not incorporated into body proteins, but is essential for pancreatic beta cell development. Rats on a low protein diet have offspring with impaired pancreatic insulin secretion. Supplementation of the maternal low protein diet with taurine alone reverses the effect on the fetal pancreatic beta cells, whereas adding taurine to the medium in which the beta cells are cultured does not achieve this effect.[60] Maternal undernutrition around the time of conception in sheep results in elevated maternal and fetal taurine levels in late gestation and is associated with increased insulin secretion in response to a glucose, but not an arginine challenge.[61] These data suggest that the higher taurine levels are associated with earlier maturation of the pancreatic beta cells.

MECHANISMS LINKING NUTRITION TO LATER DISEASE RISK

Although it is not at all clear how maternal nutrition might link size at birth and later disease risk, a number of main hypotheses have been proposed (Table 2.2). There is experimental evidence to support each of these, but whether any or all of them apply in any given situation in human populations is not yet clear.

Nutrient supply

The simplest potential link between maternal nutrition and adult disease concerns the supply of nutrients as the raw materials for growth of the relevant organ systems and their regulatory control mechanisms.

Table 2.2 Possible mechanisms by which altered maternal nutrition may lead to altered disease risk in the offspring

Mechanism	Effects	Examples
Nutrient supply	Reduced raw materials for tissue growth	Fewer nephrons leading to hypertension
Nutrient partitioning	Maternal demand compromises fetal supply	Growing adolescent mothers
Nutrient balance	Maternal high fat diet leading to endothelial dysfunction	Hypertension and altered glucose homeostasis in offspring
Fetal glucocorticoid exposure	Altered fetal HPA axis regulation	Synthetic glucocorticoid exposure leading to hypertension
Altered fetal insulin secretion	Reduced fetal growth and also postnatal insulin resistance	Glucokinase mutation
Periconceptional undernutrition	Altered cell number or cell allocation in developing embryo Altered cell cycle length Imprinting disorders Altered nutrition to oocyte/blastocyst	Dutch Hunger Winter Many examples in animal experiments, with or without alterations in fetal growth

Inadequate protein supply, for example, at the time that the kidney is developing in late gestation, might lead to impaired fetal kidney growth resulting in fewer nephrons and subsequent hypertension. There is some evidence that this sequence of events may occur: humans with hypertension have on average fewer nephrons than those who do not in adulthood.[62] Infants born SGA have also been found to have fewer nephrons.[63] Experimentally, reduced nephron number in early life has been shown to result in later hypertension.[42,64] However, such a direct link between maternal nutrition and organ growth cannot explain the long-term effects of undernutrition very early in pregnancy, when fetal nutrient demand for organ growth is so small that it cannot possibly exceed nutrient availability along the supply line. Nevertheless, many aspects of fetal development are changed by this period of undernutrition, suggesting that direct nutrient supply cannot be the whole answer.

Nutrient partitioning

Available maternal nutrients must be partitioned between the mother, the placenta, and the fetus. The regulation of this partitioning is not well understood, but includes pregnancy-related hormones such as placental lactogen and growth hormone, which is produced by the placenta during human pregnancy. These hormones contribute in part to maternal insulin resist-ance during pregnancy, thus increasing the availability of glucose and fatty acids for the nutrition of the feto-placental unit. Insulin-like growth factor I (IGF-I) also contributes to nutrient partitioning during pregnancy. Maternal IGF-I contributes to the regulation of glucose and amino acid uptake into the placenta,[65] while fetal IGF-I contributes to the regulation of glucose and amino acid uptake from placenta to fetus.[66] IGF-I also regulates the distribution of nutrients, particularly amino acids, within the feto-placental unit and between fetal viscera and carcass.[67]

Since all of these hormones are at least in part regulated by nutritional intake, some effects of maternal nutrition may be mediated via changes in nutrient partitioning and hence nutrient availability for the growing fetus. This partitioning may be a particular issue in mothers who are still growing themselves and, therefore, have a greater demand for the nutrients that might otherwise be available for the feto-placental unit. Adolescent mothers are at greater risk of delivering low birth weight babies.[68] In sheep, adolescent mothers even on a high plane of nutrition produce small lambs with small placentas.[69] This effect is associated with reduced growth hormone and high levels of placental lactogen and IGF-I in the mother.[70] The effect on lamb growth can be partly reversed by lowering the maternal nutrition plane after the first trimester,[71] or by supplementation with growth hormone at the time of maximal placental growth.[72]

Glucocorticoid exposure

The fetus is normally protected from high levels of glucocorticoids in maternal circulation by the placental enzyme 11β-hydroxysteroid dehydrogenase type 2 (11β-HSD2), which reduces the biologically active glucocorticoids to their inactive metabolites. Fetal exposure to excess glucocorticoids results in impaired fetal growth[73] and, as after birth, also results in increased blood pressure[74] and impaired insulin sensitivity.[75] In human populations, reduced fetal and placental size have been associated with reduced placental activity of 11β-HSD2.[76,77] In rats, maternal undernutrition is also associated with reduced levels of this enzyme and with increased exposure of the fetus to maternal glucocorticoids.[78] Prevention of this exposure by maternal adrenalectomy prevents the effects on the offspring's blood pressure and pancreatic beta cell mass.[78,79] Conversely, administration of a synthetic glucocorticoid which is not inactivated by the placental enzyme also reduces offspring size at birth and results in later hypertension in the offspring.[80–82] It is thus proposed that fetal exposure to excess levels of maternal glucocorticoids may be a core mechanism underlying the relationship between maternal undernutrition, fetal growth, and later hypertension.[83]

It has long been assumed that this link between maternal glucocorticoids, fetal glucocorticoid exposure and later hypertension might explain the effects of global maternal undernutrition, on the basis that undernutrition could constitute a 'stress', which would elevate maternal glucocorticoids.[84] However, the direct link between maternal undernutrition and fetal glucocorticoid exposure has been difficult to establish. In sheep, chronic undernutrition results in only a transient rise in maternal glucocorticoids, and circulating levels are then profoundly suppressed.[27,85] Thus, it seems unlikely that exposure to excess maternal glucocorticoids can explain the effects of global undernutrition in sheep, at least in early pregnancy.

Insulin sensitivity

Insulin has important effects on vascular tone and, therefore, insulin resistance has been postulated to provide another likely mechanism linking size at birth to both glucose intolerance and altered cardiovascular outcomes in the offspring. The fetal insulin hypothesis proposes that a fetus with insulin resistance of genetic origin will grow poorly, since insulin is critically involved in fetal growth.[86] Such a fetus will be born small, and as the insulin resistance persists after birth, it will result in impaired glucose tolerance and hypertension, thus explaining the link between small size at birth and later disease risk. The existence of genetic polymorphisms that provide substantial evidence for this hypothesis is well established.[86,87] However, these still account for only a small proportion of the population who demonstrate the link between low birth weight and later disease risk.

An alternative hypothesis based on the same principle of insulin resistance suggests that fetal undernutrition results in decreased insulin sensitivity of the fetus.[88] This effect would reduce fetal glucose uptake in the face of reduced fetal nutrient supply and, therefore, would conserve available nutrients for growth of insulin-insensitive tissues, such as brain and heart, which are essential for survival. If this insulin resistance persisted after birth, then again it would provide a link between low birth weight and later glucose intolerance and cardiovascular disease. However, the mechanisms by which fetal insulin resistance was initially established in response to undernutrition are not yet clear.

Endothelial dysfunction

Endothelial dysfunction may be another important process mediating the links between maternal nutrition and postnatal hypertension, glucose intolerance, and disease risk. The endothelium serves multiple roles in vascular function, including regulation of vascular tone, cellular proliferation, and thrombus formation. Activation of the endothelium results in expression of a variety of adhesion molecules and chemokines, which can result in local inflammation.[89] In rats, both undernutrition[90] and a high fat diet[45] have been demonstrated to result in endothelial dysfunction, along with postnatal obesity, insulin resistance, and hypertension. Altered endothelial function has been reported to occur very early in the pathogenesis of atherosclerosis, and there is accumulating evidence that endothelial dysfunction and insulin resistance may be intricately linked.[91]

Effects of nutrition around the time of conception

It is increasingly apparent that nutrition around the time of conception can have critical effects on fetal development and long-term disease risk. In rats, maternal exposure to a low protein diet only in the 4 days before implantation results in hypertension in the offspring.[92] In sheep, maternal undernutrition before and only up to the first month after mating alter fetal metabolism,[32] IGF-I regulation,[93] insulin secretion,[61] and function of the HPA axis in late gestation.[29,94]

There are many pathways by which these effects of very early nutrition could be mediated.[95]

It is well established that nutrient concentrations in the environment of the developing blastocyst have marked effects on early embryonic growth and development.[96] Distribution of cells between the inner and outer cell mass is altered resulting in potentially disproportionate fetal and placental growth. Rate of cell division can also be affected so that there are fewer cells or smaller cells, in the developing embryo.[92] During the very early division of the zygote and up to the blastocyst stage, DNA also undergoes demethylation and remethylation; a process which involves 'labelling' of some genes as of maternal or paternal origin, and marks these genes for subsequent inactivation. This epigenetic process of imprinting is thought to particularly affect many of the genes regulating fetal and placental growth.[97] Perturbation of epigenetic marking is associated with a number of disorders of fetal growth.[97] Even more intriguingly, this process of methylation can be altered by maternal diet, at least in the mouse.[98] Also in the mouse, methylation of DNA in the fetal liver is altered when a mother is on a low protein diet during pregnancy.[99] Thus, there are a number of mechanisms whereby nutrition can alter early embryo development, leading to long-term effects on fetal growth and development. Although not yet linked to risk for later disease within the normal range of birth weights, it seems likely that at least some of the same processes are involved.

CONCLUSIONS

Maternal nutrition may have important effects on the risk of certain diseases in her offspring. These effects may or may not also alter fetal growth and size at birth, and are mediated by a number of distinct and potentially overlapping mechanisms. Further work is required to understand the particular aspects of maternal nutrition that underlie these effects, and to develop the most effective interventions to optimize the long-term health of the offspring.

REFERENCES

1. Forsdahl A. Are poor living conditions in childhood and adolescence an important risk factor for arteriosclerotic heart disease? Br J Prev Soc Med 1977; 31: 91–5.
2. Barker DJ, Osmond C. Low birth weight and hypertension. BMJ 1988; 297: 134–5.
3. Barker DJ, Osmond C. Infant mortality, childhood nutrition, and ischaemic heart disease in England and Wales. Lancet 1986; 1: 1077–81.
4. Hales CN, Barker DJ, Clark PM et al. Fetal and infant growth and impaired glucose tolerance at age 64. BMJ 1991; 303: 1019–22.
5. Barker DJ, Hales CN, Fall CH et al. Type 2 (non-insulin-dependent) diabetes mellitus, hypertension and hyperlipidaemia (syndrome X): relation to reduced fetal growth. Diabetologia 1993; 36: 62–7.
6. Barker DJ, Martyn CN, Osmond C, Hales CN, Fall CH. Growth in utero and serum cholesterol concentrations in adult life. BMJ 1993; 307: 1524–7.
7. Huxley R, Neil A, Collins R. Unravelling the fetal origins hypothesis: is there really an inverse association between birthweight and subsequent blood pressure? Lancet 2002; 360: 659–65.
8. Huxley RR, Shiell AW, Law CM. The role of size at birth and postnatal catch-up growth in determining systolic blood pressure: a systematic review of the literature. J Hypertens 2000; 18: 815–31.
9. Curhan GC, Willett WC, Rimm EB et al. Birth weight and adult hypertension, diabetes mellitus, and obesity in US men. Circulation 1996; 94: 3246–50.
10. Joanette EA, Reusens B, Arany E et al. Low-protein diet during early life causes a reduction in the frequency of cells immunopositive for nestin and CD34 in both pancreatic ducts and islets in the rat. Endocrinology 2004; 145: 3004–13.
11. Langley SC, Jackson AA. Increased systolic pressure in adult rats induced by fetal exposure to maternal low protein diets. Clin Sci (Colch) 1994; 86: 217–22.
12. Kind KL, Clifton PM, Grant PA et al. Effect of maternal feed restriction during pregnancy on glucose tolerance in the adult guinea pig. Am J Physiol Regul Integr Comp Physiol 2003; 284: R140–52.
13. Kind KL, Roberts CT, Sohlstrom AI et al. Chronic maternal feed restriction impairs growth but increases adiposity of the fetal guinea pig. Am J Physiol Regul Integr Comp Physiol 2005; 288: R119–26.
14. Kind KL, Simonetta G, Clifton PM, Robinson JS, Owens JA. Effect of maternal feed restriction on blood pressure in the adult guinea pig. Exp Physiol 2002; 87: 469–77.
15. Roseboom TJ, van der Meulen JH, Ravelli AC et al. Effects of prenatal exposure to the Dutch famine on adult disease in later life: an overview. Mol Cell Endocrinol 2001; 185: 93–8.
16. Ravelli AC, van der Meulen JH, Michels RP et al. Glucose tolerance in adults after prenatal exposure to famine. Lancet 1998; 351: 173–7.
17. Lumey LH. Decreased birthweights in babies after maternal in utero exposure to the Dutch famine of 1944–1945. Paediatr Perinat Epidemiol 1992; 6: 240–53.
18. Roseboom TJ, van der Meulen JH, Osmond C et al. Plasma lipid profiles in adults after prenatal exposure to the Dutch famine. Am J Clin Nutr 2000; 72: 1101–6.
19. Roseboom TJ, van der Meulen JH, Osmond C et al. Coronary heart disease after prenatal exposure to the Dutch famine, 1944–45. Heart 2000; 84: 595–8.
20. Alvarez C, Martin MA, Goya L et al. Contrasted impact of maternal rat food restriction on the fetal endocrine pancreas. Endocrinology 1997; 138: 2267–73.
21. Whorwood CB, Firth KM, Budge H, Symonds ME. Maternal undernutrition during early to midgestation programs tissue-specific alterations in the expression of the glucocorticoid receptor, 11beta-hydroxysteroid dehydrogenase isoforms, and type 1 angiotensin ii receptor in neonatal sheep. Endocrinology 2001; 142: 2854–64.

22. Gopalakrishnan GS, Gardner DS, Rhind SM et al. Programming of adult cardiovascular function after early maternal undernutrition in sheep. Am J Physiol Regul Integr Comp Physiol 2004; 287: R12–20.

23. Gardner DS, Pearce S, Dandrea J et al. Peri-implantation undernutrition programs blunted angiotensin II evoked baroreflex responses in young adult sheep. Hypertension 2004; 43: 1290–6.

24. Mellor DJ, Murray L. Effects on the rate of increase in fetal girth of refeeding ewes after short periods of severe undernutrition during late pregnancy. Res Vet Sci 1982; 32: 377–82.

25. Bloomfield FH, Oliver MH, Giannoulias CD et al. Brief undernutrition in late-gestation sheep programs the hypothalamic-pituitary-adrenal axis in adult offspring. Endocrinology 2003; 144: 2933–40.

26. Harding JE. The nutritional basis of the fetal origins of adult disease. Int J Epidemiol 2001; 30: 15–23.

27. Bloomfield FH, Oliver MH, Hawkins P et al. Periconceptional undernutrition in sheep accelerates maturation of the fetal hypothalamic-pituitary-adrenal axis in late gestation. Endocrinology 2004; 145: 4278–85.

28. Edwards LJ, McMillen IC. Impact of maternal undernutrition during the periconceptional period, fetal number, and fetal sex on the development of the hypothalamo-pituitary adrenal axis in sheep during late gestation. Biol Reprod 2002; 66: 1562–9.

29. Bloomfield FH, Oliver MH, Hawkins P et al. A periconceptional nutritional origin for non-infectious preterm birth. Science 2003; 300: 606.

30. Gluckman PD, Hanson MA. Developmental origins of disease paradigm: a mechanistic and evolutionary perspective. Pediatr Res 2004; 56: 311–17.

31. Harding JE. Periconceptual nutrition determines the fetal growth response to acute maternal undernutrition in fetal sheep of late gestation. Prenat Neonat Med 1997; 2: 310–19.

32. Oliver MH, Hawkins P, Harding JE. Periconceptional undernutrition alters growth trajectory, endocrine and metabolic responses to fasting in late-gestation fetal sheep. Pediatr Res 2005; 57: 591–8.

33. Kramer MS. Balanced protein/energy supplementation in pregnancy (Cochrane review). In: The Cochrane Library. Oxford: Update Software, 2003.

34. Kramer MS. High protein supplementation in pregnancy (Cochrane review). In The Cochrane Library. Oxford: Update Software, 2003.

35. Godfrey K, Robinson S, Barker DJ, Osmond C, Cox V. Maternal nutrition in early and late pregnancy in relation to placental and fetal growth. BMJ 1996; 312: 410–14.

36. Moore VM, Davies MJ, Willson KJ, Worsley A, Robinson JS. Dietary composition of pregnant women is related to size of the baby at birth. J Nutr 2004; 134: 1820–6.

37. Mitchell EA, Robinson E, Clark PM et al. Maternal nutritional risk factors for small for gestational age babies in a developed country: a case-control study. Arch Dis Child Fetal Neonatal Ed 2004; 89: F431–5.

38. Rao S, Yajnik CS, Kanade A et al. Intake of micronutrient-rich foods in rural Indian mothers is associated with the size of their babies at birth: Pune Maternal Nutrition Study. J Nutr 2001; 131: 1217–24.

39. Shiell AW, Campbell-Brown M, Haselden S et al. High-meat, low-carbohydrate diet in pregnancy: relation to adult blood pressure in the offspring. Hypertension 2001; 38: 1282–8.

40. Herrick K, Phillips DI, Haselden S et al. Maternal consumption of a high-meat, low-carbohydrate diet in late pregnancy: relation to adult cortisol concentrations in the offspring. J Clin Endocrinol Metab 2003; 88: 3554–60.

41. Roseboom TJ, van der Meulen JH, van Montfrans GA et al. Maternal nutrition during gestation and blood pressure in later life. J Hypertens 2001; 19: 29–34.

42. Langley-Evans SC, Welham SJ, Jackson AA. Fetal exposure to a maternal low protein diet impairs nephrogenesis and promotes hypertension in the rat. Life Sci 1999; 64: 965–74.

43. Buckley AJ, Jaquiery AL, Harding JE. Nutritional programming of adult disease. Cell Tissue Res 2005; D01: 10.1007/s00441-005-1095-7.

44. Taylor PD, McConnell J, Khan IY et al. Impaired glucose homeostasis and mitochondrial abnormalities in offspring of rats fed a fat-rich diet in pregnancy. Am J Physiol Regul Integr Comp Physiol 2005; 288: R134–9.

45. Khan IY, Dekou V, Douglas G et al. A high-fat diet during rat pregnancy or suckling induces cardiovascular dysfunction in adult offspring. Am J Physiol Regul Integr Comp Physiol 2005; 288: R127–33.

46. Khan I, Dekou V, Hanson M, Poston L, Taylor P. Predictive adaptive responses to maternal high-fat diet prevent endothelial dysfunction but not hypertension in adult rat offspring. Circulation 2004; 110: 1097–102.

47. Aerts L, Van Assche FA. Is gestational diabetes an acquired condition? J Dev Physiol 1979; 1: 219–25.

48. Holemans K, Aerts L, Van Assche FA. Lifetime consequences of abnormal fetal pancreatic development. J Physiol 2003; 547(Pt 1): 11–20.

49. Gillman MW, Rifas-Shiman SL, Kleinman KP, Rich-Edwards JW, Lipshultz SE. Maternal calcium intake and offspring blood pressure. Circulation 2004; 110: 1990–5.

50. Belizan JM, Villar J, Bergel E et al. Long-term effect of calcium supplementation during pregnancy on the blood pressure of offspring: follow up of a randomised controlled trial. BMJ 1997; 315: 281–5.

51. Steer P, Alam MA, Wadsworth J, Welch A. Relation between maternal haemoglobin concentration and birth weight in different ethnic groups. BMJ 1995; 310: 489–91.

52. Beischer NA, Sivasamboo R, Vohra S, Silpisornkosal S, Reid S. Placental hypertrophy in severe pregnancy anaemia. J Obstet Gynaecol Br Commonw 1970; 77: 398–409.

53. Barker DJ, Bull AR, Osmond C, Simmonds SJ. Fetal and placental size and risk of hypertension in adult life. BMJ 1990; 301: 259–62.

54. Rasmussen K. Is there a causal relationship between iron deficiency or iron-deficiency anemia and weight at birth, length of gestation and perinatal mortality? J Nutr 2001; 131: 590S–601S; discussion 601S–603S.

55. Ramakrishnan U, Gonzalez-Cossio T, Neufeld LM, Rivera J, Martorell R. Multiple micronutrient supplementation during pregnancy does not lead to greater infant birth size than does iron-only supplementation: a randomized controlled trial in a semirural community in Mexico. Am J Clin Nutr 2003; 77: 720–5.

56. Jackson AA. The glycine story. Eur J Clin Nutr 1991; 45: 59–65.

57. Brawley L, Torrens C, Anthony FW et al. Glycine rectifies vascular dysfunction induced by dietary protein imbalance during pregnancy. J Physiol 2004; 554(Pt 2): 497–504.

58. Jackson AA, Dunn RL, Marchand MC, Langley-Evans SC. Increased systolic blood pressure in rats induced by a maternal low-protein diet is reversed by dietary supplementation with glycine. Clin Sci (Lond) 2002; 103: 633–9.

59. van Zijl PL, Oliver MH, Harding JE. Periconceptual under-nutrition in sheep leads to longterm changes in maternal amino acid concentrations. Proceedings of the 6th Annual Congress of the Perinatal Society of Australia and New Zealand, Christchurch, 2002: p. 190.

60. Cherif H, Reusens B, Ahn MT, Hoet JJ, Remacle C. Effects of taurine on the insulin secretion of rat fetal islets from dams fed a low-protein diet. J Endocrinol 1998; 159: 341–8.

61. Oliver MH, Hawkins P, Breier BH et al. Maternal under-nutrition during the periconceptual period increases plasma taurine levels and insulin response to glucose but not argi-nine in the late gestational fetal sheep. Endocrinology 2001; 142: 4576–9.

62. Jensen BL. Reduced nephron number, renal development and 'programming' of adult hypertension. J Hypertens 2004; 22: 2065–6.

63. Amann K, Plank C, Dotsch J. Low nephron number – a new cardiovascular risk factor in children? Pediatr Nephrol 2004; 19: 1319–23.

64. Ingelfinger JR. Pathogenesis of perinatal programming. Curr Opin Nephrol Hypertens 2004; 13: 459–64.

65. Liu L, Harding JE, Evans PC, Gluckman PD. Maternal insulin-like growth factor-I infusion alters feto-placental carbohydrate and protein metabolism in pregnant sheep. Endocrinology 1994; 135: 895–900.

66. Harding JE, Liu L, Evans PC, Gluckman PD. Insulin-like growth factor 1 alters feto-placental protein and carbohy-drate metabolism in fetal sheep. Endocrinology 1994; 134: 1509–14.

67. Jensen EC, van Zijl P, Evans PC, Harding JE. The effect of IGF-I on serine metabolism in fetal sheep. J Endocrinol 2000; 165: 261–9.

68. Fraser AM, Brockert JE, Ward RH. Association of young maternal age with adverse reproductive outcomes. N Engl J Med 1995; 332: 1113–17.

69. Wallace JM, Aitken RP, Milne JS, Hay WW Jr. Nutritionally mediated placental growth restriction in the growing adoles-cent: consequences for the fetus. Biol Reprod 2004; 71: 1055–62.

70. Gadd TS, Aitken RP, Wallace JM, Wathes DC. Effect of a high maternal dietary intake during mid-gestation on com-ponents of the utero-placental insulin-like growth factor (IGF) system in adolescent sheep with retarded placental development. J Reprod Fertil 2000; 118: 407–416.

71. Wallace JM, Bourke DA, Aitken RP, Cruickshank MA. Switching maternal dietary intake at the end of the first trimester has profound effects on placental development and fetal growth in adolescent ewes carrying singleton fetuses. Biol Reprod 1999; 61: 101–10.

72. Wallace JM, Milne JS, Aitken RP. Maternal growth hor-mone treatment from day 35 to 80 of gestation alters nutri-ent partitioning in favor of uteroplacental growth in the overnourished adolescent sheep. Biol Reprod 2004; 70: 1277–85.

73. Fowden AL, Szemere J, Hughes P, Gilmour RS, Forhead AJ. The effects of cortisol on the growth rate of the sheep fetus during late gestation. J Endocrinol 1996; 151: 97–105.

74. Jensen EC, Gallaher BW, Breier BH, Harding JE. The effect of a chronic maternal cortisol infusion on the late-gestation fetal sheep. J Endocrinol 2002; 174: 27–36.

75. Gurrin LC, Moss TJ, Sloboda DM et al. Using WinBUGS to fit nonlinear mixed models with an application to pharmaco-kinetic modelling of insulin response to glucose challenge in sheep exposed antenatally to glucocorticoids. J Biopharm Stat 2003; 13: 117–39.

76. Stewart PM, Rogerson FM, Mason JI. Type 2 11 beta-hydroxysteroid dehydrogenase messenger ribonucleic acid and activity in human placenta and fetal membranes: its relationship to birth weight and putative role in fetal adrenal steroidogenesis. J Clin Endocrinol Metab 1995; 80: 885–90.

77. Kajantie E, Dunkel L, Turpeinen U et al. Placental 11 beta-hydroxysteroid dehydrogenase-2 and fetal cortisol/cortisone shuttle in small preterm infants. J Clin Endocrinol Metab 2003; 88: 493–500.

78. Lesage J, Bondeau B, Grino M, Breant B, Dupouy JP. Maternal undernutrition during late gestation induces fetal overexposure to glucocorticoids and intrauterine growth retardation, and disturbs the hypothalamo-pituitary-adrenal axis in the newborn rat. Endocrinology 2001; 142: 1692–702.

79. Blondeau B, Lesage J, Czernichow P, Dupouy JP, Breant B. Glucocorticoids impair fetal beta-cell development in rats. Am J Physiol Endocrinol Metab 2001; 281: E592–9.

80. Levitt NS, Lindsay RS, Holmes MC, Seckl JR. Dexamethasone in the last week of pregnancy attenuates hippocampal glucocorticoid receptor gene expression and elevates blood pressure in the adult offspring in the rat. Neuroendocrinology 1996; 64: 412–18.

81. Dodic M, May CN, Wintour EM, Coghlan JP. An early pre-natal exposure to excess glucocorticoid leads to hypertensive offspring in sheep. Clin Sci 1998; 94: 149–55.

82. Moss TJ, Sloboda DM, Gurrin LC et al. Programming effects in sheep of prenatal growth restriction and gluco-corticoid exposure. Am J Physiol Regul Integr Comp Physiol 2001; 281: R960–70.

83. Benediktsson R, Lindsay RS, Noble J, Seckl JR, Edwards CRW. Glucocorticoid exposure in utero: a new model for adult hypertension. Lancet 1993; 341: 339–41.

84. Edwards LJ, Coulter CL, Symonds ME, McMillen IC. Prenatal undernutrition, glucocorticoids and the program-ming of adult hypertension. Clin Exp Pharmacol Physiol 2001; 28: 938–41.

85. Bispham J, Gopalakrishnan GS, Dandrea J et al. Maternal endocrine adaptation throughout pregnancy to nutritional manipulation: consequences for maternal plasma leptin and cortisol and the programming of fetal adipose tissue development. Endocrinology 2003; 144: 3575–85.

86. Hattersley AT, Tooke JE. The fetal insulin hypothesis: an alternative explanation of the association of low birth-weight with diabetes and vascular disease. Lancet 1999; 353: 1789–92.

87. Hattersley AT, Beards F, Ballantyne E et al. Mutations in the glucokinase gene of the fetus result in reduced birth weight. Nat Genet 1998; 19: 268–70.

88. Barker DJP. Mothers, Babies and Disease in Later Life, 1st edn. London: BMJ Publishing Group, 1994.

89. Egashira K. Clinical importance of endothelial function in arteriosclerosis and ischemic heart disease. Circ J 2002; 66: 529–33.

90. Torrens C, Brawley L, Barker AC et al. Maternal protein restriction in the rat impairs resistance artery but not con-duit artery function in pregnant offspring. J Physiol 2003; 547 (Pt 1): 77–84.

91. Shinozaki K, Ayajiki K, Kashiwagi A, Masada M, Okamura T. Malfunction of vascular control in lifestyle-related diseases: mechanisms underlying endothelial dys-function in the insulin-resistant state. J Pharmacol Sci 2004; 96: 401–5.

92. Kwong WY, Wild AE, Roberts P, Willis AC, Fleming TP. Maternal undernutrition during the preimplantation period

of rat development causes blastocyst abnormalities and programming of postnatal hypertension. Development 2000; 127: 4195–202.

93. Gallaher BW, Oliver MH, Eichhorn K et al. Circulating insulin-like growth factor II/mannose-6-phosphate receptor and insulin-like growth factor binding proteins in fetal sheep plasma are regulated by glucose and insulin. Eur J Endocrinol 1994; 131: 398–404.

94. Bloomfield FH, Oliver MH, Hawkins P, Challis JRG, Harding JE. Periconceptual undernutrition in the sheep causes premature activation of the hypothalamic-pituitary-adrenal (HPA) axis resulting in preterm birth. Endocrine Abstracts 2001; 2: OC21.

95. Waterland RA, Garza C. Potential mechanisms of metabolic imprinting that lead to chronic disease. Am J Clin Nutr 1999; 69: 179–97.

96. Thompson JG, Gardner DK, Pugh PA, McMillan WH, Tervit HR. Lamb birth weight is affected by culture system utilized during in vitro pre-elongation development of ovine embryos. Biol Reprod 1995; 53: 1385–91.

97. Constancia M, Kelsey G, Reik W. Resourceful imprinting. Nature 2004; 432: 53–7.

98. Wolff GL, Kodell RL, Moore SR, Cooney CA. Maternal epigenetics and methyl supplements affect agouti gene expression in Avy/a mice. FASEB J 1998; 12: 949–57.

99. Rees WD, Hay SM, Brown DS, Antipatis C, Palmer RM. Maternal protein deficiency causes hypermethylation of DNA in the livers of rat fetuses. J Nutr 2000; 130: 1821–6.

3

Prenatal stress influences human fetal development and birth outcomes: implications for developmental origins of health and disease

Pathik D Wadhwa and Ilona S Federenko

INTRODUCTION

Epidemiological studies of human populations across the world suggest that markers of an individual's birth phenotype, such as low birth weight and small body size, are associated with a significantly increased risk of physical and mental diseases in adult life, including hypertension, coronary artery disease, type 2 diabetes mellitus, endocrine cancers, depression, and other cognitive and affective disorders.[1–5] These associations are independent of adult size and other established disease risk factors, such as obesity, unfavorable lipid profile, or smoking.[6,7] Moreover, these observed effects extend continuously across the normal range of distribution of birth phenotype, and are not just a function of adverse birth outcomes, such as low birth weight or small-for-gestational age (SGA) birth.[7,8] It is unlikely that birth phenotype, *per se*, plays a causal role in increasing risk of adult disease.[7,9] Instead, birth phenotype is more likely a crude reflection of developmental processes in intrauterine life that also may influence the structure and function of physiological systems that underlie health and disease risk in later life.[7,9,10] Two major evolutionary forces that act upon and shape the development of living organisms are those related to the availability and utilization of energy substrate (nutrition) and those involved in adaptation to physical or psychological challenges or threats to homeostasis (stress). Disruption of mammalian reproductive function and development is, in fact, a well-known consequence of stress. In the first part of this chapter, the evidence linking prenatal

stress with human fetal development and adverse birth outcomes is discussed, and putative physiological mechanisms that may mediate these effects are described. In the second part, the implications of these findings with regard to the issue of the developmental origins of health and disease are discussed.

MATERNAL PRENATAL STRESS AND ADVERSE BIRTH OUTCOMES IN HUMAN PREGNANCY: REVIEW OF EPIDEMIOLOGICAL STUDIES

The distribution of adverse birth outcomes, such as preterm birth and low birth weight, in the population is characterized by persistent and large disparities that reflect social disadvantage (low socioeconomic status)[11] and minority racial/ethnic status.[12–14] The causes of these disparities are not well understood. Lack of prenatal care availability/utilization, poor diet and nutrition, lack of or excessive physical activity, and unhealthy behaviors, such as smoking and alcohol/drug use, have been shown to play only a limited role in accounting for these sociodemographic and racial/ethnic disparities.[15,16] This has led to the hypothesis that high levels of maternal stress may, in part, account for these disparities because a) the experience of social disadvantage and minority racial/ethnic status is associated with increased stress and lack of psychosocial resources,[17] and b) stress is known to play a causal role in a wide array of adverse developmental and health outcomes.[18–20]

Studies examining the effects of maternal stress on birth outcomes first appeared in the scientific literature in the mid-1950s. Much of the earlier research, however, was limited by conceptual and methodological problems.[21,22] Over the past decade or so, larger, better-designed studies have been published. A growing body of empirical evidence, based on these prospective, methodologically rigorous, population-based studies in pregnant women of different racial/ethnic, socioeconomic, and national backgrounds, now provides substantial support for the premise that women experiencing high levels of psychological or social stress during pregnancy are at significantly increased risk for shorter gestation/preterm delivery and reduced fetal growth/low birth weight/small for gestational age (SGA) birth, even after adjusting for the effects of other established biomedical, sociodemographic, and behavioral risk factors.[23-33] In terms of effect size, pregnant women reporting high levels of stress are at approximately doubled risk for preterm birth or fetal growth restriction as compared to women reporting low levels of stress.[29,34,35] The effects of prenatal stress are not restricted to only the ends of the distribution of length of gestation and fetal growth (i.e. preterm birth, low birth weight), but are associated with a shift to the left of the entire distribution of these outcomes, indicating a generalized effect. 'Subjective' measures of stress appraisals are more strongly related to birth outcomes than 'objective' measures of stress exposure,[23,36-40] suggesting that individual differences in appraisals and responses to potentially negative events or conditions are a crucial determinant of susceptibility for adverse birth outcomes. Moreover, in a number of studies, the trimester during which stress is assessed has been found to moderate the effects of psychosocial stress on birth outcomes.[26-28] Based on studies with multiple assessments, there is evidence of a larger effect for stress in the first trimester than for stress in the second or third trimesters. These findings, thus, suggest that the earlier stage of gestation may represent a period of increased susceptibility with respect to the potentially detrimental effects of prenatal stress on birth outcomes. Finally, in many instances, the effects of maternal psychosocial stress are *moderated* by factors such as body mass index (BMI), smoking,[34] occupational status,[41] coping style,[42] ethnicity,[43] and maternal age,[44,45] thus underscoring the importance of ascertaining the individual/contextual factors that either protect or increase susceptibility for risk of adverse birth outcomes among women reporting high levels of stress.

In summary, maternal stress is a significant risk factor for a shortened gestation/preterm birth and reduced fetal growth, low birth weight or SGA births.

The magnitude of the effect size of stress on risk of adverse birth outcomes in population-based, epidemiological studies is similar to that of most other established obstetric and sociodemographic risk factors. However, it also is clear that not all women reporting high levels of stress during pregnancy proceed to deliver early or deliver a smaller infant (i.e. the specificity and sensitivity of stress as a predictor of adverse birth outcomes in any individual pregnancy is, at best, modest). Thus, before these research findings can be translated into a public health framework with clinical applications and effective interventions, it is important to identify which subgroup(s) of pregnant women are especially vulnerable to the potentially deleterious effects of maternal stress on reproductive and birth outcomes, under what circumstances (context), and at what stage(s) in pregnancy.

For any individual, the probability of a stress-related adverse health outcome is a combined function of not only cumulative stress exposure, but also that individual's biological responsivity to stress.[46] Stress responsivity refers to an individual's propensity for biological perturbation upon stress exposure. Two major limitations of the maternal stress and birth outcome literature are that a) previous studies have considered only the stress exposure side of the above equation, but not the issue of individual differences in responsivity to stress, and b) the measurement of maternal stress has relied exclusively on self-report, retrospective recall measures of psychological state or affect over time.[47] Self-report, summary measures of an individual's states and experiences over time, rely on autobiographical memory (as opposed to semantic memory), which is as much a matter of reconstruction as of accurate recall, and is known to be highly susceptible to numerous systematic biases that impact on accuracy (e.g. effects of recency, maximum saliency, and valence of affect at the time of reporting).[48-51] Recent technological and methodological advances in behavioral medicine now afford the opportunity to obtain longitudinal and repeated collection of information simultaneously about respondents' current biological and psychological state, affect, experience, and behavior in real time (also referred to as experience-sampling methods, or ecological momentary assessment (EMA).[52] Besides providing more accurate summary measures of stress over time, this methodology allows for the computation of indices of other important dimensions of stress such as variability and context-specific measures of temporal linkages between psychosocial state/affect and biological processes of interest. Moreover, EMA methods provide greater ecological validity because they are collected in natural settings as respondents go about their day-to-day activities. Thus, we suggest that an important future direction in this area is to obtain more accurate and valid measures of psychosocial, behavioral and biological states by importing and adapting EMA methodologies into the area of human perinatology research.

ANIMAL MODELS OF PRENATAL STRESS AND FETAL DEVELOPMENT

Experimental studies in animals provide convincing evidence to support a causal role for prenatal stress in negatively influencing critical developmental and health outcomes over the lifespan, including brain structure and function, sexual differentiation, (re)activity of the autonomic nervous, neuroendocrine, immune and reproductive systems, physical and mental health, and longevity.[22,53–55] For example, the application of prenatal stress in rodents has been found to alter baseline and stress-induced responsivity of the hypothalamic-pituitary-adrenal (HPA) axis and levels and distribution of regulatory neurotransmitters, including norepinephrine, dopamine, serotonin, and acetylcholine, and to modify key limbic structures. These prenatal stress-induced alterations have been shown to affect cognition (decreased learning), emotionality (increased anxiety), and social behavior (increased withdrawal).[53] Similarly, the application of prenatal stress in non-human primates has been shown to alter endocrine, immune, and neurobehavioral outcomes in offspring.[56,57] Such animal studies have also offered valuable insights into putative physiological mechanisms that may be involved in mediating the effects of stressful maternal and intrauterine environments on the developing organism. However, the generalizability of some of these findings from animals to humans may be limited by the existence of inter-species differences in physiology and the developmental time line. Perhaps no single system exemplifies the magnitude of these inter-species physiological differences as vividly as the reproductive system, even between otherwise very closely related species such as humans and non-human primates.[58,59] For example, primates are the only species that produce corticotropin-releasing hormone (CRH) by the placenta during pregnancy. The timing of maturation of the HPA axis relative to birth is also highly species-specific and is closely linked to important landmarks of brain development.[60] In animals that give birth to precocious offspring (sheep, guinea pigs, primates), maximal brain growth and a large proportion of neuroendocrine maturation takes place *in utero*. By contrast, in species that give birth to altricial offspring (rats, rabbits, mice), much of

neuroendocrine development occurs in the postnatal period.[61] Hence, it is critical to consider human development within this context.

A BIOBEHAVIORAL APPROACH TO THE STUDY OF PRENATAL STRESS, FETAL DEVELOPMENT, AND BIRTH OUTCOMES IN HUMANS

From a biological perspective, the term 'stress' is used to describe any physical or psychological challenge that threatens or is perceived to have the potential to threaten the stability or homeostasis of the internal milieu of the organism. The autonomic nervous, neuroendocrine, immune, and vascular systems play a major role in adaptation to stress. The principal effectors of these adaptive responses are the corticotropin-releasing hormone (CRH) and locus ceruleus-noradrenaline (LC/NA) neurons in the hypothalamus and brainstem, which regulate the peripheral activities of the HPA axis and the systemic/adrenomedullary sympathetic nervous system (SNS), respectively. Activation of the HPA axis and LC-NA/autonomic system results in the systemic elevation of glucocorticoids (cortisol) and catecholamines, respectively, which act in concert on target tissues to mobilize and redistribute available resources and maintain or effect a return to the state of homeostasis.[46]

There are no *direct* neural, vascular or other connections between the mother and her developing fetus. All communication between the maternal and fetal compartments is mediated via the placenta, an organ of fetal origin, through one or both of two mechanisms: the actions of maternal factors on placental activity, or via transplacental exchange of blood-borne substances. Based on the evidence linking maternal stress to earlier delivery and reduced fetal growth, and on our understanding of the physiology of stress, fetal growth, and parturition, we have proposed a biobehavioral framework of prenatal stress and adverse birth outcomes.[22,47,62] This framework proposes that chronic maternal stress may exert a significant influence on fetal developmental outcomes (Figure 3.1). The effects of maternal stress may be mediated through biological and/or behavioral mechanisms. Maternal stress may act via neuroendocrine, immune/inflammatory, and vascular pathways to ultimately result in premature and/or greater degree of activation of the maternal-placental-fetal (MPF) systems that regulate fetal growth and parturition. We further suggest that placental CRH plays a key role in coordinating the effects of endocrine, immune, and vascular processes on fetal growth and parturition.

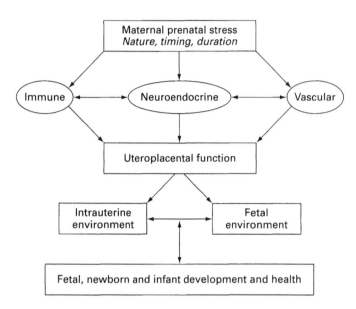

Figure 3.1 Biobehavioral model of prenatal stress and human fetal development and health outcomes.

Human fetal development and parturition involve the time- and context-dependent interplay of several systems and signaling molecules within the maternal, placental, and fetal tissues. Events that underlie fetal development and lead to parturition start early in pregnancy, occur sequentially, and involve feedback systems.[59,63–66] Clinical and experimental evidence broadly support the concept that adverse birth outcomes are heterogeneous, multifactorial entities, determined by multiple genetic and environmental factors that reflect the interactions among one or more of several pathophysiological processes, which may share common biological pathways, including: a) early or excessive activation of the MPF neuroendocrine axis; b) decidual/chorioamniotic/fetal inflammation caused by ascending genitourinary tract or systemic infection; and c) uteroplacental vascular lesions caused by coagulopathy, hypertension, or abruption/decidual hemorrhage.[67] These pathways certainly do not represent *all* potential routes to adverse birth outcomes. Moreover, these pathways may not be mutually exclusive and distinct, and there may be substantial overlap and interaction between them.

PRENATAL STRESS AND MATERNAL-PLACENTAL-FETAL (MPF) NEUROENDOCRINE PROCESSES

The major elements of the mammalian MPF neuroendocrine system are the maternal and fetal HPA axes,

respectively, and the placenta (see Figure 3.2). In all mammals, processes underlying parturition and fetal development are coordinated to ensure that birth occurs after the developing fetus is sufficiently mature for survival outside the uterus. Though the exact biological mechanisms underlying parturition are not fully understood, it is widely accepted that one important pathway involves the activation of the maternal, fetal, and placental neuroendocrine systems that simultaneously play a critical role in fetal maturation and parturition. The onset of parturition is believed to result from a transition in the control of the MPF neuroendocrine axis from a system promoting uterine quiescence in early gestation to one promoting uterine contractility in late gestation. This shift in the balance from a progesterone-dominant to an estrogen-dominant milieu over the course of gestation results in a sequence of events in the gestational tissues (myometrium) to promote labor, including gap junction formation, expression of oxytocin receptors, and synthesis of prostaglandins.[59,63–66]

In humans, placental CRH plays a central role in the control of the MPF neuroendocrine system in pregnancy, and CRH-mediated activation has been characterized as a 'placental clock' that determines or alters the timing of onset of parturition.[68,69] In this model, CRH is produced by the placenta and promotes fetal cortisol and DHEA-S production by the fetal adrenal gland. These steroids return via the umbilical circulation to the placenta, where cortisol promotes further CRH secretion (the positive feedback circuit outlined

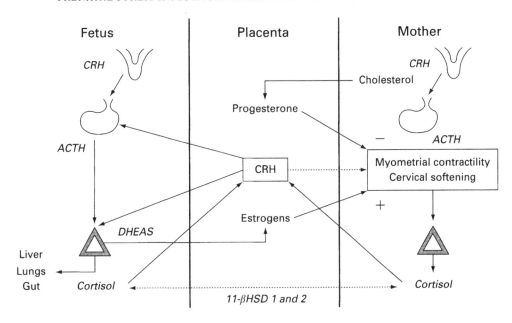

Figure 3.2 Maternal-placental-fetal neuroendocrine axis in human pregnancy and fetal development.

in Figure 3.2), and DHEA-S serves as the immediate precursor for the production of estriol (E_3, influencing the state of uterine activity). Plasma concentrations of placental CRH are low during the first trimester. As a result of the positive feedback loop, they rise exponentially from mid-gestation to term reaching concentrations that are 1000-fold greater than those found in nonpregnant women. Once established, this positive feedback loop is progressively amplified and drives the fetal–placental unit towards the outcomes of fetal maturation and delivery. In this model, plasma CRH level and its activity are associated with the timing of gestation, including the outcomes of preterm, term, and post-term delivery.[59,63–66,69]

Converging lines of evidence suggest that placental CRH plays an important role in coordinating and regulating the physiology of fetal development and parturition. Women in preterm labor have significantly elevated levels of CRH compared with gestational age-matched controls, and these elevations of CRH, assessed in some studies as early as 15 weeks gestation, precede the onset of spontaneous preterm labor.[22,68–78] Studies that conducted serial assessments of CRH over the course of gestation have found that compared to term deliveries, women delivering preterm had not only significantly elevated CRH levels, but also a significantly accelerated rate of CRH increase over the course of their gestation.[68,72,79] Conversely, women delivering post term (>41 weeks) have lower CRH levels and a slower rate of CRH increase over the course of gestation.[68,69] Several concepts have arisen from this

work. First, it establishes that, for at least a proportion of pregnant women, it is possible to predict the rate of fetal growth and the timing of delivery in advance. Second, it suggests that events early in pregnancy have an influence on the later timing of parturition. Understanding the regulation and activity of the MPF neuroendocrine system may, therefore, provide insights into the determination of fetal growth and length of gestation.

Regulation of CRH production has been explored in human placental tissue.[80] CRH is produced by syncytial cells, which can be created *in vitro* by fusion of purified cytotrophoblast cells. Using cultured placental cells and radioimmunoassays, a consistent effect has been demonstrated of the stress hormone cortisol in stimulation of CRH secretion.[81] Interestingly, the exponential increase observed in human pregnancy can be reproduced using a model that incorporates a positive feed forward relationship between cortisol and CRH.[82] This finding was surprising, because glucocorticoids are known to inhibit CRH secretion within the hypothalamus. Using transfections of CRH promoter constructs, the stimulatory mechanism has been partially elucidated. In placental tissue, glucocorticoids stimulate CRH gene expression by interacting with proteins that bind to the cAMP response site of the CRH promoter,[83] and the difference in behavior of the CRH gene in the placenta and hypothalamus is due to the expression of different transcription factors, co-activators and co-repressors in these two tissues.[84]

Placental CRH is stress-sensitive. Clinical evidence suggests that the trajectory of placental CRH production over the course of gestation may be increased by an adverse intrauterine environment characterized by physiological stress. For example, elevated CRH in the maternal and/or fetal compartments has been observed in pregnancies complicated by pre-eclampsia, reduced uteroplacental perfusion, intrauterine infection, and in cases where fetal distress has led to elective preterm delivery.[85] A series of *in vitro* studies by Petraglia and colleagues has shown that CRH is released from cultured human placental cells in a dose-response manner in response to *all* the major biological effectors of stress, including cortisol, catecholamines, and proinflammatory cytokines.[80,86–88] *In vivo* studies have found significant correlations among maternal pituitary-adrenal stress hormones (ACTH, cortisol) and placental CRH levels.[72,88–91] Moreover, maternal psychosocial stress is significantly correlated with maternal pituitary-adrenal hormone levels (ACTH, cortisol)[92] that are known to stimulate placental CRH secretion. Some,[71,72] but not all studies,[93] also have reported direct associations between maternal psychosocial stress and placental CRH function. Thus, depending on the interaction between the genetic makeup of the fetus and mother and the chronicity of physiological or psychological stress, the resultant alternations in CRH production may be an important factor that contributes to the early initiation of spontaneous labor and also impaired fetal growth.[67,94]

Recent advances in the elucidation of molecular events that unfold just before and during labor have implicated local inflammation in the gestational tissues as an important mediator in the final process in both term and preterm labor,[95] and several studies suggest that activation of a DNA binding protein – nuclear factor-kappa B (NF-κB) – plays an essential role to trigger the transcription of inflammatory genes and corresponding proteins in human fetal membranes in labor.[96] The MPF neuroendocrine system, and particularly steroid-receptor signaling pathways, are known to potently interact with NF-κB.[97] Yet another recent study has provided provocative experimental evidence that in the mouse a signal for initiation of parturition originates from the maturing fetal lung – lung surfactant protein A (SP-A).[98] The MPF neuroendocrine system also is known to interact with SP-A. For example, fetal lung tissue is known to produce CRH, and in baboon fetal lung explants, locally produced CRH has been shown to strongly induce the synthesis of surfactant proteins.[99]

PRENATAL STRESS AND IMMUNE/INFLAMMATORY PROCESSES

Normal pregnancy is an immunological balancing act, wherein alterations are produced in the maternal immune system to tolerate paternal major histocompatibility (MHC) antigens (the embryo and fetus is a semi-allograft for the mother because it shares one-half of its genomic complement with the father) and yet to also maintain adequate immune competence for defense against microorganisms. The mechanisms underlying this process are complex and not yet completely clarified, but are known to involve systemic as well as local changes at the MPF interface.[100] It has long been recognized that over the course of gestation lymphocytes from pregnant women exhibit a progressive decline in their ability to proliferate in response to mitogenic stimuli[101,102] – a hallmark of general immunosuppression. More recent studies indicate that in addition to a decreased proliferative response, there is a change in the normal pattern of cytokine production from a T-helper cell 1 (Th1) to a Th2 cytokine profile in pregnancy, which would favor humoral over cellular immune responses.[103] Some studies have suggested that normal full-term delivery is associated with a predominance of Th2 cytokine production, whereas preterm delivery is associated with an important maintenance of a Th1 cytokine profile.[104–107]

Microbial infection and inflammation in the gestational tissues have emerged as major risk factors associated with adverse fetal developmental and health outcomes. For example, preterm labor, premature rupture of membranes and fetal white matter brain damage in the setting of infection are believed to result from the actions of proinflammatory cytokines secreted as part of the fetal and/or maternal host response to microbial invasion.[108,109] Maternal infections may trigger parturition by the activation of the monocyte and macrophage system in peripheral blood and human decidua, resulting in release of inflammatory cytokines. Such inflammatory cytokines have been detected in elevated concentrations in the amniotic fluid and plasma of women with preterm labor/preterm rupture of membranes (PROM), and human gestational tissues are potentially rich sources of inflammatory cytokines. Also, maternal decidua and fetal membranes produce mRNA for inflammatory cytokines in the setting of infection-associated preterm labor and normal term labor. Animal models indicate that preterm labor can be stimulated by bacteria, bacterial cell wall products, and proinflammatory cytokines, such as IL-1 and tumor necrosis factor.[110] There is strong evidence that the production of the prostaglandins E2 and F2α (PGE2 and PGF2α) –

involved in the initiation and maintenance of human parturition – can be stimulated by a number of cytokines and in infection-induced preterm labor by bacterial endotoxin.[111] Romero and colleagues have argued that infection-related preterm labor and premature rupture of membranes are expressions of the same basic phenomenon: activation of the host defense macrophage system.[112] Intrauterine infection causes preterm labor in some cases if the preferential response of the host favors secretion of uterotonic agents (i.e. prostaglandins), and preterm rupture of membranes if the host response results predominantly in the production of proteases (i.e. leukocyte elastase and MMPs). A growing body of work also suggests that a systemic fetal proinflammatory cytokine response, accompanied by activation of the fetal HPA axis, is followed by the onset of spontaneous parturition.[108,112,113]

Many issues remain unanswered about the role of infection in adverse fetal developmental outcomes. Two questions of particular interest are: first, what are the factors that modulate susceptibility to developing reproductive tract or intrauterine infections during pregnancy, and second, based on the findings that not all women with infection during pregnancy proceed to have adverse outcomes, what are the risk factors that account for susceptibility to pathophysiological outcomes in the presence of infection? A large body of empirical evidence suggests that chronic stress and stress hormones are associated with immunosuppression and changes in the normal pattern of cellular (Th1) and humoral (Th2) responses to antigens.[114] For example, depression is known to directly stimulate the production of proinflammatory cytokines and downregulate the cellular immune response.[115] We have hypothesized that stress and stress biology may play an important role in increasing the susceptibility for developing reproductive tract infection in pregnancy and have published a report in support of this premise. In a sample of 454 pregnant women assessed at 14 weeks gestation, high levels of chronic maternal psychosocial stress were associated with a 2.2-fold increase in the prevalence of bacterial vaginosis (the most common reproductive tract infection) after adjusting for the effects of established risk factors.[116] We have further suggested that the effect of stress on the prevalence of reproductive tract infection may be mediated by maternal immunosuppression. A report of particular relevance to this hypothesis examined the association between immunosuppression and risk of developing infection in women of reproductive age. This study prospectively followed a cohort of 1288 women (HIV+ and HIV−) over a period of 5 years with assessments every 6 months. In this sample, immunocompromised women had a 40% higher prevalence of reproductive tract infection than women who were not immunocompromised, and the effect of immunocompromise was larger than that of even HIV status.[117]

Although maternal stress and infection have been separately implicated as risk factors for adverse fetal developmental outcomes, very little research has examined the nature of the stress-infection-immune relationship in human pregnancy to date. In fact, our review of the relevant literature found only two studies of stress and immunity in human pregnancy. A cross-sectional investigation of a sample of 72 pregnant women showed that high levels of maternal psychological stress and low levels of social support were significantly associated with depression of lymphocyte activity.[118] In the second study, psychosocial stress was assessed in 94 women with a confirmed diagnosis of first trimester spontaneous abortion. The decidua of women with high stress scores was found to have altered immune parameters, including higher numbers of MCT^+, $CD8^+$ T cells and tumor necrosis factor-α (TNF-α) cells (immune mediators of miscarriage), than women with low stress scores.[119] Furthermore, an *in vivo* study reported that women in preterm labor with microbial invasion of the amniotic cavity had significantly higher placental CRH levels than those in preterm labor without infection.[76]

INTERACTIONS BETWEEN STRESS-RELATED MPF NEUROENDOCRINE AND IMMUNE-INFLAMMATORY PATHWAYS IN PREGNANCY

As discussed earlier, fetal development and birth outcomes are complex, multifactorial processes involving several physiological pathways. Although distinct neuroendocrine and immune/inflammatory pathways have been described, growing evidence suggests that these and other physiological systems involved in pregnancy are highly inter-related, and that they extensively regulate and counter-regulate one another. It has been known for decades that stress, whether physical, psychological or inflammatory, is associated with activation of the HPA axis. In the early 1990s, it also became apparent that cytokines and other humoral mediators of inflammation are potent activators of the central stress response, constituting the afferent limb of a feedback loop through which the immune/inflammatory system and the central nervous system communicate.[120] All major inflammatory cytokines, including TNF-α, interleukin (IL)-1β and IL-6, stimulate the HPA axis directly as well as indirectly via central catecholaminergic pathways. Other inflammatory mediators, such as eicosanoids, platelet-activating factor and serotonin also participate in the activation of the HPA axis via auto/paracrine and/or endocrine effects. Conversely, activation of the HPA axis has profound inhibitory effects on inflammatory and immune responses, because virtually all components of the immune response are inhibited by cortisol, including alterations of leukocyte traffic and function, and on production of cytokines and other mediators of inflammation, with an inhibition of the latter's effects on target tissues. The potential complexity of the inter-relationships among these physiologic systems is seen when considering the role of infection in the etiology of adverse fetal developmental and birth outcomes (see Figure 3.3). For example, inflammatory cytokines that are produced in response to infection, such as TNF-α, IL-1β and IL-6, can activate components of the MPF-neuroendocrine system that also increase the risk of premature birth.[108,121-123] Conversely, it is also known that HPA hormones such as CRH and cortisol influence the production of cytokines and modulate the inflammatory response to infection.[124-126] Central CRH, acting via glucocorticoids and catecholamines, inhibits inflammation, whereas CRH directly secreted by peripheral nerves and mast cells stimulates local inflammation.[120] Moreover, it has been postulated that acute and chronic infections may be risk factors for uteroplacental vasculopathies that may be associated with premature birth.[127] Impaired nutrient and oxygen exchange associated with uteroplacental vasculopathy may stress the fetus and result in increased production of placental-fetal hormones such as CRH, while placental CRH, in turn, may influence fetal-placental circulation.[128] Thus, the relationship of a well-defined risk factor, like prenatal infection, to adverse fetal outcomes is likely to involve complex interactions between the endocrine and immune systems.

PRENATAL STRESS AND VASCULAR PROCESSES

The presence of vascular disorders in pregnancy, including pregnancy-induced hypertension and pre-eclampsia, is one of the major indications for elective preterm delivery and causes of fetal growth restriction and low birth weight.[129,130] Although a large body of research has documented a strong association between stress and increased risk for vascular disorders, relatively little work has been conducted around this question in human pregnancy. However, findings from these few studies consistently suggest that maternal psychosocial stress, specifically job strain (high job demand and low decision latitude), is significantly associated with increased risk of hypertensive disorders in pregnancy.[131-134] With respect to physiological mechanisms, a study in a sample of low-risk, primiparous women of blood pressure and heart rate responses to psychological stress (a 10-minute laboratory-based behavioral challenge during pregnancy) reported that diastolic blood pressure reactivity significantly predicted both the length of gestation and infant birth weight after controlling for resting pressure and trimester of pregnancy.[135] A couple of other studies have reported significant associations between two components of maternal psychosocial stress – state and trait anxiety – and hemodynamic processes in pregnancy. In a study of nulliparous women, maternal levels of trait anxiety were found to be significantly related to uteroplacental and fetal hemodynamics. Using measures of pulsatility index (PI) derived from Doppler flow velocimetry of the umbilical and fetal middle cerebral artery at 37–40 weeks gestation, the results indicated that fetuses of mothers with high trait anxiety scores had significantly higher PI values in the umbilical artery, significantly lower PI values in the fetal middle cerebral artery, and a significantly lower cerebro-umbilical PI ratio (signs of fetal hypoxia and compensatory redistribution of blood flow to the fetal brain).[136] Another study of pregnant women conducted at 32 weeks gestation also reported significant associations between high levels of maternal anxiety and an increased PI value in the uterine arteries.[137]

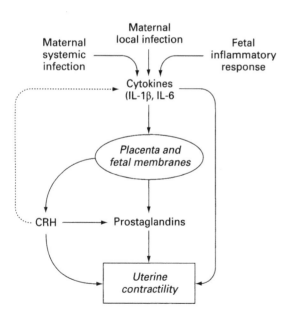

Figure 3.3 Endocrine–immune interactions in human pregnancy and fetal development.

Several cross-sectional studies have found significant gestational age-adjusted elevations of placental CRH concentrations in pregnant women with hypertensive disorders.[138–140] Moreover, a recent study reported a significant association between presence of abnormal uteroplacental flow wave forms and elevated levels of placental CRH.[85] Although the direction of causality is not clear (increased placental CRH is probably a response to vasoconstriction and hypoxia and not a cause of the hypertensive disorder), this may be another mechanism whereby stress-related vascular pathophysiology may contribute to adverse fetal developmental and birth outcomes.

STRESS VULNERABILITY IN HUMAN PREGNANCY: CRITICAL PERIODS OF SUSCEPTIBILITY

The state of pregnancy is characterized by a series of progressive biological changes. These changes over the course of gestation are associated with alterations in responsiveness to stress. For example, several studies have clearly demonstrated reduced feedback sensitivity and attenuated responsivity of the HPA axis as pregnancy advances.[141–143] These changes persist into the postpartum period,[141,142,144,145] but are then reversed to pre-pregnancy levels (IS Federenko et al, unpublished data, 2005). This attenuation of physiological responses to stimulation during pregnancy is not limited to the neuroendocrine system; a similar pattern has been reported for cardiovascular[146–149] and sympathoadrenal[146–148,150] stress responses.

This discussion about pregnancy changes is not only relevant to stress physiology, similar results have been reported for psychological stress appraisal and affect. For example, paralleling the phenomenon of an attenuation of physiological stress responses with advancing gestation, psychological appraisals of stress after a traumatic event, such as an earthquake, are reduced as pregnancy progresses.[26] Furthermore, mothers in the postpartum period report lower perceived stress in the past month and less negative mood directly after breastfeeding as compared to mothers who bottle-feed.[151] Thus, the physiological context of pregnancy and the postpartum period seems to have a stress-dampening effect through alterations in the endocrine and autonomic nervous systems. Finally, there is evidence that the pregnancy-induced changes in reproductive hormone levels, such as estrogen, affect memory[152–154] and semantic processing[155] – both of which play an important role in self-report and recall. During pregnancy, many women report memory and cognitive impairments, such as forgetfulness, confusion, and disorientation.[156–158]

Taken together, these findings suggest that the stage of pregnancy may play an important role in moderating the effects of maternal stress on birth outcomes. The notion of critical periods of susceptibility is well established in the developmental literature, and there may be critical time periods in human gestation of increased susceptibility to the effects of maternal stress. Women become less biologically and psychologically reactive as pregnancy progresses,[26,91] with likely implications for modulating maternal-fetal susceptibility to stress. Preliminary data also suggest that pregnant women who do not exhibit psychological and physiological dampening are at increased risk for elevated hormonal trajectories and at greater risk for adverse birth outcomes.

CONTEXT OF GENES

One obvious, alternate explanation for the observed association of birth phenotype and subsequent disease risk is that a common set of genes may influence both processes. However, several studies of monozygotic twins have shown that genetic effects cannot explain these effects.[159] For example, associations between birth weight and adult hypertension, seen in cohorts of (monozygotic) twins treated as individuals, have generally remained when data are analyzed within twin pairs. Similar associations are seen in animals with relative genetic homogeneity, when kept in standardized conditions. Some studies are now beginning to emerge in the literature which suggest that the effects of genes on adult health outcomes interact with processes related to fetal development. For example, the effect of a polymorphism of the gene encoding peroxisome proliferator-activated receptor $\gamma2$ (PPAR$\gamma2$), which increases tissue sensitivity to insulin and protects against type-2 diabetes mellitus, depends on birth weight, and was shown to influence only those men and women with low birth weights.[160] Similarly, with respect to the insulin response to glucose load, a significant interaction was found in the relationship between the angiotensin-1 converting enzyme (ACE) insertion/deletion (I/D) polymorphism and whether the individual was born SGA. In SGA-born adults, ACE I carriers had higher insulin than ACE DD carriers. This heterogeneity was not seen in non SGA-born adults.[161]

Genomic imprinting is an epigenetic mechanism by which certain genes become repressed on one of the two parental alleles. This parent of origin-dependent phenomenon is a notable exception to the laws of Mendelian genetics. Imprinted genes are intricately involved in fetal development.[162] The concept of imprinting was first described for insulin-like growth factors (IGFs), which play important roles in regulating and controlling placental development and growth,[163] and have a role in the etiology and consequences of placental insufficiency and fetal growth restriction. Imprinted genes have central roles in controlling both the fetal demand for, and placental supply of, maternal nutrients.[164] Specifically, deletion of the paternally imprinted gene coding IGF-II expressed in the trophoblast results in a form of placental insufficiency and reduced fetal growth,[165] a model of altered placental gene expression. Imprinting is now known to play important roles in many other aspects of mammalian development, and its dysregulation may result in disease. Recent evidence supports a role for stress in dysregulating the imprinting process during development. Studies in the mouse, for example, demonstrate that environmental stress, such as *in vitro* culture, affect the somatic maintenance of epigenetic marks at imprinted loci.[166] Other studies have shown that bovine *in vitro* (IVF)-produced and nuclear transfer (NT)-derived embryos differ from their *in vivo*-produced counterparts in a number of characteristics, including a complete lack of expression, an induced expression, or a significant up- or down-regulation of a specific gene.[167] These alterations which are considered a kind of 'stress' response of the embryos to deficient environmental conditions, are believed to be caused primarily by changes in the methylation patterns, and are associated with aberrant growth and morphology at fetal and perinatal stages of development. Nonimprinted genes can also undergo epigenetic change in response to a stressful environment. For example, a recent study in rodents reported that the choice of exon usage in the glucocorticoid receptor (GR) gene is altered by both prenatal glucocorticoid exposure and neonatal behavioral manipulation (reduced maternal care) via histone acetylation and DNA methylation in a transcriptional factor binding site, and that these changes persist throughout life as manifested in altered HPA activity.[168]

Some studies have examined the associations between several single nucleotide polymorphisms (SNPs) and stress-related neuroendocrine function. Genes that have been examined include those coding for the GR, the mineralocorticoid receptor (MR), CRH, CRH type 1 and type 2 receptors, proopiomelanocortin (POMC), ACTH (MC-2) receptor, cortisol-binding globulin (CBG), and several steroidogenic enzymes. Clinical outcomes in these studies have focused on body composition and weight, insulin resistance, leptin, lipoproteins, blood pressure, rheumatoid arthritis, and depression.[169–176] Of direct relevance in this context are studies on variations in genes coding for CRH, GR, and CRHR1. Most of these studies have described the effects of variation in the GR gene. For example, GR polymorphisms have been found to relate to dermal blanching after topical glucocorticoid exposure,[177] to cortisol responses to a nutritional load,[178] and to cortisol responses to psychosocial stress.[179] Last, CRFR1-mutant mice have been shown to have an impaired stress response and display decreased anxiety-like behavior, whereas CRFR2-mutant mice are hypersensitive to stress and display increased anxiety-like behavior.[180] We are not aware of any studies to date that have systematically examined the genomics of maternal and fetal stress-related physiological systems and pathways in human pregnancy and fetal development, and suggest this is yet another important future avenue for this line of research.

IMPLICATIONS OF PRENATAL STRESS FOR DEVELOPMENTAL ORIGINS OF HEALTH AND DISEASE

Developmental processes involved in transforming a single-cell human embryo into a fully functioning organism within a mere span of 40 weeks are exceedingly complex and fascinating; indeed, one would be hard pressed to come up with any other example in the physical or biological world that even begins to approximate the sheer elegance and scope of intrauterine development. Biologists over the ages have asked the question: Does the genetic material of the fertilized egg already contain a full set of building specifications for the organism? The answer to this question is now believed to be an unequivocal 'no'. Genes and environment are no longer considered to exert separate influences, and development is viewed not as a gradual elaboration of an architectural plan preconfigured in the genes, but rather as a dynamic interdependency of genes and environment characterized by a continuous process of interactions in a place- and time-specific dependent manner, and involving short- and long-term information storage, whereby genetic and epigenetic processes, at every step of development, become represented in the evolving structural and functional design of the organism.[181,182] (For the purpose of this discussion, we use the term 'genetic' to refer to the effects of variations in DNA sequences on protein physiology, and the term 'epigenetic' to refer to alterations in gene expression and protein physiology without changes in DNA sequences; e.g. genetic imprinting via DNA methylation.) According to this epigenetic view of development, events at one point in time have consequences that are manifested later in the developmental process, and afferent influences have a profound effect on the developmental trajectory.[183] In other words, it appears that within the constraints imposed by the heritable germ line at conception, each developing organism plays an active role in its own construction. This dynamic process is effected by evolving various systems during embryonic and fetal life to acquire information about the nature of the environment, and to use this information to guide development. In the context of this formulation, not only is the environment necessary for development to occur, but the nature of the environment may play either a supportive role for normal or optimal development, or a pernicious role to harm development.[184]

The importance of individual differences in neurobiological processes in health and diseases of the nervous, endocrine, immune, cardiovascular, reproductive, gastrointestinal, and musculoskeletal systems is well established.[185–187] With respect to the question of the origins, or determinants, of these individual differences, two kinds of models have guided theory and research. The first category of models emphasize the effect of the accumulation of adverse environmental, social, and biological conditions in producing dysregulation of normally functioning neurobiological processes (i.e. a cumulative exposure model). The second and more recent type of models emphasize the developmental origins of individual differences (i.e. a developmental trajectories model). According to these newer developmental models, individual differences in neurobiological processes evolve through a series of interactions, or conditional probabilities. The effects of genes (inherited at conception) on fetal developmental and birth outcomes are conditioned by the environment within the fetus and uterus. The effects of fetal outcomes, such as growth and other birth phenotypes, on infant developmental and health outcomes are then conditioned by the environment during childhood; and the effects of childhood factors on adult health outcomes are modified further by lifestyle and other environments in adult life. Any one influence does not have a single quantifiable risk associated with it. Its risk is shaped by events and environments at earlier, crucial stages of development (i.e. the notion of developmental switches).[188] Thus, it is the degree of congruence or discongruence between fetal, childhood, and adult environments that determines trajectories leading to either optimal or suboptimal developmental and health outcomes.[2,189]

As reviewed earlier, several epidemiological studies suggest that markers of an individual's birth phenotype, such as low birth weight and small body size, are associated with a significant and independent increase in risk of physical and mental diseases in adult life. It is unlikely that birth phenotype, *per se*, plays a causal role in increasing risk of adult disease.[7,9] Instead, birth phenotype is more likely a crude reflection of developmental processes in intrauterine life that also may influence the structure and function of the physiological systems that underlie health and disease risk in later life.[7,9,10] A model of fetal programming of adult human disease has been described. Fetal programming refers to the process whereby conditions during crucial, sensitive periods of early life have permanent effects on anatomy, physiology, and metabolism. Early programming influences factors such as metabolic set points, which define the dynamics of the adaptive range within which an individual can operate. This adaptive range influences disease susceptibilities that emerge through interaction with the environment.[2,190] According to this model, biological adaptations that enable the fetus to adapt to a period of intrauterine deprivation result in permanent (re)programming of the developmental pattern of proliferation and differentiation events within key fetal tissues and organ systems, and may have pathological consequences in adult life. This model also argues that relative to other animal species, humans may be more vulnerable to the noxious effects of an adverse intrauterine environment because organisms are most susceptible to environmental insult during phases of rapid growth, and in humans cell division occurs *in utero* at a more rapid rate than in other animal species. We have reviewed evidence suggesting that maternal stress during prenatal development is an important process with respect to its impact on birth phenotype. Moreover, we have reviewed evidence suggesting that the biological mechanisms through which prenatal stress may exert its effects on fetal development include MPF neuroendocrine, immune/inflammatory, vascular, and epigenetic processes, all of which are known to play central and critical roles in biological function, health and susceptibility to disease (see Figure 3.4).

The adoption of an epigenetic framework for early development, wherein the organism plays an active role in its own construction by adapting systems to acquire and use information about the nature of the environment to guide development, gives rise to two important questions. First, how do the fetal and maternal compartments communicate with one another? And second, in light of the fact that the fetal nervous system is itself in a state of evolution and has yet to acquire its repertoire of structural and functional capabilities, what are the modalities available to the developing fetus to receive, process and act on information acquired from the environment? As discussed

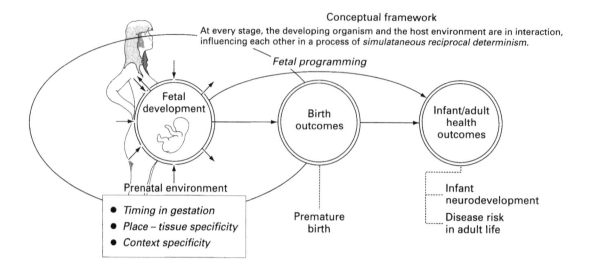

Figure 3.4 Developmental model.

earlier, there are no direct neural or vascular connections between the mother and her developing fetus, and bidirectional communication is mediated primarily via the exchange of blood-borne chemical signals such as products of the endocrine and immune systems. One of the remarkable adaptations of mammalian pregnancy is the evolution in early gestation of a transient organ of fetal origin – the placenta. In addition to the long-recognized multiple roles played by the placenta, it now appears that the placenta may also take on some functions that are usually ascribed to the central nervous system – i.e. the capability of receiving, processing and acting upon certain classes of external stimuli. Indeed, perhaps one of the important roles of the placenta is to act on behalf of the fetus as both a sensory and effector organ to facilitate the transduction and incorporation of environmental signals into the developmental process. The findings reviewed earlier support precisely such a role, mediated by the activity of the placental hormone, CRH.

A second possible stress-related pathway involves the transplacental passage of maternal cortisol to directly influence fetal growth and development.[191,192] The fetal brain and peripheral tissues are very sensitive to a number of agents, including growth factors, transcription factors, and nutrients. Steroids in particular have powerful organizational effects on the brain and peripheral tissues. Animal studies have demonstrated that during development, fetal exposure to glucocorticoids directly affects the development and subsequent function of neurotransmitter systems (and their transporter mechanisms) in the brainstem; the development of GR expression and structural components in the

hippocampus; and development and subsequent function of parvocellular neurons (CRH/AVP system). Moreover, because the brainstem neurotransmitter systems project directly to the hippocampus and paraventricular nucleus (PVN), glucocorticoid-induced changes indirectly impact the function of the hippocampus and PVN.[193] Fetal glucocorticoid exposure also delays axon myelination and has effects on the function of polyamines, which, in turn, are major regulators of neural cell replication and differentiation. In addition to the above effects in the brain, antenatal exposure to high levels of cortisol in animals has been shown to reduce offspring birth weight and produce permanent hypertension, hyperglycemia, hyperinsulinaemia, and altered behavior and neuroendocrine responses throughout the lifespan. The molecular mechanisms of these effects are believed to involve alterations in the set points of HPA axis activity and feedback sensitivity, and alterations of tissue GR expression.[194] Under normal circumstances, access to maternal cortisol by the fetus is low, because of the action of the placental enzyme, 11β-hydroxysteroid dehydrogenase type 2 (11β-HSD2), which converts cortisol to cortisone. The efficiency of 11β-HSD2, however, is both tissue- and species-specific. Although reduced 11β-HSD2 activity has been reported in intrauterine growth-restricted pregnancies, the impact of maternal stress on placental 11β-HSD2 synthesis is not known at the present time.[195]

Several of the early proponents of the notion of fetal or developmental origins of health and disease have argued that maternal malnutrition in the periconceptional and gestational period is one of the most important causal factors underlying this phenomenon.[196] However, in addition to the direct consequences of malnutrition on availability of energy substrate (calories, nutrients) for fetal growth and development, it also is possible that the observed effects of maternal malnutrition may be mediated, in part, by stress-related physiological processes, and that malnutrition, like other forms of physical, psychological, and biological insults, may serve as a trigger for the activation of stress-related biological mechanisms. For example, the offspring of pregnant rats fed a low protein diet grow up to become hypertensive. This effect has been shown to be mediated by stress and the passage of cortisol from the maternal to fetal compartment. In fact, inhibiting the activity of the enzyme 11β-HSD2 in the placenta (which converts cortisol to its inactive form, cortisone) also produced the same effect.[197a,198] Similarly, a widely cited study on the effects of malnutrition in sheep has demonstrated that a modest reduction in food intake in the periconceptional period (but not in later gestation) alters gestational length and produces earlier delivery.[199] However, fetal nutritional requirements in early gestation are extremely small, and maternal undernutrition is unlikely to have limited nutrient availability for fetal growth. Rather, the study found that the periconceptional nutritional insult produced physiological stress and led to the accelerated development of the fetal HPA axis (as indexed by precocious surges in ACTH and cortisol), which, in turn, caused earlier initiation of parturition by mechanisms discussed earlier in this chapter.[199]

SUMMARY

- Prenatal stress exerts a significant and independent influence on fetal development and birth phenotypes, which, in turn, are related to health over the lifespan and predict risk of disease in adult life.

- The biological mechanisms that mediate the effects of prenatal stress on fetal development and birth outcomes, including maternal-placental-fetal neuroendocrine, immune/inflammatory, vascular, and epigenetic processes, are also known to play central and critical roles in biological function, health, and susceptibility to disease.

- The study of the interplay between environmental, social, and biological systems in fetal life holds great challenge and promise in our efforts to arrive at a more comprehensive understanding of the determinants of health and disease.

ACKNOWLEDGMENTS

Supported, in part, by US PHS (NIH) grants HD-33506 and HD-41696 to PDW. ISF was supported by a postdoctoral fellowship from the German Academic Exchange Service (DAAD).

REFERENCES

1. Barker DJP. Mothers, Babies and Health in Later Life, 2nd edn. Edinburgh: Churchill Livingstone, 1998.
2. Gluckman PD, Hanson MA. The developmental origins of the metabolic syndrome. Trends Endocrinol Metab 2004; 15: 183–7.
3. Mellemkjaer L, Olsen J, Olsen JH, Olsen ML, Sorensen HT, Thulstrup AM. Birth weight and risk of early-onset breast cancer. Cancer Causes Control 2003; 14: 61–4.
4. Michels KB. Early life predictors of chronic disease. J Womens Health (Larchmt) 2003; 12: 157–61.
5. Sallout B, Walker M. The fetal origin of adult diseases. J Obstet Gynaecol 2003; 23: 555–60.
6. Barker DJ. Fetal programming of coronary heart disease. Trends Endocrinol Metab 2002; 13: 364–8.
7. Gluckman PD, Hanson MA. Living with the past: evolution, development, and patterns of disease. Science 2004; 305: 1733–6.
8. Osmond C, Barker DJ. Fetal, infant, and childhood growth are predictors of coronary heart disease, diabetes, and hypertension in adult men and women. Environ Health Perspect 2000; 108 (Suppl 3): 545–53.
9. Morley R, Blair E, Dwyer T, Owens J. Is birthweight a good marker for gestational exposures that increase the risk of adult disease? Pediatr Perinat Epidemiol 2002; 16: 194–9.
10. Terry MB, Susser E. Commentary: The impact of fetal and infant exposures along the life course. Int J Epidemiol 2001; 30: 95–6.
11. Denham M, Schell LM, Gallo M, Stark A. Neonatal size of low socio-economic status Black and White term births in Albany County, NYS. Ann Hum Biol 2001; 28: 172–83.
12. David RJ, Collins JW Jr. Differing birth weight among infants of U.S.-Born Blacks, African-Born Blacks, and U.S.-Born Whites. N Engl J Med 1997; 337: 1209–14.
13. Cobas J, Balcazar H, Benin MB, Keith VM, Chong Y. Acculturation and low birthweight infants among Latino women: a reanalysis of HHANES data with structural equation models. Am J Public Health 1996; 86: 394–6.
14. Cervantes A, Keith L, Wyshak G. Adverse birth outcomes among native-born and immigrant women: replicating national evidence regarding Mexicans at the local level. Matern Child Health J 1999; 3: 99–109.
15. McGrady G, Sung J, Rowley D, Hogue C. Preterm delivery and low birth weight among first-born infants of black and white college graduates. Am J Epidemiol 1992; 136: 266–76.
16. Schoendorf KC, Hogue C, Kleinman JC, Rowley D. Mortality among infants of black as compared with white college-educated parents. N Engl J Med 1992; 326: 1522–6.
17. Zambrana RE, Scrimshaw SC, Collins N, Dunkel-Schetter C. Prenatal health behaviors and psychosocial risk factors in pregnant woman of Mexican origin: the role of acculturation. Am J Public Health 1997; 87: 1022–6.
18. Barnett PA, Spence JD, Manuck SB, Jennings JR. Psychological stress and the progression of carotic artery disease. J Hypertens 1997; 15: 49–55.

19. Chrousos GP. Stress, chronic inflammation, and emotional and physical well-being: concurrent effects and chronic sequelae. J Allergy Clin Immunol 2000; 106 (5 Suppl): S275–S291.

20. Heim C, Ehlert U, Hellhammer DH. The potential role of hypocortisolism in the pathophysiology of stress-related bodily disorders. Psychoneuroendocrinology 2000; 25: 1–35.

21. Lobel M. Conceptualizations, measurement, and effects of prenatal maternal stress on birth outcomes. J Behav Med 1994; 17: 225–72.

22. Wadhwa PD, Porto M, Chicz-DeMet A, Sandman CA. Maternal CRH levels in early third trimester predict length of gestation in human pregnancy. Am J Obstet Gynecol 1998; 179: 1079–85.

23. Copper RL, Goldenberg RL, Das A et al. The preterm prediction study: maternal stress is associated with spontaneous preterm birth at less than thirty-five weeks gestation. National Institute of Child Health and Human Development Maternal-Fetal Medicine Units Network. Am J Obstet Gynecol 1996; 175: 1286–92.

24. Dole N, Savitz DA, Hertz-Picciotto I et al. Maternal stress and preterm birth. Am J Epidemiol 2003; 157: 14–24.

25. Feldman PJ, Dunkel-Schetter C, Sandman CA, Wadhwa PD. Maternal social support predicts birth weight and fetal growth in human pregnancy. Psychosom Med 2000; 62: 715–25.

26. Glynn L, Wadhwa PD, Dunkel-Schetter C, Sandman CA. When stress happens matters: the effects of earthquake timing on stress responsivity in pregnancy. Am J Obstet Gynecol 2001; 184: 637–42.

27. Hedegaard M, Henriksen TB, Sabroe S, Secher NJ. Psychological distress in pregnancy and preterm delivery. BMJ 1993; 307: 234–9.

28. Hedegaard M, Henriksen TB, Secher NJ, Hatch MC, Sabroe S. Do stressful life events affect duration of gestation and risk of preterm delivery? Epidemiology 1996; 7: 339–45.

29. Misra DP, O'Campo P, Strobino D. Testing a sociomedical model for preterm delivery. Pediatr Perinat Epidemiol 2001; 15: 110–22.

30. Nordentoft M, Lou HC, Hansen D et al. Intrauterine growth retardation and premature delivery: the influence of maternal smoking and psychosocial factors. Am J Public Health 1996; 86: 347–54.

31. Pritchard CW, Teo PY. Preterm birth, low birthweight and the stressfulness of the household role for pregnant women. Soc Sci Med 1994; 38: 89–96.

32. Rini CK, Dunkel-Schetter C, Wadhwa PD, Sandman CA. Psychological adaptation and birth outcomes: the role of personal resources, stress, and sociocultural context in pregnancy. Health Psychol 1999; 18: 333–45.

33. Wadhwa PD, Dunkel-Schetter C, Garite TJ, Porto M, Sandman CA. The association between prenatal stress and infant birth weight and gestational age at birth: a prospective investigation. Am J Obstet Gynecol 1993; 169: 858–65.

34. Cliver SP, Goldenberg RL, Cutter GR et al. The relationships among psychosocial profile, maternal size, and smoking in predicting fetal growth retardation. Obstet Gynecol 1992; 80: 262–7.

35. Dejin-Karlsson E, Hanson BS, Ostegren PO et al. Association of a lack of psychosocial resources and the risk of giving birth to small for gestational age infants: a stress hypothesis. BJOG 2000; 107: 89–100.

36. Abell TD, Baker LC, Clover RD, Ramsey CN Jr. The effects of family functioning on infant birthweight. J Fam Pract 1991; 32: 37–44.

37. Bhagwanani SG, Seagraves K, Dierker LJ, Lax M. Relationship between prenatal anxiety and perinatal outcome in nulliparious women: a prospective study. J Natl Med Assc 1997; 89: 93–8.

38. Da Costa D, Dritsa M, Larouche J, Brender W. Psychosocial predictors of labor/delivery complications and infant birth weight: a prospective multivariate study. J Psychosom Obstet Gynaecol 2000; 21: 137–48.

39. Dye TD, Tollivert NJ, Lee RV, Kenney CJ. Violence, pregnancy, and birth outcome in Appalachia. Paediatr Perinat Epidemiol 1995; 9: 35–47.

40. Lou HC, Hansen D, Nordentoft M et al. Prenatal stress of human life affects fetal brain development. Dev Med Child Neurol 1994; 36: 826–32.

41. Hoffman S, Hatch MC. Depressive symptomatology during pregnancy: evidence for an association with decreased fetal growth in pregnancies of lower social class women. Health Psychol 2000; 19: 535–43.

42. Demyttenaere K, Maes A, Nijs P, Odendael H, Van Assche FA. Coping style and preterm labor. J Psychosom Obstet Gynaecol 1995; 16: 109–15.

43. Orr ST, James SA, Miller CA et al. Psychosocial stressors and low birthweight in an urban population. Am J Prev Med 1996; 12: 459–66.

44. Sawchuk LA, Burke SD, Benady S. Assessing the impact of adolescent pregnancy and the premarital conception stress complex on birth weight among young mothers in Gibraltar's civilian community. J Adolesc Health 1997; 21: 259–66.

45. Steer RA, Scholl TO, Hediger ML, Fischer RL. Self-reported depression and negative pregnancy outcomes. J Clin Epidemiol 1992; 45: 1093–9.

46. Chrousos GP, Gold PW. The concepts of stress and stress system disorders. Overview of physical and behavioral homeostasis. JAMA 1992; 267: 1244–52.

47. Wadhwa PD, Glynn L, Sandman CA, Chicz-DeMet A, Hobel C. Racial/ethnic differences in maternal-placental stress physiology over the course of gestation. J Soc Gynecol Investig 2002; 19: 198A.

48. Gorin AA, Stone AA. Recall biases and cognitive errors in retrospective self-reports. In: Handbook of Health Psychology. (Baum A, Revenson T, Singer J eds). Mahwah NJ: Lawrence Erlbaum Associates, 2000, 405–13.

49. Kihlstrom JF, Eich E, Sandbrand D, Tobias BA. Emotion and memory: implications for self-report. In: The Science of Self-Report: Implications for Research and Practice. (Stone AA, Turkkan JJ, Bachrach CA et al., eds). Mahwah NJ: Lawrence Erlbaum Associates, 2000.

50. Shiffman S. Real-time self-report of momentary states in the natural environment: computerized ecological momentary assessment. In: The Science of Self-Report: Implications for Research and Practice. (Stone AA, Turkkan JJ, Bachrach CA et al., eds.). Mahwah, NJ: Lawrence Erlbaum Associates, 2000.

51. Kahneman D, Krueger AB, Schkade DA, Schwarz N, Stone AA. A survey method for characterizing daily life experience: the day reconstruction method. Science 2004; 306: 1776–80.

52. Stone AA, Shiffman S. Ecological momentary assessment (EMA) in behavioral medicine. Ann Behav Med 1994; 16: 199–202.

53. Kofman O. The role of prenatal stress in the etiology of developmental behavioural disorders. Neurosci Biobehav Rev 2002; 26: 457–70.

54. Maccari S, Darnaudery M, Morley-Fletcher S et al. Prenatal stress and long-term consequences: implications of glucocorticoid hormones. Neurosci Biobehav Rev 2003; 27: 119–27.

55. Weinstock M. Alterations induced by gestational stress in brain morphology and behaviour of the offspring. Prog Neurobiol 2001; 65: 427–51.

56. Coe CL, Lubach GR. Prenatal influences on neuroimmune set points in infancy. Ann N Y Acad Sci 2000; 917: 468–77.

57. Schneider ML, Moore CF, Roberts AD, Dejesus O. Prenatal stress alters early neurobehavior, stress reactivity and learning in non-human primates: a brief review. Stress 2001; 4: 183–93.

58. Smith R. The timing of birth. Sci Am 1999; 3: 68–75.

59. Smith R. The Endocrinology of Parturition. Newcastle, Australia: Karger, 2001.

60. Dobbing J, Sands J. Comparative aspects of the brain growth spurt. Early Hum Dev 1979; 3: 79–83.

61. Dent GW, Smith MA, Levine S. Rapid induction of corticotropin-releasing hormone gene transcription in the paraventricular nucleus of the developing rat. Endocrinology 2000; 141: 1593–8.

62. Wadhwa PD, Culhane JF, Rauh V et al. Stress, infection and preterm birth: a biobehavioral perspective. Pediatr Perinat Epidemiol 2001; E15: 17–29.

63. Grammatopoulos DK, Hillhouse EW. Role of corticotropin-releasing hormone in onset of labour. Lancet 1999; 354: 1546–9.

64. Challis JRG, Matthew SG, Gibb W, Lye SJ. Endocrine and paracrine regulation of birth at term and preterm. Endocr Rev 2000; 21: 514–50.

65. Majzoub JA, Karalis KP. Placental corticotropin-releasing hormone: function and regulation. Am J Obstet Gynecol 1999; 180: S242–S246.

66. Petraglia F, Florio P, Nappi C, Genazzani AR. Peptide signaling in human placenta and membranes: autocrine, paracrine, and endocrine mechanisms. Endocr Rev 1996; 17: 156–86.

67. Lockwood CJ, Kuczynski E. Risk stratification and pathological mechanisms in preterm delivery. Pediatr Perinat Epidemiol 2001; 15 (S2): 78–89.

68. McLean M, Bisits A, Davies J et al. A placental clock controlling the length of human pregnancy. Nat Med 1995; 1: 460–3.

69. Wadhwa PD, Chicz-DemMet A, Dunkel-Schetter C et al. Placental corticotropin-releasing hormone (CRH), spontaneous preterm birth, and fetal growth restriction: a prospective investigation. Am J Obstet Gynecol 2004; 191: 1063–9.

70. Campbell EA, Linton EA, Wolfe CD et al. Plasma corticotropin-releasing hormone concentrations during pregnancy and parturition. J Clin Endocrinol Metabol 1987; 64: 1054–9.

71. Erickson K, Thorsen P, Chrousos G et al. Preterm birth: associated neuroendocrine, medical, and behavioral risk factors. J Clin Endocrinol Metab 2001; 86: 2544–52.

72. Hobel CJ, Dunkel-Schetter C, Roesch SC, Castro LC, Arora CP. Maternal plasma corticotropin-releasing hormone associated with stress at 20 weeks gestation in pregnancies ending in preterm delivery. Am J Obstet Gynecol 1999; 180 (1 Pt 3): S257–S263.

73. Holzman C, Jetton J, Siler-Khodr T, Fisher R, Rip T. Second trimester corticotropin-releasing hormone levels in relation to preterm delivery and ethnicity. Obstet Gynecol 2001; 97: 657–63.

74. Korebrits C, Ramirez MM, Watson L et al. Maternal CRH is increased with impending preterm birth. J Clin Endocrinol Metab 1998A; 83: 1585–91.

75. Kurki T, Laatikainen T, Salminen-Lappalainen K, Ylikorkala O. Maternal plasma corticotrophin-releasing hormone – elevated in preterm labour but unaffected by indomethacin or nylidrin. BJOG 1991; 98: 685–91.

76. Petraglia F, Aguzzoli L, Florio P et al. Maternal plasma and placental immunoreactive corticotrophin-releasing factor concentrations in infection-associated term and pre-term delivery. Placenta 1995; 16: 157–64.

77. Warren WB, Patrick SL, Goland RS. Elevated maternal and plasma corticotropin-releasing hormone levels in pregnancies complicated by preterm labor. Am J Obstet Gynecol 1992; 166: 1198–207.

78. Wolfe CDA, Patel SP, Linton EA et al. Plasma corticotrophin-releasing factor (CRF) in abnormal pregnancy. BJOG 1988; 95: 1003–6.

79. McGarth S, McLean M, Smith D et al. Maternal plasma corticotropin-releasing hormone trajectories vary depending on the etiology of preterm birth. Am J Obstet Gynecol 2002; 186: 257–60.

80. Petraglia F, Sutton S, Vale W. Neurotransmitters and peptides modulate the release of immunoreactive corticotropin-releasing factor from cultured human placental cells. Am J Obstet Gynecol 1989; 160: 247–51.

81. Robinson BG, Emanuel RL, Frim DM, Majzoub JA. Glucocorticoid stimulates expression of corticotropin-releasing hormone gene in human placenta. Proc Natl Acad Sci USA 1988; 85: 5244–8.

82. Emanuel RL, Robinson BG, Seely EW et al. Corticotrophin releasing hormone levels in human plasma and amniotic fluid during gestation. Clin Endocrinol (Oxf) 1994; 40: 257–62.

83. Cheng YH, Nicholson RC, King B et al. Glucocorticoid stimulation of corticotropin-releasing hormone gene expression requires a cyclic adenosine $3',5'$-monophosphate regulatory element in human primary placental cytotrophoblast cells. J Clin Endocrinol Metab 2000; 85: 1937–45.

84. King BR, Smith R, Nicholson RC. Novel glucocorticoid and cAMP interactions on the CRH gene promoter. Mol Cell Endocrinol 2002; 194: 19–28.

85. Giles WB, McLean M, Davies JJ, Smith R. Abnormal umbilical artery doppler waveforms and cord blood corticotropin-releasing hormone. Obstet Gynecol 1996; 87: 107–11.

86. Petraglia F, Sawchenko PE, Rivier J, Vale W. Evidence for local stimulation of ACTH secretion by corticotropin-releasing factor in human placenta. Nature 1987; 328: 717–19.

87. Petraglia F, Volpe A, Genazzani A et al. Neuroendrocrinology of the human placenta. Front Neuroendocrinol 1990; 11: 6–37.

88. Chan EC, Smith R, Lewin T et al. Plasma corticotropin-releasing hormone, β-endorphin and cortisol inter-relationships during human pregnancy. Acta Endocrinol 1993; 128: 339–44.

89. Goland RS, Conwell IM, Warren WB, Wardlaw SL. Placental corticotropin-releasing hormone and pituitary-adrenal function during pregnancy. Neuroendocrinology 1992; 56: 742–9.

90. Sasaki A, Shinkawa O, Yoshinaga K. Placental corticotropin-releasing hormone may be a stimulator of maternal pituitary adrenocorticotropic hormone secretion in humans. J Clin Invest 1989; 84: 1997–2001.

91. Wadhwa PD, Dunkel-Schetter C, Porto M, Chicz-DeMet A, Sandman CA. Psychobiological processes and prenatal stress in human pregnancy. Ann Behav Med 1997; 19S: 39.

92. Wadhwa PD, Dunkel-Schetter C, Chicz-DeMet A, Porto M, Sandman CA. Prenatal psychosocial factors and the neuroendocrine axis in human pregnancy. Psychosom Med 1996; 58: 432–46.

93. Petraglia F, Hatch MC, Lapinski R et al. Lack of effect of psychosocial stress on maternal corticotropin-releasing factor and catecholamine levels at 28 weeks gestation. J Soc Gynecol Investig 2001; 8: 83–8.
94. Challis JR, Matthews SG, Van Meir C, Ramirez MM. Current topic: the placental corticotrophin-releasing hormone-adrenocorticotrophin axis. Placenta 1995; 16: 481–502.
95. Loudon JA, Groom KM, Bennett PR. Prostaglandin inhibitors in preterm labour. Best Pract Res Clin Obstet Gynecol 2003; 17: 731–44.
96. Elliott CL, Allport VC, Loudon JA, Wu GD, Bennett PR. Nuclear factor-kappa B is essential for up-regulation of interleukin-8 expression in human amnion and cervical epithelial cells. Mol Hum Reprod 2001; 7: 787–90.
97. McKay LI, Cidlowski JA. Molecular control of immune/inflammatory responses: interactions between nuclear factor-κB and steroid receptor-signaling pathways. Endocr Rev 1999; 20: 435–59.
98. Condon JC, Jeyasuria P, Faust JM, Mendelson CR. Surfactant protein secreted by the maturing mouse fetal lung acts as a hormone that signals the initiation of parturition. Proc Natl Acad Sci USA 2004; 101: 4978–83.
99. Emanuel RL, Torday JS, Asokananthan N, Sunday ME. Direct effects of corticotropin-releasing hormone and thyrotropin-releasing hormone on fetal lung explants. Peptides 2000; 21: 1819–29.
100. Spina V, Aleandri V, Pacchiarotti A, Salvi M. Immune tolerance in pregnancy. Maternal-fetal interactions. Minerva Ginecol 1998; 50: 533–7.
101. Strelkauskas AJ, Davis IJ, Dray S. Longitudinal studies showing alternations in the levels and functional response of T and B lymphocytes in human pregnancy. Clin Exp Immunol 1978; 32: 531–9.
102. Gehrz RC, Christianson WR, Linner KM et al. A longitudinal analysis of lymphocyte proliferative responses to mitogens and antigens during pregnancy. Am J Obstet Gynecol 1981; 104: 665–70.
103. Lin H, Mosmann TR, Guilbert L, Tuntipopipat S, Wegmann TG. Synthesis of T helper 2-type cytokines at the maternal-fetal interface. J Immunol 1993; 151: 4562–73.
104. Piccinni MP, Romagnani S. Regulation of fetal allograft survival by a hormone-controlled Th1 and Th2-type cytokines. Immunol Res 1996; 15: 141–50.
105. Shaarawy M, Nagui AR. Enhanced expression of cytokines may play a fundamental role in the mechanisms of immunologically mediated recurrent spontaneous abortion. Acta Obstet Gynecol Scand 1997; 76: 205–11.
106. Szereday L, Varga P, Szekeres-Bartho J. Cytokine production by lymphocytes in pregnancy. Am J Reprod Immunol 1997; 38: 418–22.
107. Marzi M, Vigano A, Trabattoni D et al. Characterization of type 1 and type 2 cytokine production profile in physiologic and pathologic human pregnancy. Clin Exp Immunol 1996; 106: 127–33.
108. Romero R, Gomez R, Ghezzi F et al. A fetal systemic inflammatory response is followed by the spontaneous onset of preterm parturition. Am J Obstet Gynecol 1998; 179: 186–93.
109. Dudley DJ. Preterm labor: an intrauterine inflammatory response? J Reprod Immunol 1997; 36: 93–109.
110. Goldenberg RL, Hauth JC, Andrews WW. Intrauterine infection and premature delivery. N Engl J Med 2000; 342: 1500–7.
111. Brown NL, Alvi SA, Elder MG, Bennett PR, Sullivan MH. Interleukin-1beta and bacterial endotoxin change the

metabolism of prostaglandins E2 and F2alpha in intact fetal membranes. Placenta 1998; 19: 625–30.
112. Gomez R, Romero R, Edwin SS, David C. Pathogenesis of preterm labor and preterm premature rupture of membranes associated with intraamniotic infection. Infect Dis Clin North Am 1997; 11: 135–76.
113. Falkenberg ER, Davis RO, DuBard M, Parker CR. Effects of maternal infections on fetal adrenal steroid production. Endocr Res 1999; 25: 239–49.
114. Elenkov IJ, Chrousos GP. Stress hormones, Th1/Th2 patterns, pro/anti-inflammatory cytokines and susceptibility to disease. Trends Endocrinol Metab 1999; 10: 359–368.
115. Kiecolt-Glaser JK, Glaser R. Depression and immune function. Central pathways to morbidity and mortality. J Psychosom Res 2002; 53: 873–6.
116. Culhane JF, Rauh V, Farley-McCollum K et al. Maternal stress is associated with bacterial vaginosis in human pregnacy. Matern Child Health J 2001; 5: 127–34.
117. Jamieson DJ, Duerr A, Klein RS et al. Longitudinal analysis of bacterial vaginosis: findings from the HIV epidemiology research study. Obstet Gynecol 2001; 98: 656–63.
118. Herrera JA, Alvarado JP, Matrinez JE. The psychosocial environment and cellular immunity in the pregnant patient. Stress Med 1998; 4: 49–56.
119. Arck PC, Rose M, Hertwig K et al. Stress and immune mediators in miscarriage. Hum Reprod 2001; 6: 1505–11.
120. Tsigos C, Chrousos GP. Hypothalamic-pituitary-adrenal axis, neuroednocrine factors and stress. J Psychosom Res 2002; 53: 865–71.
121. Athayde N, Edwin SS, Romero R et al. A role for matrix metalloproteinase-9 in spontaneous rupture of the fetal membranes. Am J Obstet Gynecol 1998; 197: 1248–53.
122. Yoon BH, Romero R, Jun JK et al. An increase in fetal plasma cortisol but not dehydroepiandrosterone sulfate is followed by the onset of preterm labor in patients with preterm premature rupture of the membranes. Am J Obstet Gynecol 1998; 179: 1107–14.
123. Yoon BH, Romero R, Park JS et al. Microbial invasion of the amniotic cavity with Ureaplasma urealyticum is associated with a robust host response in fetal, amniotic, and maternal compartments. Am J Obstet Gynecol 1998; 179: 1254–60.
124. Chrousos GP. Stressors, stress and the neuroendocrine integration of the adaptive response: the 1997 Hans Selye Memorial Lecture. Ann N Y Acad Sci 1998; 851: 311–35.
125. Haddad JJ, Saade NE, Safieh-Garabedian B. Cytokines and neuro-immune-endocrine interactions: a role for the hypothalamic-pituitary-adrenal revolving axis. J Neuroimmunol 2002; 133: 1–19.
126. McEwen BS, Biron CA, Brunson KW et al. The role of adrenocorticoids as modulators of immune function in health and disease: neural, endocrine and immune interactions. Brain Res Rev 1997; 23: 79–133.
127. Thorp JM. Placental vascular compromise: unifying the etiologic pathways of perinatal compromise. Curr Probl Obstet Gynecol Fertil 2001; 24: 203–20.
128. Clifton VL, Wallace EM, Smith R. Short-term effects of glucocorticoids in the human fetal-placental circulation in vitro. J Clin Endocrinol Metab 2002; 87: 2838–42.
129. Meis PJ, Goldenberg RL, Mercer BM et al. The preterm prediction study: risk factors for indicated preterm births. Maternal-Fetal Medicine Units Network of the National Institute of Child Health and Human Development. Am J Obstet Gynecol 1998; 178: 562–7.

130. Samadi AR, Mayberry RM. Maternal hypertension and spontaneous preterm births among black women. Obstet Gynecol 1998; 91: 899–904.

131. Klonoff-Cohen HS, Cross JL, Pieper CF. Job stress and preeclampsia. Epidemiology 1996; 7: 245–9.

132. Marcoux S, Berube S, Brisson C, Mondor M. Job strain and pregnancy-induced hypertension. Epidemiology 1999; 10: 376–82.

133. Landsbergis PA, Hatch MC. Psychosocial work stress and pregnancy-induced hypertension. Epidemiology 1996; 7: 346–51.

134. Wergeland E, Strand K. Working conditions and prevalence of pre-eclampsia, Norway 1989. Int J Gynaecol Obstet 1997; 58: 189–96.

135. McCubbin JA, Lawson EJ, Cox S et al. Prenatal maternal blood pressure response to stress predicts birth weight and gestational age: a preliminary study. Am J Obstet Gynecol 1996; 175: 706–12.

136. Sjostrom K, Valentin L, Thelin T, Marsal K. Maternal anxiety in late pregnancy and fetal hemodynamics. Eur J Obstet Gynecol Reprod Biol 1997; 74: 149–55.

137. Teixeira JM, Fisk NM, Glover V. Association between maternal anxiety in pregnancy and increased uterine artery resistance index: cohort based study. BMJ 1999; 318: 153–7.

138. Jeske W, Soszynski P, Lukaszewicz E et al. Enhancement of plasma corticotropin-releasing hormone in pregnancy-induced hypertension. Acta Endocrinol (Copenh) 1990; 122: 711–14.

139. Perkins AV, Linton EA, Eben F et al. Corticotrophin-releasing hormone and corticotrophin-releasing hormone binding protein in normal and pre-eclamptic human pregnancies. Br J Obstet Gynaecol 1995; 102: 118–22.

140. Warren WB, Gurewitsch ED, Goland RS. Corticotropin-releasing hormone and pituitary-adrenal hormones in pregnancies complicated by chronic hypertension. Am J Obstet Gynecol 1995; 172: 661–6.

141. Kammerer M, Adams D, Von Castelberg B, Glover V. Pregnant women become insensitive to cold stress. BMC Pregnancy Childbirth 2002; 2: 8.

142. Owens, PC, Smith R, Brinsmead MW et al. Postnatal disappearance of the pregnancy-associated reduced sensitivity of plasma cortisol to feedback inhibition. Life Sci 1987; 41: 1745–50.

143. Schulte, HM, Weisner D, Allolio B. The corticotrophin releasing hormone test in late pregnancy: lack of adrenocorticotrophin and cortisol response. Clin Endocrinol (Oxf) 1990; 33: 99–106.

144. Altemus M, Redwine LS, Leong YM et al. Responses to laboratory psychosocial stress in postpartum women. Psychosom Med 2001; 63: 814–21.

145. Magiakou MA, Mastorakos G, Rabin D et al. Hypothalamic corticotropin-releasing hormone suppression during the postpartum period: implications for the increase in psychiatric manifestations at this time. J Clin Endocrinol Metab 1996; 81: 1912–17.

146. Nisell H, Hjemdahl P, Linde B, Lunell NO. Sympatho-adrenal and cardiovascular reactivity in pregnancy-induced hypertension. I. Responses to isometric exercise and a cold pressor test. Br J Obstet Gynecol 1985; 92: 722–31.

147. Nisell H, Hjemdahl P, Linde B, Lunell NO. Sympathoadrenal and cardiovascular reactivity in pregnancy-induced hypertension II. Responses to tilting. Am J Obstet Gynecol 1985; 152: 554–60.

148. Barron WM, Mujais SK, Zinaman M, Bravo EL, Lindheimer MD. Plasma catecholamine responses to physiologic stimuli in normal human pregnancy. Am J Obstet Gynecol 1986; 154: 80–4.

149. Matthews KA, Rodin J. Pregnancy alters blood pressure responses to psychological and physical challenge. Psychophysiology 1992; 29: 232–40.

150. Whittaker PG, Gerrard J, Lind T. Catecholamine responses to changes in posture during human pregnancy. Br J Obstet Gynaecol 1985; 92: 586–92.

151. Mezzacappa ES, Katlin ES. Breast-feeding is associated with reduced perceived stress and negative mood in mothers. Health Psychol 2002; 21: 187–93.

152. Drake EB, Henderson VW, Stanczyk FZ et al. Associations between circulating sex steroid hormones and cognition in normal elderly women. Neurology 2000; 54: 599–603.

153. Phillips SM, Sherwin BB. Variations in memory function and sex steroid hormones across the menstrual cycle. Psychoneuroendocrinology 1992; 17: 497–506.

154. Rosenberg L, Park S. Verbal and spatial functions across the menstrual cycle in healthy young women. Psychoneuroendocrinology 2001; 27: 835–41.

155. Ussher JM, Wilding JM. Performance and state changes during the menstrual cycle conceptualised within a broad band testing framework. Soc Sci Med 1991; 32: 525–34.

156. Poser CM, Kassirer MR, Peyser JM. Benign encephalopathy of pregnancy: preliminary clinical observations. Acta Neurol Scand 1986; 73: 39–43.

157. Crawley RA, Dennison K, Carter C. Cognition in pregnancy and the first year post-partum. Psychol Psychother 2003; 76 (Pt 1): 69–84.

158. Brett M, Baxendale S. Motherhood and memory: a review. Psychoneuroendocrinology 2001; 26: 339–62.

159. Ozanne SE, Hales CN. Early programming of glucose-insulin metabolism. Trends Endocrinol Metab 2002; 13: 368–73.

160. Eriksson JG, Lindi V, Uusitupa M et al. The effects of the Pro12Ala polymorphism of the peroxisome proliferator-activated receptor-gamma2 gene on insulin sensitivity and insulin metabolism interact with size at birth. Diabetes 2002; 51: 2321–4.

161. Cambien F, Leger J, Mallet C et al. Angiotensin I-converting enzyme gene polymorphism modulates the consequences of in utero growth retardation on plasma insulin in young adults. Diabetes 1998; 47: 470–5.

162. Falls JG, Pulford DJ, Wylie AA, Jirtle RL. Genomic imprinting: implications for human disease. Am J Pathol 1999; 154: 635–47.

163. Han VK, Carter AM. Spatial and temporal patterns of expression of messenger RNA for insulin-like growth factors and their binding proteins in the placenta of man and laboratory animals. Placenta 2000; 21: 289–305.

164. Reik W, Constância M, Fowden A et al. Regulation of supply and demand for maternal nutrients in mammals by imprinted genes. J Physiol 2003; 547: 35–44.

165. Constancia M, Hemberger M, Hughes J et al. Placental-specific IGF-II is a major modulator of placental and fetal growth. Nature 2002; 417: 945–8.

166. Thompson SL, Konfortova G, Gregory RI et al. Environmental effects on genomic imprinting in mammals. Toxicol Lett 2001; 120: 143–50.

167. Niemann H, Wrenzycki C, Lucas-Hahn A et al. Gene expression patterns in bovine in vitro-produced and nuclear transfer-derived embryos and their implications for early development. Cloning Stem Cells 2002; 4: 29–38.

168. Weaver IC, Cervoni N, Champagne FA et al. Epigenetic programming by maternal behavior. Nat Neurosci 2004; 7: 847–54. Epub 2004 Jun 27.

169. Baerwald CG, Mok CC, Tickly M et al. Corticotropin releasing hormone (CRH) promoter polymorphisms in various ethnic groups of patients with rheumatoid arthritis. Z Rheumatol 2000; 59: 29–34.

170. Buemann B, Vohl MC, Chagnon M et al. Abdominal visceral fat is associated with a Bc1I restriction fragment length polymorphism at the glucocorticoid receptor gene locus. Obes Res 1997; 5: 186–92.

171. Derijk RH, Schaaf MJ, Turner G et al. A human glucocorticoid receptor gene variant that increases the stability of the glucocorticoid receptor beta-isoform mRNA is associated with rheumatoid arthritis. J Rheumatol 2001; 28: 2383–8.

172. Hixson JE, Almasy L, Cole S et al. Normal variation in leptin levels is associated with polymorphisms in the pro-opiomelanocortin gene, POMC. J Clin Endocrinol Metab 1999; 84: 3187–91.

173. Rosmond R, Bouchard C, Bjorntrop P et al. A Glucocorticoid receptor gene marker is associated with abdominal obesity, leptin, and dysregulation of the hypothalamic-pituitary-adrenal axis. Obes Res 2000; 8: 211–18.

174. Ukkola O, Rosmond R, Tremblay A, Bouchard C. Glucocorticoid receptor Bcl I variant is associated with an increased atherogenic profile in response to long-term overfeeding. Atherosclerosis 2001; 157: 221–4.

175. Villafuerte SM, Del-Favero J, Adolfsson R et al. Gene-based SNP genetic association study of the corticotropin-releasing hormone receptor-2 (CRHR2) in major depression. Am J Med Genet 2002; 114: 222–6.

176. Weaver JU, Hitman GA, Kopelman PG. An association between a Bcl1 restriction fragment length polymorphism of the glucocorticoid receptor locus and hyperinsulinaemia in obese women. J Mol Endocrinol 1992; 9: 295–300.

177. Panarelli M, Holloway CD, Graser R et al. Glucocorticoid receptor polymorphism, skin vasoconstriction, and other metabolic intermediate phenotypes in normal human subjects [see comments]. J Clin Endocrinol Metab 1998; 83: 1846–52.

178. Rosmond R, Chagnon YC, Chagnon M et al. A polymorphism of the 5'-flanking region of the glucocorticoid receptor gene locus is associated with basal cortisol secretion in men. Metabolism 2000; 49: 1197–9.

179. Wüst S, van Rossum EFC, Federenko IS et al. Common polymorphisms in the glucocorticoid receptor gene are associated with adrenocortical responses to psychosocial stress. J Clin Endocrinol Metab 2004; 89: 565–73.

180. Bale TL, Picetti R, Contarino A et al. Mice deficient for both corticotropin-releasing factor receptor 1 (CRFR1) and CRFR2 have an impaired stress response and display sexually dichotomous anxiety-like behavior. J Neurosci 2002; 22: 193–9.

181. Arenander AT, de Vellis J. Development of the nervous system. In: Basic Neurochemistry: Molecular, Cellular and Medical Aspects. (Siegel GJ, Agranoff BW, Albers RW, Molinoff PB, eds). New York: Raven Press, 1989.

182. Smotherman WP, Robinson SR. Tracing developmental trajectories into the prenatal period. In: Fetal Development: A Psychobiological Perspective. (Lecanuet JP, Fifer WP, Krasnegor NA, Smotherman WP eds). Hillsdale, NJ: Laurence Erlbaum Associates, 1995.

183. Kolb B. Brain Plasticity and Behavior. Mahwah, NJ: Lawrence Erlbaum Associates, 1995.

184. Bornstein MH. Sensitive periods in development: structural characteristics and casual interpretations. Psychol Bull 1989; 105: 179–97.

185. McEwen BS. Protective and damaging effects of stress mediators. N Engl J Med 1998; 338: 171–9.

186. Sapolsky RM, Romero LM, Munck AU. How do glucocorticoids influence stress responses? Integrating permissive, suppressive, stimulatory, and preparative actions. Endocr Rev 2000; 21: 55–89.

187. Lupien SJ, Lepage M. Stress, memory, and the hippocampus: can't live with it, can't live without it. Behav Brain Res 2001; 127: 137–58.

188. Barker DJ. Fetal programming of coronary heart disease. Trends Endocrinol Metab 2002; 13: 364–8.

189. Wadhwa PD, Culhane JF, Rauh V, Barve SS. Stress and preterm birth: neuroendocrine, immune/inflammatory, and vascular mechanisms. Matern Child Health J 2001; 5: 119–25.

190. Davies MJ, Norman RJ. Programming and reproductive functioning. Trends Endocrinol Metabol 2002; 13: 386–92.

191. Matthews SG. Early programming of the hypothalamo-pituitary-adrenal axis. Trends Endocrinol Metab 2002; 13: 373–80.

192. Matthews SG, Owen D, Banjanin S, Andrews MH. Glucocorticoids, hypothalamo-pituitary-adrenal (HPA) development, and life after birth. Endocr Res 2002; 28: 709–18.

193. Welberg LA, Seckl JR. Prenatal stress, glucocorticoids and the programming of the brain. J Neuroendocrinol 2001; 13: 113–28.

194. Seckl JR. Glucocorticoid programming of the fetus; adult phenotypes and molecular mechanisms. Mol Cell Endocrinol 2001; 185: 61–71.

195. McTernan CL, Draper N, Nicholson H et al. Reduced placental 11beta-hydroxysteroid dehydrogenase type 2 mRNA levels in human pregnancies complicated by intrauterine growth restriction: an analysis of possible mechanisms. J Clin Endocrinol Metab 2001; 86: 4979–83.

196. Ravelli AC, van der Meulen JH, Michels RP et al. Glucose tolerance in adults after prenatal exposure to famine. Lancet 1998; 351: 173–7.

197. Langley-Evans SC, Gardner DS, Jackson AA. Maternal protein restriction influences the programming of the rat hypothalamic-pituitary-adrenal axis. J Nutr 1996; 126: 1578–85.

198. Langley-Evans SC. Hypertension induced by foetal exposure to a maternal low-protein diet, in the rat, is prevented by pharmacological blockade of maternal glucocorticoid synthesis. J Hypertens 1997; 15: 537–44.

199. Bloomfield FH, Oliver MH, Hawkins P et al. A periconceptional nutritional origin for noninfectious preterm birth. Science 2003; 300: 606.

Section II – Prenatal programming of the neuroendocrine system – links to type 2 diabetes, obesity and cardiovascular disease

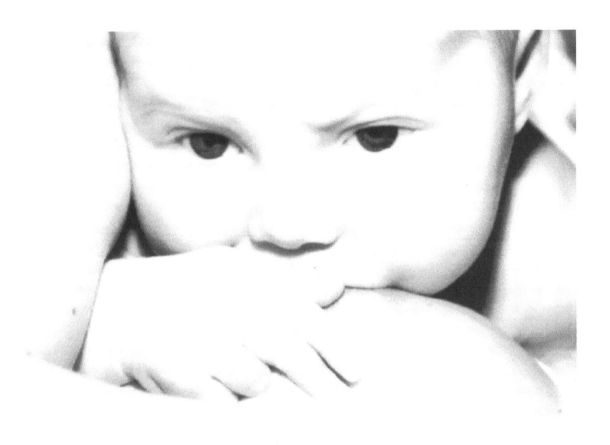

'The seeds of great discoveries are constantly floating around us, but they only take root in minds well prepared to receive them'
Joseph Henry

4

Prenatal glucocorticoid exposure and adult pathophysiology

Moffat J Nyirenda and Jonathan R Seckl

INTRODUCTION

Traditionally the common cardiovascular and metabolic diseases of middle age, such as hypertension, ischemic heart disease, and type 2 diabetes mellitus, are thought to be caused by specific lifestyle risk factors acting in adult life upon an individual's genetic background to determine disease occurrence. However, over the last decade, a plethora of epidemiological studies have suggested that factors operating in early life are also important determinants of the risk of cardiovascular and metabolic disorders in adulthood. Data from several distinct populations in Europe, Asia, Australia, and North America have shown that low birth weight or thinness at birth strongly predicts the subsequent occurrence of hypertension, hyperlipidemia, insulin resistance, type 2 diabetes, and ischemic heart disease deaths in adult life.[1-6] These relationships are largely independent of traditional adult lifestyle factors (smoking, adult weight, social class, excess alcohol intake, sedentariness), which are additive risks to the effects of birth weight.[1,2] Moreover, the association between birth weight and adult disease is continuous and includes birth weights even within the normal range, rather than severely undersized, multiple, or premature babies.[2,6] The concept of early life physiological 'programming' or 'imprinting' has been advanced to explain the associations between prenatal environmental events, altered fetal growth and development, and later pathophysiology.[2,7]

EARLY LIFE PROGRAMMING

Programming reflects the action of an environmental factor during a sensitive developmental period or 'window' to affect the development and organization of specific tissues, producing effects that persist throughout life. The individual organ system affected is determined by its unique vulnerability, based on the timing of the exposure and the systems developing during that time 'window'. It has long been known that the environment plays a fundamental part in providing cues that regulate development of the organism, and that altering environmental parameters can have significant phenotypic consequences. For example, more than a century ago, Weisman noted that butterflies that hatched during different seasons were colored differently, and that this season-dependent coloration could be mimicked by incubating larvae at different temperatures.[8] Programming has since been examined in several mammalian systems. Many agents, including homeotic genes, transcription factors, growth factors, hormones, and nutrients, are known to exert programming actions. These effects are often found with steroidal hormones, and one of the best characterized programming effects involves the action of androgens. Neonatal exposure to androgens programs the expression of steroid-metabolizing enzymes in the liver, as well as the development of sexually dimorphic structures in the brain and facilitates male typical sexual behavior.[9,10] These effects persist throughout life, irrespective of subsequent hormonal manipulation or the genetic sex of the animal.

The molecular mechanisms for the association between low birth weight and later disease are unknown, but two major environmental hypotheses have been proposed to underlie mammalian fetal programming: fetal undernutrition[2] and overexposure of the fetus to glucocorticoids[7] (see Figure 4.1). Here we review the programming effects of glucocorticoids.

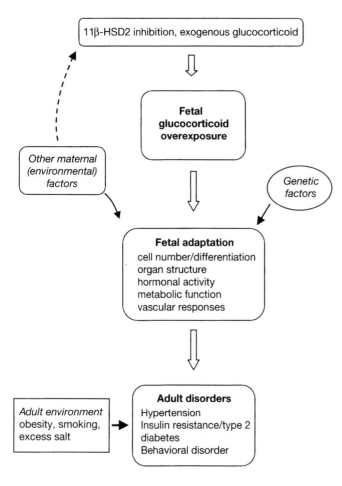

Figure 4.1 Programming by glucocorticoids. Excessive fetal glucocorticoid exposure, either from inhibition of feto-placental 11β-HSD2 activity or through exogenous administration of synthetic glucocorticoids, influences the development of many physiological systems and programs tissue responses leading to later disease. Genetic and environmental factors will influence these effects in the developing offspring.

GLUCOCORTICOID ACTION

Glucocorticoids (adrenocorticosteroid hormones) are produced by the adrenal cortex and exert their effects by binding glucocorticoid receptors (GR), which act in the cell nucleus to regulate the expression of target genes[11] (see Figure 4.2). In adult mammals glucocorticoids are involved in the control of several physiological processes that maintain homeostasis, including coordination of responses to stress. Excessive glucocorticoids, either from endogenous overproduction in Cushing's syndrome or as a result of exogenous administration, have well-characterized diabetogenic and hypertensive effects.[12]

Glucocorticoids and fetal development

During development, glucocorticoids are important for growth, tissue development, and maturation of various organs to prepare the organism for an extra-uterine life.[13] Thus, surfactant production by the lungs, activity of the enzyme systems in the fetal gut, retina, pancreas, thyroid, brain, and liver are stimulated by glucocorticoids. GR null mice die within the first few hours after birth of respiratory failure due to severe lung atelectasis.[14] The development of adrenergic chromaffin cells and maturation of hepatic gluconeogenic enzymes are also severely retarded.[14] The ability of glucocorticoids to accelerate maturation of organs, notably the lung, accounts for their widespread use in obstetric and neonatal practice in threatened or actual preterm delivery to improve neonatal viability.[15] However, supraphysiological levels of glucocorticoids cause fetal growth retardation in mammalian models and in humans.[16,17] Human intrauterine growth retardation is associated with high maternal and fetal concentrations of glucocorticoids.[17] Moreover, *in utero* levels of glucocorticoids are also increased in response to most challenges known to have programming effects, such as maternal undernutrition, placental insufficiency, and restriction of placental blood flow.[18] Thus, glucocorticoids may

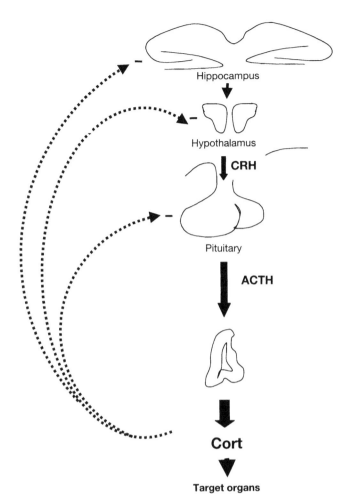

Figure 4.2 A schematic diagram of the HPA axis. Corticotrophin-releasing hormone (CRH) is synthesized in neurons of the paraventricular nucleus (PVN) of the hypothalamus and released into the hypophyseal portal circulation. CRH stimulates adrenocorticotropic hormone (ACTH) synthesis and release from corticotrophs in the anterior pituitary gland. ACTH, in turn, stimulates secretion of glucocorticoids from the adrenal cortex. Glucocorticoids are important for maintenance of homeostasis and induce a variety of metabolic changes that allow the body to respond to the stress. They also provide negative feedback on the HPA axis by inhibiting CRH and ACTH secretion at numerous levels.

signal an adverse intrauterine environment and thus adapt fetal development to maximize the chances of survival at birth. Indeed, glucocorticoids may be one of a limited number of common pathways through which diverse agents (such as maternal malnutrition and placental insufficiency) mediate their programming effects. In support of this notion, the programming of hypertension by maternal protein restriction during pregnancy in the rat can be prevented by the inhibition of maternal corticosterone biosynthesis during pregnancy.[19]

Feto-placental 11β-hydroxysteroid dehydrogenase type 2: a physiological barrier

Glucocorticoids are highly lipophilic molecules and rapidly cross biological barriers such as the placenta. However, normally fetal glucocorticoid levels are much lower than maternal levels.[20] This gradient is achieved by feto-placental 11β-hydroxysteroid dehydrogenase type 2 (11β-HSD2), which catalyzes the rapid metabolism of cortisol and corticosterone to physiologically inert 11-keto forms (cortisone and 11-dehydrocorticosterone)[21] (see Figure 4.3). A good example of the potent action and importance of 11β-HSD2 is in regulation of glucocorticoid access to mineralocorticoid receptors in the distal nephron of the kidney.[22] Purified mineralocorticoid receptors are nonselective and bind cortisol, corticosterone, and aldosterone with high and similar affinity *in vitro*. However, *in vivo* only aldosterone exerts renal mineralocorticoid actions, despite a 100-fold molar excess of circulating cortisol. Such selective access of aldosterone *in vivo* is due to local 11β-HSD2, which potently inactivates glucocorticoids, but does not metabolize aldosterone.[23] Thus, when the enzyme is congenitally absent (the 'syndrome of apparent mineralocorticoid

Maternal circulation   *Fetal circulation*

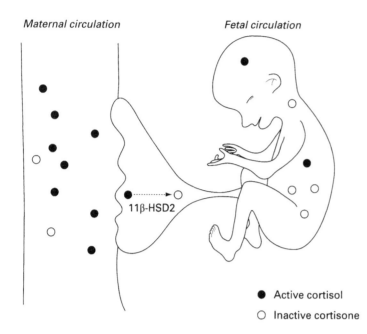

11β-HSD2

● Active cortisol

○ Inactive cortisone

Figure 4.3 Placental 11β-HSD2 rapidly inactivates physiological glucocorticoids (cortisol, corticosterone) ● to inert 11-keto forms ○. The enzyme thus ensures that excessive amounts of maternal glucocorticoid are largely excluded from the fetal compartment.

excess') or is inhibited by liquorice or its derivatives (glycyrrhetinic acid, carbenoxolone), cortisol illicitly occupies and activates renal mineralocorticoid receptors, causing sodium retention, hypokalemia, and hypertension.[24,25]

In the placenta, 11β-HSD2 forms a potent barrier to maternal glucocorticoids, although the barrier may not be complete as a minor proportion of maternal glucocorticoid crosses intact to the fetus.[26] The mechanisms involved in the regulation of placental 11β-HSD2 are largely unknown. *In vitro* studies of the human placenta have shown inhibition of 11β-HSD2 by progesterone, estrogen, and nitric oxide, and stimulation by activators of the cAMP pathway.[27] In contrast, in the baboon, estrogens synthesized locally in the placenta from fetal adrenal androgens play a role in maintaining placental 11β-HSD2 activity.[27] While no firm parallels to the *in vivo* state of human pregnancy can be drawn from these studies, it would appear that the level of expression and activity of 11β-HSD2 is determined by a delicate balance between stimulating and inhibitory influences. Indeed, studies in rats and humans indicate that the efficiency of placental 11β-HSD2 varies considerably.[28] A deficiency in 11β-HSD2 would be expected to expose the fetus to increased glucocorticoid levels from the maternal circulation, with subsequent effects on fetal development. In support of this notion, the lowest placental 11β-HSD2 activity, and presumably the highest fetal exposure to maternal glucocorticoids, is seen in babies with the smallest birth weights.[28] Moreover, patients

bearing mutations of the gene encoding 11β-HSD2 have low birth weight.[25] Fetal glucocorticoid load can be artificially increased by maternal administration of a synthetic glucocorticoid (such as dexamethasone) that is a poor substrate for 11β-HSD2 or through inhibition of placental 11β-HSD2 by liquorice or carbenoxolone.[21] Interestingly, maternal protein restriction also reduces the activity of 11β-HSD2 in the placenta,[29] which presumably results in increased fetal glucocorticoid load. This effect on an important placental enzyme provides further support that glucocorticoids may play a role in the effects of maternal undernutrition in programming later pathophysiology.

Thus, glucocorticoids play a critical role in organ maturation, and regulate major systems that are affected in the 'low birth weight baby syndrome'. These hormones are strong candidate mechanisms that may underlie the epidemiological link between low birth weight and cardiovascular and metabolic disorders in adulthood. There has been growing interest in this hypothesis, which is supported by data from several animal models and, more recently, evidence from human studies.

EFFECTS AND MECHANISMS OF GLUCOCORTICOID PROGRAMMING

Programming cardiovascular and metabolic systems

Blood pressure

The impact of prenatal glucocorticoid exposure during development on arterial blood pressure has been investigated in the offspring of several species. Treatment of pregnant rats with dexamethasone results in a lower mean birth weight (a deficit reversed by weaning at 21 days of age) and persistent elevations of arterial blood pressure in the adult offspring.[30,31] Maternal administration of carbenoxolone, a potent inhibitor of 11β-HSD2, also leads to reduced birth weight and elevated blood pressure in the adult offspring.[32] This effect requires the presence of maternal glucocorticoids, as the offspring of adrenalectomized pregnant rats are protected from carbenoxolone actions upon birth weight or adult hypertension.[32] Antenatal glucocorticoid excess, either maternally administered or through intrafetal infusion of cortisol or of the synthetic glucocorticoids betamethasone and dexamethasone, also programs adult hypertension in the sheep.[33,34] The timing of glucocorticoid exposure appears to be important; exposure to glucocorticoids during the final week of pregnancy in the rat is sufficient to produce permanent adult hypertension,[31] whereas the sensitive window for such effects in sheep is earlier in gestation.[33] The reasons for such differences are unclear but may reflect the complex species-specific patterns of expression of glucocorticoid receptors and the isoenzymes of 11β-HSD,[21] which regulate maternal glucocorticoid transfer to the fetus and modulate glucocorticoid action in individual tissues.

The mechanisms of glucocorticoid-programmed adult hypertension are not clearly understood, but probably involve a variety of processes. Infusion of glucocorticoids into the fetus elevates blood pressure in sheep[35] and baboons,[36] as well as in humans.[37] However, for programming to occur, such effects need to persist. One potential mechanism may involve a change in renal structure; prenatal glucocorticoid exposure has been shown to cause irreversible reductions in nephron number in rodents[38] and sheep.[34] In utero exposure to glucocorticoids also affects adult vascular responsivity to vasoconstrictors, enhancing endothelin-induced vasoconstriction and attenuating endothelium-dependent vasorelaxation in sheep.[39] The molecular basis for the change in vascular responsivity remains unknown. There is also evidence for an enhanced activity of the renin-angiotensin system following prenatal glucocorticoid exposure, with an increase in angiotensinogen, the angiotensin type 1 (AT1) and AT2 receptors.[34] Furthermore, prenatal dexamethasone treatment has been shown to cause alteration of the baroreceptor response in sheep.[34] Glucocorticoid exposure may also have primary effects on the heart. For example, fetal dexamethasone treatment interferes with the development of cardiac noradrenergic innervation and sympathetic activity,[40] and alters metabolic processes in the heart such as the glucose transporter 1, akt/protein kinase B, specific uncoupling proteins and PPARγ, the nuclear receptor for thiazolidinediones and fatty acids.[41] Additionally, antenatal glucocorticoid exposure increases adult calreticulin in the heart,[42] important since over-expression of cardiac calreticulin associates with cardiac dysfunction and death. Thus, increased coronary heart disease deaths in low birth weight populations may reflect a programming of primary cardiac dysfunction as well as the accrual of an increased incidence of cardiovascular risk factors such as hypertension.

Glucose–insulin homeostasis and metabolism

Prenatal overexposure to glucocorticoids also causes permanent hyperglycemia and hyperinsulinemia in the adult offspring in the rat[43,44] and sheep.[33,45] In the sheep, antenatal glucocorticoid exposure alters adult glucose metabolism whether or not there is prior fetal growth restriction,[33] suggesting that programming relates to fetal exposure to excess glucocorticoids in utero, rather than any primary effect of intrauterine growth retardation per se. Like blood pressure, the window of sensitivity for programming hyperglycaemia in the rat occurs in the last third of gestation.[44] Earlier dexamethasone exposure or postpartum treatments do not program hyperglycemia/hyperinsulinemia in the rat, suggesting that there is a tight window for this effect.[44,46] Programming of adult hyperglycemia can also be reproduced by gestational 11β-HSD inhibition with carbenoxolone.[43] These effects of carbenoxolone on birth weight and glucose tolerance are dependent on maternal glucocorticoids because maternal adrenalectomy restores both normal birth weight and normal glucose tolerance in the offspring.[43] Increasing endogenous glucocorticoid production through prenatal stress (which presumably overcomes activity of 11β-HSD2) has similar persisting effects.[47]

The mechanisms through which prenatal superphysiological levels of glucocorticoids program hyperglycemia have not been fully determined, but may involve derangements in several target organs.

Glucocorticoids regulate expression of critical hepatic metabolic enzymes, notably phosphoenolpyruvate carboxykinase (PEPCK), which develops in late gestation and catalyzes a rate-limiting step in gluconeogenesis. In rats, exposure to excess glucocorticoid *in utero* leads to offspring with permanent elevations in PEPCK mRNA and enzyme activity. The increase in PEPCK is selective to the periportal region of the hepatic acinus, the site of gluconeogenesis.[44] Increased PEPCK activity is seen in patients with type 2 diabetes,[48] and its over-expression in transgenic mice produces fasting hyperglycemia and glucose intolerance,[49] suggesting that the PEPCK may be a key mediator of hyperglycemia that results from prenatal glucocorticoid exposure. The induction of PEPCK at birth and its expression in mature hepatocytes is regulated by distinct hepatocyte-enriched nuclear transcription activators that bind their cognate DNA motifs in the PEPCK gene promoter.[50] These include family members of hepatocyte nuclear factor (HNF)1, HNF3, HNF4, HNF6, members of the CCAAT/enhancer binding protein (C/EBP) family, and GR itself. Intriguingly, livers of dexamethasone-programmed rats showed increased expression of some of these key transcription factors, notably GR,[44,51] and HNF4α (Nyirenda et al., unpublished data), suggesting that the increase in hepatic PEPCK expression may be secondary to the alterations in the transcription factor(s). Similar increases in hepatic GR are seen in the offspring of undernourished ewes,[52] suggesting a common underlying mechanism. Interestingly, the effects of prenatal dexamethasone treatment are not only observed in the immediate offspring as adults, but the second generation offspring also show elevated PEPCK and insulin levels, without further dexamethasone exposure.[53] The mechanisms for this transgenerational transmission of the phenotype are unknown, but may involve epigenetic processes.[53]

Relatively little is known about the effects of prenatal exposure to glucocorticoids on the development of the endocrine functions of the pancreas. However, indirect evidence suggests that excessive prenatal glucocorticoid levels may cause long term beta cell dysfunction. Prenatal undernutrition causes marked impairment of glucose-stimulated insulin secretion in the adult rat offspring. *In vitro* the isolated pancreatic islets have decreased insulin content and show impaired secretory response to glucose and arginine.[54] This effect depends on elevation of maternal and fetal corticosterone levels, and preventing the corticosterone increase in food-restricted dams restores beta cell mass. Indeed, fetal pancreatic insulin content correlates inversely with fetal corticosterone levels.[55] The mechanisms by which glucocorticoids modulate pancreatic development are not fully understood, but *in vitro* data suggest that this may involve interaction with transcription factors that control proliferation and/or differentiation of the pancreas.[56]

Antenatal dexamethasone exposure in rats has been shown to program fat metabolism. Thus, adult offspring of dams exposed to dexamethasone in pregnancy have increased intra-abdominal fat depots, with a parallel increase in leptin levels.[57] Moreover, *in utero* exposure to dexamethasone cause a marked increase in GR expression selectively in visceral adipose tissue in adult rats[51] and sheep.[52] Elevated GR expression in visceral adipose tissue may contribute to both adipose and hepatic insulin resistance. Prenatal dexamethasone treatment may also affect skeletal muscle glucose metabolism by altering the expression of GR.[51]

Programming of the central nervous system (CNS)

GR and MR are highly expressed in the developing brain, but the ontogeny of the expression of these receptors is complex in order to allow for selectivity of effects.[58] Glucocorticoids are important for normal maturation in most regions of the developing CNS, and are involved in initiating terminal maturation, remodelling axons and dendrites, and ensuring cell survival.[59] There is also high expression of 11β-HSD2 in the CNS at mid-gestation,[60] which presumably 'protects' vulnerable developing cells from excessive glucocorticoid action. However, 11β-HSD2 expression is dramatically switched off at the end of mid-gestation in the rat and mouse brain, coinciding with the terminal stage of neurogenesis.[60] Similarly, in human fetal brain 11β-HSD2 appears to be silenced between gestational weeks 19 and 26.[61] Thus, there appears to be an exquisitely timed system of protection and then exposure of developing brain regions to circulating glucocorticoids. Maternal and/or fetal stressors alter developmental trajectories of specific brain structures with persistent effects.[62,63] Exposure to glucocorticoids *in utero* has widespread acute effects upon neuronal structure and synapse formation and results in permanent alteration in brain structure.[62] Thus, sheep exposed to glucocorticoids *in utero* have reduced brain weight at birth and show delayed maturation of neurons, myelination, glia, and vasculature.[64] In rhesus monkeys, treatment with antenatal dexamethasone caused a dose-dependent neuronal degeneration of hippocampal neurons with persistent reduction in hippocampal volume.[65] Human and animal studies have demonstrated that altered hippocampal structure may be associated with a number of consequences for memory and behavior.[66]

Programming of the hypothalamic-pituitary-adrenal (HPA) axis

The hypothalamic-pituitary-adrenal (HPA) axis (Figure 4.2), and its key limbic regulator, the hippocampus, are particularly sensitive to glucocorticoids. This neuroendocrine system is exquisitely sensitive to environmental programming.[62] In the rat, prenatal stress or glucocorticoid exposure permanently elevates basal plasma corticosterone levels and increases the responsiveness of the HPA axis in adult rats[31,62] or primates.[67] This enhancement is thought to result from a permanent decrease in the expression of both types of corticosteroid receptor, GR and MR, in the hippocampus, which attenuates HPA axis feedback sensitivity.[62] Maternal undernutrition in rats and sheep also affects adult HPA axis function,[62] suggesting that HPA programming may be a common outcome of prenatal environmental challenge. As noted above, the programming effects of maternal dietary constraint may, at least in part, be mediated via selective down-regulation of placental 11β-HSD2 activity, with a consequent increase in fetal glucocorticoid load.[29,68] The effects of prenatal stress or glucocorticoid exposure in programming the HPA axis may be sex-specific, as female rats appear to have substantially more marked outcome than males.[69]

The GR gene: a common programming target?

GR is critical for cell function, and transgenic mice with a reduction of 30–50% in tissue levels of GR have striking neuroendocrine, metabolic, and immunological abnormalities.[70] GR gene expression shows marked tissue-specific regulation. The GR promoter is complex, with multiple tissue-specific alternate untranslated first exons in rats and mice, most within a transcriptionally active 'CpG island'.[71] All these mRNA species give rise to the same receptor protein, as only exons 2–9 encode the protein. The alternate untranslated first exons are spliced onto the common translated sequence beginning at exon 2. In the rat, two of the alternate exons are present in all tissues which have been studied; however, others are tissue-specific.[71] This variation permits considerable tissue-specific flexibility in the control of GR expression without allowing any tissue to become GR deplete. In the rat, early environmental enrichment through neonatal handling permanently programs increased expression of only one of the six alternate first exons (exon 1_7) utilized in the hippocampus.[71] Similar effects are seen in the offspring of mothers that show particularly 'attentive' forms of maternal care.[72] Exon 1_7 contains binding sites for AP-2 and NGF1-A, key transcription factors that are induced by the neonatal

manipulation.[73] In the peripheral tissues, such as the liver and visceral adipose tissue, prenatal glucocorticoid exposure or maternal malnutrition causes a permanent increase in GR expression,[44,51,68] and this up-regulation is paralleled by increased glucocorticoid sensitivity in these tissues.[44,51] A critical question that remains largely unanswered is how discrete perinatal environmental events such as glucocorticoid exposure can permanently alter gene expression. Recent evidence suggests that it may involve selective methylation/demethylation of specific promoters of the GR gene.[74] For example, the putative NGFI-A site around exon 1_7 is subject to differential and permanent methylation/demethylation in association with variations in maternal care.[74] The changes in the GR promoter DNA methylation pattern associate with altered histone acetylation and transcription factor (NGFI-A) binding to the GR promoter.[74] Treatment of the adult offspring brain with a histone deacetylase inhibitor removes the epigenetic differences in histone acetylation and DNA methylation and hence the NGFI-A binding changes. This results in a normalization of hippocampal GR expression and HPA responses to stress. These findings suggest a causal relation between the epigenetic modifications induced by early life events upon the GR gene promoter and the permanent programming of GR expression in the adult hippocampus. Similarly, this process may produce parallel tissue-specific effects in peripheral organs. Indeed, in liver-derived cells GR may mediate differential demethylation of target gene promoters, effects which persist after steroid withdrawal.[75] During development, such target promoter demethylation occurs before birth and may fine-tune the promoter to 'memorize' regulatory events occurring during development. This novel mechanism of gene control by environmental events early in life, which then persists throughout the lifespan, remains to be confirmed in other systems.

Programming behavior

Overexposure to glucocorticoids *in utero* can also lead to alterations in adult behavior. Prenatally stressed rodents exhibit increased 'anxious' behavior as adults and increased 'emotionality' in response to behavioral tests and novel environments.[62] Likewise, prenatal dexamethasone exposure late in gestation in rats impairs coping in aversive situations later in life.[62] These observations suggest that prenatal stress or glucocorticoid overexposure might influence susceptibility of humans to depression and anxiety disorders as adults. The molecular mechanisms through which adverse prenatal environment might mediate such behavioral changes are largely unknown. However, the adult offspring of dams exposed to prenatal stress or dexamethasone treatment have permanently increased corticotrophin-releasing hormone (CRH) expression in limbic structures, notably the amygdala. The amygdala plays a key role in the expression of emotional responses (fear and anxiety)[62] and CRH is known to have anxiogenic effects.[76] Moreover, corticosteroids facilitate CRH mRNA expression in the amygdala and increase GR and MR in this structure.[62] The amygdala also stimulates the HPA axis via a CRH signal.[77] Thus, an elevated corticosteroid signal in the amygdala due to hypercorticosteronemia in the adult offspring of dexamethasone-treated dams, may produce increased CRH levels in adulthood. A direct relationship between brain corticosteroid receptor levels and anxiety-like behavior is supported by the phenotype of transgenic mice with selective loss of GR gene expression in the brain, which show markedly reduced anxiety.[78] Prenatal glucocorticoid exposure also affects the developing dopaminergic system,[79] which may have pathophysiological implications in the development of other behavioral disorders such as schizo-affective, attention-deficit hyperactivity and extrapyramidal syndromes. Stressful events in the second trimester of human pregnancy have been associated with an increased incidence of schizophrenia in adolescent and adult offspring.[80]

Postnatal maternal deprivation or separation has also been associated with increased anxiety-related behaviors in both rodents and humans,[81,82] suggesting that the window of sensitivity in programming behavior extends into the early postnatal period. In rats, this is associated with increased CRH content in limbic structures, such as the amygdala, and increased activity of the HPA axis.[83] In contrast, in the 'neonatal handling' paradigm,[59] where the neonatal environment is moderately stimulated by short (15 minutes daily) handling of rat pups during the first 2 weeks of life, there is a permanent potentiation of the HPA axis sensitivity to glucocorticoid negative feedback, with lower plasma glucocorticoid levels throughout life[62] – a state compatible with better adjustments to environmental stress. The enhanced negative feedback sensitivity is mediated via increased hippocampal GR levels. The effects of neonatal handling are thought to be facilitated through the ascending serotonergic (5HT) pathways from the mid-brain raphe nuclei to the hippocampus.[74] 5HT induces GR gene expression in fetal hippocampal neurones *in vitro*, and in neonatal and adult hippocampal neurons *in vivo*.[74] The 'handling' induction of 5HT requires thyroid hormones that are elevated by the stimulation in rats and guinea pigs. At the hippocampal neuronal membrane, the ketanserin-sensitive $5HT_7$ receptor subtype, which is regulated by glucocorticoids and positively coupled to cAMP generation, is thought to play a key role in mediating the handling effects.[73] Handling stimulates hippocampal cAMP generation, which induces expression of specific transcription factors, most notably NGFI-A and AP-2.[73] NGFI-A and AP-2 bind to the GR gene promoter. This pathway might also be involved in other prenatal programming that affects the HPA axis because dexamethasone exposure in late pregnancy increases 5HT transporter expression in the rat brain,[84] an effect that would likely reduce 5HT availability in the hippocampus and elsewhere. NGFI-A has recently been shown to bind to the GR promoter and induces a specific GR transcript.[74] The 'neonatal handling' paradigm enhances maternal care-related behaviors and may be of physiological relevance because natural variation in maternal behavior is known to correlate with the offspring HPA physiology and hippocampal GR expression.[72]

EVIDENCE FOR GLUCOCORTICOID PROGRAMMING IN HUMANS

Glucocorticoids have extensive therapeutic use in obstetric practice; they are used as immunosuppressants to control various maternal conditions such as connective tissue disorders,[85] as well as for short-term treatment of the fetus to accelerate lung maturation in cases of preterm labor to prevent neonatal respiratory distress syndrome.[86] More rarely, dexamethasone is used throughout gestation from the first trimester to attenuate fetal adrenal steroid overproduction in fetuses at risk of congenital adrenal hyperplasia (CAH). Here glucocorticoid treatment reduces virilization by lowering the excessive secretion of adrenal androgen.[87] The long-term effects of fetal glucocorticoid exposure in humans have still not been comprehensively investigated. A preliminary study in children at risk for CAH who received dexamethasone in early gestation showed that prenatal dexamethasone exposure did not significantly affect cognition, but these children had increased emotional and social behavior problems.[88] Another study reported delayed psychomotor development and a failure to thrive in such patients.[89] The effects of fetal glucocorticoid exposure on cardiovascular and metabolic function in humans are unknown, but a recent report has suggested a predisposition to hypertension later in life.[90] However, the sample size in most of these studies has been small and proper evaluation of long-term effects of prenatal glucocorticoid exposure in humans awaits rigorous follow-up studies. Based upon findings in the prenatal rat model of dexamethasone exposure, low birth weight, and adult hypercorticosteronemia, recent studies have examined the relationship between birth weight and HPA function in adult humans. Intriguingly, birth weight has been shown to correlate closely with HPA measures from infancy,[91] through adolescence and young adulthood[92] to old age.[93] Low birth weight increases both basal and ACTH-stimulated cortisol levels in adulthood.[92,93] Additionally, birth weight appears to correlate linearly with adult muscle GR and insulin sensitivity (Walker et al., unpublished data). Thus, in humans, as in rodents, prenatal glucocorticoid overexposure (whether from exogenous administration or endogenous cortisol in response to maternal stress during pregnancy) appears to program an adverse adult cardiovascular, metabolic, neuroendocrine, and behavioral phenotype. Taken as a whole, these findings are compatible with the hypothesis that fetal overexposure to glucocorticoids may underlie at least in part the connection between the prenatal environment and adult disorders.

ACKNOWLEDGMENTS

Work in the authors' laboratories was supported by the Wellcome Trust, British Heart Foundation, Medical Research Council, European Union, and the Scottish Hospitals Endowments Research Trust.

REFERENCES

1. Barker DJP, Winter PD, Osmond C et al. Weight in infancy and death from ischaemic heart disease. Lancet 1989; ii: 577–80.
2. Barker DJP, Gluckman PD, Godfrey KM et al. Fetal nutrition and cardiovascular disease in adult life. Lancet 1993; 341: 938–41.
3. Curhan GC, Willett WC, Rimm EB et al. Birth weight and adult hypertension, diabetes mellitus, and obesity in US men. Circulation 1996; 94: 3246–50.
4. Leon DA, Koupilova I, Lithell HO et al. Failure to realise growth potential in utero and adult obesity in relation to blood pressure in 50 year old Swedish men. BMJ 1996; 312: 401–6.
5. Forsen T, Eriksson JG, Tuomilehto J et al. Mother's weight in pregnancy and coronary heart disease in a cohort of Finnish men: Follow up study. BMJ 1997; 315: 837–40.
6. Yajnik CS, Fall CHD, Vaidya U et al. Fetal growth and glucose and insulin metabolism in four-year-old Indian children. Diabetic Med 1995; 12: 330–6.
7. Edwards CRW, Benediktsson R, Lindsay R et al. Dysfunction of the placental glucocorticoid barrier: a link between the foetal environment and adult hypertension? Lancet 1993; 341: 355–7.
8. Weismann A. Essays on Heredity and Kindred Biological Problems. Oxford: Clarendon, 1892.
9. Arai Y, Gorski RA. Critical exposure time for androgenization of the developing hypothalamus in the female rat. Endocrinology 1968; 82: 1010–14.
10. Gustafsson JA, Mode A, Norstedt G et al. Sex steroid-induced changes in hepatic enzymes. Annu Rev Physiol 1983; 45: 51–60.
11. Yamamoto KR. Steroid receptor regulated transcription of specific genes and gene networks. Annu Rev Genet 1985; 19: 209–52.
12. Howlett TA, Rees LH, Besser GM. Cushing's syndrome. Clin Endocrinol Metab 1985; 14: 911–45.
13. Ballard PL. Glucocorticoids and differentiation. In: Glucocorticoid Hormone Action (Monographs in Endocrinology). (Rousseau GG, ed). Berlin: Springer-Verlag, 1979: 493–7.
14. Cole T, Blendy JA, Monaghan AP et al. Targeted disruption of the glucocorticoid receptor blocks adrenergic chromaffin cell development and severely retards lung maturation. Genes Dev 1995; 9: 1608–21.
15. Ward RM. Pharmacologic enhancement of fetal lung maturation. Clin Perinatol 1994; 21: 523–42.
16. Reinisch JM, Simon NG, Karwo WG et al. Prenatal exposure to prednisone in humans and animals retards intrauterine growth. Science 1978; 202: 436–8.
17. Goland RS, Josak S, Warren WB et al. Elevated levels of umbilical cord plasma corticotrophin-releasing hormone in growth-retarded fetuses. J Clin Endocrinol Metab 1993; 77: 1174–9.
18. Fowden AL, Forhead AJ. Endocrine mechanisms of intrauterine programming. Reproduction 2004; 127: 515–26.
19. Langley-Evans SC. Hypertension induced by foetal exposure to a maternal low-protein diet, in the rat, is prevented by pharmacological blockade of maternal glucocorticoid synthesis. J Hypertens 1997; 15: 537–44.
20. Campbell AL, Murphy BEP. The maternal-fetal cortisol gradient during pregnancy and at delivery. J Clin Endocrinol Metab 1977; 45: 435–40.
21. Seckl JR. Glucocorticoids, feto-placental 11beta-hydroxy-steroid dehydrogenase type 2 and the early life origins of adult disease. Steroids 1997; 62: 89–94.
22. Funder JW, Pearce PT, Smith R et al. Mineralocorticoid action: target tissue specificity is enzyme, not receptor, mediated. Science 1988; 242: 583–5.
23. Brown RW, Chapman KE, Kotelevtsev Y et al. Cloning and production of antisera to human placental 11 beta-hydroxysteroid dehydrogenase type 2. Biochem J 1996; 313 (Pt 3): 1007–17.
24. Stewart PM, Corrie JET, Shackleton CHL et al. Syndrome of apparent mineralocorticoid excess: a defect in the cortisol-cortisone shuttle. J Clin Invest 1988; 82: 340–9.
25. Mune T, Rogerson FM, Nikkilä H et al. Human hypertension caused by mutations in the kidney isozyme of 11β-hydroxysteroid dehydrogenase. Nature Gen 1995; 10: 394–9.
26. Benediktsson R, Calder AA, Edwards CRW et al. Placental 11β-hydroxysteroid dehydrogenase type 2 is the placental barrier to maternal glucocorticoids: ex vivo studies. Clin Endocrinol 1997; 46: 161–6.
27. Pepe G, Albrecht E. Actions of placental and fetal adrenal steroid hormones in primate pregnancy. Endor Rev 1995; 16: 608–48.
28. Stewart PM, Rogerson FM, Mason JI. Type 2 11β-hydroxysteroid dehydrogenase messenger RNA and activity in human placenta and fetal membranes: its relationship to birth weight and putative role in fetal steroidogenesis. J Clin Endocrinol Metab 1995; 80: 885–90.
29. Langley-Evans SC, Phillips PG, Benediktsson R et al. Protein intake in pregnancy, placental glucocorticoid metabolism

and the programming of hypertension in the rat. Placenta 1996; 17: 169–72.

30. Benediktsson R, Lindsay R, Noble J et al. Glucocorticoid exposure in utero: a new model for adult hypertension. Lancet 1993; 341: 339–41.

31. Levitt N, Lindsay RS, Holmes MC et al. Dexamethasone in the last week of pregnancy attenuates hippocampal glucocorticoid receptor gene expression and elevates blood pressure in the adult offspring in the rat. Neuroendocrinology 1996; 64: 412–18.

32. Lindsay RS, Lindsay RM, Edwards CRW et al. Inhibition of 11β-hydroxysteroid dehydrogenase in pregnant rats and the programming of blood pressure in the offspring. Hypertension 1996; 27: 1200–4.

33. Moss TJ, Sloboda DM, Gurrin LC et al. Programming effects in sheep of prenatal growth restriction and glucocorticoid exposure. Am J Physiol 2001; 281: R960–70.

34. Dodic M, Abouantoun T, O'Connor A et al. Programming effects of short prenatal exposure to dexamethasone in sheep. Hypertension 2002; 40: 729–34.

35. Tangalakis K, Lumbers ER, Moritz KM et al. Effect of cortisol on blood pressure and vascular reactivity in the ovine fetus. Exp Physiol 1992; 77: 709–17.

36. Koenen SV, Mecenas CA, Smith GS et al. Effects of maternal betamethasone administration on fetal and maternal blood pressure and heart rate in the baboon at 0.7 of gestation. Am J Obstet Gynecol 2002; 186: 812–17.

37. Kari MA, Hallman M, Eronen M et al. Prenatal dexamethasone treatment in conjunction with rescue therapy of human surfactant: a randomized placebo-controlled multicenter study. Pediatrics 1994; 93: 730–6.

38. Ortiz LA, Quan A, Weinberg A et al. Effect of prenatal dexamethasone on rat renal development. Kidney Int 2001; 59: 1663–9.

39. Molnar J, Howe DC, Nijland MJM et al. Prenatal dexamethasone leads to both endothelial dysfunction and vasodilatory compensation in sheep. J Physiol 2003; 547: 61–6.

40. Bian XP, Seidler FJ, Slotkin TA. Fetal dexamethasone exposure interferes with establishment of cardiac noradrenergic innervation and sympathetic activity. Teratology 1993; 47: 109–17.

41. Langdown ML, Holness MJ, Sugden MC. Early growth retardation induced by excessive exposure to glucocorticoids in utero selectively increases cardiac GLUT1 protein expression and Akt/protein kinase B activity in adulthood. J Endocrinol 2001; 169: 11–22.

42. Langdown ML, Holness MJ, Sugden MC. Effects of prenatal glucocorticoid exposure on cardiac calreticulin and calsequestrin protein expression during early development and in adulthood. Biochem J 2003; 371: 61–9.

43. Lindsay RS, Lindsay RM, Waddell BJ et al. Prenatal glucocorticoid exposure leads to offspring hyperglycaemia in the rat: studies with 11β-hydroxysteroid dehydrogenase inhibitor carbenoxolone. Diabetologia 1996; 39: 1299–305.

44. Nyirenda MJ, Lindsay RS, Kenyon CJ et al. Glucocorticoid exposure in late gestation permanently programs rat hepatic phosphoenolpyruvate carboxykinase and glucocorticoid receptor expression and causes glucose intolerance in adult offspring. J Clin Invest 1998; 101: 2174–81.

45. Gatford KL, Wintour EM, De Blasio MJ et al. Differential timing for programming of glucose homoeostasis, sensitivity to insulin and blood pressure by in utero exposure to dexamethasone in sheep. Clin Sci 2000; 98: 553–60.

46. Nyirenda MJ, Welberg LA, Seckl JR. Programming hyperglycaemia in the rat through prenatal exposure to glucocorticoids – fetal effect or maternal influence? J Endocrinol 2001; 170: 653–60.

47. Lesage J, Del-Favero F, Leonhardt M et al. Prenatal stress induces intrauterine growth restriction and programmes glucose intolerance and feeding behaviour disturbances in the aged rat. J Endocrinol 2004; 181: 291–6.

48. Consoli A, Nurjhan N. Contribution of gluconeogenesis to overall glucose output in diabetic and nondiabetic men. Ann Med 1990; 22: 191–5.

49. Valera A, Pujol A, Pelegrin M et al. Transgenic mice overexpressing phosphoenolpyruvate carboxykinase develop non-insulin-dependent diabetes. Proc Natl Acad Sci USA 1994; 91: 9151–4.

50. Xanthopoulos KG, Mirkovitch J. Gene regulation in rodent hepatocyte during development, differentiation and disease. Eur J Biochem 1993; 216: 353–60.

51. Cleasby ME, Kelly PA, Walker BR et al. Programming of rat muscle and fat metabolism by in utero overexposure to glucocorticoids. Endocrinology 2003; 144: 999–1007.

52. Whorwood CB, Firth KM, Budge H et al. Maternal undernutrition during early to midgestation programs tissue-specific alterations in the expression of the glucocorticoid receptor, 11 beta-hydroxysteroid dehydrogenase isoforms, and type 1 angiotensin II receptor in neonatal sheep. Endocrinology 2001; 142: 2854–64.

53. Drake AJ, Walker BR. The intergenerational effects of fetal programming: non-genomic mechanisms for the inheritance of low birth weight and cardiovascular risk. J Endocrinol 2004; 180: 1–16.

54. Garofano A, Czernichow P, Breant B. Beta-cell mass and proliferation following late fetal and early postnatal malnutrition in the rat. Diabetologia 1998; 41: 1114–20.

55. Blondeau B, Lesage J, Czernichow P et al. Glucocorticoids impair fetal beta-cell development in rats. Am J Physiol 2001; 281: E592–9.

56. Gesina E, Tronche F, Herrera P et al. Dissecting the role of glucocorticoids on pancreas development. Diabetes 2004; 53: 2322–9.

57. Dahlgren J, Nilsson C, Jennische E et al. Prenatal cytokine exposure results in obesity and gender-specific programming. Am J Physiol 2001; 281: E326–34.

58. Kitraki E, Kittas C, Stylianopoulou F. Glucocorticoid receptor gene expression during rat embryogenesis. An in situ hybridization study. Differentiation 1997; 62: 21–31.

59. Meaney MJ, Aitken DH, van Berkel C et al. Effect of neonatal handling on age-related impairments associated with the hippocampus. Science 1988; 239: 766–8.

60. Brown RW, Diaz R, Robson AC et al. The ontogeny of 11β-hydroxysteroid dehydrogenase type 2 and mineralocorticoid receptor gene expression reveal intricate control of glucocorticoid action in development. Endocrinology 1996; 137: 794–7.

61. Stewart PM, Murry BA, Mason JI. Type 2 11β-hydroxysteroid dehydrogenase in human fetal tissues. J Clin Endocrinol Metab 1994; 78: 1529–32.

62. Welberg LA, Seckl JR. Prenatal stress, glucocorticoids and the programming of the brain. J Neuroendocrinol 2001; 13: 113–28.

63. Weinstock M. Alterations induced by gestational stress in brain morphology and behaviour of the offspring. Prog Neurobiol 2001; 65: 427–51.

64. Huang WL, Harper CG, Evans SF et al. Repeated prenatal corticosteroid administration delays astrocyte and capillary tight junction maturation in fetal sheep. Int J Dev Neurosci 2001; 19: 487–93.

65. Uno H, Lohmiller L, Thieme C et al. Brain damage induced by prenatal exposure to dexamethasone in fetal rhesus macaques. I. hippocampus. Dev Brain Res 1990; 53: 157–67.

66. Sheline YI, Wang PW, Gado MH et al. Hippocampal atrophy in recurrent major depression. Proc Natl Acad Sci USA 1996; 93: 3908–13.

67. Uno H, Eisele S, Sakai A et al. Neurotoxicity of glucocorticoids in the primate brain. Horm Behav 1994; 28: 336–48.

68. Bertram C, Trowern AR, Copin N et al. The maternal diet during pregnancy programs altered expression of the glucocorticoid receptor and type 2 11beta-hydroxysteroid dehydrogenase: potential molecular mechanisms underlying the programming of hypertension in utero. Endocrinology 2001; 142: 2841–53.

69. McCormick CM, Smythe JW, Sharma S et al. Sex-specific effects of prenatal stress on hypothalamic-pituitary-adrenal responses to stress and brain glucocorticoid receptor density in adult rats. Dev Brain Res 1995; 84: 55–61.

70. Pepin MC, Pothier F, Barden N. Impaired glucocorticoid receptor function in transgenic mice expressing antisense RNA. Nature 1992; 355: 725–8.

71. McCormick J, Lyons V, Jacobson M et al. 5'-heterogeneity of glucocorticoid receptor mRNA is tissue-specific; differential regulation of variant promoters by early life events. Mol Endocrinol 2000; 14: 506–17.

72. Liu D, Diorio J, Tannenbaum B et al. Maternal care, hippocampal glucocorticoid receptors, and hypothalamic-pituitary-adrenal responses to stress. Science 1997; 277: 1659–62.

73. Meaney MJ, Diorio J, Francis D et al. Postnatal handling increases the expression of cAMP-inducible transcription factors in the rat hippocampus: the effects of thyroid hormones and serotonin. J Neurosci 2000; 20: 3926–35.

74. Weaver IC, Cervoni N, Champagne FA et al. Epigenetic programming by maternal behavior. Nature Neurosci 2004; 7: 847–54.

75. Thomassin H, Flavin M, Espinas M et al. Glucocorticoid-induced DNA demethylation and gene memory during development. EMBO J 2001; 20: 1974–83.

76. Dunn A, Berridge C. Physiological and behavioral responses to corticotropin-releasing factor administration – is CRF a mediator of anxiety or stress responses. Brain Res Rev 1990; 15: 71–100.

77. Feldman S, Weidenfeld J. The excitatory effects of the amygdala on hypothalamo-pituitary-adrenocortical responses are mediated by hypothalamic norepinephrine, serotonin, and CRF-41. Brain Res Bull 1998; 45: 389–93.

78. Tronche F, Kellendonk C, Kretz O et al. Disruption of the glucocorticoid receptor gene in the nervous system results in reduced anxiety. Nat Genet 1999; 23: 99–103.

79. Diaz R, Ögren SO, Blum M et al. Prenatal corticosterone increases spontaneous and d-amphetamine induced locomotor activity and brain dopamine metabolism in prepubertal male and female rats. Neuroscience 1995; 66: 467–73.

80. Koenig JI, Kirkpatrick B, Lee P. Glucocorticoid hormones and early brain development in schizophrenia. Neuropsychopharmacology 2002; 27: 309–18.

81. Bremne JD, Vermetten E. Stress and development: behavioral and biological consequences. Dev Psychopathol 2001; 13: 473–89.

82. Heim C, Nemeroff CB. The role of childhood trauma in the neurobiology of mood and anxiety disorders: preclinical and clinical studies. Biol Psychiatry 2001; 49: 1023–39.

83. Plotsky PM, Meaney MJ. Early, postnatal experience alters hypothalamic corticotropin-releasing factor (CRF) mRNA, median eminence CRF content and stress-induced release in adult rats. Mol Brain Res 1993; 18: 195–200.

84. Slotkin TA, Barnes GA, McCook EC et al. Programming of brainstem serotonin transporter development by prenatal glucocorticoids. Dev Brain Res 1996; 93: 155–61.

85. Rayburn W. Glucocorticoid therapy for rheumatic diseases: maternal, fetal, and breast feeding considerations. Am J Reprod Immunol 1992; 28: 138–40.

86. Kattner E, Metze B, Waiss E et al. Accelerated lung maturation following maternal steroid treatment in infants born before 30 weeks gestation. J Perinat Med 1992; 20: 449–57.

87. Speiser PW, New MI. Prenatal diagnosis and management of congenital adrenal hyperplasia. Clin Perinatol 1994; 21: 631–45.

88. Trautman PD, Meyer-Bahlburg HFL, Postelnek J et al. Effects of early prenatal dexamethasone on the cognitive and behavioral development of young children: results of a pilot study. Psychoneuroendocrinology 1995; 20: 439–49.

89. Lajic S, Wedell A, Bui TH et al. Long-term somatic follow-up of prenatally treated children with congenital adrenal hyperplasia. J Clin Endocrinol Metab 1998; 83: 3872–80.

90. Doyle LW, Ford GW, Davis NM et al. Antenatal corticosteroid therapy and blood pressure at 14 years of age in preterm children. Clin Sci 2000; 98: 137–42.

91. Clark PM, Hindmarsh PC, Shiell AW et al. Size at birth and adrenocortical function in childhood. Clin Endocrinol 1996; 45: 721–6.

92. Levitt NS, Lambert EV, Woods D et al. Impaired glucose tolerance and elevated blood pressure in low birth weight, nonobese, young South African adults: early programming of cortisol axis. J Clin Endocrinol Metab 2000; 85: 4611–18.

93. Reynolds RM, Walker BR, Syddall HE et al. Altered control of cortisol secretion in adult men with low birth weight and cardiovascular risk factors. J Clin Endocrinol Metab 2001; 86: 245–50.

5

Neuroendocrine programming of adult disease: current perspectives and future directions

Stephen G Matthews and David IW Phillips

INTRODUCTION

There is now an increasingly compelling body of data indicating that adverse events in early life are associated with an increased prevalence of several chronic diseases of adult life including diabetes, hypertension, and cardiovascular disease. A key question is the nature of the processes which link early events with later disease, as understanding of these processes may offer prospects for intervention. Studies in both humans and animals have clearly identified a link between an adverse fetal environment and modification of neuroendocrine function throughout life. The hypothalamo-pituitary-adrenal (HPA) axis and sympathetic nervous system have become the focus of many studies in this field. However, emerging evidence indicates that other endocrine axes including the hypothalamo-pituitary-thyroid and hypothalamo-pituitary-gonadal axes are also permanently influenced by the perinatal environment. Lifelong changes in the set point of these axes may affect the predisposition to many common adult diseases.

NEUROENDOCRINE PROGRAMMING AND PHENOTYPIC PLASTICITY

Several studies show that there is a graded increase in the prevalence of cardiovascular disease with smaller size at birth and that these trends are paralleled by increases in the occurrence of major cardiovascular risk factors including hypertension, glucose intolerance, and the metabolic syndrome. These associations are robust and appear to predispose affected individu-als to the influence of established adult risk factors for these diseases. A good example is the effect of obesity; men and women who were small at birth are particularly susceptible to the metabolic syndrome and vascular disease if they gain weight in later life.

These observations have led to the hypothesis that these common disorders might originate as a consequence of 'fetal programming' or phenotypic plasticity. It is suggested that adverse environmental factors during pregnancy affect the developing fetus permanently altering its morphology and/or physiology, which in turn predisposes it to disease. The programming hypothesis is strongly supported by animal experiments which show that adverse influences such as undernutrition during gestation result in the birth of offspring with raised blood pressure or poorer glucose tolerance. It is becoming clear that one way in which the early environment can have long-term effects is by resetting key hormonal systems that control growth and development. It is well established that these systems can be programmed during development. In particular, there is compelling evidence from animal studies that the HPA axis and autonomic nervous system (see Figure 5.1) are highly susceptible to programming during development and that this is one important factor leading to disease susceptibility. It is suggested that the biological 'purpose' of programming is to adapt the organism to its environment. These adaptive benefits are most evident in animals. If a pregnant animal is exposed to a hostile environment that requires increased vigilance (e.g. high level of predation), it is logical for an appropriate signal to be transmitted to the fetus, which leads to the development of appropriate hormonal responses (for example, an increased biological response to stress)

Hypothalamic-pituitary-adrenal and sympathoadrenal system function

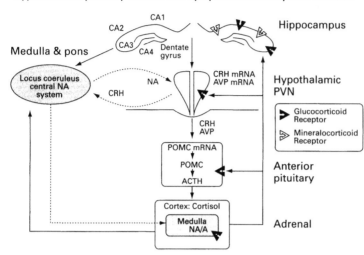

Figure 5.1 Schematic diagram illustrating the hypothalamo-pituitary-adrenocortical (HPA) axis and the major pathways of glucocorticoid feedback within the axis. The HPA axis and the sympathoadrenal system interact to regulate the biological response to stress. Broken line indicates activation, solid line indicates inhibition. A, adrenaline; ACTH, adrenocorticotrophin; AVP, vasopressin; CRH, corticotrophin-releasing hormone; NA, noradrenaline; POMC proopiomelanocortin.

and associated behaviors resulting in enhanced vigilance and, therefore an increased ability to survive after birth. Perhaps humans have also inherited a sophisticated mechanism with which to adapt our offspring to the environment in which they are to live. Thus in previous periods people born into poverty were likely to remain poor throughout their lives. However, this process may lead to disease if the environment changes and the adaptations in early life become inappropriate. This transformation may occur if, for example, people born in an adverse environment become relatively over-nourished and obese in adult life. An adaptation may also be inappropriate if it is set in motion by a compromised pregnancy (e.g. placental insufficiency, maternal stress or nutrient restriction), regardless of whether it is related to the environment into which the fetus will be born. The outcome may be a dysfunctional modification of physiological regulation.

EARLY INFLUENCES ON THE HPA AXIS

There is a large body of evidence that several different manipulations in early development can program HPA function in adult primates, cows, pigs, guinea pigs, sheep, and rats. Broadly, these can be split into prenatal and postnatal manipulations. Examples of prenatal manipulation are maternal stress,[1,2] exposure to synthetic glucocorticoids[3–5] and nutrient restriction.[6,7] Postnatal manipulations include neonatal handling,[8] modified maternal behaviour,[9] exposure to synthetic glucocorticoids,[10] and infection.[11] However, there is clearly an interaction between prenatal and postnatal environmental manipulations. For example,

maternal stress during pregnancy can modify the quality of maternal care, which in turn will also influence behavioral and neuroendocrine outcome in offspring.[12]

An important determinant of the effect of these interventions is the pace and timing of neuroendocrine development. The timing of maturation of the HPA axis relative to birth is highly species-specific, and is closely linked to developmental landmarks of brain maturation.[13] In animals that give birth to precocious young (e.g. sheep, guinea pigs, and primates) maximal brain growth and a significant proportion of neuroendocrine maturation take place *in utero*.[13,14] By contrast, in species that give birth to immature young (e.g. rats, rabbits, and mice), much brain and neuroendocrine development occurs in the postnatal period.[15] Therefore, manipulations of the fetal and neonatal environment will impact different stages of neuroendocrine development, depending on the species studied. Although prenatal and postnatal development are essentially continuous, analysis of outcome following postnatal manipulations must include consideration of alterations in maternal–infant interactions. The latter have major influences on development and subsequent function of the HPA axis.[9,16]

In late gestation there is a rapid increase in fetal HPA activity in most mammalian species.[14] It was originally thought that the primary role of this surge in fetal glucocorticoid levels was to mature the fetal lung.[17] However, it is now clear that the elevation in fetal HPA activity is critical for the development of several organ systems including the brain.[3,18] Very recent evidence from our laboratory indicates that there is a dramatic increase (800%) in the transcription factor NGFI-A in the fetal guinea pig hippocampus in the final days of gestation.[19] This rise would indicate a very profound increase in transcriptional activity at a time when fetal glucocorticoid levels are high. Indeed, maternal administration of synthetic glucocorticoid resulted in a further increase in fetal hippocampal NGFI-A, indicating possible glucocorticoid regulation.[19]

Prenatal stress during pregnancy permanently programs neuroendocrine and behavioral responses in offspring (for review see ref. 1). Most studies have been undertaken in the rat, with fewer studies in the primate, guinea pig, and cow. The prenatal stress paradigm typically involves induction of maternal stress from one to three times a day, either throughout or at selected time points during pregnancy. In the guinea pig, prenatal stress results in adult offspring with reduced basal and activated HPA function.[20] These observations are remarkable, because the pregnant guinea pigs were subjected only to a single 3-hour period of stress on day 60 of gestation (term ~70 days). An acute period (48 hours) of maternal nutrient restriction during the period of maximal fetal brain growth (day 50 of gestation) in the guinea pig, also resulted in young adult offspring with modified HPA function in adult life.[6] Restricting maternal nutrient intake (48 hours) resulted in a 50% decrease in fetal plasma glucose concentrations and intrauterine growth restriction (IUGR). This treatment significantly increased maternal cortisol secretion,[21] which in turn reached the fetus and modified fetal HPA activity.[21,22] As adults the male guinea pigs later exhibited reduced basal and stress-induced HPA activity, and the female offspring had both elevated basal and activated HPA function as young adults.[6] In a very recent study, we have demonstrated further that short focused periods of maternal psychological stress (induced by a high frequency strobe light), at critical times of fetal brain development, results in adult offspring that exhibit altered HPA regulation. Once again these effects were sexually dimorphic.[23]

In rats, maternal stress during pregnancy is generally associated with increased responsiveness of the HPA axis to stress in offspring; either an increased peak level and/or extended duration of the response. Basal plasma adrenocorticotrophin (ACTH) and corticosterone concentrations are elevated in female rats born to prenatally stressed dams,[24] and the higher hormone levels are associated with adrenal hypertrophy.[25] By contrast, some other studies have failed to find elevated basal HPA activity in offspring following prenatal stress.[26] This discrepancy between studies could result from variation in the time of day when follow-up measures were undertaken, because prenatal stress has been shown to induce a phase advance in the circadian corticosterone rhythm in offspring.[27] Few studies have carefully compared the impact of maternal stress during pregnancy on HPA activity in male and female offspring.[24,27–29] Basal ACTH, but not corticosterone, is elevated in female offspring born to prenatally stressed mothers and HPA responses to stress are also elevated.[24] In contrast, basal HPA activity is not different and responses to stress are reduced in male offspring.[24] Another study has described elevated basal and stress-stimulated corticosterone levels in adult female but not male offspring whose mothers were exposed to stress during pregnancy.[29] These studies indicate that the female HPA axis is more susceptible to prenatal stress-induced programming. It is also clear that there is considerable variability in HPA outcome in male offspring. This variation is not surprising given the wide spectrum of paradigms used to induce stress in pregnancy and the different methods used to activate HPA function in the offspring. With respect to the latter, different types of stress are known to activate distinct brain pathways.[30] The development of each of these pathways is likely to be affected in a unique fashion by prenatal stress.

The wide spectrum of experimental paradigms makes many of these studies difficult to compare. The timing of the insult is crucial, particularly if data are to be compared between species. Interpretation is also complicated because maternal stress during pregnancy alters other aspects of maternal physiology. Repeated restraint is associated with reduced maternal food intake and weight loss, which can independently modify HPA function and behavior in offspring.[6,7] Prenatal stress can also alter maternal behavior towards her offspring, and this change in care will have a major impact on offspring development.[9]

In primates, repeated maternal stress between 90 and 145 days of gestation (term ~170 days) results in offspring that exhibit abnormal social behavior and increased ACTH secretion in response to stress.[31] However, much less is known as to the extent to which these stress-induced hormone mechanisms operate in humans. One approach has been to investigate the relationship between size at birth or other indices of fetal growth (a crude measure of early adversity) and neuroendocrine function during childhood or later life. These studies suggest that size at birth is associated with alterations in both autonomic and HPA function. Fetuses with IUGR have higher pulse rates and have higher catecholamine concentrations in cord blood. In one study, small-for-gestational age (SGA) newborns had increased heart rate and reduced heart rate variability when compared with controls during sleep.[32] In a study of 266 men and women aged 50, resting pulse rate was inversely related to birth weight.[33] This finding has been confirmed in 2648 African school children.[34] A number of studies have now shown that low birth weight babies have raised cortisol concentrations in umbilical cord blood and raised urinary cortisol excretion in childhood.[35] That these effects may persist into later life has been shown by a study of men, aged 65, born in Hertfordshire, UK, where carefully timed adult cortisol concentrations were found to be inversely related to birth weight, falling from 408 nmol/l in those who weighed 5.5 lb or less to 309 nmol/l among those who weighed 9.5 lb or more. These trends were paralleled by the concentrations of 'free cortisol' estimated by the ratio of cortisol to corticosteroid binding globulin and were independent of the current levels of obesity or central obesity.[36] Although a single fasting cortisol measurement has substantial limitations, this observation suggested the possibility of an important link between birth size and adrenocortical hormone activity in adult life. A similar finding was also reported in a sample of 165 men and women born in Adelaide, South Australia, from 1975 to 1976, 199 men and women born in Preston, UK, from 1935 to 1943 and 306 women born in East Hertfordshire, UK, from 1923 to 1930. Although the fasting blood samples for the measurement of cortisol were less accurately timed than in the study of Hertfordshire men, low birth weight was associated with raised fasting plasma cortisol concentrations in all three populations.[37] A combined analysis, which allowed for differences in the gender composition, age, and body mass index between the populations showed that cortisol concentrations fell by 23.9 nmol/l per kg increase in birth weight (95% CI, 9.6 to 38.2, $p < 0.001$). More detailed studies of HPA function have been carried out in a subset of 205 men from the original Hertfordshire study. They underwent a low dose (1 μg) $ACTH_{1-24}$ stimulation test. A 24-hour urine sample was collected for analysis of cortisol metabolites by gas chromatography/electron impact mass spectrometry. Men with lower birth weight had enhanced responses of plasma cortisol to the administered ACTH and increased total urinary cortisol metabolite excretion (after adjustment for confounding effects of increased obesity and lean body mass in high birth weight men).[38] Similar results have been obtained in a study in South Africa, and have also been recently replicated in women in Hertfordshire.[39] More recent research, however, has indicated that secretion of cortisol in the unstressed state is not associated with birth weight. In a hospital-based study of 83 healthy elderly men and women, 24-hour serum cortisol profiles (sampled every 20 minutes) showed no relation to birth weight.[40] These findings suggest that the previously observed relation-

ship between birth weight and morning cortisol concentrations represents a stress response due to the combination of fasting and the novel clinic setting in which the blood samples were obtained. This is supported by studies of Swedish army recruits of low birth weight who had increased stress susceptibility to a psychological assessment, and recent evidence from a small-scale study has suggested that low birth weight is associated with increased responses to a standard psychological stressor in young adults.[41,42]

Evidence is accumulating that neuroendocrine disturbance involving the HPA axis may play an important part in the causation of the metabolic syndrome and contribute to development of cardiovascular disease. As patients with Cushing's syndrome develop a severe form of the metabolic syndrome with hypertension, insulin resistance, glucose intolerance, dyslipidemia, and central obesity, it is an attractive idea that less profound disturbances of the HPA might underlie the metabolic syndrome. Case-control and cross-sectional studies of people without pituitary or adrenal disease show that elevated plasma cortisol concentrations in morning samples are associated with high blood pressure, glucose intolerance, insulin resistance, and hyperlipidemia.

MECHANISMS OF HPA PROGRAMMING

The route by which maternal stress programs HPA activity and behavior in offspring is not entirely clear. Stress will lead to several cardiovascular and endocrine changes in the mother, including increases in the secretion of ACTH, β-endorphin, glucocorticoids, and catecholamines. The placenta forms a structural and biochemical barrier to many of these maternal hormones, although several will enter the fetus. Alternatively, there might be indirect effects on the fetus via modification of placental function. Catecholamines can constrict placental blood vessels and cause fetal hypoxia, which will activate the fetal HPA axis.[14]

Glucocorticoids have become a primary candidate for programming the fetal HPA axis during maternal stress. They are essential for normal brain development, exerting a wide spectrum of organizational effects via both GR and MR. However, sustained elevation in, or removal of, GC during development can permanently modify brain structure and function.[3] In rats, maternal and fetal plasma corticosterone are significantly elevated after maternal stress.[27] In the guinea pig, cortisol concentrations in the maternal plasma are 10-fold those in the fetus and maternal stress results in up-regulation of cortisol concentrations in both mother and fetus.[20,43] Interestingly, it has been shown that greater glucocorticoid transfer occurs across the placenta of female compared with male fetuses.[44] This difference could account, in part, for the increased effects of maternal stress in female offspring.

Under normal circumstances, access of maternal endogenous glucocorticoids to the fetus is low. This restriction is due to the expression of 11β-hydroxysteroid dehydrogenase (11β-HSD) in the placenta.[45] 11β-HSD interconverts cortisol and corticosterone to inactive products (cortisone, 11-dehydrocorticosterone). There are two isoforms, 11β-HSD type 1, which is bidirectional, and type 2, which is unidirectional (cortisol to cortisone). The efficiency of placental 11β-HSD2 varies across species: however, it is generally accepted that placental 11β-HSD2 is of primary importance in excluding maternal glucocorticoid from the fetus. The impact of maternal stress on placental 11β-HSD2 expression is not known. However, placental 11β-HSD2 activity is reduced in human intrauterine growth-restricted (IUGR) pregnancies.[46] In animal studies, it has been shown that feeding of a low protein diet to animals throughout pregnancy results in a reduction in the levels of placental 11β-HSD.[47]

Several approaches have been taken to establish the role of glucocorticoid in programming of HPA function. These have involved maternal adrenalectomy and treatment with endogenous or synthetic glucocorticoid or ACTH. Treatment of pregnant rats with ACTH results in offspring with elevated basal corticosterone, but reduced adrenocortical responses to stress.[48] As with prenatal stress, effects were larger in female than in male offspring. In another experiment, pregnant rats were adrenalectomized and basal levels of corticosterone replaced. In this group, maternal stress was without effect on HPA function in adult offspring,[49] indicating that maternal glucocorticoid, or a factor stimulated by glucocorticoid, passes to the fetus to mediate prenatal stress-induced changes in HPA function. Further support for the 'glucocorticoid driver hypothesis' has been provided by an elegant series of studies in which 11β-HSD activity has been modified. Pharmacological blockade of 11β-HSD during pregnancy, and resulting increased transfer of maternal glucocorticoid to the fetus, leads to offspring that exhibit elevated basal and stress-stimulated HPA activity.[50]

The impact of fetal glucocorticoid exposure (either synthetic or endogenously produced) is dependent on the expression of corticosteroid receptors in the fetal brain at the time of exposure. There are two forms of corticosteroid receptors in the brain: mineralocorticoid receptors (MR) and glucocorticoid receptors (GR). The expression of MR is confined primarily to limbic structures, whereas the GR is more widely distributed with highest levels in the limbic system, the hypothalamic paraventricular nucleus (PVN) and the cerebral cortex. In the brain, the affinity of MR is 10-fold higher ($K_d = 0.5$ nM) than the affinity of GR for cortisol ($K_d = 5.0$ nM).[51,52] As the hippocampus does not express high levels of 11β-HSD2, the hippocampal MR is activated by low levels of cortisol in the basal state and regulates the diurnal, basal rhythms of HPA activity.[51] However, during periods of elevated plasma glucocorticoid (i.e. during stress), there is increased occupation of the GR.

In the fetal guinea pig, GR and MR mRNA and protein are present in the cortex and all regions of the hippocampus and dentate gyrus by gestational day 40 (term ~70 days). Between day 40 and 50, there is a dramatic increase in GR, but a decrease in MR expression, indicating differential developmental regulation of the two receptors in the hippocampus. Hippocampal GR mRNA and protein levels increase to a peak near term, but there is little further change in MR, which remains low.[53] The increase in hippocampal GR expression is counterintuitive as there appears to be a reduction in glucocorticoid feedback sensitivity in the late gestation fetus, allowing sustained increases in adrenocortical activity. However, we have recently demonstrated that other aspects of steroid receptor signaling may be altered in late gestation. There is a significant decrease in the hippocampal expression of SRC-1 mRNA and protein over the second half of gestation in the fetal guinea pig.[54] Steroid receptor coactivators (SRCs) enhance transcriptional activity of the nuclear receptor through histone acetyltransferase activity and they facilitate other basal transcriptional machinery.[55] Decreasing SRC-1 levels in late gestation may contribute to increased fetal HPA activity at this time by decreasing glucocorticoid signaling in the hippocampus even in the presence of increasing GR levels.

In contrast to the situation in the hippocampus, GR mRNA levels in the hypothalamic PVN are higher at day 40 than at any other stage of fetal or postnatal life in the guinea pig. There is a dramatic decrease (50%) in GR mRNA near term.[53] A similar reduction in GR mRNA in the PVN has been noted in the fetal sheep near term.[56] Though GR immunoreactivity has been identified in the human embryo,[57,58] detailed regional and developmental profiling has not been undertaken.

In species that give birth to immature young the developmental pattern of corticosteroid receptors in the brain is quite different. GR and MR in the rat brain are low through gestation, but increase rapidly after birth, which is consistent with the postnatal nature of brain and HPA development in these species.

However, there is a distinct developmental pattern for GR and MR in the fetal rat brain.[59,60] GR mRNA is present in the hippocampus, hypothalamus, and pituitary by gestational day 13 (term ~21 days), and levels increase around term. In contrast, MR is not present in the hippocampus until gestational day 16–17.[59,61] In summary, development of GR and MR expression is highly species-specific, and differences in receptor number at the time of the experimental manipulation likely account, in part, for the inconsistent outcomes observed following prenatal treatment regimes across studies.

PRENATAL SYNTHETIC GLUCOCORTICOID EXPOSURE AND PROGRAMMING OF HPA FUNCTION

Preterm delivery occurs in approximately 7% of all births in North America and is responsible for about 75% of neonatal deaths.[62] Neonatal morbidity in surviving preterm infants is high and complications such as respiratory distress syndrome, intraventricular hemorrhage, and necrotizing enterocolitis are common. Prenatal synthetic glucocorticoid therapy reduces the frequency of these complications. In 1994 the National Institute of Health recommended treatment of all women at risk of preterm delivery, between 24 and 34 weeks of gestation, with synthetic glucocorticoid.[62] The effectiveness of synthetic glucocorticoid treatment in promoting neonatal lung function had led to many centers prescribing multiple courses of synthetic glucocorticoid in women who did not deliver early, but who remained at risk of preterm labour. By the late 1990s, emerging evidence, particularly from animal studies, suggested that there may be a long-term consequence of multiple course synthetic glucocorticoid exposure on the developing brain as well as on metabolic function.[63–65] Indeed, following an NIH Consensus Update Conference (2000), it was recommended that a single course of synthetic glucocorticoid should be administered to all women presenting in preterm labour, and that the multiple course treatment should be confined to ongoing clinical trials.[66]

Unlike the situation for endogenous glucocorticoids, 11β-HSD2 has a low affinity for synthetic glucocorticoids (dexamethasone and betamethasone), and so they pass rapidly from mother to fetus. Maternal treatment with synthetic glucocorticoid has provided a useful tool with which to investigate the impact of glucocorticoids on the development and subsequent function of the HPA axis in offspring. This is also an important line of clinical investigation, given the routine use of synthetic glucocorticoids to treat women. However, unlike endogenous glucocorticoids, synthetic glucocorticoids bind predominantly to the GR, and the effects on development following prenatal synthetic glucocorticoid administration are likely mediated at the level of this receptor alone. Therefore, care must be applied when extrapolating between pharmacological and natural hormone models.

Treatment of pregnant guinea pigs with three courses of synthetic glucocorticoid in late gestation, at doses pharmacologically equivalent to those used in pregnant women, results in decreased HPA activity in adult male offspring.[4] This decrease is associated with reduced CRH mRNA in the PVN and increased hippocampal MR mRNA; indicating increased central glucocorticoid-negative feedback sensitivity. Fetal exposure to synthetic glucocorticoid also reduces male brain weight and increases plasma testosterone concentrations in early adult life.[4] Since testosterone is known to inhibit HPA activity,[67] this secondary pathway provides an additional route of adrenocortical suppression in adult male offspring exposed to synthetic glucocorticoid in utero. A more recent study from our laboratory has shown that the effects of prenatal synthetic glucocorticoid exposure appear to change as a function of age. When male guinea pig offspring from mothers treated in a similar fashion to that described above[4] were assessed at 150 days rather than in young adulthood (~80 days), the effects on HPA function and feedback regulation were quite different. Basal plasma cortisol concentrations were not different between prenatal treatment groups and plasma testosterone concentrations were normalized. Interestingly, hippocampal MR mRNA remained elevated in animals that had been exposed to synthetic glucocorticoid in utero. Together, these observations would suggest that the increased testosterone was a major factor in the inhibition of HPA activity in the males prenatally exposed to dexamethasone.[5] Also, the older animals became hypertensive, exhibiting increased mean arterial pressure. Hippocampal MR has been implicated in cardiovascular regulation, and we suggested that the increased MR expression observed in these animals may be, in part, responsible for the increase in blood pressure. Further studies are required to explore this possibility. The fact that the effects of prenatal synthetic glucocorticoid change as a function of age indicates the importance of studying outcome at several different times during the life course.

In young adult female offspring, fetal exposure to synthetic glucocorticoid results in increased HPA activity in the follicular/early luteal phase of the estrous cycle. The increased cortisol is associated with reduced hippocampal MR mRNA, and decreased GR mRNA in the PVN and pituitary.[4] These changes are suggestive of reduced central glucocorticoid-negative feedback in these animals. Interestingly, the same animals exhibit reduced HPA activity in the late luteal phase, resembling the HPA phenotype of young adult males that had been exposed to synthetic glucocorticoid *in utero*. This cyclical variation provides some of the first evidence that glucocorticoid-induced programming of HPA function is dynamic (depending on stage of the estrous cycle), and sex-specific.[4]

The acute effects of repeated synthetic glucocorticoid exposure on MR and GR expression in the fetal brain of the guinea pig have recently been investigated. Maternal treatment results in dose-dependent inhibition of plasma cortisol levels in mother and fetus.[68] Since cortisol represents the primary MR ligand in the fetal brain, a unique situation arises, in which the GR is fully activated by synthetic glucocorticoid, and the MR is largely unoccupied. Interestingly, repeated maternal synthetic glucocorticoid treatment fails to inhibit fetal hippocampal GR mRNA. This effect is counterintuitive, because glucocorticoids act to down-regulate central GR levels in the adult. More importantly it indicates that the fetus has no way of protecting itself from excess glucocorticoid exposure.

In the rat, daily treatment with synthetic glucocorticoid (0.1 mg kg^{-1}) in the final week or throughout gestation results in elevated basal plasma corticosterone levels in adult male offspring.[65,69] This was associated with increased blood pressure in adulthood. In another study, maternal synthetic glucocorticoid treatment (0.05 mg kg^{-1}) on gestational day 17, 18, and 19, resulted in adult male offspring that mount a greater adrenocortical response to stress.[70] By contrast, treatment on gestational day 17 and 19 does not alter basal HPA function in prepubertal offspring. However, there is a difference in the arginine vasopressin (AVP):CRH ratio in the hypothalamic median eminence of these young rats,[71] suggesting that programmed changes in HPA function might develop as animals mature postnatally.

The mechanisms that underlie programming of adult HPA function are dependent on dose and timing of exposure.[69] Adult male offspring from mothers exposed to synthetic glucocorticoid in the last week of gestation exhibit reduced hippocampal GR and MR expression and increased CRH mRNA in the PVN, but no change in GR expression in the PVN. This hormone-receptor profile would indicate reduced hippocampal glucocorticoid-feedback sensitivity resulting in an elevation of HPA activity. By contrast, in offspring born to mothers treated daily with synthetic glucocorticoid throughout pregnancy, and in which HPA activity is also increased, there are no

changes in hippocampal corticosteroid receptors, but increases in MR and GR mRNA in the basolateral nucleus of the amygdala are observed. The amygdala primarily exerts a stimulatory effect on CRH neurons in the PVN,[72] and so these data would suggest that long-term fetal exposure to synthetic glucocorticoid increases forward drive to the HPA axis.[69] While the majority of rat studies have been undertaken in male offspring a recent study has indicated that, like the guinea pig,[4] there are gender differences in the endocrine, cardiovascular, and metabolic outcomes associated with prenatal exposure to synthetic glucocorticoids.[60] In this detailed study, synthetic glucocorticoid administered over the last week of gestation produced adult male, but not female offspring that exhibited elevated basal pituitary-adrenal activity. Interestingly, the effect in the male was confined to the morning nadir and was not present during the afternoon peak of HPA activity.[60]

A recent report of a study in sheep indicates that there are long-term effects of prenatal synthetic glucocorticoid exposure in late gestation on HPA activity after birth in this species, and that these effects change as a function of postnatal age.[73] This study also demonstrates that HPA outcome in offspring is different depending on the route of synthetic glucocorticoid administration (maternal or fetal), and that modification of adrenocortical sensitivity is in part responsible for the altered HPA function.[73] Another study has shown that synthetic glucocorticoid exposure at 27 days of gestation, which results in increased blood pressure in adult sheep, appears to have no long-term effect on HPA function.[74] A single study has been undertaken to establish the long-term effects of fetal exposure to synthetic glucocorticoid on HPA function in the primate.[75] Basal and stress-stimulated cortisol levels were elevated in the offspring (10 months of age) born to glucocorticoid-treated mothers.[75] To date, no studies have assessed HPA function in children who were exposed to antenatal glucocorticoid during fetal life, though a number are currently underway.

Together, these studies indicate that within a single species, timing of synthetic glucocorticoid treatment, gender, and the stage of life at which offspring are tested all influence the outcome. The gender differences are critical and this is currently an area of intensive investigation. Previous studies have shown that there are subtle differences in the development of the fetal HPA axis as well as in the response to prenatal glucocorticoid therapy in the guinea pig.[53,68] In addition, there may be differences in the levels of synthetic glucocorticoid that reach male and female fetuses. While it has become generally accepted that synthetic glucocorticoids pass across the placenta to enter the fetus, there is emerging evidence that the placenta can selectively exclude a portion of the synthetic glucocorticoids from passing to the fetus.[76] This selective blockade results from the expression of the multidrug-resistance p-glycoprotein (MDR-PgP). We have shown that the MDR gene and associated PgP are expressed at high levels in the mouse and human placenta, and that there are temporal and spatial changes in expression through pregnancy.[77,78] In late gestation, there is a reduction in MDR-PgP in both the human and mouse placenta. This potentially decreases fetal protection to many exogenous compounds including synthetic glucocorticoids. Given that the placenta is primarily of fetal origin, it also raises the possibility that gender differences in the expression of the placental MDR gene may exist.

While there appear to be a number of inconsistencies between the outcomes of prenatal exposure to synthetic glucocorticoid and maternal stress a number of similarities are emerging. Female fetuses tend to be more susceptible to the insult, and as adults, offspring tend to exhibit elevated HPA activity. In contrast, males appear less sensitive and offspring often exhibit reduced HPA activity. It is also apparent that other endocrine interactions are involved, particularly the hypothalamo-pituitary-gonadal axis, and this is likely responsible for the sex differences in outcome as well as differences in outcome across the reproductive cycle in female offspring. While substantial progress has been made, further work is required to understand the mechanisms involved in programming HPA function.

What is clear is that programming of HPA function involves modification of glucocorticoid-negative feedback at the level of the limbic system, hypothalamus, and pituitary, but that the effect at each of these sites is dependent on the duration and timing of the prenatal manipulation. An elegant series of studies in the rat has provided further insights on the mechanisms involved in HPA programming. Neonatal handling results in elevated hippocampal GR, increased glucocorticoid-negative feedback and a reduction in HPA activity. It has been established that an elevation in hippocampal serotonin is responsible for this up-regulation of hippocampal GR.[8] Serotonin can directly up-regulate GR mRNA and GR ligand-binding in primary cultures of embryonic hippocampal cells.[8,79] This effect is mediated via serotonin ($5HT_7$) receptors and appears to be permanent, involving altered methylation of the GR promoter.[9] Neonatal handling also increases thyroid activity in the neonate, and thyroid hormone increases serotonin turnover in the hippocampus. As a result, it has been suggested that the ascending serotonin neurons are stimulated by thyroid hormones to increase hippocampal serotonin

and thence GR expression.[8] Interestingly, exposure of the fetal guinea pig to synthetic glucocorticoid increases fetal thyroid hormone and up-regulates GR mRNA.[80] Further, prenatal synthetic glucocorticoid exposure advances maturation of the serotonin transporter system in the developing rat brain.[81] Together, these data indicate that the ascending serotonergic system may be involved in glucocorticoid-induced HPA programming during prenatal life.

IMPLICATIONS AND FUTURE DIRECTIONS

Despite the wealth of animal data, neuroendocrine programming in humans has been largely neglected. The mechanisms involved are clearly complex and hard to disentangle. For example, the effects of stressful influences on the mother are complex and are likely to be conditioned by other factors such as the maternal social environment, the fetal and maternal genetic backgrounds, the maternal early environment, and transgenerational effects (see Figure 5.2). However, neuroendocrine programming may be a common pathway by which a wide variety of adverse external influences has long-term effects on the fetus and through its subsequent life course. These influences include psychosocial stress, ergonomic challenges (for example, prolonged standing or carrying heavy loads), maternal diet (macro- and micronutrient intakes, dietary balance), the physical environment (heat or cold), exposure to environmental toxins or drugs, and maternal illness.

It is likely that maternal stressors affect the fetus by the transplacental passage of maternal hormones such as cortisol. The human fetal HPA axis is well developed and functional in late gestation and able to respond to external factors, especially hypoxia and nutrient restriction. Therefore, external factors that reduce uterine blood flow would restrict fetal nutrient or oxygen supply and may initiate a fetal stress response. Examples of these are likely to be ergonomic factors such as prolonged standing or carrying heavy loads or the release of maternal stress hormones that in turn reduce uterine vascular perfusion. In the human context, maternal stress may also affect the fetus by influencing maternal behaviors. These may include medication taken by pregnant women, smoking, and consumption of alcohol. Finally, it is also possible that external stressors, such as trauma and noise, which may be perceived by the fetus, could activate fetal stress responses. We have recently obtained direct evidence that maternal nutrition can influence the offspring's neuroendocrine function. A follow-up of men and women in Motherwell, UK whose mothers had

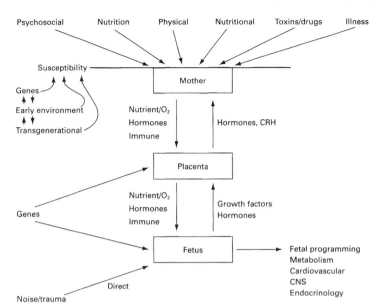

Figure 5.2 A wide variety of adverse environmental influences may impact on the mother, which in turn will affect the fetus, either by impairing fetal nutrient or oxygen delivery or by altering hormonal signaling between mother and baby. These effects cause neuroendocrine alterations in the fetus, which then may lead to a predisposition to metabolic and cardiovascular disease. Also shown is how the maternal response may be shaped by other factors, including the mother's genetic makeup, her own early environment experiences and even transgenerational factors.

been advised to eat a diet high in animal protein and low in carbohydrates during pregnancy, showed that this unusual diet was associated with higher fasting plasma cortisol levels in the adult offspring.[82]

The effects of stressors in the neonatal period and infancy, and the extent to which the neonate or infant responds to stressors, remain poorly understood. Yet, the large body of data from animal studies in a variety of species from rodent to nonhuman primates suggests that external stressors at this vulnerable developmental stage have the potential for long-term, important effects. Neonatal vulnerability to stress is likely to be enhanced by factors such as prematurity, low birth weight, multiple birth, maternal parity, and mode of delivery. These factors would be expected to increase the susceptibility to many stressors, including cold, trauma, surgery, antigenic challenge, illness, and difficulties in establishing feeding. It is important that these early influences are understood more completely, which remains a challenge for both basic and clinical research.

CONCLUSIONS

1. Adversity in the fetal environment can modify neuroendocrine function throughout later life.
2. One important consequence of these changes may be an increase in stress susceptibility in the offspring.
3. This increased reactivity may be an important mechanism accounting for the links between early life events and metabolic, cardiovascular, and neurologic disease.

REFERENCES

1. Weinstock M. Alterations induced by gestational stress in brain morphology and behaviour of the offspring. Prog Neurobiol 2001; 65: 427–51.
2. Welberg LA, Seckl JR. Prenatal stress, glucocorticoids and the programming of the brain. J Neuroendocrinol 2001; 13: 113–28.
3. Matthews SG. Antenatal glucocorticoids and programming of the developing CNS. Pediatr Res 2000; 47: 291–300.
4. Liu L, Li A, Matthews SG. Maternal glucocorticoid treatment programs HPA regulation in adult offspring: sex-specific effects. Am J Physiol Endocrinol Metab 2001; 280: E729–E739.
5. Banjanin S, Kapoor A, Matthews S. Prenatal glucocorticoid exposure alters hypothalamic-pituitary-adrenal function and blood pressure in mature male guinea pigs. J Physiol 2004; 558: 305–18.
6. Lingas R, Matthews SG. A short period of maternal nutrient restriction in late gestation modifies pituitary-adrenal function in adult guinea pig offspring. Neuroendocrinology 2001; 73: 302–11.
7. Lesage J, Dufourny L, Laborie C et al. Perinatal malnutrition programs sympathoadrenal and hypothalamic-pituitary-adrenal axis responsiveness to restraint stress in adult male rats. J Neuroendocrinol 2002;14: 135–43.
8. Meaney MJ, Diorio J, Francis D et al. Postnatal handling increases the expression of cAMP-inducible transcription factors in the rat hippocampus: the effects of thyroid hormones and serotonin. J Neurosci 2000; 20: 3926–35.
9. Weaver IC, Cervoni N, Champagne FA et al. Epigenetic programming by maternal behavior. Nat Neurosci 2004; 7: 847–54.
10. Kamphuis PJ, Gardoni F, Kamal A et al. Long-lasting effects of neonatal dexamethasone treatment on spatial learning and hippocampal synaptic plasticity: involvement of the NMDA receptor complex. FASEB J 2003; 17: 911–3.
11. Nilsson C, Jennische E, Ho HP et al. Postnatal endotoxin exposure results in increased insulin sensitivity and altered activity of neuroendocrine axes in adult female rats. Eur J Endocrinol 2002; 146: 251–60.

12. Smith JW, Seckl JR, Evans AT, Costall B, Smythe JW. Gestational stress induces post-partum depression-like behaviour and alters maternal care in rats. Psychoneuroendocrinology 2004; 29: 227–44.

13. Dobbing J, Sands J. Comparative aspects of the brain growth spurt. Early Hum Dev 1979; 3: 79–83.

14. Challis JRG, Matthews SG, Gibb W, Lye SJ. Endocrine and paracrine regulation of birth at term and preterm. Endocr Rev 2000; 21: 514–50.

15. Darlington RB, Dunlop SA, Finlay BL. Neural development in metatherian and eutherian mammals: variation and constraint. J Comp Neurol 1999; 411: 359–68.

16. Gunnar MR, Donzella B. Social regulation of the cortisol levels in early human development. Psychoneuroendocrinology 2002; 27: 199–220.

17. Liggins GC, Howie RN. A controlled trial of antepartum glucocorticoid treatment for the prevention of the respiratory distress syndrome in premature infants. Pediatrics 1972; 50: 515–23.

18. Liggins GC. The role of cortisol in preparing the fetus for birth. Reprod Fertil Dev 1994; 6: 141–50.

19. Andrews MH, Kostaki A, Setiawan E et al. Developmental regulation of the 5-HT7 serotonin receptor and transcription factor NGFI-A in the fetal guinea-pig limbic system: influence of GCs. J Physiol 2004; 555: 659–70.

20. Cadet R, Pradier P, Dalle M, Delost P. Effects of prenatal maternal stress on the pituitary adrenocortical reactivity in guinea-pig pups. J Dev Physiol 1986; 8: 467–75.

21. Lingas R, Dean F, Matthews SG. Maternal nutrient restriction (48 hours) modifies brain corticosteroid receptor expression and endocrine function in the fetal guinea pig. Brain Res 1999; 846: 236–42.

22. Go KS, Lingas R, Wheeler MB, Irwin DM, Matthews SG. Decreased CRH mRNA expression in the fetal guinea pig hypothalamus following maternal nutrient restriction. Brain Res 2001; 896: 179–82.

23. Kapoor A, Matthews SG. Short periods of focussed moderate maternal stress modifies growth, pituitary-adrenal activity and behaviour in male guinea pig offspring. Society for Neuroscience, San Diego, October 2004.

24. McCormick CM, Smythe JW, Sharma S, Meaney MJ. Sex-specific effects of prenatal stress on hypothalamic-pituitary-adrenal responses to stress and brain glucocorticoid receptor density in adult rats. Dev Brain Res 1995; 84: 55–61.

25. Ward HE, Johnson EA, Salm AK, Birkle DL. Effects of prenatal stress on defensive withdrawal behavior and corticotropin releasing factor systems in rat brain. Physiol Behav 2000; 70: 359–66.

26. Kay G, Tarcic N, Poltyrev T, Weinstock M. Prenatal stress depresses immune function in rats. Physiol Behav 1998; 63: 397–402.

27. Koehl M, Darnaudéry M, Dulluc J et al. Prenatal stress alters circadian activity of hypothalamo-pituitary-adrenal axis and hippocampal corticosteroid receptors in adult rats of both gender. J Neurobiol 1999; 40: 302–15.

28. Weinstock M, Matlina E, Maor GI, Rosen H, McEwen BS. Prenatal stress selectively alters the reactivity of the hypothalamic-pituitary adrenal system in the female rat. Brain Res 1992; 595: 195–200.

29. Szuran TF, Pliska V, Pokorny J, Welzl H. Prenatal stress in rats: effects on plasma corticosterone, hippocampal glucocorticoid receptors, and maze performance. Physiol Behav 2000; 71: 353–62.

30. Pacak K, Palkovits M. Stressor specificity of central neuroendocrine responses: implications for stress-related disorders. Endocr Rev 2001; 22: 502–48.

31. Schneider ML, Moore CF, Kraemer GW, Roberts AD, DeJesus OT. The impact of prenatal stress, fetal alcohol exposure, or both on development: perspectives from a primate model. Psychoneuroendocrinology 2002; 27: 285–98.

32. Spassov L, Curzi-Dascalova L, Clairambault J et al. Heart rate and heart rate variability during sleep in small-for-gestational age newborns. Pediatr Res 1994; 35 (4 Pt 1): 500–5.

33. Phillips DI, Barker DJ. Association between low birthweight and high resting pulse in adult life: is the sympathetic nervous system involved in programming the insulin resistance syndrome? Diabetic Med 1997; 14: 673–7.

34. Longo-Mbenza B, Ngiyulu R, Bayekula M, et al. Low birth weight and risk of hypertension in African school children. J Cardiovasc Risk 1999; 6: 311–14.

35. Fujimori O. A double protein A-gold-silver staining method for tissue antigens in lightmicroscopy. Histochem J 1992; 24: 61–6.

36. Phillips DI, Barker DJ, Fall CH et al. Elevated plasma cortisol concentrations: a link between low birthweight and the insulin resistance syndrome. J Clin Endocrinol Metab 1998; 83: 757–60.

37. Phillips DI, Walker BR, Reynolds RM et al. Low birth weight predicts elevated plasma cortisol concentrations in adults from 3 populations. Hypertension 2000; 35: 1301–6.

38. Reynolds RM, Walker BR, Syddall HE et al. Altered control of cortisol secretion in adult men with low birth weight and cardiovascular risk factors. J Clin Endocrinol Metab 2001; 86: 245–50.

39. Levitt NS, Lambert EV, Woods D et al. Impaired glucose tolerance and elevated blood pressure in low birth weight, nonobese, young South African adults: early programming of cortisol axis. J Clin Endocrinol Metab 2000; 85: 4611–18.

40. Fall CH, Dennison E, Cooper C et al. Does birth weight predict adult serum cortisol concentrations? Twenty-four-hour profiles in the United Kingdom 1920–1930 Hertfordshire Birth Cohort. J Clin Endocrinol Metab 2002; 87: 2001–7.

41. Nilsson PM, Nyberg P, Ostergren PO. Increased susceptibility to stress at a psychological assessment of stress tolerance is associated with impaired fetal growth. Int J Epidemiol 2001; 30: 75–80.

42. Ward AM, Moore V, Steptoe A et al. Size at birth and cardiovascular responses to psychological stressors: evidence for fetal programming in women. J Hypertens 2004; 22: 2295–301.

43. Dauprat P, Monin G, Dalle M, Delost P. The effects of psychosomatic stress at the end of pregnancy on maternal and fetal plasma cortisol levels and liver glycogen in guinea-pigs. Reprod Nutr Dev 1984; 24: 45–51.

44. Montano MM, Wang M-H, Vom Saal FS. Sex differences in plasma corticosterone in mouse fetuses are mediated by differential placental transport from the mother and eliminated by maternal adrenalectomy or stress. J Reprod Fertil 1993; 99: 283–90.

45. Burton PJ, Waddell BJ. Dual function of 11β-hydroxysteroid dehydrogenase in placenta: modulating placental glucocorticoid passage and local steroid action. Biol Reprod 1999; 60: 234–40.

46. McTernan CL, Draper N, Nicholson H et al. Reduced placental 11beta-hydroxysteroid dehydrogenase type 2 mRNA levels in human pregnancies complicated by intrauterine growth restriction: an analysis of possible mechanisms. J Clin Endocrinol Metab 2001; 86: 4979–83.

47. Langley-Evans SC, Phillips GJ, Benediktsson R et al. Protein intake in pregnancy, placental glucocorticoid metabolism

and the programming of hypertension in the rat. Placenta 1996; 17: 169–72.

48. Fameli M, Kitraki E, Stylianopoulou F. Effects of hyperactivity of the maternal hypothalamic-pituitary-adrenal (HPA) axis during pregnancy on the development of the HPA axis and brain monoamines of the offspring. Int J Dev Neurosci 1994; 12: 651–9.

49. Barbazanges A, Piazza PV, Le Moal M, Maccari S. Maternal glucocorticoid secretion mediates long-term effects of prenatal stress. J Neurosci 1996; 16: 3943–9.

50. Seckl JR, Cleasby M, Nyirenda MJ. Glucocorticoids, 11β-hydroxysteroid dehydrogenase, and fetal programming. Kidney Int 2000; 57: 1412–17.

51. De Kloet ER, Vreugdenhil E, Oitzl MS, Joels M. Brain corticosteroid receptor balance in health and disease. Endocr Rev 1998; 19: 269–301.

52. Reul JM, De Kloet ER. Two receptor systems for corticosterone in rat brain: microdistribution and differential occupation. Endocrinology 1985; 117: 2505–11.

53. Owen D, Matthews SG. Glucocorticoids and sex-dependent development of brain glucocorticoid and mineralocorticoid receptors. Endocrinology 2003; 144: 2775–84.

54. Setiawan E, Owen D, McCabe L et al. Glucocorticoids do not alter developmental expression of hippocampal or pituitary steroid receptor coactivator-1 and -2 in the late gestation fetal guinea pig. Endocrinology 2004; 145: 3796–803.

55. Meijer OC. Coregulator proteins and corticosteroid action in the brain. J Neuroendocrinol 2002; 14: 499–505.

56. Andrews MH, Matthews SG. Regulation of glucocorticoid receptor mRNA and heat shock protein 70 mRNA in the developing sheep brain. Brain Res 2000; 878: 174–82.

57. Costa A, Rocci MP, Arisio R et al. Glucocorticoid receptors immunoreactivity in tissue of human embryos. J Endocrinol Invest 1996; 19: 92–8.

58. Condon J, Gosden C, Gardener D et al. Expression of type 2 11beta-hydroxysteroid dehydrogenase and corticosteroid hormone receptors in early human fetal life. J Clin Endocrinol Metab 1998; 83: 4490–7.

59. Diaz R, Brown RW, Seckl JR. Distinct ontogeny of glucocorticoid and mineralocorticoid receptor and 11β-hydroxysteroid dehydrogenase types I and II mRNAs in the fetal rat brain suggest a complex control of glucocorticoid actions. J Neurosci 1998; 18: 2570–80.

60. O'Regan D, Kenyon CJ, Seckl JR, Holmes MC. Glucocorticoid exposure in late gestation in the rat permanently programs gender-specific differences in adult cardiovascular and metabolic physiology. Am J Physiol Endocrinol Metab 2004; 287: E863–70.

61. Kretz O, Schmid W, Berger S, Gass P. The mineralocorticoid receptor expression in the mouse CNS is conserved during development. Neuroreport 2001; 12: 1133–7.

62. NIH Consensus development conference. Effect of corticosteroids for fetal maturation and perinatal outcomes. Am J Obstet Gynecol 1995; 173: 253–344.

63. Cleasby ME, Kelly PA, Walker BR, Seckl JR. Programming of rat muscle and fat metabolism by in utero overexposure to glucocorticoids. Endocrinology 2003; 144: 999–1007.

64. Matthews SG. Early programming of the hypothalamo-pituitary-adrenal axis. Trends Endocrinol Metab 2002; 13: 373–80.

65. Levitt NS, Lindsay RS, Holmes MC, Seckl JR. Dexamethasone in the last week of pregnancy attenuates hippocampal glucocorticoid receptor gene expression and elevates blood pressure in the adult offspring in the rat. Neuroendocrinology 1996; 64: 412–18.

66. Antenatal corticosteroids revisited: Repeat courses – National Institutes of Health consensus development conference statement, Aug 17–18, 2000. Obstet Gynecol 2001; 98: 144–50.

67. Viau V, Soriano L, Dallman MF. Androgens alter corticotropin releasing hormone and arginine vasopressin mRNA within forebrain sites known to regulate activity in the hypothalamic-pituitary-adrenal axis. J Neuroendocrinol 2001; 13: 442–52.

68. McCabe L, Marash D, Li A, Matthews SG. Repeated antenatal glucocorticoid treatment decreases hypothalamic corticotropin releasing hormone mRNA but not corticosteroid receptor mRNA expression in the fetal guinea-pig brain. J Neuroendocrinol 2001; 13: 425–31.

69. Welberg LA, Seckl JR, Holmes MC. Prenatal glucocorticoid programming of brain corticosteroid receptors and corticotrophin-releasing hormone: possible implications for behaviour. Neuroscience 2001; 104: 71–9.

70. Muneoka K, Mikuni M, Ogawa T et al. Prenatal dexamethasone exposure alters brain monoamine metabolism and adrenocortical response in rat offspring. Am J Physiol 1997; 273: R1669–R1675.

71. Bakker JM, Schmidt ED, Kroes H et al. Effects of short-term dexamethasone treatment during pregnancy on the development of the immune system and the hypothalamo-pituitary adrenal axis in the rat. J Neuroimmunol 1995; 63: 183–91.

72. Herman JP, Prewitt CM, Cullinan WE. Neuronal circuit regulation of the hypothalamo-pituitary-adrenocortical stress axis. Crit Rev Neurobiol 1996; 10: 371–94.

73. Sloboda DM, Moss TJ, Gurrin LC, Newnham JP, Challis JR. The effect of prenatal betamethasone administration on postnatal ovine hypothalamic-pituitary-adrenal function. J Endocrinol 2002; 172: 71–81.

74. Dodic M, Peers A, Moritz K, Hantzis V, Wintour EM. No evidence for HPA reset in adult sheep with high blood pressure due to short prenatal exposure to dexamethasone. Am J Physiol Regul Integr Comp Physiol 2002; 282: R343–R350.

75. Uno H, Eisele S, Sakai A et al. Neurotoxicity of glucocorticoids in the primate brain. Horm Behav 1994; 28: 336–48.

76. Schinkel AH. The physiological function of drug-transporting P-glycoproteins. Semin Cancer Biol 1997; 8: 161–70.

77. Kalabis GM, Kostaki A, Andrews MH, Gibb W, Matthews SG. Dramatic changes in multidrug resistance phospho-glycoprotein (mdr1a and mdr1b) mRNA expression in the mouse placenta during pregnancy. Endocrine Society, New Orleans P3–351. 2004.

78. Sun M, Kingdom J, Baczyk D, Matthews SG, Gibb W. Expression and localization of human placental multidrug resistance protein during gestation. Endocrine Society, New Orleans, pp. 3–352. 2004.

79. Erdeljan P, MacDonald JF, Matthews SG. Glucocorticoids and serotonin alter glucocorticoid receptor (GR) but not mineralocorticoid receptor MR mRNA levels in fetal mouse hippocampal neurons, in vitro. Brain Res 2001; 896: 130–6.

80. Dean F, Matthews SG. Maternal dexamethasone treatment in late gestation alters glucocorticoid and mineralocorticoid receptor mRNA in the fetal guinea pig brain. Brain Res 1999; 846: 253–9.

81. Slotkin TA, Barnes GA, McCook EC, Seidler FJ. Programming of brainstem serotonin transporter development by prenatal glucocorticoids. Dev Brain Res 1996; 93: 155–61.

82. Herrick K, Phillips DI, Haselden S et al. Maternal consumption of a high-meat, low-carbohydrate diet in late pregnancy: relation to adult cortisol concentrations in the offspring. J Clin Endocrinol Metabol 2003; 88: 3554–60.

6

Prenatal programming of postnatal obesity

I Caroline McMillen, Jaime A Duffield, and Beverly S Muhlhausler

INTRODUCTION

Given the marked increase in the global prevalence of obesity and the association between a high fat mass and the metabolic syndrome, type 2 diabetes, and cardiovascular disease, there is intense interest in determining those factors which contribute to and amplify obesity and the specific contribution of visceral adiposity to the pathology of insulin resistance. In this context it is of particular interest that it has been shown that there are associations between the nutritional environment experienced before and immediately after birth, different patterns of postnatal growth and body fat mass in adult life. The extent to which such associations program an 'intergenerational cycle of obesity' and the extent to which they contribute to and amplify insulin resistance and the other pathologies of the metabolic syndrome are currently being debated. This chapter first reviews the evidence for the relationship between prenatal and postnatal growth patterns and adult fat mass. The impact of varying nutritional exposure during early life on the development of the adipocyte and the neural network within the brain that regulates appetite and energy balance in later life is then discussed. Such studies are important to help define those critical windows during an individual's lifespan when nutritional or other intervention strategies will have the maximum benefit for preventing the development of obesity.

THE EARLY ORIGINS OF ADULT OBESITY

During the past 20 years, there has been a marked increase in the global prevalence of being overweight or obese and currently more than half of all adults in the USA and the UK are overweight, i.e. have a body mass index (BMI) over 25 kg/m^2.[1-4] With an increase in obesity (BMI $>$ 30 kg/m^2) also comes an increase in the prevalence of the associated disorders, type 2 diabetes, high blood pressure, and ischemic heart disease and a significant increase in health care costs.[1] Abdominal or visceral obesity, in particular, is associated with the clustering of pathologies, which defines the 'insulin resistance' or metabolic syndrome (insulin resistance with or without glucose intolerance, raised blood pressure, atherogenic dyslipidemia, and prothrombotic and proinflammatory states).[5] Given the increase in and impact of adult obesity, there is currently intense interest in determining the factors which contribute to and amplify obesity, as well as in the critical windows during an individual's lifespan when intervention strategies will have maximum benefit and do minimum harm. The difficulty of effective intervention in obesity is well known. In part, this difficulty relates to the complexities of the physiological systems that regulate energy balance. This regulation includes evolved features reflecting the requirement present for most of human history to protect and maintain energy stores in order to survive long periods of famine, rather than feasting.

In this context it is of interest that epidemiological, clinical, and experimental studies have shown that there are associations between the prenatal nutritional environment, patterns of postnatal growth and the amount and distribution of adipose tissue in adult life.[6-9] The extent to which such associations have contributed or will contribute to the increase in the global prevalence of obesity through an 'intergenerational cycle of obesity', and the extent to which they contribute to and amplify insulin resistance and the other pathologies of the metabolic syndrome, are currently being debated. This chapter reviews the evidence for the relationship between birth weight and adult fat mass and the interactions between early growth, the functional characteristics of adipose tissue, and the development of insulin resistance. We also discuss the potential impact of early nutritional experience on the development of the endocrine and neuroendocrine systems that regulate energy balance.

High birth weight and adult obesity

The relationship between birth weight and fatness, measured in childhood or adulthood, is generally positive, although a number of studies have reported that there is a J-shaped or U-shaped relationship between birth weight and adult fat mass, with a higher prevalence of later obesity occurring at both low and high birth weights (Figure 6.1). Birth weight is also positively related to both maternal and paternal birth weight and where adjustments for maternal BMI have been able to be made,[10–13] the relationship between birth weight and adult BMI has diminished. A recent study in a large British cohort found a weak but positive relationship between birth weight and BMI at age 33, and determined that this relationship was largely accounted for by maternal weight, i.e. heavier mothers had heavier babies and these babies went on to have a high BMI in adult life.[13] It has been suggested that the influence of maternal weight on the relationship between birth weight and subsequent BMI may operate through an impact of a high maternal and hence fetal nutrient supply. This conclusion is supported by studies of infants of mothers who are diabetic or glucose intolerant. In these pregnancies, maternal and fetal blood glucose levels are higher and this results in offspring who are heavier at birth and who are at risk of developing obesity and glucose intolerance in later life.[14,15] The findings suggest that an increase in fetal nutrient supply, as a consequence of an increase in maternal

energy intake or resulting from maternal glucose intolerance, may program childhood and later obesity (Figure 6.2). While there are positive associations between birth weight and later BMI, it is not necessarily the case, however, that the higher BMI reflects an increased fat mass. There is recent evidence that a high birth weight may program a relatively greater proportion of lean mass in children and adolescents, suggesting that the positive associations between birth weight and later BMI may represent an association of birth weight with lean, rather than fat tissue.[16] Such an increase in lean mass in high birth weight infants might explain the paradoxical associations of a high birth weight with adult BMI (positive) and cardiovascular disease (negative).

Low birth weight and central obesity

While people who were small babies tend to have a lower BMI in adult life than people who were larger at birth, these individuals have a more abdominal distribution of obesity, a significantly reduced muscle mass, and a high body fat content in adolescent and adult life.[16–22] As summarized in other chapters, being small at birth is also associated with impaired insulin sensitivity and an increased prevalence of the metabolic syndrome later in life. In general, after adjustment for current BMI, there is an inverse relationship between birth weight and these outcomes. Exposure to a reduced nutrient supply in early pregnancy, as occurred in the Dutch Winter Famine in 1944–1945, also resulted in increased fat mass in later life. In people exposed to this famine during early gestation, there was an increase in body weight, BMI, and waist circumference at 50 years of age.[23] Interestingly, Parsons and colleagues[13] have shown that those low birth weight babies who were most vulnerable to developing obesity were men who had been light and thin at birth and had experienced a period of rapid childhood growth. Thus, men with a lower birth weight who had achieved more of their adult height by age 7 had a risk of obesity comparable with that for men with the highest birth weights. Furthermore, several studies have shown that people who were thin at birth but who developed obesity in childhood or adulthood have the highest risk of insulin resistance and cardiovascular disease.[24,25]

Although there are clear associations between birth weight, early childhood growth, and the pattern of adult obesity, the mechanisms underlying these associations are still unknown. The two primary targets for the 'programming' of adult obesity are the developing fat cell – the adipocyte – and the neural network which regulates appetite and energy balance in adult life (Figure 6.3).

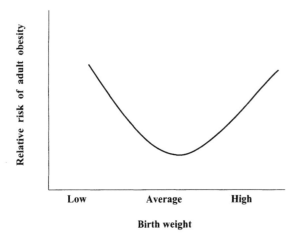

Figure 6.1 The U-shaped relationship between birth weight and subsequent body mass index (BMI) in adult life.

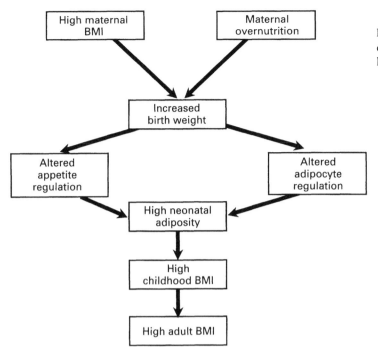

Figure 6.2 Potential pathways explaining the relationship between high birth weight and adult obesity.

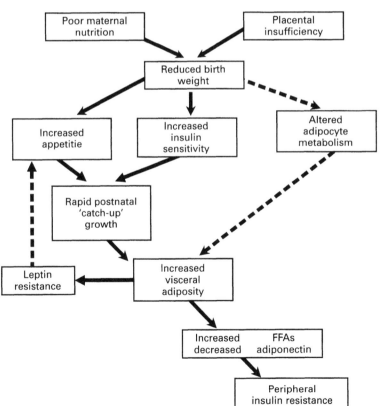

Figure 6.3 Potential pathways explaining the relationship between low birth weight, visceral adiposity, and insulin resistance.

TARGETS FOR PROGRAMMING: THE ADIPOCYTE AND ADIPOKINES

Development of the adipocyte and the role of leptin in obesity

The early formation of fat cells is a complex process, regulated by a suite of genes that are activated in sequence during development. The adipocyte lineage is derived from an embryonic stem cell precursor, which has the capacity to differentiate into the mesodermal cell types of adipocytes, chondrocytes, osteoblasts, and myocytes.[26,27] Preadipocytes arise from this mesenchymal precursor pool and, given appropriate environmental cues, they undergo clonal expansion and subsequent terminal differentiation to form adipocytes. The progression of adipose cells through the differentiation pathway is under the control of a series of transcription factors. There is considerable evidence, predominantly derived from *in vitro* culture of cell lines, that CCAAT/enhancer-binding protein β (C/EBPβ) acts as a transcriptional activator for both the C/EBPα and the peroxisome proliferator-activated receptor γ (PPARγ) genes and that following their expression, C/EBPα and PPARγ appear to serve as transcriptional activators and coordinately induce expression of a range of adipocyte specific genes. Genes such as lipoprotein lipase (LPL) and the adipocyte glucose transporter (GLUT-4) are activated resulting in the final differentiation of the lipid-filled adipocyte.[26]

Studies modulating PPARγ expression or action in rodent cell lines have confirmed that the receptor is both essential and, in the presence of PPARγ agonists,

sufficient for adipogenesis.[27] Furthermore it has been demonstrated that fusion of PPARγ null mutant and normal embryonic stem cells overcomes the embryonic lethality of PPARγ knockouts but results in the birth of an animal with no discernible adipose tissue.[26] Whilst activation of PPARγ influences the expression of genes involved in the regulation of adipose tissue mass, it is also important in the signaling of adipose tissue to other tissues to result in an increase in whole body insulin sensitivity. The predominant effect of PPARγ activation on peripheral insulin sensitivity is most likely mediated through an up-regulation of adiponectin, and through a decrease in circulating free fatty acid (FFA) levels.[26] Activation of LPL increases the uptake of FFAs from circulating lipoprotein particles into the adipocyte. The efflux of FFAs from the adipocyte is also reduced by the induction of genes that promote their storage in the form of triglyceride, e.g. glycerol-3-phosphate dehydrogenase. Thus, PPARγ has a central role in the regulation of adipogenesis (formation of fat cells), lipogenesis (*de novo* synthesis of lipid), and lipid storage in fat and in the control of the synthesis and secretion of adipokines (factors secreted by adipocyte into the circulation), such as adiponectin, which in turn regulate peripheral insulin sensitivity.

Another adipokine, leptin, is also synthesized and secreted by adipose tissue into circulation. Leptin is a signal of fat mass and acts through classic negative feedback mechanisms to ensure that fat mass is maintained at relatively constant levels (Figure 6.4). Leptin acts through binding to specific leptin receptors at central and peripheral sites, which results in a decrease in food intake and an increase in energy utilization.[28] Leptin deficiency in human populations is relatively

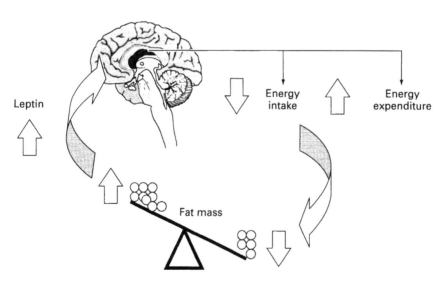

Figure 6.4 Role of leptin as a signal of fat mass.

rare and in humans, obesity is associated with high, rather than low, circulating leptin concentrations.[29,30] It has been suggested that an increased fat mass and exposure to elevated plasma levels of leptin may lead to the disruption of leptin signaling at its receptor resulting in a 'leptin resistance'. Resistance to the actions of leptin would result in a relative inability of high circulating leptin concentrations to suppress appetite and increase energy utilization.[31] The presence of functional leptin receptors on pancreatic beta cells and the observation that leptin directly inhibits insulin secretion led to the concept of an 'adipoinsular axis'[32] whereby insulin stimulates adipogenesis and the synthesis of leptin, and in turn leptin inhibits the production of insulin in the pancreas. It has also been proposed, therefore, that pancreatic leptin resistance may be a mechanism underlying the hyperinsulinism frequently associated with obesity and that it may contribute to the subsequent development of diabetes in obese individuals.[33]

Early nutrition and programming of adipose tissue and leptin in the human

Newborn infants who are small for gestational age (SGA) have a marked reduction in body fat mass at birth, which mainly reflects a decreased accumulation of lipid in the adipocytes.[34] Children born SGA, who grow rapidly in infancy have an increased body fat mass, however, with a more central distribution of adipose tissue when compared with children born at normal birth weight. Interestingly, in adults who were SGA at birth, adipose tissue appears to be resistant to the antilipolytic actions of insulin in later life such that FFA production is not suppressed to the same extent by insulin.[34] Furthermore, there are interactions between the effects of low birth weight and the Pro12Ala polymorphisms of the PPARγ gene on insulin resistance.[35,36] This finding suggests that there may be a potential role for altered regulation of PPARγ expression in adipose tissue, either in the genesis of obesity and/or in the emergence of insulin resistance in low birth weight individuals in later life.

In the human infant, there is a positive relationship between cord blood concentrations of leptin at delivery and either birth weight or neonatal adiposity.[37–40] While plasma leptin concentrations are low in growth-restricted infants at birth, they increase to become higher in these infants at 1 year of age when compared with normal birth weight counterparts.[41] People with a low birth weight also go on to have higher leptin concentrations in adult life when compared with individuals with a higher birth weight at the same BMI.[42]

There is also evidence that nutrition in the early postnatal period may be an important determinant of the future leptin synthetic capacity of adipose cells. One study reported that the ratio of leptin to fat mass in adolescents was significantly greater in those who had received a nutrient-enriched formula than in those who received a standard formula or banked breast milk after preterm delivery.[43] Human milk intake was also associated with lower leptin concentrations relative to fat mass in adolescence.[43] It has been suggested, therefore, that programming of leptin synthesis or secretion in adipocytes by early nutritional exposure may be one mechanism that links early nutrition with later obesity.[43]

Early nutrition and programming of adipose tissue and leptin in animal models

Rat

The development of the adipocyte and leptin synthesis and secretion have been investigated in the rodent in a number of models in which the early nutritional experience has been manipulated. The most common manipulations of fetal nutrition in the rodent are through exposure of the pregnant dam to either a low protein diet (generally 9% vs 18% protein content) or to a global undernutrition through a 30–50% reduction in energy intake. Also of relevance are models in which mild maternal diabetes is induced through treatment of the mother with the drug, streptozotocin, which ablates pancreatic endocrine function and results in exposure of the fetal rat to increased glucose concentrations.

Restriction of maternal protein intake during pregnancy and lactation results in an increased glucose tolerance and an increased expression of insulin receptors in epididymal adipocytes in the rat offspring at 6 weeks of age.[44] The improved glucose tolerance is maintained into young adult life and, consistent with an increase in insulin sensitivity, the offspring have lower circulating triglyceride concentrations and reduced circulating β-hydroxybutyrate concentrations, despite higher circulating FFA concentrations.[45,46] In early adult life, mesenteric adipocytes from offspring exposed to a low protein diet during gestation show an enhanced sensitivity to insulin, and insulin receptor expression is increased in epididymal and intra-abdominal, but not subcutaneous, adipocytes at 3 months of age.[47] Basal glucose uptake was higher in adipocytes from epididymal, intra-abdominal and subcutaneous fat depots; however, insulin-stimulated uptake of glucose into these adipocytes was smaller in low protein offspring when compared with controls. By 15 months of age, the magnitude of insulin inhibition of isoproterenol-stimulated lipolysis was also smaller in epididymal and intra-abdominal adipocytes from low protein offspring, suggesting a selective resistance to insulin in these adipocytes.[47–49] There was no difference, however, in the level of expression of the insulin receptor in adipocytes from offspring exposed to the low protein diet *in utero* and control animals, suggesting that the molecular alteration that leads to insulin resistance must therefore be at the postreceptor level.[49] At 3 and 15 months of age, insulin-stimulated phosphatidylinositol 3-kinase (PI3-kinase) activity was reduced and this was associated with a reduction in the level of the p110β subunit in adipocytes from low protein offspring.[49] It may be that this catalytic subunit of PI3-kinase is required to mediate the antilipolytic action of insulin. At 15 months, insulin-stimulated protein kinase B was also reduced in the adipocytes from low protein offspring, which may explain the insulin resistance observed in the adipocyte at this age.[49] Thus, there is a complex relationship between the effects of exposure to a low protein diet *in utero* and the development of subsequent insulin resistance in the rat, with an initial period during which insulin sensitivity is increased, followed by the development of insulin resistance.

In rodents, the capacity of fetal adipocytes to synthesize leptin is low until relatively late in gestation. The rodent placenta synthesizes little if any leptin, but there is significant transplacental transfer of maternal leptin to the fetus and this transfer increases during late pregnancy.[50] Maternal protein restriction results in a significant decrease in maternal, but not fetal, leptin concentrations during late gestation.[51] It has been shown that administration of leptin to rats fed a protein-restricted diet during late pregnancy and lactation makes their male offspring less susceptible to weight gain and insulin resistance when fed a high fat diet.[52] This effect may be an example of an experimental induction of a 'maternal predictive adaptation', i.e. an increase in maternal leptin normally associated with an increase in body fat programs the ability of the offspring to respond better to a high fat diet in the postnatal period.

Exposure of rats to a global maternal undernutrition (30% of normal energy intake) during gestation leads to an increase in relative adiposity and hyperleptinemia in adult offspring.[53] The combination of prenatal undernutrition together with an increase in postnatal nutrition leads to a major amplification of the hyperleptinemia. The amplified hyperleptinemia in the presence of hyperinsulinism in the offspring on the hypercaloric diet suggests that there may be development of leptin resistance both at the hypothalamus and the pancreas, which explains the hyperphagia and hyperinsulinism, respectively.

When fetal macrosomia is induced by administration of streptozotocin to the pregnant rat at day 5 of gestation,[54] the offspring are obese and hyperinsulinemic at 70 days of age and the adipocytes of the epididymal fat from obese males and periovarian fat from obese females had a higher lipid content and significantly larger cell size when compared with control rats. The adipocytes of the macrosomic pups also showed an attenuated response to insulin in terms of glucose conversion to lipid and fatty acid when compared with controls. The authors concluded that a postreceptor deficit most likely accounted for the abnormality in glucose metabolism in these obese rats.[54]

Thus, in the rat, exposure to either fetal undernutrition or to fetal hyperglycemia during critical windows of development can each result in abnormalities in insulin signaling within the adipocytes of the offspring. One possibility is that a period of relative overnutrition – experienced either in the immediate postnatal period in the rat which experienced undernutrition *in utero*, or in late gestation following maternal administration of streptozotocin model – may represent a common element in the programming of the adipocyte and obesity.

Large animal models

In the sheep and pig in which fat is deposited before birth, leptin is synthesized in fetal adipose tissue and is present in the fetal circulation through late gestation. Circulating leptin concentrations are lower in the fetus than the pregnant ewe throughout late gestation.[55,56] Intrafetal leptin infusion in the presence of normoglycemia and normoinsulinemia results in a decrease in the proportion of the larger lipid locules stored in perirenal adipose tissue and in the abundance of leptin mRNA in this tissue.[57] These findings suggest that leptin may act as a signal of energy supply and have a 'lipostatic' role before birth. It is possible, therefore, that leptin in the fetal circulation derived either from the maternal circulation (as in the rat in late gestation and potentially the sheep in early gestation) or fetal adipose tissue (as in the sheep and human in late gestation) acts centrally via leptin receptors located on neurons within the fetal hypothalamus and peripherally on leptin receptors on the adipocyte or pancreatic beta cell. There has been relatively little work to date on whether adipokines secreted from fetal adipose tissue can play a role in the subsequent programming of obesity. Future studies are clearly required to determine whether fetal adipokines, such as leptin or adiponectin, can play a role along with adipocyte growth factors, such as the insulin-like growth factors (IGFs), in the programming of postnatal obesity in animal models including sheep or pig, in which fat is deposited and adipoctye hormones are expressed within fat depots before birth.

TARGETS FOR PROGRAMMING: THE APPETITE REGULATORY NEURAL NETWORK

The appetite regulatory system in the adult

In the adult, appetite and energy balance homeostasis are regulated primarily by a complex neuronal network located within the hypothalamus, which receives nutrient, hormonal, and neural signals from a range of sources including fat cells, the pancreas, the gastrointestinal tract, and other brain regions. There are a range of appetite regulatory neuropeptides that either stimulate appetite, e.g. neuropeptide Y (NPY) and agouti-related protein (AgRP), or inhibit it, pro-opiomelanocortin (POMC) and cocaine- and amphetamine-regulated transcript (CART).[58] NPY is a 36 amino acid neuropeptide, which markedly stimulates appetite and is predominantly localized in the arcuate nucleus of the hypothalamus (ARC). NPY neurons project to hypothalamic regions which play important roles in energy balance including the paraventricular nucleus (PVN), DMN, periformical region, and the lateral hypothalamic area.[59] The blood-brain barrier is effectively reduced within the area of the arcuate nucleus and NPY neurons are therefore able to sense and respond to a range of peripheral metabolic signals, including insulin, glucose, ghrelin, and leptin. NPY expression is down-regulated by nutrient and hormonal signals of increased energy stores, such as insulin and leptin. The leptin receptor is highly expressed on cell bodies in the ARC and DMN, and increases in circulating leptin concentrations during periods of increased food intake result in a decrease in hypothalamic NPY mRNA and a subsequent fall in energy intake.[58] AgRP is an appetite stimulatory peptide, which is coexpressed with NPY in the ARC, and is an endogenous antagonist of the anorexigenic melanocortin receptors, MC3 and MC4R in the PVN and other hypothalamic regions. The POMC-derived peptide, α-MSH, is an endogenous appetite inhibitor, which acts at these melanocortin receptors to suppress food intake. Leptin increases POMC expression within the arcuate nucleus, which results in a decrease in energy intake.[58] The neuropeptide, CART, is colocalized within POMC neurons in the hypothalamus and also acts to suppress food intake.

Central administration of NPY into the PVN significantly increases feeding activity, increases LPL activity in fat cells, decreases sympathetic nerve activity and thermogenesis in brown adipose tissue and can lead to obesity.[58] Fasting or food restriction markedly increases NPY expression in the arcuate nuclei and NPY release into the PVN both *in vivo* and *in vitro*.

Early undernutrition and the programming of appetite

When rats are undernourished during the first 2 weeks of pregnancy, but refed during the third week, the male offspring develop significant increase in appetite (hyperphagia) and obesity when maintained on a high fat diet.[60–62] The obesity has a delayed onset (~50 days of age) and is characterized by increases in the proportion of body fat and adipocyte hypertrophy in the epididymal and retroperitoneal fat pads. At this level of maternal undernutrition, refeeding during the third week of pregnancy is critical for the induction of postnatal obesity.[63] When maternal nutrition is restricted to 30% of control intake throughout the whole of gestation, the offspring are smaller throughout postnatal life, but there is an increase in the relative mass of the retroperitoneal fat pad in these animals at 100 days of age.[53] Food intake in the offspring of the undernourished rats (cross-fostered on to mothers fed *ad libitum*) was increased early in postnatal life, increased with increasing age, and was amplified by postnatal hypercaloric nutrition.[53] Interestingly in these offspring, locomotor activity was also decreased before the development of maturity onset obesity and was significantly reduced in male as compared with female offspring.[64]

In the rat brain, neurons expressing the appetite regulatory peptides develop in the hypothalamus at around 14.5 days gestation (term = ~21 days) and NPY mRNA expression rapidly increases during the first 2 weeks after birth.[59] POMC, AgRP, and MC4R mRNA are also all present within the rat hypothalamus through this postnatal period. While NPY is present within the arcuate nucleus from late fetal life, connections between these neurons and the neurons that act to regulate appetite are not complete until 2 weeks after birth.[59] During the first week after birth, there appears to be a relative dominance of NPY and α-MSH innervation of the PVN by efferents derived from the brainstem, rather than the arcuate nucleus. It has been suggested therefore that information relating to gut fullness may be the dominant influence on feeding behavior in the rat pup in this early period before the appetite regulatory system fully matures.[59]

Even though the appetite regulatory system is relatively immature at birth in the rat, a series of early studies demonstrated that the amount of food consumed during the suckling period plays an important role in determining subsequent food intake in the rat.[65] When postnatal overnutrition is induced in rats by rearing in small litters of only three pups, they show an increased early weight gain and fat deposition, followed by an increased appetite (hyperphagia), obesity, hyperleptinemia, hyperglycemia, hyperinsulinemia, and insulin resistance.[66–68] Leptin has a lower inhibitory effect on the appetite stimulatory neurons of the hypothalamus in these animals as young adults.[69,70] When mild hyperglycemia is induced by streptozotocin-induced diabetes in pregnant rats from early pregnancy, pups are large at birth and grow rapidly during the first 10 weeks of life.[71] In these offspring as adults, there is also a significant increase in the number of NPY-containing neurons in the hypothalamus.[72,73] Both a reduction in litter size and mild gestational diabetes are associated with high circulating insulin concentrations, and it may be that exposure to hyperinsulinemia during fetal or early postnatal life results in increased fat mass and altered development of the appetite regulating system in the hypothalamus.[74–77]

Interestingly, a recent study has reported that neural projection pathways from the arcuate nucleus are permanently disrupted in leptin-deficient (Lep^{ob}/Lep^{ob}) mice and that treatment of these mice with leptin in neonatal, but not in adult life, rescues the development of projections from the arcuate nucleus.[78] These data provide direct evidence that leptin promotes formation of hypothalamic pathways that will have a role in later life in regulating food intake and energy consumption. These actions of leptin appear to be specific for projections from the arcuate nucleus and occur only during a critical window of time that corresponds to a neonatal period when leptin concentrations are usually high. This neonatal 'critical period' also corresponds to the period when the axons from the arcuate neurons are guided to their targets.[78]

Thus, it appears that in the rat, glucose, insulin, and leptin derived from the maternal circulation or present in breast milk may each exert an important influence on the development of the appetite regulatory neural network and that the immediate postnatal period is of particular importance for the long-term programming of food intake.

While there have been a substantial number of studies that have investigated the relationship between the level of nutritional exposure before and immediately after birth and changes in the appetite regulatory system in the rat, there have been relatively few in other animal models. It is the case, however, that the role of maternal metabolic and hormonal signals and the critical windows during which programming of appetite may occur in the litter-bearing, altricial rodent are likely to be different from those in nonlitter-bearing, precocial species such as sheep and humans.

Development and programming of the appetite regulatory system in the human and sheep

In contrast to the rodent, NPY immunoreactivity has been found to be present in the human hypothalamus in early fetal life (21 weeks gestation) and, at this stage of pregnancy, there are already projections between the arcuate nucleus and the PVN.[79] It is possible, therefore, that in the human, nutritional exposure during fetal or early neonatal life may be important in determining the subsequent development of the appetite regulatory system. Similar to the human and in contrast to the rat, the appetite regulating neuropeptides, NPY, AGRP, POMC, and CART and the leptin receptor are each highly expressed in the fetal sheep hypothalamus in late gestation.[80] In this species, it has been demonstrated that intrafetal infusion of glucose in late gestation resulted in a significant increase in POMC mRNA in the ARC of the fetal sheep hypothalamus.[81] This change occurred in the absence of an increase in circulating leptin, indicating that during fetal life, POMC mRNA expression in the hypothalamus may be responsive to increases in glucose or insulin, acting either alone or in combination. Interestingly, there was no effect of intrafetal glucose infusion on the expression of the orexigenic neuropeptides NPY and AgRP in the fetal sheep hypothalamus.[81] This is surprising given that circulating glucose and insulin concentrations in the fetus are relatively low compared with those measured in adult life and that fetal hypothalamic NPY content is increased following maternal undernutrition in sheep.[82] Fetal hypothalamic expression of NPY and AgRP may therefore be relatively insensitive to an increase in fetal glucose or insulin concentrations and indeed the preservation of orexigenic drive may be an important survival strategy for the neonate immediately after birth. In the sheep, intrafetal leptin infusion in the presence of normoglycemia and normoinsulinemia results in a decrease in the proportion and relative mass of unilocular tissue in the perirenal adipose depot and a decrease in the relative abundance of leptin mRNA in perirenal adipose tissue in fetal sheep.[57] The precise site of this action of leptin, either within the fetal hypothalamus or peripherally within the adipoinsular axis, remains to be determined. It is possible, therefore, that leptin in the fetal circulation derived either from the maternal circulation (as in the rat in late gestation and potentially the sheep in early gestation) or fetal adipose tissue (as in the sheep and human in late gestation) acts centrally via leptin receptors located on neurons within the fetal hypothalamus to have a 'lipostatic' role. Despite the role played by leptin in regulating the structural and functional characteristics of the developing adipocyte *in utero*, it is also possible that exposure to high or low leptin concentrations during critical windows of development of the neural network that regulates appetite may have longer-term consequences for this network and for the regulation of energy balance after birth.

In summary, a series of studies have provided significant evidence that changes in perinatal nutrition program the development of the hypothalamic neural network that regulates appetite in adult life. These studies have been primarily carried out in the rodent utilizing maternal undernutrition imposed at different stages of pregnancy or manipulation of litter size in postnatal life in conjunction with the measurement of the expression, localization, and activity of hypothalamic neuropeptides. Such research has provided a neuroanatomical and functional framework for the often mentioned hypothalamic body weight 'set point' hypothesis,[83] and this can now be interrogated in animal models in which the appetite regulatory network develops before birth to determine the extent to which there could be perinatal programming of this network in humans.

SUMMARY

There is substantial evidence from epidemiological studies that either being of high birth weight or being of low birth weight and growing rapidly in postnatal life can each be associated with an increased BMI in later life. There is also evidence which indicates that maternal body composition and the level of maternal nutrition may contribute to the programming of obesity in her offspring. In the face of the epidemic of global obesity, there is the potential for an intergenerational transmission of obesity as women enter pregnancy with a higher BMI, have heavier babies, who are then programmed to be heavier in adult life.[84] Findings from experimental studies also highlight that exposure to relative overnutrition in either late gestation, or in early postnatal life following a period of gestational undernutrition, can permanently alter the responses of the adipocyte and the appetite regulatory network within the brain to subsequent nutrient and hormonal

signals. In the face of the compelling epidemiological and clinical evidence, it is now important to define the initiating mechanisms within the 'fat-brain' axis in early life which precede the development of adult obesity. In addition, we urgently need to determine the critical windows during which nutritional 'interventions' will have maximum benefit to ensure a lifelong resilience to the effects of an increased body fat mass.

REFERENCES

1. James WP. The epidemiology of obesity. Ciba Found Symp 1996; 201: 1–11.
2. Campfield LA, Smith FJ, Burn P. Strategies and potential molecular targets for obesity treatment. Science 1998; 280: 1383–7.
3. Flegal KM, Carroll MD, Ogden CL, Johnson CL. Prevalence and trends in obesity among US adults, 1999–2000. JAMA 2002; 288: 1723–7.
4. Ogden CL, Flegal KM, Carroll MD, Johnson CL. Prevalence and trends in overweight among US children and adolescents, 1999–2000. JAMA 2002; 288: 1728–32.
5. Reaven G. Banting lecture 1988. Role of insulin resistance in human disease. Diabetes 1988; 37: 1595–607.
6. Fall CHD, Vijayakumar M, Barker DJP, Osmond C, Duggleby S. Weight in infancy and prevalence of coronary heart disease in adult life. BMJ 1995; 310: 17–19.
7. Sorensen HT, Sabroe S, Rothman KJ et al. Relation between weight and length at birth and body mass index in young adulthood: cohort study. BMJ 1997; 315: 1137.
8. Loos RJ, Fagard R, Beunen G, Derom C, Vlietinck R. Birth weight and blood pressure in young adults: a prospective twin study. Circulation 2001; 104: 1633–8.
9. Yajnik CS. Nutrition, growth, and body size in relation to insulin resistance and type 2 diabetes. Curr Diab Rep 2003; 3: 108–14.
10. Maffeis C, Micciolo R, Must A, Zaffanello M, Pinelli L. Parental and perinatal factors associated with childhood obesity in north-east Italy. Int J Obes Relat Metab Disord 1994; 18: 301–5.
11. Curhan GC, Willett WC, Rimm EB et al. Birth weight and adult hypertension, diabetes mellitus and obesity in US men. Circulation 1996; 94: 3246–50.
12. Curhan GC, Chertow GM, Willett WC et al. Birth weight and adult hypertension and obesity in women. Circulation 1996; 94: 1310–15.
13. Parsons TJ, Power C, Manor O. Fetal and early life growth and body mass index from birth to early adulthood in 1958 British cohort: longitudinal study. BMJ 2001; 323: 1331–5.
14. Dorner G, Plagemann A. Perinatal hyperinsulinism as possible predisposing factor for diabetes mellitus, obesity and enhanced cardiovascular risk in later life. Horm Metab Res 1994; 26: 213–21.
15. Silverman BL, Rizzo T, Green OC et al. Long-term prospective evaluation of offspring of diabetic mothers. Diabetes 1991; 40 (Suppl 2): 121–5.
16. Singhal A, Wells J, Cole TJ, Fewtrell M, Lucas A. Programming of lean body mass: a link between birth weight, obesity, and cardiovascular disease? Am J Clin Nutr 2003; 77: 726–30.
17. Law CM, Barker DJP, Osmond C, Fall CHD, Simmonds SJ. Early growth and abdominal fatness in adult life. J Epidemiol Community Health 1992; 46: 184–6.

18. Fall CHD, Osmond C, Barker DJP et al. Fetal and infant growth and cardiovascular risk factors in women. BMJ 1995; 310: 428–32.

19. Malina RM, Katzmarzyk PT, Beunen G. Birth weight and its relationship to size attained and relative fat distribution at 7 to 12 years of age. Obes Res 1996; 4: 385–90.

20. Okosun IS, Liao Y, Rotimi CN, Dever GE, Cooper RS. Impact of birth weight on ethnic variations in subcutaneous and central adiposity in American children aged 5–11 years. A study from the Third National Health and Nutrition Examination Survey. Int J Obes Relat Metab Disord 2000; 24: 479–84.

21. Loos RJ, Beunen G, Fagard R, Derom C, Vlietinck R. Birth weight and body composition in young adult men – a prospective twin study. Int J Obes Relat Metab Disord 2001; 25: 1537–45.

22. Loos RJ, Beunen G, Fagard R, Derom C, Vlietinck R. Birth weight and body composition in young women: a prospective twin study. Am J Clin Nutr 2002; 75: 676–82.

23. Ravelli GP, Stein ZA, Susser MW. Obesity in young men after famine exposure in utero and early infancy. N Engl J Med 1976; 295: 349–53.

24. Bavdekar A, Yajnik C, Fall C et al. Insulin resistance syndrome in 8-year-old Indian children: small at birth, big at 8 years, or both? Diabetes 1999; 48: 2422–9.

25. Eriksson JG, Forsen T, Tuomilehto J et al. Effects of size at birth and childhood growth on the insulin resistance syndrome in elderly individuals. Diabetologia 2002; 45: 342–8.

26. Gregoire FM, Smas CM, Sul HS. Understanding adipocyte differentiation. Physiol Rev 1998; 78: 783–809.

27. Rangwala SM, Lazar MA. Peroxisome proliferator-activated receptor gamma in diabetes and metabolism. Trends in Pharmacological Sciences 2004; 25: 331–6.

28. Friedman JM, Halaas JL. Leptin and the regulation of body weight in mammals. Nature 1998; 395: 763–70.

29. Chessler SD, Fujimoto WY, Shofer JB, Boyko EJ, Weigle DS. Increased plasma leptin levels are associated with fat accumulation in Japanese Americans. Diabetes 1998; 47: 239–43.

30. Lissner L, Karlsson C, Lindroos AK et al. Birth weight, adulthood BMI, and subsequent weight gain in relation to leptin levels in Swedish women. Obes Res 1999; 7: 150–4.

31. Ahima RS, Flier JS. Adipose tissue as an endocrine organ. Trends Endocrinol Metab 2000; 11: 327–32.

32. Kieffer TJ, Habener JF. The adipoinsular axis: effects of leptin on pancreatic beta-cells. Am J Physiol Endocrinol Metab 2000; 278: E1–14.

33. Seufert J, Kieffer TJ, Leech CA et al. Leptin suppression of insulin secretion and gene expression in human pancreatic islets: implications for the development of adipogenic diabetes mellitus. J Clin Endocrinol Metab 1999; 84: 670–6.

34. Levy-Marchal C, Jaquet D, Czernichow P. Long term metabolic consequences of being born small for gestational age. Semin Neonatol 2004; 9: 67–74.

35. Jaquet D, Tregouet DA, Godefroy T et al. Combined effects of genetic and environmental factors on insulin resistance associated with reduced fetal growth. Diabetes 2002; 51: 3473–8.

36. Eriksson JG, Lindi V, Uusitupa M et al. The effects of the Pro12Ala polymorphism of the peroxisome proliferator-activated receptor-γ2 gene on insulin sensitivity and insulin metabolism interact with size at birth. Diabetes 2002; 51: 2321–4.

37. Jaquet D, Leger J, Levy-Marchal C, Oury JF, Czernichow P. Ontogeny of leptin in human fetuses and newborns: effect of intrauterine growth retardation on serum leptin concentrations. J Clin Endocrinol Metab 1998; 83: 1243–6.

38. Koistinen HA, Koivisto VA, Andersson S et al. Leptin concentration in cord blood correlates with intrauterine growth. J Clin Endocrinol Metab 1997; 82: 3328–30.

39. Shekhawat PS, Garland JS, Shivpuri C et al. Neonatal cord blood leptin: its relationship to birth weight, body mass index, maternal diabetes, and steroids. Pediatr Res 1998; 43: 338–43.

40. Cetin I, Morpurgo PS, Radelli T et al. Fetal plasma leptin concentrations: relationship with different intrauterine growth patterns from 19 weeks to term. Pediatr Res 2000; 48: 646–51.

41. Jaquet D, Leger J, Tabone MD, Czernichow P, Levy Marchal C. High serum leptin concentrations during catch-up growth of children born with intrauterine growth retardation. J Clin Endocrinol Metab 1999; 84: 1949–53.

42. Phillips DIW, Fall CHD, Cooper C et al. Size at birth and plasma leptin concentrations in adult life. Int J Obes Relat Metab Disord 1999; 23: 1025–9.

43. Singhal A, Farooqi IS, O'Rahilly S et al. Early nutrition and leptin concentrations in later life. Am J Clin Nutr 2002; 75: 993–9.

44. Shepherd PR, Crowther NJ, Desai M, Hales CN, Ozanne SE. Altered adipocyte properties in the offspring of protein malnourished rats. Br J Nutr 1997; 78: 121–9.

45. Lucas A, Baker BA, Desai M, Hales CN. Nutrition in pregnant or lactating rats programs lipid metabolism in the offspring. Br J Nutr 1996; 76: 605–12.

46. Ozanne SE, Wang CL, Petry CJ, Smith JM, Hales CN. Ketosis resistance in the male offspring of protein-malnourished rat dams. Metabolism 1998; 12: 1450–4.

47. Ozanne SE, Dorling MW, Wang CL, Petry CJ. Depot-specific effects of early growth retardation on adipocyte insulin action. Horm Metab Res 2000; 32: 71–5.

48. Ozanne SE, Wang CL, Dorling MW, Petry CJ. Dissection of the metabolic actions of insulin in adipocytes from early growth-retarded male rats. J Endocrinol 1999; 162: 313–19.

49. Ozanne SE, Dorling MW, Wang CL, Nave BT. Impaired PI 3-kinase activation in adipocytes from early growth-restricted male rats. Am J Physiol Endocrinol Metab 2001; 280: E534–9.

50. Smith JT, Waddell BJ. Leptin distribution and metabolism in the pregnant rat: transplacental leptin passage increases in late gestation but is reduced by excess glucocorticoids. Endocrinology 2003; 144: 3024–30.

51. Fernandez-Twinn DS, Ozanne SE, Ekizoglou S et al. The maternal endocrine environment in the low-protein model of intra-uterine growth restriction. Br J Nutr 2003; 90: 815–22.

52. Stocker C, O'Dowd J, Morton NM et al. Modulation of susceptibility to weight gain and insulin resistance in low birth-weight rats by treatment of their mothers with leptin during pregnancy and lactation. Int J Obes Relat Metab Disord 2004; 28: 129–36.

53. Vickers MH, Breier BH, Cutfield WS, Hofman PL, Gluckman PD. Fetal origins of hyperphagia, obesity, and hypertension and postnatal amplification by hypercaloric nutrition. Am J Physiol Endocrinol Metab 2000; 279: E83–7.

54. Gelardi NL, Cha CJ, Oh W. Glucose metabolism in adipocytes of obese offspring of mild hyperglycemic rats. Pediatr Res 1990; 28: 641–5.

55. Ehrhardt RA, Bell AW, Boisclair YR. Spatial and developmental regulation of leptin in fetal sheep. Am J Physiol Regul Integr Comp Physiol 2002; 282: R1628–35.

56. Yuen BSJ, Owens PC, McFarlane JR et al. Circulating leptin concentrations are positively related to leptin messenger RNA expression in the adipose tissue of fetal sheep in the pregnant ewe fed at or below maintenance energy requirements during late gestation. Biol Reprod 2002; 67: 911–16.

57. Yuen BSJ, Owens PC, Muhlhausler BS et al. Leptin alters the structural and functional characteristics of adipose tissue before birth. FASEB J 2003; 17: 1102–4.

58. Schwartz MW. Brain pathways controlling food intake and body weight. Exp Biol Med 2001; 226: 978–81.

59. Grove KL, Smith MS. Ontogeny of the hypothalamic neuropeptide Y system. Physiol Behav 2003; 79: 47–63.

60. Jones AP, Friedman MI. Obesity and adipocyte abnormalities in offspring of rats undernourished during pregnancy. Science 1982; 215: 1518–19.

61. Anguita RM, Sigulem DM, Sawaya AL. Intrauterine food restriction is associated with obesity in young rats. J Nutr 1993; 123: 1421–8.

62. Jones AP, Assimon SA, Friedman MI. The effect of diet on food intake and adiposity in rats made obese by gestational undernutrition. Physiol Behav 1996; 37: 381–6.

63. Stephens DN. Growth and development of dietary obesity in adulthood of rats which have been undernourished during development. Br J Nutr 1980; 44: 215–27.

64. Vickers MH, Breier BH, McCarthy D, Gluckman PD. Sedentary behavior during postnatal life is determined by the prenatal environment and exacerbated by postnatal hypercaloric nutrition. Am J Physiol Regul Integr Comp Physiol 2003; 285: R271–3.

65. Oscai LB, McGarr JA. Evidence that the amount of food consumed in early life fixes appetite in the rat. Am J Physiol Regul Integr Comp Physiol 1978; 235: R141–4.

66. Plagemann A, Heidrich I, Gotz F, Rohde W, Dorner G. Obesity and enhanced diabetes and cardiovascular risk in adult rats due to early postnatal overfeeding. Exp Clin Endocrinol 1992; 99: 154–8.

67. Plagemann A, Harder T, Rake A et al. Observations on the orexigenic hypothalamic neuropeptide Y-system in neonatally overfed weanling rats. J Neuroendocrinol 1999; 11: 541–6.

68. Plagemann A, Harder T, Rake A et al. Perinatal elevation of hypothalamic insulin, acquired malformation of hypothalamic galaninergic neurons, and syndrome X-like alterations in adulthood of neonatally overfed rats. Brain Res 1999; 836: 146–55.

69. Davidowa H, Plagemann A. Decreased inhibition by leptin of hypothalamic arcuate neurons in neonatally overfed young rats. Neuroreport 2000; 21: 2795–8.

70. Davidowa H, Plagemann A. Inhibition by insulin of hypothalamic VMN neurons in rats overweight due to postnatal overfeeding. Neuroreport 2001; 12: 3201–4.

71. Oh W, Gelardi NL, Cha CJ. Maternal hyperglycemia in pregnant rats: its effect on growth and carbohydrate metabolism in the offspring. Metabolism 1988; 37: 1146–51.

72. Plagemann A, Harder T, Rake A et al. Hypothalamic insulin and neuropeptide Y in the offspring of gestational diabetic mother rats. Neuroreport 1998; 9: 4069–73.

73. Plagemann A, Harder T, Melchior K et al. Elevation of hypothalamic neuropeptide Y-neurons in adult offspring of diabetic mother rats. Neuroreport 1999; 10: 3211–16.

74. Jones AP, Pothos EN, Rada P, Olster DH, Hoebel BG. Maternal hormonal manipulations in rats cause obesity and increase medial hypothalamic norepinephrine release in male offspring. Brain Res Dev Brain Res 1995; 88: 127–31.

75. Jones AP, Olster DH, States B. Maternal insulin manipulations in rats organize body weight and noradrenergic innervation of the hypothalamus in gonadally intact male offspring. Brain Res Dev Brain Res 1996; 97: 16–21.

76. Harder T, Plagemann A, Rohde W, Dorner G. Syndrome X-like alterations in adult female rats due to neonatal insulin treatment. Metabolism 1998; 47: 855–62.

77. Harder T, Rake A, Rohde W, Doerner G, Plagemann A. Overweight and increased diabetes susceptibility in neonatally insulin-treated adult rats. Endocr Regul 1999; 33: 25–31.

78. Bouret SG, Draper SJ, Simerly RB. Trophic action of leptin on hypothalamic neurons that regulate feeding. Science 2004; 304: 108–10.

79. Koutcherov Y, Mai JK, Ashwell KW, Paxinos G. Organization of human hypothalamus in fetal development. J Comp Neurol 2002; 446: 310–24.

80. Muhlhausler BS, McMillen IC, Rouzaud G et al. Appetite regulatory neuropeptides are expressed in the sheep hypothalamus before birth. J Neuroendocrinol 2004; 16: 502–7.

81. Mühlhäusler BS, Adam CL, Marrocco EM et al. Impact of glucose infusion on the structural and functional characteristics of adipose tissue and on hypothalamic gene expression for appetite regulatory neuropeptides in the sheep fetus during late gestation. J Physiol 2005; 565 (Pt 1): 185–95.

82. Warnes KE, Morris MJ, Symonds ME et al. Effects of increasing gestation, cortisol and maternal undernutrition on hypothalamic neuropeptide Y expression in the sheep fetus. J Neuroendocrinol 1998; 10: 51–7.

83. Elmquist JK, Flier JS. The fat-brain axis enters a new dimension. Science 2004; 304: 63–4.

84. Kral JG. Preventing and treating obesity in girls and young women to curb the epidemic. Obes Res 2004; 12: 1539–46.

7

Programming the fetal pancreatic axes

Deborah M Sloboda, John P Newnham, and John RG Challis

INTRODUCTION

Over the last 20 years, it has become clear that subtle changes in the intrauterine environment are important in determining the health and development of the fetus, effects that may be seen much later in adulthood. A key factor is the occurrence of intrauterine growth restriction (IUGR) and the association between fetal growth and the incidence of developing diseases, such as type 2 diabetes. Described elsewhere in this book are the associations between low birth weight and the increased incidence of poor glucose regulation and insulin resistance related to type 2 diabetes. The specific mechanisms underlying these associations are unclear, although studies have suggested that an alteration in pancreatic function and the prevalence of impaired beta cell growth and function are important. This chapter will briefly describe prenatal pancreatic development and the consequences for the endocrine activity of the pancreas when the intrauterine environment is altered. Some mechanisms regulating abnormal pancreatic development are examined.

THE DEVELOPMENTAL ORIGINS OF METABOLIC DYSFUNCTION

It is now well established that intrauterine factors are important determinants of the risk of developing a variety of adult diseases and these factors interact with lifestyle and social class in postnatal life.[1–4] Low birth weight has been associated with impaired glucose tolerance and insulin resistance and linked to alterations in pancreatic function.[5–9] The developmental programming hypothesis has been proposed to explain these associations.[10]

Human evidence and epidemiological studies

More than a decade ago, Professor David Barker and his colleagues described the association between low birth weight and the increased incidence of glucose intolerance, insulin resistance, and noninsulin-dependent diabetes (NIDDM; type 2 diabetes mellitus).[6,7,11,12] In early studies, this group demonstrated that the risk of developing glucose intolerance and diabetes later in life was two-fold greater among men who had low birth weights.[6] Similar reports described a strong negative relationship between birth size and the prevalence of impaired glucose tolerance in adult life, independent of the gestational age.[7] Evidence now suggests that the association between IUGR and postnatal metabolic dysfunction is influenced by inappropriate postnatal 'catch-up' growth.[13] Recent reports have observed that small for gestational age (SGA) children were more insulin-resistant than children born at an appropriate weight for gestational age, and that this effect was more pronounced in SGA children that demonstrated catch-up growth in height and had elevated body mass indices (BMIs).[14,15]

Among the numerous postnatal metabolic derangements associated with alterations in fetal growth, metabolic syndrome X is one that has serious lifelong consequences. Many studies have reported that low birth weight is associated with a higher incidence of syndrome X,[1,4,16] which comprises several physiological alterations including insulin resistance, glucose intolerance, hyperinsulinemia, hypertriglyceridemia, decreased high-density lipoprotein cholesterol, and hypertension. This syndrome appears to be important in the genesis of many cases of coronary artery disease.[17]

The relationship between reduced fetal growth and postnatal metabolic dysfunction has been demonstrated in a number of models, although the regulatory mechanisms are not yet clear. Fetal undernutrition (resulting from either maternal or fetal malnutrition or maternal, fetal or placental pathology) has been shown to have long-term consequences on metabolic function. Ravelli et al. described the effects of maternal malnutrition in the study of the Dutch Hunger Winter of 1944. In this previously well-fed population, individuals (including pregnant women) were forced into severe starvation due to the extreme conditions of World War II. Offspring of women who were malnourished in their third trimester suffered the most profound effects, evincing significant increases in the incidence of glucose intolerance, type 2 diabetes, and cardiovascular disease as adults.[9,18]

The mechanisms underlying the association between the prenatal environment and postnatal metabolic disease are incompletely understood, although it is now apparent that low birth weight can be viewed as one type of fetal adaptation to an 'adverse' intrauterine environment or portends of prenatal programming for an intended postnatal life of thrift.[19] Animal models have demonstrated that the development of the fetal pancreas is sensitive to prenatal programming and alterations in beta cell development contribute to postnatal metabolic dysfunction. Although pancreatic beta cell dysfunction is a strong predictor of diabetes, attempts to show the presence of a beta cell defect that is attributable to programming in human populations have been controversial. Studies have shown that either low birth weight is correlated with a reduction in pancreatic function[6,11] or that no relationship exists.[8,12] In animal models, however, poor fetal nutrition has been associated with the prevalence of impaired beta cell growth and function, and it appears that fetal adaptations to the adverse intrauterine environment contribute to permanent alterations in pancreatic function.[5,19–21]

THE ENDOCRINE PANCREAS

To understand the possible mechanisms by which changes in the intrauterine environment could influence beta cell programming, knowledge of normal pancreatic development and the factors driving morphological change and differentiation of endocrine cells is required.

The endocrine cells of the pancreas reside in the islets of Langerhans and account for approximately 2% of the total volume of the pancreas. Four islet cell types have been identified; alpha (α) cells primarily secrete glucagon, beta (β) cells secrete insulin, delta (δ) cells secrete somatostatin, and PP cells secrete pancreatic polypeptide. The beta cells are the most common endocrine cell type and account for 60–75% of the cells in the islets. Beta cells are generally located in the center of each islet surrounded by other endocrine cells. Insulin and glucagon are powerful regulators of metabolism, coordinating levels of endogenous glucose, free fatty acids and amino acids (for review see ref. 22).

Ontogeny of the endocrine pancreas

During embryologic development, the pancreas arises from the outpouching of the midgut endoderm as two pancreatic buds, dorsal and ventral, in the duodenal area.[23] As the duodenum rotates and becomes C-shaped, the ventral bud migrates and ventral and dorsal buds fuse to form the final pancreas with the formation of highly branched acini and ducts.[24] Endocrine cells are present at early stages of pancreatic bud development; within the first 10 embryonic days of development in the mouse and at approximately 5 weeks of gestation in the human. Initially the immature islet cells are arranged individually or in small clusters, in close proximity to the pancreatic ducts. In general, endocrine cells in many species, including primates and rodents, develop from duct-like cells in the embryo, fetus and neonate, leading to the formation of primitive islets in the mesenchyme adjacent to the ducts.[25] Once maturity is reached the islets differentiate into an outer mantle of alpha cells and an inner mass of beta and delta cells, surrounded by connective tissue and distinctly separated from the ducts.[26] In the human fetus, this maturational process nears completion by early in the third trimester. Lineage progression of endocrine cells in the developing pancreas has been described in a number of reviews.[22,27,28] In the mouse, the first endocrine precursor cells expressing glucagon are present in the dorsal pancreatic bud as early as 9.5 days of gestation, followed by insulin-expressing cells a day later. After branching, somatostatin-positive cells appear and the exocrine acini become branched. Later in gestation, PP-positive cells appear.[28–30] Although endocrine cells are apparent very early in gestation, islets do not form until the end of gestation.[31,32]

The ability to increase beta cell mass is critical for the increasing insulin demands of the growing fetus late in gestation.[33–35] The ontogeny of islet cells in early life involves a balance between beta cell replication, neogenesis, and programmed cell death (apoptosis). A transient wave of apoptosis occurs in neonatal rat islets between 9 and 16 days of postnatal age and has been localized to the beta cells.[36,37] A new population of beta cells compensates for this loss. This remodeling event also occurs in the human fetal pancreas in the perinatal period.[38] Interestingly, in rats this apoptotic event coincides with a significant decrease in insulin-like growth factor II (IGF-II) expression in rat pancreatic tissue 2 weeks after birth.[39] Overexpression of IGF-II in transgenic mice resulted in a significantly lower number of apoptotic cells in the beta cells of mice pancreata and greater mean islet area,[40] suggesting that IGF-II is a growth factor that protects beta cells from apoptosis. This balance between neogenesis and apoptosis represents a period in which pancreatic remodeling is occurring, with apoptotic cells being replaced through the neogenesis of beta cells from the ductal epithelium. This partial replacement of beta cells is proposed to create a new cell population of 'adult phenotype' beta cells, which are nonproliferative and suited to metabolic control later in life.[26,31] Although some regenerative ability remains during neonatal life, the ability to further remodel pancreatic islets declines with age to the point where only low levels of replication are possible in the adult pancreas.[25,26] Any environmental modification that adversely affects the maturing beta cell popula-

tion before completion of pancreatic development could have lasting effects on the offspring's ability to meet insulin requirements into adult life.

Transcription factors regulating fetal pancreatic development

Recent reviews have described the role of a number of transcription factor families that signal differentiation of islet cells.[26,28,30,41–43] Of particular interest to this chapter are those transcription and growth factors that influence beta cell proliferation and differentiation.

In the rodent, pancreatic endocrine cells are derived from a common precursor stem cell.[44,45] This concept is supported by the coexistence of pancreatic hormone immunoreactivities in the islet cells of human, mice, and guinea pig pancreata.[45,46] The development of endocrine precursor cells is regulated by a number of transcription factor and growth factor families that interact together to regulate endocrine and exocrine tissue differentiation (Figure 7.1).[31,32] Endoderm in the region of the ventral pancreatic precursor cell line has

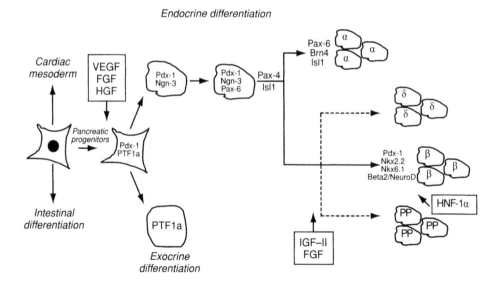

Figure 7.1 Endoderm in the region of the ventral pancreatic precursor cell line has three potential fates: cardiac mesoderm, intestinal differentiation, and pancreatic progenitor cells. Ptf1a and Pdx-1 positive progenitors give rise to all mature pancreatic cell types. Islet progenitors differentiate from the pools of Ptf1a and Pdx-1 positive cells through the induction of transcription factor neurogenin-3 (Ngn-3), and the repression of others, and all mature islet cells arise from these progenitors. Exocrine tissue differentiation occurs through the repression of Ngn-3 expression and continued expression of Ptf1a. Pax-6 is initially expressed in all pancreatic endocrine cells and in its absence the development of all endocrine lineages is affected. Pax-4 is required for the formation of alpha (α) and beta (β) cells. Recent hypotheses suggest that alpha cell differentiation is brought about through the expression of Brn4, Isl1, and Pax-6 and the repression of other factors. The differentiation of beta cells is determined by a sequence of events involving the expression of Pax-6 and Isl1, inactivation of Ngn-3 and the subsequent expression of Pdx-1, Nkx2.2, Nkx6.1, and Pax-4. (Figure based on data adapted from refs 30, 32, 42, 43, 48, 49.)

three potential fates: cardiac mesoderm, intestinal differentiation, and pancreatic progenitor cells. Ptf1a- and Pdx-1-positive progenitors give rise to all mature pancreatic cell types. Duct cells arise from a distinct cell lineage. Pdx-1 is one of the earliest markers of pancreatic bud cells and is necessary for the development of all three types of pancreatic tissue: exocrine, endocrine, and ductal.[30,47,48] Pdx-1 expression is also known to transactivate the insulin gene promoter to enhance insulin secretion of beta cells in the adult pancreas. It is found more diffusely in the pancreas during differentiation but later becomes restricted to mature beta cells. In animal experiments with a targeted deletion of Pdx-1, pancreatic ducts form, but no further endocrine differentiation or morphological changes occur.[49]

Islet progenitors differentiate from the pools of Ptf1a- and Pdx-1-positive cells through the induction of transcription factor neurogenin-3 (Ngn-3) (and the repression of others; see ref. 43 for review) and all mature islet cells arise from these progenitors. Exocrine tissue differentiation occurs through the repression of Ngn-3 and continued expression of Ptf1a.[30,43] It appears that the presence of early factors is sufficient for alpha cell differentiation (in the presence of Ngn-3), but differentiation of the other three cell types (beta, delta, and PP) is determined by transcription factors expressed later in gestation.[43] The Pax gene family is a group of nine transcription factors, which are essential to endocrine cell differentiation. Pax-6 is initially expressed in all pancreatic endocrine cells and, in its absence, the development of all endocrine lineages is affected.[30] Targeted Pax-6 deletions in mice result in a decrease in the numbers of all islet cells, although alpha cells in particular are completely abolished. Mutations of the Pax-4 gene in mice cause a complete loss of pancreatic beta and delta cells but an increased number of alpha cells. If both genes are absent, then no mature endocrine cells develop.[26,30] Recent hypotheses suggest that alpha cell differentiation is brought about through the expression of Brn4, Isl1, and Pax-6 and the repression of other factors. The differentiation of beta cells is determined by a sequence of events involving the expression of Pax-6 and Isl1, inactivation of Ngn-3 and the subsequent expression of Pdx-1, Nkx2.2, Nkx6.1, and Pax-4.[42,43]

Endocrine and growth factors regulating fetal pancreatic development

Proliferation and differentiation of beta cells is dependent upon a number of growth factors including IGFs.[25,31] IGFs have been identified as cellular mito-gens and differentiation factors during development in many fetal tissues.[50] Two isomers of IGFs exist, IGF-I and IGF-II.[51,52] IGF-II mRNA and protein are highly expressed in islet cells and some ductal epithelial cells in late fetal and early neonatal life in rats and humans.[51,53] Over-expression of IGF-II in transgenic mice caused a marked increase in the mean islet size at birth (affecting all endocrine cell types) but without affecting the number of islets, suggesting that IGF-II, while promoting replication does not affect neogenesis of islet cells.[40,54] Both IGF-I and IGF-II are associated with inhibiting apoptosis in other differentiating cell lineages and IGFs also act as survival factors in the pancreas. These actions probably explain the reduction in IGF-II expression that is known to be associated with the wave of apoptosis occurring in the neonatal rat.

The fibroblast growth factors (FGFs) are a family of related peptides, which are mitogenic, angiogenic, and morphogenic for a wide range of tissues in fetal development. Multiple FGFs are present throughout pancreatic development localized to different cell types and expressed at different periods of development. Their expression is associated with sites of beta cell neogenesis and vascular development.[55] FGF-7 appears to have the strongest ability to potentiate beta cell growth, inducing pancreatic duct hyperplasia in adult rats and beta cell neogenesis in mouse embryos.[26,56] Other growth factors also influence pancreatic endocrine development. Vascular endothelial growth factor (VEGF), a potent mitogen for endothelial cells, has been located in pancreatic ductal epithelium and vascular endothelium and has been shown to increase ductal cell replication and insulin content.[57,58] Hepatocyte growth factor (HGF) has been shown in vitro to act as a mitogen for pancreatic ductal epithelial cells as well as beta cells.[26]

Glucocorticoids have been implicated in beta cell mass and phenotype regulation. Glucocorticoid receptors are present in the beta cells of the rat pancreas[59] and glucocorticoid binding sites increase in the neonatal rat pancreas at postnatal day 15, at a time when plasma corticosterone levels rise sharply.[60] Glucocorticoids have been shown to decrease Pdx-1 expression[61] as well as decrease IGF-II expression.[62,63] Therefore, exposure to elevated glucocorticoid concentrations similar to those seen in the neonatal rat at the time of pancreatic remodeling[64] may precipitate a reduction in pancreatic IGF-II and a wave of apoptosis in beta cells within the islet.[26] The availability of glucocorticoids in the pancreas can be regulated by 11β-hydroxysteroid dehydrogenase type 2 (11β-HSD2), which catalyzes the conversion of bioactive glucocorticoids to biologically inactive 11-keto metabolites.

11β-HSD2 is expressed in the pancreas,[65] raising the possibility that altered activity of this enzyme might permit control of local tissue levels of glucocorticoids.

Development of fetal insulin responses to glucose

Data concerning whether or not the fetus is capable of responding to glucose with increased insulin secretion appear conflicting. A number of reports suggest that in the human and rat fetus, insulin release is independent of plasma glucose concentrations. Moreover, insulin release appears to be relatively unresponsive to glucose, but highly responsive to amino acids and agents that increase cAMP levels in the absence of glucose.[23,66] Others suggest that fetal insulin secretion is directly related to fetal glucose concentrations.[34,67] Insulin has been detected in fetal sheep plasma very early in gestation (~40–50 days of gestation) and is present until term (150 days).[67] In vitro and in vivo studies have demonstrated that insulin release can be stimulated by glucose in fetal sheep pancreatic cells and a positive correlation exists between plasma glucose and insulin concentrations.[68–70]

The onset of pancreatic responsiveness appears to be species-specific. It has been suggested in the rodent model that insulin release from the fetal type of islets (prior to the apoptotic event) are poorly responsive to glucose. Shortly after birth in rodents, apoptosis appears to remove fetal-type beta cells, which are replaced with a new adult-type of cells following neogenesis. This new population of cells is now sensitive to glucose with normal insulin release. This development may then prepare the pancreas for postnatal metabolism (for review see ref. 31). The mechanisms regulating these events are unclear, and whether this occurs in other species warrants further investigation.

EXPERIMENTAL MODELS OF DEVELOPMENTAL PROGRAMMING OF THE FETAL PANCREAS

The developmental mechanisms that underlie the relationship between fetal adaptation to intrauterine events and postnatal metabolic dysfunction are clearly multifactorial. Two major models of developmental programming have emerged to explain the increased risk of developing long-term metabolic dysfunction; prenatal undernutrition (reduction in total caloric intake or protein restriction) and prenatal exposure to glucocorticoids.

Undernutrition

One of the most well-studied models of nutrient restriction in animals is maternal protein restriction. Early studies investigating the effects of maternal protein restriction in rats demonstrated that the developing fetal pancreas suffers long-term consequences as a result of the prenatal manipulation. Maternal protein restriction throughout pregnancy has been reported to cause fetal growth reduction, altered glucose tolerance, and hypertension in adult offspring[71–74] and abnormal pancreatic development that includes reduced insulin content and islet size, reduced islet vascularization and blood flow, beta cell number and insulin content, and impaired secretory responses to glucose and arginine.[75–79]

Maternal protein restriction has been demonstrated to alter pancreatic remodeling as well. Offspring of rats fed a low protein diet during pregnancy had significantly greater levels of pancreatic islet apoptosis and diminished levels of IGF-II mRNA levels.[80] Protein restriction may contribute, therefore, to changes in the balance of beta cell replication and apoptosis in fetal and neonatal life, and thus contribute to impaired insulin release observed later in life.

More recent studies have begun to unravel some of the regulatory processes underlying these alterations in pancreatic, and more specifically, beta cell development and function. Glucose-induced first and second phases of insulin secretion were drastically reduced in cultured islets from offspring of protein-restricted pregnant rats. The insulin response to individual amino acids was also significantly reduced. These poor secretory responses were associated with altered calcium handling of the protein restricted islets.[81] Intrauterine protein restriction may also influence long-term pancreatic glucose sensing. A recent study demonstrated that islets of offspring exposed to low protein in utero have reduced glucokinase (low affinity glucose phosphorylating enzyme) expression levels and affinity, resulting in effects on glucose homeostatic mechanisms.[82]

Some advances have been made in regards to the understanding of nutritional regulation of pancreatic programming. In early studies, Professor Joseph Hoet and colleagues proposed the importance of taurine in pancreatic programming and function. Taurine, a sulfur-containing amino acid found in most mammalian tissue, plays an integral role in fetal development (for review see ref. 83). A low protein diet in pregnant rats modifies the levels of specific amino acids, such as taurine, in the mother and the fetus.[84,85] Plasma levels of taurine in the fetus appear to be the main predictor of fetal plasma insulin levels.[85] Cherif et al. demonstrated that a low protein diet during pregnancy in the rat resulted in a reduction in the *in vitro* release of insulin upon stimulation with a secretagogue (leucine). The addition of taurine increased the release of insulin from the control islets in response to arginine or leucine, but it did not restore the reduced responsiveness of low protein islets to these amino acids. However, when taurine was added to the drinking water of low protein-fed dams throughout gestation, circulating taurine concentrations of dams and fetuses were increased and the release of insulin was restored to control levels.[86] In a similar study, Merezak et al. demonstrated that taurine supplementation of pregnant rats fed a low protein diet was protective against interleukin and nitric oxide-induced apoptosis.[87] These observations suggest that specific nutritional components influence the developmental programming of the endocrine pancreas.

The regulation of transcription factors is also influenced by intrauterine protein deficiency. Pdx-1 protein levels were significantly decreased in neonatal rat pancreatic tissue after exposure to a low protein diet during gestation. This reduction was associated with a reduction in islet area and a reduction in *in vitro* stimulated insulin secretion. Interestingly, the reintroduction of a normal diet early in life restored islet area and insulin secretion.[88] These observations suggest that in the period immediately following birth, neonatal rat pancreatic islets are still adaptable and can be 'rescued' by nutritional manipulation. It is possible that nutrient supplementation to pregnant mothers could have long-term benefits for the developing fetus and impact on later metabolic capacity.

Pancreatic endocrine cell lineage may also be vulnerable to developmental programming. Recently, Joanette and colleagues published an elegant study investigating the effects of a low protein diet during pregnancy on the development of pancreatic progenitor cells and pancreatic endocrine cell lineage. In this study, pregnant rats were exposed to either a control or low protein diet for 20 days during gestation. Additional groups of control or low protein-fed animals were supplemented with taurine. Pancreatic progenitor cells or cells contributing to the endocrine pancreas were identified using cellular markers known to be associated with endocrine cells: nestin, CD34 and c-kit. Nestin is an intermediate filament protein known to be involved with the development of the central nervous system and is expressed in neuroepithelial stem cells, developing human myocytes, and in the gastrointestinal tract.[89] It has been suggested that nestin is expressed in putative endocrine progenitor cells in the pancreas.[90] In low protein-fed animals, islet area was smaller due to a reduction in beta cells.

Nestin-positive cell number was associated with the area of beta cells. Significantly lower numbers of nestin-positive cells and a reduction in nestin mRNA levels were found in endocrine cells of fetal and postnatal pancreatic tissue of low protein offspring. CD34-positive and Pdx-1-positive cells were similarly reduced. Supplementation of pregnant and lactating rats fed a low protein diet with taurine resulted in a recovery of mean islet area and the number of cells immunopositive for nestin (Figures 7.2 and 7.3).[91] These data further indicate a role for specific nutrients in programming the pancreas during development.

Glucocorticoids

Glucocorticoid exposure *in utero* may also be a contributing factor to the programming of the fetal pancreas and beta cell development.[26] In addition to acting directly on ductal epithelial cells and beta cell proliferation,[31] glucocorticoids have been shown to regulate important transcription factors involved in pancreatic growth and remodeling, such as Pdx-1.[25,92] Moreover, glucocorticoids have been shown to regulate fetal IGF-II,[63] contributing to changes in pancreatic beta cell apoptosis and remodeling (as described previously).

A number of studies have suggested that fetal glucocorticoid exposure can alter pancreatic development and contribute to changes in metabolic function. Administration of dexamethasone to female sheep early in pregnancy (40–41 days of gestation), resulted in elevated basal and stimulated insulin levels in the fetus at 135 days of gestation.[93] Maternal treatment with carbenoxolone, a placental 11β-HSD2 inhibitor, allows increased passage of maternal glucocorticoids to the fetus,[94] and resulted in reduced birth weight in rats.[95] Adult male offspring in this study had altered glucose tolerance. Lindsay and colleagues were able to demonstrate that maternal adrenalectomy prevented this effect, supporting the role of fetal exposure to maternally derived glucocorticoids in the programming of metabolic function.[95]

Over the last decade, our group has conducted a series of experiments designed to evaluate the maturational effect of prenatal glucocorticoids on postnatal lung function and on fetal and postnatal HPA function and glucose tolerance. In our model, pregnant ewes are randomized to receive either single or multiple doses of 0.5 mg/kg betamethasone or saline placebo at 7-day intervals from 104 to 118 and 124 days of gestation (term is 150 days). This protocol was designed to mimic clinical administration of synthetic glucocorticoids. These studies have shown that prenatal exposure to betamethasone significantly improves neonatal

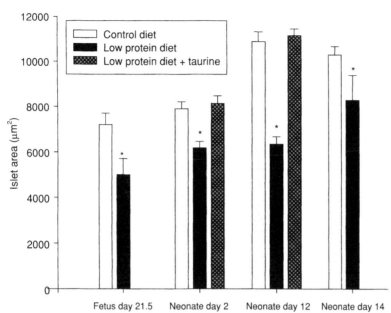

Figure 7.2 Mean area of pancreatic islets in offspring of pregnant rats fed a low protein diet (8%) throughout pregnancy (striped bars) compared to offspring of pregnant rats fed a control diet (20%) (gray bars). Exposure to low protein throughout pregnancy resulted in a significant reduction in the mean islet area of pancreatic tissue in fetuses and infants postpartum. * $p < 0.05$. Offspring of mothers fed a low protein diet with taurine supplementation in the drinking water showed a significant recovery in mean islet area (crosshatched bars). Values are presented as mean +/− SEM. * represents control vs low protein diet ($p < 0.05$). (Data adapted from ref. 91.)

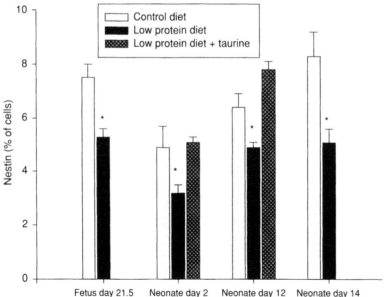

Figure 7.3 Frequency of islet cells immunopositive for nestin in fetal and neonatal pancreatic islets in offspring of pregnant rats fed a low protein diet (8%) throughout pregnancy (striped bars) compared to offspring of pregnant rats fed a control diet (20%) (gray bars). Exposure to low protein throughout pregnancy resulted in a significant reduction in the mean percentage of cells positive for nestin in pancreatic islets in fetal and postnatal offspring. Offspring of mothers fed a low protein diet with taurine supplementation in the drinking water had a significant recovery in nestin staining cells (crosshatched bars). Values are presented as mean +/− SEM. * represents control vs low protein diet ($p < 0.05$). (Data adapted from ref. 91.)

lung function in a dose-dependent manner.[96] However, despite these improvements, birth weight was decreased by 15% after one dose, by 19% after two doses, and by 27% after three doses of maternal betamethasone. Furthermore, offspring that received either single or multiple (four) doses prenatally had increased insulin responses to glucose challenge at 1 year of age, as well as significantly higher insulin to

glucose ratios.[97] These data resemble patterns of insulin resistance observed in humans who later go on to develop type 2 diabetes.

Although there is currently no information regarding fetal or neonatal pancreatic development in sheep, or the effects of prenatal glucocorticoid exposure on this development, it seems likely that the fetal pancreas is programmed by glucocorticoids in a way that predisposes offspring to altered metabolism. In other studies, we observed two populations of islets in fetal sheep pancreatic sections; large irregular immuno-positive islets in addition to smaller conventional type islets. Mean islet area was significantly reduced with advancing gestation in control animals (Figure 7.4). The fetuses of betamethasone-treated ewes did not demonstrate any changes in islet size with advancing gestation (Figure 7.4). Moreover, fetal islet area stained for insulin was significantly elevated in fetuses of mothers treated with betamethasone compared with controls.[98] We have also observed that Pdx-1 expression in islets is suppressed in ovine fetuses of mothers treated with betamethasone (unpublished observations). We speculate that maternal betametha-sone treatment may result in a fetal islet phenotype that may be suboptimal for postnatal metabolism. Shen and colleagues in rat studies have also demon-strated significant alterations in pancreatic beta cell development following fetal glucocorticoid expo-sure.[99] In this study, pregnant rats were treated with dexamethasone during the last week of gestation. Beta cells from offspring at 3 weeks of age had lower insulin expression than controls. Further, Shen et al. demonstrated that *in vitro* treatment of dorsal pancre-atic buds from mouse embryos with dexamethasone resulted in a reduction in the proportion of cells expressing both the transcription factor Pdx-1 and insulin and that after removal of dexamethasone from culture for 4 days there was some recovery of insulin and Pdx-1 cells.[99] It appears, therefore, that prenatal dexamethasone exposure in this model inhibits pan-creatic insulin expression, most likely through the inhibition of Pdx-1 expression.

CLINICAL IMPLICATIONS AND CONCLUSIONS

The relationship between low birth weight and the emergence of chronic disease later in life has led to the development of the 'thrifty phenotype hypothesis'.[19] This concept proposes that the fetus is programmed for the metabolic life the mother signals that it may live. For example, in an environment of poor nutri-tion, adaptations are made to the metabolic function-ing of the fetus which would optimize its survival in a postnatal world requiring thrift. This concept also describes the process by which individuals and cul-tures are impacted by a transition from traditional

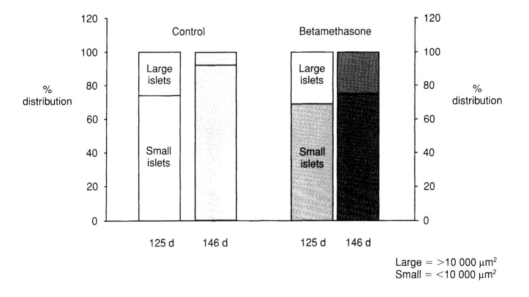

Figure 7.4 Histograms representing islet size distribution according to area in fetuses of pregnant sheep treated with three doses of betamethasone during late gestation compared to mothers treated with saline. Small islets were defined as < 10 000 μm² and large islets as ≥ 10 000 μm². Fetuses of saline-treated mothers are presented on the left and fetuses of betamethasone-treated mothers on the right. Values are presented as percentage distribution. Islet size distribution was significantly altered with advancing gestation in fetuses of saline-treated mothers, but this difference was not found in fetuses of mothers that received betamethasone treatment. d, days of gestation. (Data from ref. 98.)

lives of 'thrift' to more sedentary lives of 'plenty'. In postnatal life, the predisposition conferred by prenatal programming is then amplified or minimized by lifestyle (environment) influences, such as diet and inactivity. It is essential that research begins to unravel the mechanisms underlying the developmental origins of the 'thrifty phenotype', because many developing populations around the world are now undergoing the transition from lives of thrift to lives of plenty, with the associated increased risk for metabolic disease.

Epidemiological and experimental studies show that type 2 diabetes is a chronic disease that perfectly fits this paradigm. The incidence of type 2 diabetes is increasing worldwide and developing countries making the transition from traditional to modern lifestyles have experienced the highest rate of increase.[100] It is predicted that the number of people in India with diabetes could increase from 19 million to 60 million by the year 2025.[101] The increasing rates of type 2 diabetes in developing countries are likely the result of developmental programming for a life of thrift followed by exposure after birth to increased levels of nutrition and inactivity. The transition from a traditional diet (high in carbohydrates) to a modern diet (high in fat) in Pima Indians has been associated with a decrease in oral glucose tolerance, higher plasma cholesterol levels, and lower beta cell sensitivity to glucose. This effect was also seen in Caucasians on a high fat diet within the same environment, but to a lesser extent.[102]

It may be that simple interventions, such as the addition or substraction of micronutrients (perhaps taurine supplementation), or alterations to postnatal lifestyle, can influence developmental programming and the occurrence of chronic disease. However, the application of these interventions awaits the development of more complete understanding of the mechanisms responsible for these associations.

REFERENCES

1. Barker DJP, Hales CN, Fall CHD et al. Type 2 (non-insulin-dependent) diabetes melllitus, hypertension and hyperlipidemia (syndrome X): relation to reduced fetal growth. Diabetologia 1993; 36: 62–7.
2. Barker DJP. In utero programming of chronic disease. Clin Sci 1998; 95: 115–28.
3. Osmond C, Barker DJP, Winter PD, Fall CHD, Simmonds SJ. Early growth and death from cardiovascular disease in women. BMJ 1993; 307: 1519–24.
4. McCance DR, Pettitt DJ, Hanson RL et al. Birth weight and non-insulin dependent diabetes: thrifty genotype, thrifty phenotype, or surviving small baby genotype. BMJ 1994; 308: 942–5.
5. Van Assche AF, De Prins F, Aerts L, Verjans M. The endocrine pancreas in small for dates infants. BJOG 1977; 84: 751–3.
6. Hales CN, Barker DJP, Clark PMS et al. Fetal and infant growth and impaired glucose tolerance at age 64. BMJ 1991; 303: 1019–22.
7. Phipps K, Barker DJP, Hales CN, Fall CHD, Osmond C, Clark PMS. Fetal growth and impaired glucose tolerance in men and women. Diabetologia 1993; 36: 225–8.
8. Lithell HO, McKeigue PM, Berglund L et al. Relation of size at birth to non-insulin dependent diabetes and insulin concentrations in men aged 50–60 years. BMJ 1996; 312: 406–10.
9. Ravelli ACJ, van der Meulen JHP, Michels RPJ et al. Glucose tolerance in adults after prenatal exposure to famine. Lancet 1998; 351: 173–7.
10. Barker DJ. The developmental origins of adult disease. Eur J Epidemiol 2003; 18: 733–6.
11. Robinson S, Walton RJ, Clark PMS et al. The relation of fetal growth to plasma glucose in young men. Diabetologia 1992; 35: 444–6.
12. Phillips DIW, Hirst S, Clark PMS, Hales CN, Osmond C. Fetal growth and insulin secretion in adult life. Diabetologia 1994; 37: 592–6.
13. Hales CN, Ozanne SE. The dangerous road of catch-up growth. J Physiol (Lond) 2003; 547: 5–10.
14. Veening MA, van Weissenbruch MM, Delemarre-van de Waal HA. Glucose tolerance, insulin sensitivity, and insulin secretion in children born small for gestational age. J Clin Endocrinol Metab 2002; 87: 4657–61.
15. Veening MA, van Weissenbruch MM, Heine RJ, Delemarre-van de Waal HA. β-Cell capacity and insulin sensitivity in prepubertal children born small for gestational age: influence of body size during childhood. Diabetes 2003; 52: 1756–60.
16. Levitt NS, Lambert EV, Woods D et al. Impaired glucose tolerance and elevated blood pressure in low birth weight, nonobese, young South African adults: early programming of cortisol axis. J Clin Endocrinol Metab 2000; 85: 4611–18.
17. Reaven GM. Role of insulin resistance in human disease. Diabetes 1988; 37: 1595–607.
18. Roseboom TJ, van der Meulen JH, Ravelli AC et al. Effects of prenatal exposure to the Dutch famine on adult disease in later life: an overview. Mol Cell Endocrinol 2001; 185: 93–8.
19. Hales CN, Barker DJP. Type 2 (non-insulin-dependent) diabetes mellitus: the thrifty phenotype hypothesis. Diabetologia 1992; 35: 595–601.
20. Holemans K, Aerts L, Assche FAV. Lifetime consequences of abnormal fetal pancreatic development. J Physiol (Lond) 2003; 547: 11–20.
21. Hoet JJ. Influence of dietary changes on the development of the fetal pancreas – consequences later in life. Isr J Med Sci 1991; 27: 423–4.
22. Murtaugh LC, Melton DA. Genes, signals, and lineages in pancreas development. Annu Rev Cell Dev Biol 2003; 19: 71–89.
23. Dubois PM. Ontogeny of the endocrine pancreas. Horm Res 1989; 32: 53–60.
24. Blackburn ST, Loper DL. Maternal, Fetal and Neonatal Physiology. A Clinical Perspective. 1st edn. Philadelphia: WB Saunders, 1992.
25. Hill DJ, Petrik J, Arany E. Growth factors and the regulation of fetal growth. Diabetes Care 1998; 21(2S): 60B–69B.
26. Hill DJ. Fetal programming of the pancreatic β cells and the implications for postnatal diabetes. Semin Neonatol 1999; 4: 99–113.

27. Bouwens L. Islet morphogenesis and stem cell markers. Cell Biochem Biophys 2004; 40 (3 Suppl): 81–8.

28. Teitelman G. Islet-derived multipotential cells/progenitor cells. Cell Biochem Biophys 2004; 40 (3 Suppl): 89–102.

29. Herrera PL, Huarte J, Sanvito F et al. Embryogenesis of the murine endocrine pancreas; early expression of pancreatic polypeptide gene. Development 1991; 113: 1257–65.

30. Merino PL. Developmental biology of the pancreas. Cell Biochem Biophys 2004; 40 (3 Suppl): 127–42.

31. Hill DJ, Duvillie B. Pancreatic development and adult diabetes. Pediatr Res 2000; 48: 269–74.

32. Sander M, German MS. The β cell transcription factors and development of the pancreas. J Mol Med 1997; 75: 327–40.

33. Hay WW, Sparks JW. Placental, fetal, and neonatal carbohydrate metabolism. Clin Obstet Gynecol 1985; 28: 473–85.

34. Fowden AL. The role of insulin in prenatal growth. J Dev Physiol 1989; 12: 173–82.

35. Dornhorst A, Nicholls JS, Ali K et al. Fetal proinsulin and birth weight. Diabetes Med 1994; 11: 177–81.

36. Finegood DT, Scaglia L, Bonner-Weir S. Dynamics of β-cell mass in the growing rat pancreas: estimation with a simple mathematical model. Diabetes 1995; 44: 249–56.

37. Scaglia L, Cahill CJ, Finegood DT, Bonner-Weir S. Apoptosis participates in the remodeling of the endocrine pancreas in the neonatal rat. Endocrinology 1997; 138: 1736–41.

38. Kassem SA, Ariel I, Thornton PS, Scheimberg I, Glaser B. Beta-cell proliferation and apoptosis in the developing normal human pancreas and in hyperinsulinism of infancy. Diabetes 2000; 49: 1325–33.

39. Petrik J, Arany E, McDonald TJ, Hill DJ. Apoptosis in the pancreatic islet cells of the neonatal rat is associated with a reduced expression of insulin-like growth factor II that may act as a survival factor. Endocrinology 1998; 139: 2994–3004.

40. Hill DJ, Strutt B, Zaina AS, Coukell S, Graham CF. Increased and persistent circulating insulin-like growth factor II in neonatal transgenic mice suppresses developmental apoptosis in the pancreatic islets. Endocrinology 2000; 141: 1151–7.

41. Schwitzgebel VM. Programming of the pancreas. Mol Cell Endocrinol 2001; 185: 99–108.

42. Wilson ME, Scheel D, German MS. Gene expression cascades in pancreatic development. Mech Dev 2003; 120: 65–80.

43. Ball SG, Barber TM. Molecular development of the pancreatic beta cell: implications for cell replacement therapy. Trends Endocrinol Metab 2003; 14: 349–55.

44. Sanchez D, Moriscot C, Marchand S et al. Developmental gene expression and immunohistochemical study of the human endocrine pancreas during fetal life. Horm Res 1998; 50: 258–63.

45. De Krijger RR, Aanstoot HJ, Kranenburg G et al. The midgestational human fetal pancreas contains cells co-expressing islet hormones. Dev Biol 1992; 153: 368–75.

46. Reddy S, Biddy NJ, Elliott RB. An immunocytochemical study of endocrine cell development in the early fetal guinea pig pancreas. Gen Comp Endocrinol 1992; 86: 275–83.

47. Slack JM. Developmental biology of the pancreas. Development 1995; 121: 1569–80.

48. Gu G, Dubauskaite J, Melton DA. Direct evidence for the pancreatic lineage: NGN3+ cells are islet progenitors and are distinct from duct progenitors. Development 2002; 129: 2447–57.

49. Ahlgren U, Jonsson J, Jonsson L, Simu K, Edlund H. Beta-cell-specific inactivation of the mouse Ipf1/Pdx1 gene results in loss of the beta-cell phenotype and maturity onset diabetes. Genes Dev 1998; 12: 1763–8.

50. D'Ercole AJ. Somatomedins/insulin-like growth factors and fetal growth. J Dev Physiol 1987; 9: 481–95.

51. Hogg J, Hill DJ, Han VKM. The ontology of insulin-like growth factor (IGF) and IGF-binding protein gene expression in the rat pancreas. J Mol Endocrinol 1994; 13: 49–58.

52. Hogg J, Han VKM, Clemmons DR, Hill DJ. Interactions of nutrients, insulin-like growth factors (IGFs) and IGF-binding proteins in the regulation of DNA synthesis by isolated fetal rat islets of Langerhans. J Endocrinol 1993; 138: 401–12.

53. Han VKM, Lund PK, Lee DC, D'Ercole AJ. Expression of somatomedin/insulin-like growth factor messenger ribonucleic acids in the human fetus: identification, characterization, and tissue distribution. J Clin Endocrinol Metab 1988; 66: 422–9.

54. Petrik J, Pell JM, Arany E et al. Over expression of insulin-like growth factor-II in transgenic mice is associated with pancreatic islet cell hyperplasia. Endocrinology 1999; 140: 2353–63.

55. Arany E, Hill DJ. Ontogeny of fibroblast growth factors in the early development of the rat endocrine pancreas. Pediatr Res 2000; 48: 389–403.

56. Fowden AL, Hill DJ. Intra-uterine programming of the endocrine pancreas. Br Med Bull 2001; 60: 123–42.

57. Oberg-Welsh C, Sandler S, Andersson A, Welsh M. Effects of vascular endothelial growth factor on pancreatic duct cell replication and the insulin production of fetal islet-like cell clusters in vitro. Mol Cell Endocrinol 1997; 126: 125–32.

58. Kuroda M, Oka T, Oka Y et al. Colocalization of vascular endothelial growth factor (vascular permeability factor) and insulin in pancreatic islet cells. J Clin Endocrinol Metab 1995; 80: 3196–200.

59. Fischer B, Rausch U, Wollny P et al. Immunohistochemical localization of the glucocorticoid receptor in pancreatic β-cells of the rat. Endocrinology 1990; 126: 2635–41.

60. Lu RB, Lebenthal E, Lee PC. Developmental changes of glucocorticoid receptors in the rat pancreas. J Steroid Biochem Mol Biol 1987; 26: 213–18.

61. Sharma S, Jhala US, Johnson T et al. Hormonal regulation of an islet specific enhancer in the pancreatic homeobox gene STF-1. Mol Cell Biol 1997; 17: 2598–604.

62. Price WA, Stiles AD, Moats-Staats BM, D'Ercole AJ. Gene expression of insulin-like growth factors (IGFs), the type 1 IGF receptor, and IGF binding proteins in dexamethasone induced fetal growth retardation. Endocrinology 1992; 130: 1424–32.

63. Li J, Saunders JC, Gilmour RS, Silver M, Fowden AL. Insulin-like growth factor II messenger ribonucleic acid expression in fetal tissues of the sheep during late gestation: effects of cortisol. Endocrinology 1993; 132: 2083–9.

64. Sapolsky RM, Meaney M. Maturation of the adrenocortical stress response: neuroendocrine control mechanisms and the stress hyporesponsive period. Brain Res Rev 1986; 11: 65–76.

65. Albiston AL, Obeyesekere VR, Smith RE, Krozowski Z. Cloning and tissue distribution of the human 11 beta-hydroxysteroid dehydrogenase type 2 enzyme. Mol Cell Endocrinol 1994; 105: R11–R17.

66. Simpson AM, Tuch BE. Control of insulin biosynthesis in the human fetal beta cell. Pancreas 1995; 11: 48–54.

67. Alexander DP, Britton HG, Cohen NM, Nixon DA, Parker RA. Insulin concentrations in the fetal plasma and fetal fluids of the sheep. J Endocrinol 1968; 40: 389–90.

68. Bassett JM, Thorburn GD. The regulation of insulin secretion by the ovine foetus in utero. J Endocrinol 1971; 50: 59–74.
69. Philipps AF, Carson RS, Meschia G, Battaglia FC. Insulin secretion in fetal and newborn sheep. Am J Physiol 1978; 235: E467–E474.
70. Gresores A, Anderson S, Hood D, Zerbe GO, Hay WW. Separate and joint effects of arginine and glucose on ovine fetal insulin secretion. Am J Physiol 1997; 272: E68–E73.
71. Langley-Evans SC. Hypertension induced by fetal exposure to a maternal low protein diet in the rat is prevented by pharmacological blockade of maternal glucocorticoid synthesis. J Hypertens 1997; 15: 537–44.
72. Holness MJ. Impact of early growth retardation on glucoregulatory control and insulin action in mature rats. Am J Physiol 1996; 270: E946–E954.
73. Langley-Evans SC, Phillips GJ, Benediktsson R et al. Protein intake in pregnancy, placental glucocorticoid metabolism and the programming of hypertension in the rat. Placenta 1996; 17: 169–72.
74. Langley-Evans SC, Nwagwu M. Impaired growth and increased glucocorticoid sensitive enzyme activities in tissues of rat fetuses exposed to maternal low protein diets. Life Sci 1998; 63: 605–15.
75. Dahri S, Snoek A, Reusens-Billen B, Remacle C, Hoet JJ. Islet function in offspring of mothers on low-protein diet during gestation. Diabetes 1991; 40 (Suppl 2): 115–20.
76. Snoeck A, Remacle C, Reusens B, Hoet JJ. Effect of a low-protein diet during pregnancy and the fetal rat endocrine pancreas. Biol Neonate 1990; 57: 107–18.
77. Dahri S, Reusens B, Remacle C, Hoet JJ. Nutritional influences on pancreatic development and potential links with non-insulin-dependent diabetes. Proc Nutr Soc 1995; 54: 345–56.
78. Iglesias-Barreira V, Ahn MT, Reusens B, Dahri S, Hoet JJ, Remacle C. Pre- and postnatal low protein diet affect pancreatic islet blood flow and insulin release in adult rats. Endocrinology 1996; 137: 3797–801.
79. Berney DM, Desai M, Greenwald S et al. The effects of maternal protein deprivation on the fetal rat pancreas: major structural changes and their recuperation. J Pathol 1997; 183: 109–15.
80. Petrik J, Reusens B, Arany E et al. A low protein diet alters the balance of islet cell replication and apoptosis in the fetal and neonatal rat and is associated with a reduced pancreatic expression of insulin-like growth factor-II. Endocrinology 1999; 140: 4861–73.
81. Latorraca MQ, Mello EMCAR, Boschero AC. Reduced insulin secretion in response to nutrients in islets from malnourished young rats is associated with a diminished calcium uptake. J Nutr Biochem 1999; 10: 37–43.
82. Heywood WE, Mian N, Milla PJ, Lindley KJ. Programming of defective rat pancreatic beta-cell function in offspring from mothers fed a low-protein diet during gestation and the suckling periods. Clin Sci (Lond) 2004; 107: 37–45.
83. Sturman JA. Taurine in development. Physiol Rev 1993; 73: 119–47.
84. Reusens B, Dahri S, Bennis-Taleb N, Remacle C, Hoet JJ. Long term consequences of diabetes and its complications may have a fetal origin: experimental and epidemiological evidence. Diabetes 1995; 35: 187–98.
85. Bertin E, Gangnerau M-N, Bellon G et al. Development of beta-cell mass in fetuses of rats deprived of protein and/or energy in last trimester of pregnancy. Am J Physiol Regul Integr Comp Physiol 2002; 283: R623–630.

86. Cherif H, Reusens B, Ahn M, Hoet J, Remacle C. Effects of taurine on the insulin secretion of rat fetal islets from dams fed a low-protein diet. J Endocrinol 1998; 159: 341–8.
87. Merezak S, Hardikar A, Yajnik C, Remacle C, Reusens B. Intrauterine low protein diet increases fetal beta-cell sensitivity to NO and IL-1 beta: the protective role of taurine. J Endocrinol 2001; 171: 299–308.
88. Arantes VC, Teixeira VP, Reis MA et al. Expression of PDX-1 is reduced in pancreatic islets from pups of rat dams fed a low protein diet during gestation and lactation. J Nutr 2002; 132: 3030–5.
89. Humphrey RK, Bucay N, Beattie GM et al. Characterization and isolation of promoter-defined nestin-positive cells from the human fetal pancreas. Diabetes 2003; 52: 2519–25.
90. Yashpal NK, Li J, Wang R. Characterization of c-Kit and nestin expression during islet cell development in the prenatal and postnatal rat pancreas. Dev Dyn 2004; 229: 813–25.
91. Joanette EA, Reusens B, Arany E et al. Low-protein diet during early life causes a reduction in the frequency of cells immunopositive for nestin and CD34 in both pancreatic ducts and islets in the rat. Endocrinology 2004; 145: 3004–13.
92. Sander M, Neubuser A, Kalamaras J, Ee HC, Martin GR, German MS. Genetic analysis reveals that PAX-6 is required for normal transcription of pancreatic hormone genes and islet development. Genes Dev 1997; 11: 1662–73.
93. Cox DB, Brubaker P, Fraser M, Whittle W, Challis JRG. The effect of maternal dexamethasone during early pregnancy on fetal growth, HPA development and the control of glucose homeostasis. J Soc Gynecol Investig 1999; 6 (1 Suppl): 110A.
94. Whorwood CB, Sheppard MC, Stewart PM. Licorice inhibits 11β hydroxysteroid dehydrogenase messenger ribonucleic acid levels and potentiates glucocorticoid hormone action. Endocrinology 1993; 132: 2287–92.
95. Lindsay RS, Lindsay RM, Waddell BJ, Seckl JR. Prenatal glucocorticoid exposure lead to offspring hyperglycemia in the rat: studies with the 11β hydroxysteroid dehydrogenase inhibitor carbenoxolone. Diabetologia 1996; 39: 1299–305.
96. Ikegami M, Jobe AH, Newnham J et al. Repetitive prenatal glucocorticoids improve lung function and decrease growth in preterm lambs. Am J Respir Crit Care Med 1997; 156: 178–84.
97. Moss TJ, Sloboda DM, Gurrin LC et al. Programming effects in sheep of prenatal growth restriction and glucocorticoid exposure. Am J Physiol 2001; 281: R960–R970.
98. Sloboda DM, Newnham J, Challis JR. Maternal betamethasone administration and fetal pancreatic development. Journal of the Society for Gynecological Investigation 2002; 9: 290A.
99. Shen CN, Seckl JR, Slack JM, Tosh D. Glucocorticoids suppress beta-cell development and induce hepatic metaplasia in embryonic pancreas. Biochem J 2003; 375 (Pt 1): 41–50.
100. Abate N, Chandalia M. Ethnicity and type 2 diabetes: focus on Asian Indians. J Diabetes Complications 2001; 15(6): 320–7.
101. Chatterjee P. India sees parallel rise in malnutrition and obesity. Lancet 2002; 360(9349): 1948.
102. Swinburn BA, Nyomba BL, Saad MF et al. Insulin resistance associated with lower rates of weight gain in Pima Indians. J. Clin Invest 1991; 88(1): 168–73.

8

Perinatal programming of metabolic homeostasis

Julie A Owens, Kathryn L Gatford, Miles J De Blasio, Dane M Horton, Karen L Kind, and Jeffrey S Robinson

INTRODUCTION

The incidence of noninsulin-dependent diabetes or type 2 diabetes and obesity is rapidly increasing in Australia and globally.[1,2] These are the most common disorders of metabolic homeostasis and are major contributors to the development of cardiovascular disease. It is increasingly understood that development of type 2 diabetes requires inadequate insulin secretion, as well as insulin resistance, and that obesity contributes to the development of both of these defects. Factors known to influence the risk of type 2 diabetes include the levels of physical activity and caloric intake, while monogenic causes are rare and genetic contributions remain poorly defined. A recent life course study found that in mature adults at least, markers of early life experiences, including fetal and infant growth, could account for a similar proportion of the incidence of the metabolic syndrome as do lifestyle factors, and more than putative genetic factors.[3] Much of the recent global increase in type 2 diabetes and obesity undoubtedly reflects changes in lifestyle.[4] Nevertheless, in developing countries and in particular communities in developed countries with a high prevalence of restricted fetal growth, an interaction between early life and lifestyle factors may be exacerbating the increase in the burden of metabolic disease.

A recent systematic review found that small size at birth for gestational age, indicated by low weight or thinness at birth, is consistently associated with increased risk of type 2 diabetes in populations from developed countries.[5] Obesity is also associated with small size at birth albeit less consistently, but usually positively or, in some cases, in a J- or U-shaped pattern with birth weight, in children and young adults, suggesting that individuals who were heavy at birth are also at risk of obesity.[6] Individuals of low birth weight do have altered body composition, however, with reduced lean tissue mass and increased and altered fat deposition, with more central or abdominal fat.[6] The latter is a stronger predictor of cardiovascular disease than total fat.[7] While both genetic and environmental factors affect size at birth, being small for gestational age (SGA), reflects the failure of a fetus to achieve its genetic potential for growth. This outcome most commonly results from alterations in maternal and placental environmental factors that determine the fetal substrate supply, which lead to restricted oxygen and nutrient delivery and growth of the fetus (Figure 8.1).[8] The prenatal environment and poor substrate supply, in particular, are implicated therefore as initiating factors in development of impaired metabolic homeostasis in later life. In addition to the risks of later disease directly associated with small size at birth, the majority

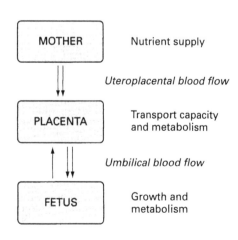

Figure 8.1 Determinants of fetal growth.

of intrauterine growth restricted (IUGR) infants undergo accelerated growth (catch-up growth) from the first few weeks of postnatal life.[9–12] This infant or childhood catch-up growth is an independent risk factor for later development of insulin resistance,[13] type 2 diabetes,[14] obesity,[13,15,16] the central metabolic syndrome[4] and cardiovascular disease.[17,18] There is also evidence that pre- and postnatal factors act synergistically to increase the risk of later metabolic disease, so that the individual who grew poorly before birth is most susceptible to the impact of adverse adult lifestyle factors and obesity (Figure 8.2).[19] These findings have led to the concept that a mismatch between the prenatal and postnatal environments, especially between prenatal deprivation programming of the individual's capacity and subsequent exposure to postnatal abundance, will have the most adverse outcomes. Understanding the initiating factors and causal pathways linking poor fetal growth, infant catch-up growth, and impaired metabolic homeostasis in later life is essential to enable the development of strategies to reduce the impact of these diseases. Here we review what has been learned from human and experimental studies about the nature and mechanistic basis for poor metabolic homeostasis following restricted fetal growth and infant catch-up growth, and comment on future research directions in this area.

CAN THE PERINATAL ENVIRONMENT INFLUENCE ADULT METABOLIC HOMEOSTASIS?

The concept that events in early life might be causally related to later outcomes for health and disease has gained widespread acceptance, since the studies in humans by Barker and others in particular, although the phenomenon had in fact been recognized earlier.[20] Lucas defined this process as 'programming', where an event occurring at a critical period in development has long-lasting effects.[21] This hypothesis has been extended to take account of the potential impact of events before and around conception, to be described as the developmental origins of later disease. Thus, it is proposed that disturbance of the environment in early life at critical stages in the maturation of regulatory systems and their target tissues or their precursors, alters development and affects functional capacity, predisposing or increasing vulnerability to disease in later life.

Some of the earliest evidence that the intrauterine environment could affect subsequent metabolic health derived from geographical associations between high rates of neonatal death and subsequent high rates of coronary heart disease and stroke in the survivors of the same cohort.[22] Subsequent studies in the UK assessed blood pressure and markers of metabolic homeostasis in individuals of known birth weight. Most found that individuals who were light or thin at birth had increased rates of death from cardiovascular disease and also an increased incidence of risk factors for cardiovascular disease, including high blood pressure and type 2 diabetes or markers of insulin resistance.[20] Much larger epidemiological studies,[23,24] originally designed to disprove the 'developmental origins' hypothesis, also reported strong negative associations between size at birth and risks of heart disease and of diabetes. Although the research clearly demonstrated that small size at birth was a risk factor for metabolic and cardiovascular disease in later life, most

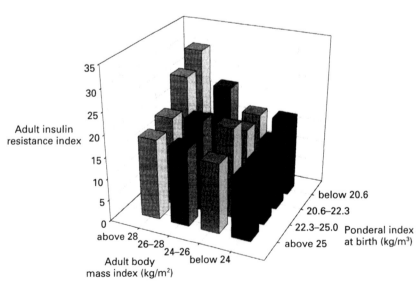

Figure 8.2 Thinness at birth, adult body mass index, and adult insulin resistance. Across the population range in adult fatness (body mass index) in the Preston cohort studied by Phillips, Barker and colleagues, the increase in the insulin resistance index from the thinnest to the fattest adults was 71% in adults who were thinnest at birth but only 31% in adults who were fattest at birth. (Adapted from Phillips et al. 1994.[19])

lacked information on gestational age at birth, and therefore could not distinguish between restricted fetal growth and prematurity as causes of small size at birth and later consequences. The inclusion of gestational age data and information on fetal growth trajectories in contemporary cohorts is assisting in resolving this issue, although many of these cohorts are presently children or young adults, and it will be several decades before their risks for metabolic and cardiovascular disease in later life can be fully assessed. Nevertheless, both small size at birth for gestational age and prematurity are emerging as independent risk factors for later disorders.

The mother's environment, her ability to acquire oxygen and nutrients from this and to transport them to the placenta and in turn, the placenta's functional capacity to deliver these resources to the fetus, all determine substrate supply growth of the fetus (Figure 8.1).[8] Maternal and placental factors are implicated, therefore, in the initiation of developmental programming of later impairment of metabolic homeostasis. Clearly, maternal or placental factors cannot be deliberately perturbed in humans to assess their causal links to later consequences. Experiments of history, however, do offer some insight into these processes. Severe acute maternal undernutrition during the first half of pregnancy in women during the Dutch famine of World War II increased rates of obesity in their offspring as young adult men, and increased body mass index (BMI) in the female but not male offspring in middle age.[25,26] In contrast, offspring of mothers exposed to famine during the last trimester of pregnancy had a reduced incidence of obesity as young men, while BMI in middle-age was unaffected in either sex.[25,26] Maternal exposure to famine in the middle or third trimesters impaired glucose tolerance in offspring as middle-aged

men and women.[27] While fetal exposure to such a delimited and severe maternal undernutrition has few, if any, contemporary equivalents, it does support associations between perturbations of the early life environment and later disease as being causal in nature in the human. These findings also suggest that different aspects of physiological control and homeostasis have a different sensitivity to the timing of at least some perturbations in early life in humans. Both these conclusions are confirmed by extensive experimental studies in other species described below, which demonstrated that interventions in early life that alter or restrict fetal growth, including restriction of maternal feed or protein intake during pregnancy and/or induction of placental insufficiency, will impair metabolic homeostasis in the progeny.

HOW COULD THE PERINATAL ENVIRONMENT INFLUENCE ADULT METABOLIC HOMEOSTASIS?

Perturbations of the fetal environment, such as restriction of substrate supply, induce various metabolic, neural, and endocrine responses by the fetus and placenta, aimed at reducing metabolic demand by slowing growth and redirecting scarce substrates to the most vital organs in order to ensure survival. This altered metabolic and hormonal milieu has consequences for the development and differentiation of key regulatory systems including their effector tissues and targets, and may lead to altered functional capacity longer term. There are a number of potential targets of this developmental programming that could affect insulin action and metabolic control and risk of type 2 diabetes (Table 8.1). Metabolic and glucose homeostasis is determined primarily by insulin action, which is the product of insulin secretion by beta cells of the endocrine pancreas and insulin sensitivity of skeletal muscle and liver and indirectly by that of adipose tissue (Table 8.1). These key processes are affected by the activity of other regulatory axes and systems, including the adipoinsular axis, the hippocampal-hypothalamo-pituitary adrenal (HPA) axis, sympathetic nervous system and appetite regulatory networks, including the leptin axis (Table 8.1). Thus, at the systemic level, there may be changes in production and abundance of circulating hormones related to these axes[5] or in the activation of the sympathetic nervous system,[28] possibly reflecting changes to the sensitivity of endocrine or nerve tissues and cells to their own regulatory signals. In turn, sensitivity of their target or effector tissues and organs may be altered, contributing to an overall impairment of

---

Table 8.1 Known and likely targets of developmental programming mechanisms

Determinants of metabolic homeostasis
- Insulin axis
- Adipoinsular axis
- Hippocampal hypothalamo-pituitary-adrenal axis
- Sympathetic nervous system
- Appetite control and leptin axis

Behaviors affected
- Glucose homeostasis
- Food intake
- Energy expenditure and thermogenesis
- Body composition and adiposity

insulin action. The behaviors and aspects of homeostasis affected by these processes either directly or indirectly impair blood glucose control, including food intake, energy expenditure, thermogenesis and body composition and adiposity (Table 8.1).

The next question is how events in early life can continue to affect the behavior of these body systems throughout life and in humans, decades later? There may be changes in the tissue and cellular components of regulatory systems and their targets, including alterations in cell number, type, and the proportions of different cell types. Changes may occur in tissue structure and vascularity, which has an impact on functional capacity. Finally, there may also be changes in the intrinsic capacity of cells through altered gene expression, which are permanent and add to the consequences of altered extrinsic signals and determinants. The processes that may be involved include altered cell kinetics in early life, such as different rates of cell proliferation and apoptosis. In this way, perturbations of the fetal environment might alter organ size or structure or the proportions of different cell types, as shown in some limited human studies and in many experimental studies.[29] There may also be clonal selection of cells with differing phenotypes arising from spontaneous variegation and hence varying in their metabolic capacity and in their sensitivity to regulatory inputs.[30] Within cells, there may be heritable epigenetic modifications, such as in DNA methylation state, the histone code and in chromatin structure, which alter expression of particular genes and thereby cellular metabolic capacity and sensitivity. The candidate targets of such processes include imprinted genes, metastable alleles or other susceptible genes that are normally developmentally modulated. There is increasing evidence that these mechanisms may also operate in early postnatal life, which may explain the independent associations of markers of this stage of development with outcomes in later life. The aspects of physiological capacity and homeostasis, which are programmed via such mechanisms, may also vary depending on the sensitivity of the developing tissues, the timing and duration of exposure to an adverse intrauterine environment, as well as the severity and type of insult imposed.[31,32] Assessing the developmental programming of metabolic regulation and other aspects of homeostasis is currently the focus of experimental studies in a range of species and increasingly in human cohorts.

MECHANISTIC BASIS FOR PROGRAMMING OF METABOLIC HOMEOSTASIS – EVIDENCE FROM HUMAN STUDIES

What is currently known of the systemic, tissue, or cellular changes underlying metabolic disease that is related to size at birth in humans? Indicators of impaired glucose tolerance or diabetes are consistently negatively associated with size at birth in the majority of studies in children, young and old adults (Table 8.2).[5,33–38] Small size at birth is also associated with indirect measures of insulin resistance, such as fasting plasma insulin, in children and adults in most studies (Table 8.2). Fewer studies have more directly measured insulin sensitivity in relation to size at birth, and a negative relationship between birth weight and insulin sensitivity is present consistently in older adults, but less so in young adults and children (Table 8.2). Furthermore, there is some evidence that insulin sensitivity might actually be increased in the neonate that is clinically growth restricted (Table 8.2). This finding is important in that it suggests that prenatally induced insulin resistance is not present before birth and therefore is unlikely to have a genetic basis and also identifies a gradual emergence postnatally as part of its etiology. Unlike insulin resistance, failure of insulin secretion, which must occur concomitantly with insulin resistance before progression to type 2 diabetes occurs, was not consistently associated with size at birth in a recent systematic review (Table 8.2). Indeed, children and adults of low birth weight had elevated fasting or glucose-stimulated plasma insulin concentrations in most studies (Table 8.2), probably indicating some degree of compensatory hyperinsulinemia. The difficulty here is that unequivocal evaluation of insulin secretion is not possible unless insulin sensitivity is also evaluated within the same individual.[39] Thus, an individual may exhibit hyperinsulinemia, but still have inadequate and impaired insulin secretion *for their level of insulin sensitivity*, in terms of what is needed to maintain good glucose control. The insulin disposition index (product of insulin secretion and insulin sensitivity, each measured independently) provides a more accurate and unbiased assessment of insulin secretory capacity than indirect measures, such as plasma insulin concentrations, because it provides a measure of whether insulin secretion is appropriate given the individual's insulin sensitivity.[39] Use of the disposition index in biological studies has been limited because independent and direct measures of each parameter are required and this is technically demanding in the case of insulin sensitivity. Nevertheless, two of four recent studies suggested that the level of insulin secretion in IUGR individuals might be lower

Table 8.2 Associations of metabolic disease with small size at birth in humans

Defect	Relationship with birth weight
Indicators of glucose intolerance and noninsulin-dependent diabetes	
Fasting plasma glucose concentration	Negative (15 of 25 studies of children and adults)[5]
Plasma glucose 2 h after glucose load	Negative (20 of 25 studies of children and adults)[5]
Prevalence of type 2 diabetes	Negative (13 of 16 studies of children and adults)[5]
Whole-body insulin resistance	
Indirect measures of insulin sensitivity	Negative (17 of 22 studies of children and adults)[5]
	Reduced[33] or increased[34] in SGA cf. AGA neonates
Direct measure of insulin sensitivity by hyperinsulinemic euglycemic clamp	Negative (2 of 4 studies), inverted U-shaped (1 of 4 studies), or not related (1 of 4 studies of children and adults)[5]
Insulin secretion	
Fasting plasma insulin concentration	Negative (20 of 26 studies of children and adults)[5]
	Reduced[33] or increased[34] in SGA cf. AGA neonates
Insulin secretion after glucose load	Negative (16 of 24 studies), not related (6 of 24 studies), positive (7 of 24 studies of children and adults)[5]
Insulin secretion relative to sensitivity	
Slope of secretion versus sensitivity	Negative in all children; steeper in children of normal cf. low birth weight[35]
Insulin disposition index	30% lower in 19-year-old men of low birth weight cf. normal birth weight[36]
	Not different between SGA and AGA prepubertal children[35,37]
	Not different between IUGR and controls in 25-year-old men and women[38]

SGA, small for gestational age; AGA, appropriate for gestational age; IUGR, intrauterine growth restriction.

than appropriate for their level of insulin resistance, indicating impaired beta cell capacity for compensatory insulin hypersecretion (Table 8.2). Further studies of IUGR individuals with independent measures of insulin secretion and sensitivity are needed to determine whether prenatally induced beta cell defects indeed play an additional role in their increased susceptibility to diabetes. Thus, we do not know whether beta cell defects are programmed directly by the fetal environment or result from the long-term challenge imposed by insulin resistance and the consequent need to maintain compensatory hyperinsulinemia. However, in at least one study, insulin secretion was impaired in young adults with IUGR prior to the onset of whole body or peripheral insulin resistance, consistent with independent programming of a defect.[36] Overall, the outcomes of studies of size at birth and long-term metabolic homeostasis in humans implicate defects in both insulin secretion and insulin sensitivity as a common mechanism leading to type 2 diabetes and associated disorders following poor intrauterine growth.

Rather less is known about the mechanisms underlying the increased risks of metabolic and cardiovascular disease associated with infant catch-up growth or rapid growth later in childhood. It is important to distinguish this type of growth, as the latter is not catch-up growth, which is a particular phenomenon defined as taking place immediately following a period of restricted growth. Catch-up growth in terms of length, but not in terms of weight, in the first year of life was positively associated with fasting insulin and insulin secretion during an IVGTT in 1-year old children,[40] but it is not clear to what extent this reflects compensatory insulin secretion in response to resistance. In children who were SGA at birth, a rapid increase in BMI between 2 and 9 years of age predicted reduced whole-body insulin sensitivity and increased first and second phase insulin secretion or hyperinsulinemia at 9 years of age.[37] In children of normal birth weight, the rate of BMI gain during this period was not related to either insulin sensitivity or secretion.[37] Two other studies[13,41] have reported that relative gains in weight or ponderal index during childhood are positively associated with the HOMA insulin resistance index across the range of population birth weights, and not only following IUGR. Thus, catch-up after IUGR or simply accelerated growth in early life, are associated with insulin resistance in children. To date, insulin secretion in older children, and insulin sensitivity and secretion in adults have not been examined in relation to their patterns of growth as infant and children. Whether any impairment of insulin secretion is present at any age following accelerated early growth is also not clear, as independent direct measures of both secretion and sensitivity have not been conducted. However, two studies have taken the approach of examining size at birth and the infant and childhood patterns of growth in those adults who developed diabetes.[14] Interestingly, these investigators found that poor growth rather than catch-up growth in the first year of life, followed by accelerated growth in childhood, is characteristic of adult onset of diabetes. These are older cohorts born early last century in one instance and whether this accounts for the inconsistency with other studies is unclear.[14,40]

What is known about the systemic, tissue or cellular basis of impaired insulin sensitivity and secretion following restricted fetal growth? Decreased whole-body insulin sensitivity might reflect decreased sensitivity in peripheral tissues, predominantly skeletal muscle, but also in adipose tissue, or in liver. Individuals who were small at birth have reduced muscle mass as adults.[42] Since muscle is a major insulin-sensitive tissue in the control of blood glucose, reduced muscle mass might contribute to decreased glucose uptake in response to insulin on a whole-body basis. Some but not all studies have demonstrated that insulin sensitivity of peripheral tissues, specifically that of muscle, is reduced in low birth weight individuals, which would also decrease the action of insulin per unit mass of muscle (Table 8.3).[43–51] As discussed earlier, this variability may reflect the different ages of the subjects under study, with insulin resistance found more consistently in older individuals of low birth weight. Insulin appears to stimulate endothelial-mediated vasodilation in muscle normally, concomitant with impaired insulin stimulation of glucose uptake, in individuals of low birth weight,[43] suggesting cell and functional specificity in the site of prenatally induced insulin resistance within skeletal muscle (Table 8.3). The available evidence in humans suggests that a signaling defect downstream of the insulin receptor impairs insulin stimulation of glucose transport and hence glucose uptake in skeletal muscle and in adipose tissue (Table 8.3). There are more limited and inconsistent reports of effects of birth weight on hepatic insulin sensitivity, with either increased or decreased suppression of endogenous glucose production by insulin in low birth weight individuals compared with those of normal birth weight (Table 8.3). The structural changes that might affect insulin secretion by the pancreas have been little studied, with one but not another study reporting decreases in the proportions of islet tissue and numbers of beta cells in IUGR babies (Table 8.3). Altered activity of systemic regulation may contribute to these defects in insulin action, as there is evidence for moderate increases in the activity of the HPA axis in adults of low birth weight, with increased morning plasma cortisol and a recent report of increased stress-activated cortisol responses.[20] This increase could impair both insulin sensitivity in liver and peripheral tissues and insulin secretion by reducing beta cell numbers. In addition, increased sympathetic nervous system activity may account for some impairment of insulin secretion in adults of low birth weight.[28] Clearly, further studies in humans are required to confirm the presence and timing of onset of insulin resistance in peripheral tissues and liver, of impaired insulin secretion following fetal growth restriction, and the roles of extrinsic versus intrinsic factors.

USE OF EXPERIMENTAL MODELS IN THE INVESTIGATION OF PROGRAMMING OF METABOLIC HOMEOSTASIS IN HUMANS

Since much of the contemporary data in humans relates size at birth to later outcomes, relevant experimental paradigms are likely to be those that perturb the determinants of fetal growth. Although genetic factors determine the expected size of the fetus, the intrauterine environment regulates the extent to which this is achieved or exceeded.[8,31,52] Thus, the supply of nutrients and oxygen to the fetus depends on maternal factors that affect their availability, but also on placental metabolism and capacity to transport nutrients to the fetus and placental utilization and competition for these (Figure 8.1). Placental weight and function are major predictors of fetal growth and size at birth in humans and other mammalian species.[8,52] A range of factors that limit maternal capacity to supply nutrients and those that impact on placental growth or function are associated with small size at birth or IUGR in humans (Table 8.4).[52,53] This includes total food or energy availability to the mother, but also the composition of the maternal diet, although detailed studies of their effects on fetal growth are limited. Recently, Moore et al.[54] reported that birth weight and placental weight were positively related to the percentage of energy derived from

---

Table 8.3 Effects of clinical fetal growth restriction and size at birth on tissue and cellular characteristics that might underlie metabolic disease in humans

Defects that might underlie whole-body insulin resistance

- Insulin resistance of peripheral tissue (**yes**):
  - Young adults who were IUGR had:
    - Decreased forearm glucose uptake in response to insulin[43]
    - Reduced up-regulation of GLUT4 expression by insulin in muscle and adipose tissue[44]
    - Normal basal and insulin-stimulated gene expression of insulin receptor and signaling pathway components in muscle[44]
  - Variable size at birth:
    - No relationship with postprandial glycogen synthase activity in muscle in middle-aged women[45]

- Decreased insulin stimulation of muscle blood flow (**no**):
  - Adults and children who were light or thin at birth had:
    - Normal forearm basal and insulin-stimulated endothelium-dependent vasodilation[43]
    - Normal skeletal muscle capillary density and resting blood flow[46]
    - Faster muscle re-oxygenation[46,47]
  - Variable size at birth:
    - No relationship with endothelium-dependent and -independent vasodilation in prepubertal children
    - Positive relationship with post-occlusive capillary recruitment in prepubertal children[48]

- Changes in muscle fibre composition (**no**):
  - Thinness at birth did not predict skeletal muscle fibre density and proportions of type 1 and 2 fibres in middle-aged women[46]

- Hepatic insulin resistance (**?**):
  - Low birth weight INCREASED insulin suppression of endogenous glucose production and glycolytic flux in young men[36]
  - Low birth weight DECREASED insulin suppression of endogenous glucose production in Pima Indians as young adults[49]

Defects that might underlie impaired insulin secretion

- Decreased numbers of islets or beta cells (**?**):
  - IUGR decreased[50] or did not change[51] islet density and beta cell fraction in pancreas of late gestation fetuses and term neonates

- Decreased perfusion of beta cells (**?**):
  - 'Less pronounced vasculature', in pancreas from IUGR infants than in those of normal weight[50]

---

protein in the maternal diet in early pregnancy in a population in Australia, demonstrating that even in contemporary Western societies, nutrient composition affects fetal growth. The metabolic characteristics of the nutrients consumed even within a macronutrient class may also be important. For example, iso-energetic diets containing most carbohydrates in high glycemic index produce larger babies and placenta than diets in which the carbohydrates were predominantly of low glycemic index.[55] The placenta itself presents significant nutrient demands related to its own growth and also plays an important role in modifying maternally and even fetally derived factors for fetal consumption, for example in the interconversion of amino acids.[56,57] The peri-conceptual environment is also emerging as an important factor impacting on subsequent placental and fetal development, and possibly programming postnatal metabolic capacity and homeostasis. The use of assisted reproductive technology (ART), and hence extra-uterine culture in the first few cycles of cell division, is associated with lower average birth weights and increased rates of clinical IUGR, as well as with increased perinatal mortality.[58,59] Whether this reflects the effects of ART itself rather than factors that may have contributed to the decision to use ART is unclear, as a history of infertility is itself associated with decreased birth weight and an increased incidence of IUGR.[60]

These known risk factors and influences on size at birth in humans have been used as the basis for the development of various experimental paradigms to demonstrate the long-term consequences for metabolic homeostasis and to define the mechanisms involved. These can be classed as: (1) involving manipulations of maternal or placental factors, or (2) mimicking of clinical scenarios and interventions.

Maternal factors

In much of the world, chronic undernutrition or malnutrition is significant and associated with high rates of IUGR. Imposition of mild or moderate maternal global feed restriction from before and/or during pregnancy in the rat[61-64] and guinea pig[65,66] reduces fetal growth and size at birth and induces obesity and insulin resistance in offspring after birth (Table 8.4). In the guinea pig, progeny of feed-restricted mothers are also glucose intolerant despite increased insulin secretion,[66] and have an impaired capacity to maintain cholesterol homeostasis when subjected to a dietary challenge.[65] The latter also exhibit atherosclerotic changes in blood vessels, suggesting greater susceptibility to the development of cardiovascular disease

following fetal growth restriction due to maternal undernutrition.[65] One inconsistency in outcomes between human IUGR and experimental food restriction throughout pregnancy in nonhuman species is the failure of neonatal progeny in many of the latter to undergo catch-up growth. Moderate food restriction has also been imposed for only part of pregnancy in several species. While it is difficult to identify a common human exposure that this relates to, it does help address the question of critical periods of sensitivity of different body systems to perturbation, and where it occurs in the second half of pregnancy, possibly that of onset of placental restriction.[67-74] These perturbations have variable effects on birth weight and do not consistently impair glucose homeostasis in the progeny (Table 8.5).[30,61-66,69-108] Although its prevalence in various human communities is unclear, the metabolic programming effects of restricted maternal protein intake have been explored in far greater detail than those of restricted maternal feed intake. Protein restriction (6–8% cf. 20%) throughout pregnancy in the rat, reduces birth weight and may decrease insulin secretory capacity of progeny, but does not impair adult glucose tolerance, and unlike the human is not characterized by neonatal catch-up growth[79-83] (Table 8.5). Prolonging protein restriction (8% cf. 20%) throughout lactation as well as pregnancy in the rat does impair adult insulin sensitivity, although the

---

Table 8.4 Factors associated with small size at birth and/or clinical IUGR in humans

Maternal factors
    Small or underweight mother
    First pregnancy
    Multiple pregnancy (twins or higher multiples)
    Chronic undernutrition or severe undernutrition in late gestation
    Adolescent pregnancy
    Smoking
    Socio-economic disadvantage
    Infection

Placental factors
    Small placental size
    Low uteroplacental blood flow
    Impaired placental transport of amino acids
    Pre-eclampsia

Clinical interventions
    Assisted reproductive technology, including *in vitro* fertilization
    Repeated corticosteroid treatment for threatened premature delivery[53]

Adapted from Robinson et al.[52]

Table 8.5 Size at birth and metabolic programming in experimental perturbations of the fetal environment*

Intervention and species	Reported effect	Size at birth	Neonatal growth rates	Adult size	Obesity	Outcome					
						Basal glucose	Basal insulin	Glucose intolerance	Insulin secretion	Insulin sensitivity of glucose metabolism	Elevated plasma cholesterol
Constraints to maternal supply											
Food restriction – whole pregnancy											
Rat (fed 30% or 50% of *ad libitum*)[61-64]	Effect of nutrition	→	↓ AGR ↓ FGR	↔	↑	↔	↓ at birth ↔ neonates and juveniles ↑↓ adults	NR	NR	→	NR
Guinea pig (fed 60–85%) of *ad libitum*)[65,66,75]	Effect of nutrition	↔↓	↓ AGR FGR	↔↓	↑	↔	↑	↑	↑	NR	↔↑ basal ↔↑ post-challenge
	Relationship to/effect of size at birth	...	AGR + ve FGR – ve	↔↓ in LBW	NR	none	↑ in LBW	none	none	NR	↔ basal ↔↑ post-challenge in LBW
Food restriction – part of pregnancy											
Rat (fed 50% of *ad libitum* in early pregnancy)[67,76]	Effect of nutrition	↔	↑ males ↔ females	↑ males ↔ females	↑ males ↔ females	NR	NR	NR	NR	NR	NR
Rat (fed 50% of *ad libitum* for first ⅔ of pregnancy)[68]	Effect of nutrition	↔	↔ AGR	↑	NR	↔	↔	↔	↔	↔	NR
Rat (fed 30% of *ad libitum* for last ⅔ of pregnancy)[69]	Effect of nutrition	↔	NR	NR	NR	NR	NR	NR	NR	NR	↑ post-challenge
Rat (fed 50% of *ad libitum* for last ⅓ of pregnancy)[70-72]	Effect of nutrition	→	↓ AGR	↔	NR	↔ juveniles ↑ adults	↓ juveniles ↔ adults	↔	↔↓	↑ young adults	NR

Table 8.5 *continued*

Intervention and species	Reported effect	Size at birth	Neonatal growth rates	Adult size	Obesity	Basal glucose	Outcome Basal insulin	Glucose intolerance	Insulin secretion	Insulin sensitivity of glucose metabolism	Elevated plasma cholesterol
Guinea pig (fed 50% of *ad libitum* for second ½ of pregnancy)[73]	Effect of nutrition	→	↓ AGR	NR	↑	NR	NR	NR	NR	NR	NR
Sheep (fed 2–3% of *ad libitum* for 10 or 20 days in late pregnancy)[74]	Effect of nutrition	→	NR	↕	NR	↕	↕	↕	↕	↕	NR
	Relationship to size at birth	...	NR	NR	NR	none	none	– ve at 5 mo ↔ at 30 mo	none	NR	NR
Food restriction – whole of pregnancy and lactation											
Rat (fed 50% of *ad libitum*)[61,77,78]	Effect of nutrition	→	↓ AGR	→	NR	↕ juveniles ↑ adults	↕ juveniles ↓ adults	↕ juveniles ↑ adults	→ juveniles and adults	→	NR
Protein restriction – whole of pregnancy											
Rat (maternal dietary protein range 6–20%)[79–83]	Effect of low protein	→	↓ ↔ AGR	→ ↔	NR	↕	→ juveniles ↔ adults	↓ ↕ juveniles ↔ adults	→	NR	↓ basal
Pig (maternal diet 0.5% vs 13% protein)[84]	Effect of low protein	→	↓ AGR	→	↕	NR	NR	NR	NR	NR	NR
Protein restriction – whole of pregnancy and lactation											
Rat (maternal diet 8 vs 20% protein)[30,80,82,85–88]	Effect of low protein	→	↓ AGR	→	↕	↕	↔↓↑	↓ young adults ↔↑ old adults	↔↓↑	↓ whole body ↓ muscle and liver	↓ basal

Table 8.5 continued

Intervention and species	Reported effect	Size at birth	Neonatal growth rates	Adult size	Obesity	Basal glucose	Outcome — Basal insulin	Outcome — Glucose intolerance	Outcome — Insulin secretion	Outcome — Insulin sensitivity of glucose metabolism	Outcome — Elevated plasma cholesterol
Restricted placental size or function											
Natural variation in litter size											
Guinea pig[89,90]	Effect of large litter size	→	↑ FGR	NR	NR	NR	NR	NR	NR	NR	NR
Pig[91,92]	Relationship to size at birth	...	↓ AGR ↑ FGR	NR	+ ve	– ve	NR	NR	NR	+ ve	NR
	Effect of LBW	...	↓ AGR ↑ FGR	↓ females	NR	→	↓ males ↔ females	↑	↑	males ↓ females	NR
Sheep[93,94]	Relationship to size at birth	...		+ ve females	NR	NR	+ ve	– ve	NR	– ve males	NR
	Effect of LBW	...	↓ AGR ↓↑ FGR	NR	↑	↔	↔ at birth ↑ juveniles	NR	NR	NR	NR
Surgical restriction of placental growth or function											
Sheep (surgical removal of most placental implantation sites)[95–97]	Effect of placental restriction	→	↔ AGR ↑ FGR	↓ females	↑ neonates	↔	↑	↑	↑ absolute ↓ insulin disposition in neonates	↓ juvenile males ↑ adult females	NR
	Relationship to size at birth	...	+ ve	NR	+ ve	NR	NR	NR	+ ve for insulin disposition in adult males	NR	NR
Rat (surgical restriction of uterine blood flow in late pregnancy)[98]	Effect of restricted blood flow	→	↓ AGR	↑	↑	↑	↑	↑	→	→	NR

Table 8.5 *continued*

Intervention and species	Reported effect	Size at birth	Neonatal growth rates	Adult size	Obesity	Basal glucose	Basal insulin	Glucose intolerance	Insulin secretion	Insulin sensitivity of glucose metabolism	Elevated plasma cholesterol
Modeling of clinical scenarios and interventions											
Maternal gestational diabetes											
Rat (mild maternal hyperglycemia after streptozotocin in early pregnancy)[99,100]	Effect of streptozotocin	↑	↑	→	↑	↕	↕	↑	↑	→	NR
Rat (moderate maternal hyperglycemia during glucose infusion in late pregnancy)[101,102]	Effect of maternal glucose infusion	↑	NR	→	NR	↕	↕	↑	→	NR	NR
Maternal glucocorticoid treatment											
Sheep (single dose of dexamethasone to mother in early or mid pregnancy)[103,104]	Effect of glucocorticoid	↕	NR	↕	NR	↕	↕	↕	↕	↕	NR
Sheep (single dose of dexamethasone to mother in late pregnancy)[105]	Effect of glucocorticoid	↕	NR	↕	NR	↕	↕	↔ in juveniles ↑ in adults	↑	NR	NR
Rat (multiple doses of dexamethasone to mother in early or mid pregnancy)[106,107]	Effect of glucocorticoid	↕	↑ AGR	↑↕	↑	↕	↕	↕	↕	↕	NR

Table 8.5 *continued*

Intervention and species	Reported effect	Outcome									
		Size at birth	Neonatal growth rates	Adult size	Obesity	Basal glucose	Basal insulin	Glucose intolerance	Insulin secretion	Insulin sensitivity of glucose metabolism	Elevated plasma cholesterol
Sheep (multiple doses of dexamethasone to mother in late pregnancy)[105]	Effect of glucocorticoid	↓	NR	↔	NR	↔ in juveniles ↑ in adults	↔ in juveniles ↑ in adults	↔	↑	NR	NR
Rat (multiple doses of dexamethasone to mother in late pregnancy)[106]	Effect of glucocorticoid	↓	NR	↔	NR	↑	↔	↑	↑	NR	NR
Guinea pig (multiple doses of dexamethasone to glucocorticoid mother in late pregnancy)[108]	Effect of glucocorticoid	↔	NR	↔	NR	NR	NR	NR	NR	NR	NR

*↓, decreased; ↑, increased; ↔, unchanged; AGR, absolute growth rate; FGR, fractional growth rate; NR not reported; + ve, positive; − ve, negative; LBW, low birth weight; mo, months old.

effects on glucose tolerance and insulin secretion are more variable[30,80,82,85–88] (Table 8.5). Some inconsistencies between outcomes following human IUGR and in progeny of dams subject to food or protein restriction during pregnancy may limit extrapolation of the information on specific mechanisms obtained in these paradigms. Nevertheless, they have been critical in clearly substantiating the programming phenomenon.

Placental factors

Small size at birth occurring due to spontaneous variation in litter size in guinea pigs[89,90] and pigs[91,92] produces postnatal consequences for progeny that are similar to those seen after human IUGR (Table 8.5). This spontaneous fetal growth restriction appears to have a substantial placental component, as fetal and neonatal birth weights are highly correlated with placental weight in these species as in humans. The postnatal outcomes include early catch-up growth and later onset obesity, glucose intolerance, increased insulin secretion in response to a glucose challenge, and insulin resistance, although some of these responses differ between genders (Table 8.5). Multiple pregnancy, which is characterized by reduced placental size and function in the sheep,[93,94] also produces obesity, variable catch-up growth depending on neonatal nutrition, and elevated fasting insulin in the offspring as young lambs, but the consequences for glucose homeostasis have not been determined (Table 8.5). Surgical restriction of placental implantation and subsequent placental growth and function in sheep[95–97] reduces progeny birth weight, and results in neonatal catch-up growth, increased fat deposition even in neonatal life, and elevated fasting and post-glucose insulin secretion, although insulin secretion was impaired when adjusted for the level of insulin sensitivity (Table 8.5). Surgical restriction of uterine blood flow and placental function in late pregnancy in rats[98] has a more severe effect on progeny phenotype. The adult progeny of these rats show elevated fasting glucose and impaired post-glucose insulin secretion in addition to obesity, glucose intolerance, and insulin resistance (Table 8.5). These consequences of placental restriction for progeny in the rat resemble the late stages in the development of diabetes, including failure of insulin secretion as well as insulin resistance. In the three species where outcomes of experimental restriction of placental growth and function for insulin sensitivity of offspring have been characterized, only in the rat do offspring also exhibit overt insulin secretory deficiency. The insulin secretory response to glucose in absolute terms is increased in small pigs from large litters and in placentally

restricted sheep, although secretion relative to sensitivity is in fact impaired in the latter paradigm. These results suggest that placental restraint in late pregnancy in the rat affects the development and/or function of the pancreas more severely than placental restraint imposed by large litter size or restricted implantation in the pig and sheep. Overall, these studies clearly show that placental restraint of oxygen and nutrient supply impairs both insulin secretion and sensitivity to adversely impact on glucose homeostasis in offspring postnatally, consistent with a common cause of fetal growth restriction in humans causing later metabolic disease.

Clinical scenarios and interventions

It is not only restricted supply before birth that leads to later metabolic disease in offspring, however. Maternal diabetes, including gestational diabetes as well as obesity, increases birth weight and is increasingly linked to programming of metabolic disease in offspring. Maternal hyperglycemia induced by maternal streptozotocin treatment and consequent mild maternal hyperglycemia throughout pregnancy in rats[99,100] increases size at birth and results in progeny with increased adiposity, glucose intolerance, and insulin resistance, but no changes in fasting glucose. These experimental paradigms, therefore, may provide useful information about the mechanisms underlying the development of diabetes and obesity in children who were exposed to gestational diabetes in fetal life.[109] Maternal glucocorticoid treatment to mature fetal lungs in threatened premature delivery is a common obstetric exposure. However, relatively few studies of the metabolic consequences of corticosteroid exposure in humans or experimentally in other species have been carried out (Table 8.5). Exposure to a single dose of maternally administered dexamethasone during late gestation in sheep,[105] which does not affect birth weight, increases insulin secretion after a glucose challenge (Table 8.5). This finding suggests that a single exposure to glucocorticoid during fetal life may cause insulin resistance in sheep, although it has not yet been measured directly, and these animals are able to maintain normal glucose tolerance. Progeny of ewes given multiple maternally administered doses of dexamethasone in late pregnancy[105] also have exaggerated insulin responses to glucose, and develop glucose intolerance with aging (Table 8.5). Repeated doses of glucocorticoids decrease fetal growth to a greater extent in sheep[105] than that suggested in limited human trials to date,[53] suggesting that the sheep may be more sensitive to glucocorticoid exposure.

Nevertheless, the data available from sheep studies indicate that repeated fetal exposure to glucocorticoids may program metabolic homeostasis and this possible effect is being further investigated in human cohorts.

MECHANISTIC BASIS FOR PROGRAMMING OF METABOLIC HOMEOSTASIS – EVIDENCE FROM EXPERIMENTAL MODELS

What additional information have experimental studies in nonhuman species provided about the mechanisms that underlie the onset of impaired insulin action and metabolic homeostasis following restriction of fetal growth in humans?

One interesting feature that emerges from a review of experimental observations is that progeny outcomes appear to relate more closely to size at birth than to treatment effects. For example, in our studies in sheep[95–97] we found that size at birth is a stronger predictor of neonatal growth rates and adult insulin sensitivity than whether the mother was a control ewe or had undergone surgery to restrict placental implantation. Similarly, measures of glucose homeostasis were more closely related to size at birth than to litter size in the guinea pig with spontaneous variation in size at birth.[89,90] These observations might suggest that many factors, such as maternal undernutrition or protein deprivation and even glucocorticoid exposure may act via a common mechanism to induce fetal programming. It could include an element of impaired placental function, which restricts oxygen as well as nutrient supply, which is a strong determinant of fetal growth rate and size at birth. Commonalities in the neuroendocrine and endocrine responses of the fetus to various challenges before birth may also contribute, including increases in catabolic hormones and decreases in anabolic hormones in response to restraint. Changes in fetal glucocorticoid exposure, with increases accelerating differentiation while reducing proliferation of cells within a range of tissues, have been suggested as one common mechanism that might mediate the effects of multiple environmental factors on the fetus.[31] Certainly, maternal glucocorticoid administration in rats[106,107] and sheep[105] produce progeny with some similarities to outcomes following human IUGR. Direct demonstration of the importance of particular factors in the initiation or amplification of developmental programming of metabolic homeostasis is still somewhat limited.

Rather less is known about the systematic tissue or cellular changes and the mechanisms underlying changes in postnatal growth and the related consequences for metabolic homeostasis following experimental manipulations of the prenatal environment. Several experimental paradigms of constraints to placental size or function produce progeny with reduced size at birth followed by neonatal catch-up growth (Table 8.5). Increased neonatal appetite appears to be a central feature of catch-up growth,[93] although the underlying mechanism is largely unknown. In rats, fetal growth restriction induced by maternal undernutrition during pregnancy increases the appetite of progeny after weaning, which may contribute to the later development of obesity and metabolic dysfunction.[64] Neonatal catch-up growth is also associated with increased whole-body sensitivity to the actions of insulin and insulin-like growth factor, important anabolic hormones for neonatal growth, in sheep and guinea pigs that were small at birth.[110–112] Despite increased insulin sensitivity as neonates, insulin resistance develops with aging, as young adults who were small at birth are insulin-resistant in both experimental models.[110,113,114] At least in the guinea pig that was small at birth, whole-body insulin resistance is primarily peripheral[90] and we have preliminary data to show that this occurs in muscle (JA Owens et al., unpublished data). Impairment of glucose tolerance with aging probably also reflects a reduced capacity for compensatory insulin secretion, as in our studies insulin disposition is positively related to size at birth in young adult male sheep.[97] Further studies are needed to delineate the mechanistic basis of catch-up growth and increased appetite, and how these contribute to later disease.

The specific structural, cellular, and molecular changes, which underlie impaired insulin sensitivity in various tissues and impaired secretory capacity following perinatal challenge, are increasingly being defined. While space limitations prevent a detailed review, the molecular defects within insulin-sensitive tissues and in the endocrine pancreas of offspring of rats subjected to protein deprivation and following placental restriction have been defined to some extent.[30,86,87] These effects have been relatively little explored in other paradigms and species. Defining the time of onset of changes in various determinants of insulin action in key tissues in relation to the emergence of functional deficits will help to delineate the causal pathways of developmental programming.

CONCLUSIONS

The experimental characterization of prenatal perturbations that restrict fetal growth and lead to similar pre- and postnatal phenotypes as human IUGR does, has demonstrated that these phenomena can be causally linked. Human and experimental studies consistently implicate whole-body and skeletal muscle insulin resistance as primary defects underlying the association of metabolic disease with small size at birth. Evidence from experimental studies also supports the more limited evidence of impaired insulin secretory capacity in humans of low birth weight. Relevant experimental paradigms will allow a more detailed and hopefully more rapid exploration of the systemic, tissue, and cellular changes underlying altered insulin resistance and impaired secretion, their timing of onset and the initiating factors and mediating pathways involved, than may be possible in humans. The real power of experimental paradigms, however, may be that they allow us to more readily test pre- and postnatal interventions to prevent or ameliorate the deleterious consequences of exposure to an adverse fetal environment. Finally, there is increasing recognition of the value of utilizing long-term follow-up of relevant trials of obstetric and pediatric interventions, to directly test the developmental programming paradigm and possible therapies in humans.

ACKNOWLEDGMENTS

The authors wish to acknowledge the support of the National Health and Medical Research Council of Australia and the National Heart Foundation of Australia. Kathryn L Gatford currently holds the Hilda Farmer Medical Research Associateship awarded by the Faculty of Health Sciences, University of Adelaide.

REFERENCES

1. Fagot-Campagna A. Emergence of type 2 diabetes mellitus: epidemiological evidence. J Pediatr Endocrinol Metab 2000; 13: 1395–402.
2. Aye T, Levitsky LL. Type 2 diabetes: an epidemic disease in childhood. Curr Opin Pediatr 2003; 15: 411–15.
3. Parker L, Lamont DW, Unwin N et al. A lifecourse study of risk for hyperinsulinaemia, dyslipidaemia and obesity (the central metabolic syndrome) at age 49–51 years. Diabetic Med 2003; 20: 406–15.
4. Schulze MB, Hu FB. Primary prevention of diabetes: what can be done and how much can be prevented? Annu Rev Public Health 2005; Review in advance: doi: 10.1146/annurev.publhealth.26.021304.144532.
5. Newsome CA, Shiell AW, Fall CHD et al. Is birth weight related to later glucose and insulin metabolism? – a systemic review. Diabetic Med 2003; 20: 339–48.
6. Rogers I, Group E-BS. The influence of birthweight and intrauterine environment on adiposity and fat distribution in later life. Int J Obes 2003; 27: 755–77.
7. Pi-Sunyer FX. The epidemiology of central fat distribution in relation to disease. Nutr Rev 2004; 62: S120–S126.
8. Robinson JS, Owens JA. Pathophysiology of intrauterine growth failure. In: Pediatrics and Perinatology. The Scientific Basis, 2 edn. (Gluckman PD, Heymann MA, eds). London: Arnold, 1996: 290–7.
9. Fitzhardinge PM, Steven EM. The small-for-date infant I. Later growth patterns. Pediatrics 1972; 49: 671–81.
10. Tenovuo A, Kero P, Piekkala P et al. Growth of 519 small for gestational age infants during the first two years of life. Acta Paediatr Scand 1987; 76: 636–46.
11. Albertsson-Wikland K, Wennergren G, Wennergren M et al. Longitudinal follow-up of growth in children born small for gestational age. Acta Paediatr 1993; 82: 438–43.
12. Hokken-Koelega ACS, De Ridder MAJ, Lemmen RJ et al. Children born small for gestational age: do they catch up? Pediatr Res 1995; 38: 267–71.
13. Crowther NJ, Cameron N, Trusler J et al. Association between poor glucose tolerance and rapid post natal weight gain in seven-year-old children. Diabetologia 1998; 41: 1163–7.
14. Forsén T, Eriksson J, Tuomilehto J et al. The fetal and childhood growth of persons who develop type 2 diabetes. Ann Intern Med 2000; 133: 176–82.
15. Ong KKL, Ahmed ML, Emmett PM et al. Association between postnatal catch-up growth and obesity in childhood: prospective cohort study. BMJ 2000; 320: 967–71.
16. Parsons TJ, Power C, Manor O. Fetal and early life growth and body mass index from birth to early adulthood in 1958 British cohort: longitudinal study. BMJ 2001; 323: 1331–5.
17. Eriksson JG, Forsen T, Tuomilehto J et al. Catch-up growth in childhood and death from coronary heart disease: longitudinal study. BMJ 1999; 318: 427–31.
18. Forsén T, Eriksson JG, Tuomilehto J et al. Growth in utero and during childhood among women who develop coronary heart disease: longitudinal study. BMJ 1999; 319: 1403–7.
19. Phillips DIW, Barker DJP, Hales CN et al. Thinness at birth and insulin resistance in adult life. Diabetologia 1994; 37: 150–4.
20. Barker DJP. Mothers, Babies and Health in Later Life, 2 edn. Edinburgh: Churchill Livingstone, 1998.
21. Lucas A. Programming by early nutrition in man. In: The Childhood Environment and Adult Disease (Bock GR, Whelan J, eds). Chicester: Wiley, 1991: 38–55.
22. Barker DJP, Osmond C. Infant mortality, childhood nutrition, and ischaemic heart disease in England and Wales. Lancet 1986; 1: 1077–81.
23. Rich-Edwards JW, Stampfer MJ, Manson JE et al. Birth weight and risk of cardiovascular disease in a cohort of women followed up since 1976. BMJ 1997; 315: 396–400.
24. Rich-Edwards JW, Colditz GA, Stampfer MJ et al. Birthweight and the risk for type 2 diabetes mellitus in adult women. Ann Intern Med 1999; 130: 322–4.
25. Ravelli G-P, Stein ZA, Susser MW. Obesity in young men after famine exposure in utero and early infancy. N Engl J Med 1976; 295: 349–53.
26. Ravelli ACJ, ven der Meulen JHP, Osmond C et al. Obesity at the age of 50 y in men and women exposed to famine prenatally. Am J Clin Nutr 1999; 70: 811–16.
27. Ravelli ACJ, van der Meulen JHP, Michels RPJ et al. Glucose tolerance in adults after prenatal exposure to famine. Lancet 1998; 351: 173–7.
28. Flanagan DE, Vaile JC, Petley GW et al. The autonomic control of heart rate and insulin resistance in young adults. J Clin Endocrinol Metab 1999; 84: 1263–7.

29. Fowden AL, Hill DJ. Intra-uterine programming of the endocrine pancreas. Br Med Bull 2001; 60: 123–42.

30. Ozanne SE, Nave BT, Wang CL et al. Poor fetal nutrition causes long-term changes in expression of insulin-signaling components in adipocytes. Am J Physiol 1997; 273: E46–E51.

31. Fowden AL, Forhead AJ. Endocrine mechanisms of intrauterine programming. Reproduction 2004; 127: 515–26.

32. Gluckman PD, Hanson MA. Living with the past: evolution, development, and patterns of disease. Science 2004; 305: 1733–6.

33. Bazaes RA, Salazar TE, Pittaluga E et al. Glucose and lipid metabolism in small for gestational age infants at 48 hours of age. Pediatrics 2003; 111: 804–9.

34. Wang X, Cui Y, Tong X et al. Effects of the Trp64Arg polymorphism in the β3-adrenergic receptor gene on insulin sensitivity in small for gestational age neonates. J Clin Endocrinol Metab 2004; 89: 4981–5.

35. Li C, Johnson MS, Goran MI. Effects of low birth weight on insulin resistance syndrome in Caucasian and African-American children. Diabetes Care 2001; 24: 2035–42.

36. Jensen CB, Storgaard H, Dela F et al. Early differential defects of insulin secretion and action in 19-year-old Caucasian men who had low birth weight. Diabetes 2002; 51: 1271–80.

37. Veening MA, van Weissenbruch MM, Heine RJ et al. β-cell capacity and insulin sensitivity in prepubertal children born small for gestational age. Influence of body size during childhood. Diabetes 2003; 52: 1756–60.

38. Jaquet D, Gaboriau A, Czernichow P et al. Insulin resistance early in adulthood in subjects born with intrauterine growth retardation. J Clin Endocrinol Metab 2000; 85: 1401–6.

39. Bergman RN, Ader M, Huecking K et al. Accurate assessment of β-cell function. The hyperbolic correction. Diabetes 2002; 51 (Suppl 1): S212–S220.

40. Soto N, Bazaes RA, Pena V et al. Insulin sensitivity and secretion are related to catch-up growth in small-for-gestational-age infants at age 1 year: results from a prospective cohort. J Clin Endocrinol Metab 2003; 88: 3645–50.

41. Whincup PH, Cook DG, Adshead F et al. Childhood size is more closely related than size at birth to glucose and insulin levels in 10–11-year-old children. Diabetologia 1997; 40: 319–26.

42. Phillips DIW. Relation of fetal growth to adult muscle mass and glucose tolerance. Diabetic Med 1995; 12: 686–90.

43. Hermann TS, Rask-Madsen C, Ihlemann N et al. Normal insulin-stimulated endothelial function and impaired insulin-stimulated muscle glucose uptake in young adults with low birth weight. J Clin Endocrinol Metab 2003; 88: 1252–7.

44. Jaquet D, Vidal H, Hankard R et al. Impaired regulation of glucose transporter 4 gene expression in insulin resistance associated with in utero undernutrition. J Clin Endocrinol Metab 2001; 86: 3266–71.

45. Phillips DIW, Borthwick AC, Stein C et al. Fetal growth and insulin resistance in adult life: relationship between glycogen synthase activity in adult skeletal muscle and birthweight. Diabetic Med 1996; 13: 325–9.

46. Thompson CH, Sanderson AL, Sandeman D et al. Fetal growth and insulin resistance in adult life: role of skeletal muscle morphology. Clinical Science 1997; 92: 291–6.

47. Arrowsmith F, Ward J, Ling A et al. Fetal nutrition and muscle oxygen supply in childhood. Metabolism 2002; 51: 1569–72.

48. IJzerman RG, van Weissenbruch MM, Voordouw JJ et al. The association between birth weight and capillary recruitment is independent of blood pressure and insulin sensitivity: a study in prepubertal children. J Hypertens 2002; 20: 1957–63.

49. Stefan N, Weyer C, Levy-Marchal C et al. Endogenous glucose production, insulin sensitivity, and insulin secretion in normal glucose-tolerant Pima Indians with low birth weight. Metabolism 2004; 53: 904–11.

50. Van Assche FA, De Prins F, Aerts L et al. The endocrine pancreas in small-for-dates infants. BJOG 1977; 84: 751–3.

51. Béringue F, Blondeau B, Castellotti MC et al. Endocrine pancreas development in growth-retarded human fetuses. Diabetes 2002; 51: 385–91.

52. Robinson JS, Moore VM, Owens JA et al. Origins of fetal growth restriction. Eur J Obstet Gynecol Reprod Biol 2000; 92: 13–19.

53. Crowther C, Harding J. Repeat doses of prenatal corticosteroids for women at risk of preterm birth for preventing neonatal respiratory disease. The Cochrane Database of Systematic Reviews 2003; Issue 2(2): Art. No.: CD003935. DOI: 10.1002/14651858.CD003935.

54. Moore VM, Davies MJ, Willson KJ et al. Dietary composition of pregnant women is related to size of the baby at birth. J Nutr 2004; 134: 1820–6.

55. Clapp JFr. Maternal carbohydrate intake and pregnancy outcome. Proc Nutr Soc 2002; 61: 45–50.

56. Battaglia FC. Fetal liver and the placenta: an interactive system. In: Placental Function and Fetal Nutrition (Battaglia FC, ed). Philadelphia: Lippincott-Raven Publishers, 1997: 47–57.

57. Meschia G. Placental delivery of amino acids. Utilization and production vs. transport. In: Placental Function and Fetal Nutrition (Battaglia FC, ed). Philadelphia: Lippincott-Raven Publishers, 1997: 21–30.

58. Helmerhorst FM, Perquin DA, Donker D et al. Perinatal outcome of singletons and twins after assisted conception: a systematic review of controlled studies. BMJ 2004; 328: 261.

59. Jackson RA, Gibson KA, Wu YW et al. Perinatal outcomes in singletons following in vitro fertilization: a meta-analysis. Obstet Gynecol 2004; 103: 551–63.

60. Ghazi HA, Speilberger C, Kallen B. Delivery outcome after infertility – a registry study. Fertil Steril 1991; 55: 726–32.

61. Holemans K, Verhaeghe J, Dequeker J et al. Insulin sensitivity in adult female rats subjected to malnutrition during the perinatal period. J Soc Gynecol Investig 1996; 3: 71–7.

62. Woodall SM, Breier BH, Johnston BM et al. A model of intrauterine growth retardation caused by chronic maternal undernutrition in the rat: effects on the somatotrophic axis and postnatal growth. J Endocrinol 1996; 150: 231–42.

63. Woodall SM, Johnston BM, Breier BH et al. Chronic maternal undernutrition in the rat leads to delayed postnatal growth and elevated blood pressure of offspring. Pediatr Res 1996; 40: 438–43.

64. Vickers MH, Breier BH, Cutfield WS et al. Fetal origins of hyperphagia, obesity, and hypertension and postnatal amplification by hypercaloric nutrition. Am J Physiol 2000; 279: E83–E87.

65. Kind KL, Clifton PM, Katsman AI et al. Restricted fetal growth and the response to dietary cholesterol in the guinea pig. Am J Physiol 1999; 277: R1675–R1682.

66. Kind KL, Clifton PM, Grant PA et al. Effect of maternal feed restriction during pregnancy on glucose tolerance in the adult guinea pig. Am J Physiol 2003; 284: R140–R152.

67. Jones AP, Simson EL, Friedman MI. Gestational undernutrition and the development of obesity in rats. J Nutr 1984; 114: 1484–92.

68. Portha B, Kergoat M, Blondel O et al. Underfeeding of rat mothers during the first two trimesters of gestation does not alter insulin action and insulin secretion in the progeny. Eur J Endocrinol 1995; 133: 475–82.

69. Szitanyi P, Hanzlova J, Poledne R. Influence of intrauterine undernutrition on the development of hypercholesterolemia in an animal model. Physiol Res 2000; 49: 721–4.

70. Garofano A, Czernichow P, Bréant B. In utero undernutrition impairs rat beta-cell development. Diabetologia 1997; 40: 1231–4.

71. Garofano A, Czernichow P, Bréant B. Beta-cell mass and proliferation following late fetal and early postnatal malnutrition in the rat. Diabetologia 1998; 41: 1114–20.

72. Bertin E, Gangnerau MN, Bailb D et al. Glucose metabolism and beta-cell mass in adult offspring of rats protein and/or energy restricted during the last week of pregnancy. Am J Physiology 1999; 277: E11–E17.

73. Ashwell M, Purkins L, Cowen T et al. Pre- and postnatal development of adipose tissue at four sites in the guinea pig: effect of maternal diet restriction during the second half of pregnancy. Ann Nutr Metab 1987; 31: 197–210.

74. Oliver MH, Breier BH, Gluckman PD et al. Birth weight rather than maternal nutrition influences glucose tolerance, blood pressure, and IGF-I levels in sheep. Pediatr Res 2002; 52: 516–24.

75. Dwyer CM, Madgwick AJA, Ward SS et al. Effect of maternal undernutrition in early gestation on the development of fetal myofibres in the guinea-pig. Reprod Fertil Dev 1995; 7: 1285–92.

76. Jones AP, Friedman MI. Obesity and adipocyte abnormalities in offspring of rats undernourished during pregnancy. Science 1982; 215: 1518–19.

77. Bedi KS, Birzgalis AR, Mahon M et al. Early life undernutrition in rats 1. Quantitative histology of skeletal muscles from underfed young and refed adult animals. Br J Nutr 1982; 47: 417–31.

78. Garofano A, Czernichow P, Bréant B. Effect of aging on beta-cell mass and function in rats malnourished during the perinatal period. Diabetologia 1999; 42: 711–18.

79. McLeod KI, Goldrick RB, Whyte HM. The effect of maternal malnutrition on the progeny of the rat. Aust J Exp Biol Med Sci 1972; 50: 435–46.

80. Dahri S, Snoeck A, Reusens-Billen B et al. Islet function in offspring of mothers on low-protein diet during gestation. Diabetes 1991; 40 (Suppl 2): 115–20.

81. Langley SC, Browne RF, Jackson AA. Altered glucose tolerance in rats exposed to maternal low protein diets in utero. Comp Biochem Physiol 1994; 109A: 223–9.

82. Lucas A, Baker BA, Desai M et al. Nutrition in pregnant or lactating rats programs lipid metabolism in the offspring. Br J Nutr 1996; 76: 605–12.

83. Muaku SM, Beauloye V, Thissen J-P et al. Long-term effects of gestational protein malnutrition on postnatal growth, insulin-like growth factor (IGF)-I, and IGF-binding proteins in rat progeny. Pediatr Res 1996; 39: 649–55.

84. Schoknecht PA, Pond WG, Mersmann HJ et al. Protein restriction during pregnancy affects postnatal growth in swine progeny. J Nutr 1993; 123: 1818–25.

85. Hales CN, Desai BM, Ozanne SE et al. Fishing in the stream of diabetes: from measuring insulin to the control of fetal organogenesis. Biochem Soc Trans 1996; 24: 341–50.

86. Ozanne SE, Smith GD, Tikerpae J et al. Altered regulation of hepatic glucose output in the male offspring of protein-malnourished rat dams. Am J Physiol 1996; 2701: E559–E564.

87. Ozanne SE, Wang CL, Coleman N et al. Altered muscle insulin sensitivity in the male offspring of protein-malnourished rats. Am J Physiol 1996; 271: E1128–E1134.

88. Sugden MC, Holness MJ. Gender-specific programming of insulin secretion and action. J Endocrinol 2002; 175: 757–67.

89. Horton DM, Kind KL, Thavaneswaran P et al. Large size at birth and neonatal catch-up growth independently predict increased adiposity and reduced muscle mass in the guinea pig. Paper presented at the Perinatal Society of Australia and New Zealand 6th Annual Congress, Christchurch, New Zealand, 2002.

90. Horton DM, Kind KL, Walker MR et al. Fetal growth restriction and accelerated postnatal growth independently predict insulin resistance in the adult guinea pig. Am J Physiol 2005; in press.

91. Poore K, Fowden AL. The effect of birth weight on glucose tolerance in pigs at 3 and 12 months of age. Diabetologia 2002; 45: 1247–54.

92. Poore K, Fowden AL. Insulin sensitivity in juvenile and adult Large White pigs of low and high birthweight. Diabetologia 2004; 47: 340–8.

93. Greenwood PL, Hunt AS, Hermanson JW et al. Effects of birth weight and postnatal nutrition on neonatal sheep: I. Body growth and composition, and some aspects of energetic efficiency. J Anim Sci 1998; 76: 2354–67.

94. Greenwood PL, Hunt AS, Slepetis RM et al. Effects of birth weight and postnatal nutrition on neonatal sheep: III. Regulation of energy metabolism. J Anim Sci 2002; 80: 2850–61.

95. Gatford KL, Clarke IJ, De Blasio MJ et al. Perinatal growth and plasma GH profiles in adolescent and adult sheep. J Endocrinol 2002; 173: 151–9.

96. De Blasio MJ, Gatford KL, Fielke SL et al. Placental restriction of fetal growth reduces size at birth and increases postnatal growth and adiposity in the young lamb. Am J Physiol 2005; in press.

97. Gatford KL, De Blasio MJ, Walker M et al. Restriction of placental and fetal growth impairs insulin secretory capacity in the sheep postnatally. Paper presented at the 12th International Congress of Endocrinology, Lisbon, Portugal, 2004.

98. Simmons RA, Templeton LJ, Gertz SJ. Intrauterine growth retardation leads to the development of type 2 diabetes in the rat. Diabetes 2001; 50: 2279–86.

99. Gelardi NL, Cha C-JM, Oh W. Glucose metabolism in adipocytes of obese offspring of mild hyperglycemic rats. Pediatr Res 1990; 28: 641–5.

100. Holemans K, van Bree R, Verhaeghe J et al. Maternal semi-starvation and streptozotocin-diabetes in rats have different effects on the in vivo glucose uptake by peripheral tissues in their female adult offspring. J Nutr 1997; 127: 1371–6.

101. Bihoreau M-T, Ktorza A, Kinebanyan MF et al. Impaired glucose homeostasis in adult rats from hyperglycemic mothers. Diabetes 1986; 35: 979–84.

102. Gauguier D, Bihoreau M-T, Ktorza A et al. Inheritance of diabetes mellitus as consequence of gestational hyperglycemia in rats. Diabetes 1990; 39: 734–9.

103. Dodic M, May CN, Wintour EM et al. An early prenatal exposure to excess glucocorticoid leads to hypertensive offspring in sheep. Clin Sci 1998; 94: 149–55.

104. Gatford KL, Wintour EM, De Blasio MJ et al. Differential timing for programming of glucose homeostasis, metabolic sensitivity to insulin and blood pressure by in utero exposure to dexamethasone in sheep. Clin Sci 2000; 98: 553–60.

105. Moss TJM, Sloboda DM, Gurrin LC et al. Programming effects in sheep of prenatal growth restriction and glucocorticoid exposure. Am J Physiol 2001; 281: R960–R970.

106. Nyirenda MJ, Lindsay RS, Kenyon CJ et al. Glucocorticoid exposure in late gestation permanently programs rat hepatic phosphoenolpyruvate carboxykinase and glucocorticoid receptor expression and causes glucose intolerance in adult offspring. J Clin Investig 1998; 101: 2174–81.

107. Dahlgren J, Nilsson C, Jennische E et al. Prenatal cytokine exposure results in obesity and gender-specific programming. Am J Physiol 2001; 281: E326–E334.

108. Banjanin S, Kapoor A, Matthews SG. Prenatal glucocorticoid exposure alters hypothalamic-pituitary-adrenal function and blood pressure in mature male guinea pigs. J Physiol (Lond) 2004; 558: 305–18.

109. Weintrob N, Karp M, Hod M. Short- and long-range complications in offspring of diabetic mothers. J Diabetes Complications 1996; 10: 294–301.

110. De Blasio MJ, Gatford KL, Fielke SL et al. Fetal growth restriction increases growth rate and insulin sensitivity in the postnatal lamb. Paper presented at the 11th International Congress of Endocrinology, Sydney, Australia, 2000.

111. De Blasio MJ, Bradbury MR, Adams DH et al. Placental restriction increases postnatal growth rate and sensitivity to IGF-I in the neonatal lamb. Paper presented at the Endocrine Society of Australia Annual Scientific Meeting, Gold Coast, Australia, 2001.

112. Lloyd NK, Thavaneswaran P, Grover S et al. IGF-1 sensitivity and catch-up growth following intrauterine growth restriction in the weanling guinea pig. Paper presented at the Second World Congress on Fetal Origins of Adult Disease, Brighton, UK, 2003.

113. Horton DM. Prenatal growth and postnatal insulin sensitivity in the guinea pig. Paper presented at the Perinatal Origins of Adult Disease Workshop, Melbourne, Australia, 1999.

114. Gatford KL, De Blasio MJ, McMillen IC et al. Placental restriction and ontogeny of insulin-regulated glucose homeostasis in sheep. Paper presented at the Endocrine Society of Australia Annual Scientific Meeting, Adelaide, Australia, 2002.

9

Development of domestic animal models for the study of the ontogeny of human disease

Johanna de Groot, Wim JA Boersma, Franz Josef van der Staay, Theo Niewold, Norbert Stockhofe, Sietse Jan Koopmans, Tette van der Lende, and Teun Schuurman

INTRODUCTION: DOMESTIC ANIMALS IN BIOMEDICAL RESEARCH

Animal models can clarify many pathological mechanisms in humans and contribute enormously to disease understanding and treatment. Most animal models have been developed using inbred rodent strains. They are characterized by low variability, can be bred easily, and reduce costs of experiments. In contrast, domestic animals have historically been studied for food production purposes. These studies have yielded a broad knowledge on nutrition, endocrinology, reproduction, immunology, and infection. Prenatal programming has been studied in sheep[1] and pigs[2,3] with a focus on production and fertility parameters. Until recently, this knowledge has hardly been utilized in biomedical research. However, due to their similarities with humans, large animals can be of great value in preclinical research.[4] Large model animals, such as pigs, sheep, dogs, horses, and nonhuman primates, have been used successfully to bridge the gap between results obtained with rodent models and observations in the clinic.[5,6]

An obvious advantage of large model animals concerns the practical possibilities for biotechnical instrumentation. Cannulation of blood and lymph vessels (e.g. thoracic ducts) allows one to sample continuously or intermittently the large number of cells in circulation. To study nutrition, metabolism, and development of the immune system in the fetus, chronic catheterization techniques are often necessary to investigate maternal and fetal blood flow in conscious animals. Blood sampling and infusion into maternal and fetal arteries and veins allow for study of the metabolic interactions between a sow, placenta, and the fetuses. Due to technical constraints, these studies are best performed in fetuses from large animal models.[7,8] In addition, the availability of multiple littermates in sheep and pigs allows for comparison of treatments in animals of the same genetic background.

Considering the different species that are in use as large model animals, the pig has two major advantages over dogs, horses, and nonhuman primates. First, they are generally used for human consumption, and the public harbors relatively little resentment about porcine research. Second, pigs are easily bred and can be manipulated genetically.[6] The expense and diversity of the large outbred pig makes them impractical for mechanistic studies. Instead, they have been used mainly to answer questions about the efficacy, safety, and toxicity of drug treatments. To reduce the amount of drug needed for testing, the Göttinger minipig,[9] Yucatan micropig, and (Sinclair) miniature swine have been bred. Based on proven similarities in biotransformation between man and minipig, it seems to be the experimental animal of choice for preclinical pharmacokinetic studies.[10] In addition, minipigs are utilized in research on the gastrointestinal tract, diabetes (including island transplants), obesity, and related vascular diseases.[11,12] For studies of immunity[13] including MHC restricted cytotoxicity, vaccines, (xeno)transplantation studies, or gene therapy, the inbreeding of the minipig lines at the level of class I and class II MHC antigens is of great importance. Pigs have also been genetically manipulated to produce knockout[14] and transgenic pigs[15] for various purposes.

The use of large model animals for studying the pathological mechanisms of disease is still limited, as compared with the small animals, particularly genetically defined mice.[6] These latter models sometimes may lead to erroneous conclusions about the mechanisms of disease in humans, and hence to the failure of therapies or interventions in clinical trials.[5] Although large model animals have the disadvantage of higher costs of studies and a longer lifespan, they offer a number of advantages in the subject area of prenatal programming:

(1) The greater similarity to humans in pregnancy and neonatal development;
(2) The size of fetus and neonate, which allows for imaging, detailed anatomic and pathological analysis, and human-like pharmacokinetics; and
(3) High face validity of models of intrauterine growth restriction (IUGR), fetal malnutrition, and intrauterine infections.

PREGNANCY IN PIGS AND MODELS OF IUGR AND FETAL MALNUTRITION

Pregnancy in pigs

Porcine embryos enter the uterus within 2 or 3 days after oocyte fertilization. By this time they have reached the three or four-cell stage. On the sixth day of gestation (DG 6), the embryos, which are then in the early blastocyst stage, emerge from the zona pellucida. The latter is a complex extracellular glycoprotein matrix that is formed around each oocyte during follicular development. Between DG 7 and DG 12, the embryos migrate through the uterine horns and subsequently redistribute themselves over the full length of both uterine horns (each uterine horn is 100–150 cm long!). This process of spacing is often accompanied by trans-uterine migration, even if the distribution of ovulations between both ovaries has been equal. Both estradiol-17β and histamine are involved in intrauterine migration of embryos. Until DG 11 or DG 12, the embryos are spherical. Their diameter increases during this period up to 10 mm. Subsequently, the embryos start to elongate. This elongation is initially due mainly to cell reorganization and not to cell division. Almost simultaneously with the onset of elongation, the embryos develop aromatase activity and start to synthesize and secrete estrogens, which is essential for maternal recognition of pregnancy. Embryonic estrogens are also important to stimulate the coordinated secretion of proteins from the endometrium. During or shortly after elongation, the embryos start to attach to the luminal epithelium of the endometrium. The blastocysts, each with a length of up to 100 cm by the end of elongation (DG 14), follow the endometrial folds. Each blastocyst occupies only a relatively short length (approximately 20 cm) of one of the two uterine horns. Concomitant with this attachment, the trophoblast (former trophectoderm) and embryoblast (former inner cell mass) differentiate to form the extra-embryonic membranes (placenta) and specialized structures of the conceptus, respectively. By DG 35 of pregnancy, placentation and embryonic organogenesis are completed. The remainder of pregnancy up to parturition at ± DG 115 is mainly characterized by placental and fetal growth.

IUGR

The pig is a good model species for studying these long-term effects on IUGR. First, and most importantly, IUGR is a natural phenomenon with a relatively high prevalence in this litter-bearing species. Thus, no pharmacological, dietary, or surgical interventions are needed to induce IUGR. Such manipulations are generally required when rats, guinea pigs or sheep are used as a model.[16,17] Second, since intrauterine growth restricted piglets are born within litters alongside normally developed littermates, the growth-restricted piglet can be studied with piglets that experienced the same prenatal environment.

Analysis of birth weight distributions in a large number of litters from different purebred and cross-bred pigs verified the presence of at least one intrauterine growth restricted piglet in 30% of all litters.[18] The relatively high incidence of IUGR in the pig is due to a large extent to a relatively high within-litter diversity in early embryonic development by the time that the embryos start implantation (reviewed in ref. 19). Implantation in the pig is actually not more than a superficial attachment of the embryonic membranes to the endometrial epithelium because the porcine placentation is of the diffuse and noninvasive epitheliochorial type.[20] Although within the uterus of the sow, preimplantation embryos distribute themselves almost equidistantly throughout both uterine horns between DG 6 and DG 9, due to the variation in stage of development by DG 11, the less well developed embryos have to compete for uterine space once trophoblast elongation starts. As a result, some embryos will ultimately have smaller, insufficient placentae and thus have a developmental disadvantage throughout pregnancy. This inequality leads to altered endocrine status and lower circulating levels of many essential amino acids during the fetal stage of pregnancy.[21] Effects at birth have been reported, for example, for gut health,[22] renal function[23] and ovarian follicular development.[24]

The reasons to suggest that the intrauterine growth-retarded piglet provides a suitable model for intrauterine growth-retarded human infants have been summarized by Bauer et al.,[25] and include developmental similarities in the growth spurt during the perinatal period, cardiovascular and central autonomic functions, energy metabolism, and oxidative brain metabolism, as well as the fact that the distinct morphometric signs in growth restricted piglets[2] are pathognomonic for intrauterine growth-retardation in humans.

Fetal growth restriction can also be induced by restricting maternal feed intake during pregnancy. For instance, a reduction in the sow's feed intake from DG 25 to DG 50 will affect the genesis of fetal tissue specificity, whereas a reduction in maternal feed intake from DG 50 to DG 80 affects growth and maturation of fetal tissues. Undernutrition *in utero* during the entire period of pregnancy causes low birth weight, a decrease in muscle fiber number, and a reduction in postnatal growth rate in pigs. More specifically, undernutrition leads to a decreased production of secondary myofibers in the fetuses, which suggests that skeletal muscle percentage in later life will be reduced. Indeed, adult pigs, which suffered from *in utero* undernutrition, showed a reduction in growth efficiency. The latter was determined by measuring the weight gain to feed intake ratio. In general, a low weight gain to feed intake ratio is indicative of increased fat (adipose tissue) accretion and decreased protein (skeletal muscle) accretion.[26]

Fetal overnutrition in pigs can be achieved by the chemical induction of maternal diabetes during pregnancy. Streptozotocin is a pancreatic beta cell toxic agent, which can be administered to sows at any time during pregnancy, to induce diabetes. Nutrient concentrations in maternal blood are increased and will chronically over-feed the developing fetuses. Effects on birth weight, body composition, and health in later life can then be investigated. Body chemical composition data showed increases in percentage lipid in the progeny of streptozotocin-induced diabetic sows,[27] but data on health parameters in later life are still not available in the literature. The pig can also provide a useful model to study the efficacy of functional foods and nutriceuticals in the development of the fetus. Highly standardized nutritional intervention studies during pregnancy to prevent obesity and to increase skeletal muscle development in the fetus can easily be performed in the pregnant sow. For instance, it has been shown that dietary daidzein (an isoflavone of plant origin) supplementation to the pregnant sow increases fetal growth, in association with higher insulin-like growth factor receptor gene expression in skeletal muscle.[28]

PROGRAMMING OF THE METABOLIC SYSTEM

Pigs are excellent models to study metabolic diseases[29] because they are omnivores and develop spontaneous atherosclerosis with increased age, and have lipoprotein profiles and metabolism similar to humans. Both pigs and humans have more high density than low density lipoproteins and carry the majority of their cholesterol in the low density lipoprotein form. When fed cholesterol- and saturated fat-containing diets (cafeteria diets), normal pigs develop atherosclerosis in most arterial beds within 3 months after diet introduction and the severity of atherosclerosis is proportional to the cholesterol and triglyceride concentrations in the blood. Moreover, in diabetic pigs, the process of atherosclerosis is accelerated and becomes, in general, twice as severe. Pigs (30–40 kg body weight) treated with streptozotocin to induce diabetes, and fed a cafeteria-style diet become hyperphagic, hyperglycemic, and dyslipidemic (with elevated cholesterol and triglyceride concentrations; Figure 9.1). In addition, these pigs show severe whole-body and moderate hepatic insulin resistance for glucose metabolism and their mean arterial blood pressure is increased compared with normal pigs on a low fat diet (S.J. Koopmans, unpublished data).

When studying the ontogeny of metabolic diseases, related to obesity, such as diabetes, cardiovascular disease, and the metabolic syndrome in a pig model, the possibility of embryo transfer allows investigation of the interaction between genetic background and nutritional conditions during *in utero* development. Embryos can be collected from the oviducts of lean donor (i.e. Yorkshire, Duroc) or obese sows (i.e. Meishan, Ossabaw) and subsequently half of the embryos from a donor can be transferred surgically to a lean recipient gilt and the other half of the embryos to an obese recipient gilt.[30]

Current knowledge about the long-term effects of IUGR in pigs is limited. Since the domesticated pig is kept for meat production, animal scientists have mainly studied the effects on muscle fiber development and growth potential until slaughter at an age of approximately 6 months and 90 kg body weight.[31,32] To our knowledge, only a few studies concerning the long-term effects on reproduction or health have been reported. The study by Poore and Fowden[33] was concerned with the effect of IUGR on insulin resistance in juvenile and adult Large White pigs. It was shown that female pigs with low birth weight were insulin-resistant at 3 months of age, as compared to female pigs with high birth weight. Male pigs with low birth weight, however, were more sensitive to insulin. Finally, irrespective of sex, early catch-up growth was associated with insulin resistance in pigs at 12 months of age. With the growing biomedical interest in the pig as a model species, more studies on the long-term pathophysiological effects of IUGR are to be expected in the near future.

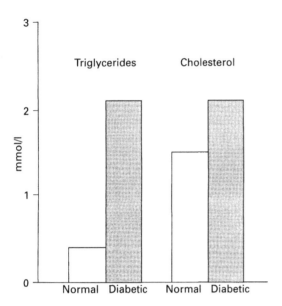

Figure 9.1 Plasma triglyceride and cholesterol concentrations in streptozotocin-induced diabetic pigs fed a cafeteria-style diet (20% fat, 0.25% cholesterol, 10% sucrose) and in normal pigs fed a standard low fat (6%) diet.

PRENATAL STRESS

Stress can have profound effects on physiologic and behavioral functions in humans and animals. Stress, especially repeated episodes and chronic stress, seems to be involved in the etiology of a number of disorders. Stress–disease relationships are evident in several neuropsychiatric disorders, such as depression and anxiety neurosis, as well as cardiovascular diseases and metabolic disorders, such as diabetes.

Studies in rats and mice have shown that prenatal stress affects growth, reproduction parameters, and health of the offspring. Scientists have also started to investigate the effects of prenatal stress in domesticated animals. However, the data about prenatal stress effects in farm animals and pets are still very limited.[34] Research in rodents shows that results vary when using different types and intensities of the stressor, and are influenced by timing of the stress during gestation. Also, variation is observed across different strains of rats.[34] Genetically outbred farm animals can provide a means to test hypotheses arising from rodent studies for their generality to human epidemiological data.

The major stressors for pregnant sows are individual housing, tethering (restraining the animal), social stress due to mixing with unfamiliar sows in group housing systems, and the stress due to restricted feeding. It has been shown that tethering sows results in the development of abnormal behaviors, such as stereotypies and apathy. This form of chronic restraint stress results in autonomic regulatory changes, changes in hypothalamus-pituitary-adrenocortical (HPA) activity (elevated cortisol levels), altered feedback control of the HPA system (increased cortisol response after a standard adrenocorticotropic hormone (ACTH) challenge) and in alterations of the endogenous opioid system (decreased opioid receptor densities in the hippocampus and hypothalamus).[35,36] Furthermore, in long-term tethered pigs, the circadian rhythm of cortisol secretion was blunted.[37] The HPA system of pigs responds very strongly to social stressors, especially social defeat. Single and repeated social defeat results in markedly elevated cortisol concentrations in the blood, increased sympathetic-adrenal medullary activity, shifts in leukocyte subsets, and decreased behavioral activity in a novel environment.[38] Other studies have shown that piglets housed in a barren environment (little space, no straw bedding, stimulus deprivation) develop signs of chronic stress. They showed retarded growth, and did not develop appropriate social behavior in adulthood (increased aggression) as compared with pigs kept previously in an enriched environment.[39,40]

Until now, only a limited number of studies on the consequences of prenatal stress for offspring have been performed in pigs. Different methods to induce prenatal stress have been employed, e.g. daily application of a nose-sling, and weekly injection with ACTH. When sows were restrained daily during the last third of gestation, offspring showed lower basal plasma cortisol and increased cortisol binding globulin concentrations at the age of 3 days. The adrenal cortex was enlarged, and thymus weight was reduced at 1 day of age. Prenatally stressed piglets showed lower IgG levels, and decreased lymphocyte proliferation. Mortality after birth was higher in prenatally stressed piglets.[41] The number of glucocorticoid receptors was also decreased in the hypothalamus, but increased in the hippocampus at the first day after birth. Brain monoamine concentrations, however, were not affected by prenatal stress.[3]

Injection of the sow with ACTH weekly from 6 to 12 weeks of gestation resulted in an increased adrenal cortex:medulla ratio, lower concentrations of hypothalamic beta-endorphin, and higher concentrations of hypothalamic corticotropin-releasing hormone. Offspring from ACTH-treated sows showed a higher cortisol response to social stress (mixing with unfamiliar pigs) than control offspring. Wound healing was slower in control pigs than in ACTH-treated pigs.[42]

Recently, we have established a model using oral administration of cortisol to pregnant sows.[43]

Hydrocortisone acetate (HCA) was administered orally from 7 until 11 weeks of gestation. Plasma and salivary cortisol concentrations were significantly elevated in sows that received 60 or 180 mg HCA, but not in sows that received 20 mg HCA. Duration of gestation was shorter in sows that received 180 mg HCA. Oral administration of 60 mg HCA (0.3 mg/kg body weight) provided a suitable model to elevate cortisol levels in pregnant sows. When this dosage of HCA was given during the first (P1), second (P2), and third period (P3) of pregnancy, it did not result in a change in the duration of gestation or number of piglets born. At birth, P1 and P3 piglets weighed less than control piglets treated only with placebo. This weight difference was no longer evident at 17 days of age. At slaughter, P2 and P3 offspring had increased backfat thickness compared with control piglets. In the open field test, P1 offspring vocalized more and P3 offspring spent more time walking and running. P2 piglets showed a shorter latency to touch the object in a novel object test.[44] We also investigated the effect of prenatal HCA treatment in sows on the sensitivity of the offspring to an inflammatory stimulus, lipopolysaccharide (LPS). Compared to control piglets, P1 and P3 offspring showed an increased febrile response to LPS, whereas the behavioral and cortisol responses to LPS were unaltered.[45]

Effects of prenatal stress have also been investigated in sheep. Isolation stress in pregnant sheep during the last 5 weeks of gestation resulted in an increased birth weight in offspring. Prenatally stressed lambs showed more exploration and locomotion in behavioral tests at 8 months of age, but not at 25 days of age. Basal cortisol concentrations were higher in prenatally stressed lambs at 25 days of age, but prenatally stressed lambs did not respond with a higher cortisol response to isolation stress or to ACTH injection.[46]

In rodents, the main effects of prenatal stress are lower birth weights, elevated HPA axis activity and higher emotional reactivity. Some of these effects are also seen in the pig and sheep studies of prenatal stress. However, it is also apparent that the timing of prenatal stress and the type of stressor are equally important in pig and sheep models.

BEHAVIOR AND CENTRAL NERVOUS SYSTEM (CNS) DYSFUNCTION

The developing brain of the human fetus shows a dramatic growth spurt during the last third of gestation. During growth spurt, the fetal brain is highly sensitive to disturbances caused by insufficient supply of oxygen and the effects of neurotoxins. These disturbances may strongly affect the physical and mental development of the neonate.[47]

A *systemic* dysfunction such as failure of the respiratory or circulatory system may cause encephalopathies. These ischemic/hypoxic encephalopathies, a heterogeneous group of genetic or acquired brain disorders, are caused by deprivation of the brain from critical oxygen supply, either through insufficient cerebral perfusion (ischemia), or due to an insufficient satiation of the blood with oxygen (hypoxia).[48] Perinatal asphyxia, i.e. an interference in gas exchange between mother and fetus, leads to impaired tissue perfusion and oxygenation of vital organs of the fetus. This may cause multiorgan damage in the neonate that affects further development. Asphyxia has an estimated incidence of 1–1.5% in neonates after normal gestation, and may increase to 9% in children delivered prematurely (≤ 36 weeks).

In addition, two main types of cerebrovascular accidents or strokes can be distinguished: rupture of cerebral vessels, which causes hemorrhage, and occlusion of large or small blood vessels in the brain by an embolus or thrombus, which induces an ischemic infarct. The neurological symptoms provide a first hint about the precise type and location of the stroke.[48,49]

Animal models of asphyxia, and/or ischemic stroke or hemorrhage are important tools to identify and characterize new therapeutics. In recent years, several animal models of cerebrovascular diseases have been developed.[50] These models employ many different techniques to induce cerebral infarcts. The main aim is to study the pathophysiology of stroke in order to identify the processes that cause the damage. In these models the efficacy of neuroprotective or recovery-promoting agents can be tested.

A prenatal condition threatening normal neurodevelopment, and consequently, normal functioning of the child, is the maternal use of drugs. Exposure to alcohol, cocaine, heroin, environmental toxins,[51] or agricultural herbicides and insecticides during pregnancy has been investigated using animal models, among them pigs. Notably, alcohol exposure during the brain growth spurt in the third trimester of pregnancy leads to more severe deficits than during other stages of gestation.[52]

The piglet has a number of advantages when studying the effects of asphyxia, hypoxia/ischemia,[53] and of neurotoxins during pregnancy on brain development. Its physiology resembles that of humans,[29] and its brain growth spurt in relation to birth is similar to that in humans[54,55] (Figure 9.2). Whereas the growth spurt of the brain in humans and pigs occurs in the third trimester of gestation,[47] the growth spurt of rodents occurs during days 1–10 postnatally.

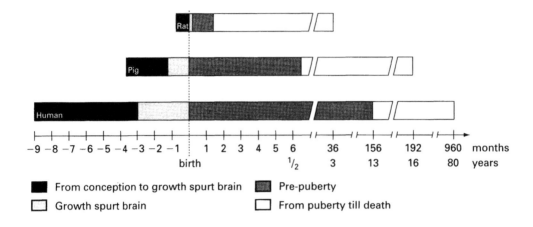

Figure 9.2 Comparison of distinct periods during the lifespan of rat, pig, and human from conception to death. The estimated mean lifespan of rats is extremely strain-dependent and refers to strains that do not develop specific age-related diseases. The estimate for pigs is taken from ref. 102, and the estimate for humans refers to the developed, industrialized countries. Note that the growth spurt period of brain in pigs and humans occurs before birth, whereas it covers the period of postnatal days 1–10 in rats.

Moreover, pigs have large brains allowing the use of noninvasive imaging techniques (e.g. magnetic resonance imaging[56]), cerebral bioimpedance for measuring cerebral edema, and electroencephalography.[57]

Pigs mature rapidly (puberty at 6–7 months of age), allowing investigations of the effects of the encephalopathies on neurodevelopmental outcome and behavioral consequences reaching into adulthood. Unfortunately, neurological and behavioral consequences of perinatal asphyxia, hypoxia/ischemia and stroke, or exposure of the developing fetus to neurotoxins have only sporadically been included in animal studies. Roohey and colleagues in their 1997 review on animal models[58] already highlighted this shortcoming for the study of perinatal hypoxia/ischemia, and the situation has not changed much since. As can be seen in Figure 9.2, the duration of pregnancy, the period of growth spurt of the brain, and the time to adulthood in pigs spans a time period that would facilitate investigations under highly controlled and standardized conditions. Pig studies can be performed in periods lasting less than 1 year.

MATERNAL INFECTION

The immunological mechanisms that govern the success of pregnancy are complex. During placental formation, the invasion of fetal cells into maternal tissue must be controlled to prevent damage to the mother. Equally, maternal recognition of the implanted embryo must be such that rejection does not occur. Suppression of paternal antigens helps to prevent rejection, but must be combined with protection from infections by pathogens.[59]

Later pre- and perinatal infections can also have strong impact on the development of the implant and may go beyond the adaptive capacity of the young. Intrauterine infection is not only a common cause of preterm onset of labour but also a trigger for lung injury, which significantly increases the risk of development of long-term respiratory disease in the newborn infant.[60] Also, there has been a suspicion of an increased incidence of schizophrenia following maternal infections, primarily from viral infections, but also bacterial pathogens during pregnancy.[61] Animal modeling can provide powerful tools to evaluate whether maternal exposure to infectious agents has long-term effects on health of offspring, and to delineate the mechanisms involved.

In humans intrauterine inflammation is most generally caused by progressing cervicovaginal infections. Similar infections have been studied in pigs as well as in cattle and sheep. In a sheep model, an inflammatory state induced by LPS administration during pregnancy led to markedly elevated fetal cortisol and prostaglandin E2 concentrations. This could be a potential protective mechanism that aids the fetus in the event of premature delivery. The fetal response was attenuated when LPS was injected into the amniotic fluid, despite a much higher dose used, which may support a role for the amniotic fluid in protecting the fetus from bacterial pathogens during pregnancy.[62] Pig models have also been developed for parasitic and congenital infections e.g. *Schistosoma*[63] and *Toxoplasma*.[64,65]

Viral infections are capable of producing a wide spectrum of abnormalities. Apparently healthy progeny can be delivered that develop a late-onset disease, months or years after birth. The ultimate outcome of a congenital infection is mainly determined by the stage at which infection occurs.[66] Pigs are suitable to study the consequences of adenovirus infections as they are one of their natural hosts. Transplacental infection with an adenovirus in pigs causes pathological changes such as severe skin cyanosis, edema of the subcutaneous tissues in the submandibular, thoracic, and abdominal regions and eosinophilic intranuclear inclusion bodies in endothelial cells of capillary and small blood vessels throughout the body.[67] In addition, transplacental transmission of porcine cytomegalovirus has been demonstrated.[68] Bacterial infections, such as *Staphylococcus* spp.[69] can also be evaluated in pig models of intrauterine infection in humans.

The similarities and differences of pestivirus infections with human hepatitis C infection and congenital rubella have been studied extensively in domestic animals. Pestiviruses include classical swine fever virus (CSFV), border disease virus of sheep (BDV), and bovine viral diarrhea virus (BVDV). There are some similarities in the pathology of all three infections. *In utero* transmission to the fetus can cause early losses, severe congenital abnormalities and, particularly with BVDV, lifelong persistent infections.[70,71] The pathology may not be due to BVDV but is rather caused by a host response to the virus, particularly the production of proinflammatory cytokines.[72] Infections with these pathogens in animals and man cause similar pathology, especially during pregnancy. However, there are also some important differences. Human fetuses exposed to rubella virus raise an antibody response to the virus, whereas domestic animals frequently fail to respond immunologically to a congenital pestivirus infection. After congenital rubella infection, the virus usually disappears from the host by 1–2 years after birth. However, congenital pestivirus infections are characterized by a lifelong and widespread persistence of virus even in symptom-free healthy animals.[66]

In conclusion, several models of maternal infection are available in domestic animals. The pathology of these models is well described and information regarding the mechanisms of these diseases is growing. Several of these models are useful analogs to human maternal infections with regard to the infectious agent, maternal immune response, and congenital pathology.

PROGRAMMING OF THE IMMUNE SYSTEM

Much less is known about prenatal programming of the immune system in large animals.[73] Immunocompetence in neonates is dependent on the development of the fetal immune system, the exchange of elements between the maternal and fetal immune system, and maternal antigen exposure.[29,74] In some species including humans, aspects of maternal immunity may be transferred transplacentally including both cells and antibodies, while in other species the epitheliochorial placenta limits the transfer of maternal immune factors to colostrum and milk.[75] The pig is an example of the latter type of animal. The double placental membrane in the sow effectively prevents the transfer of immunoglobulins prenatally.[29] In cattle and pigs, ingestion of colostrum provides the protective maternal antibodies that are taken up in the circulation of the newborn via the gut. Nevertheless, the kinetics and order of appearance of innate immunity, humoral and cellular immune responses show a similar sequence of development to that observed in humans.[76–78] The ontogeny of the different lines of T and B lymphocytes in the blood and organs of the porcine embryo and fetus is well documented.[79] Pigs attain mature immune responses of the adults by 6–8 weeks of age.

The gastrointestinal (GI) tract and airways, and their associated mucosal immune responses, play an important role as these surfaces and tissues are the major entrance for invasive microorganisms. In pigs, the development of the intestinal immune system in the postnatal period has been studied in detail.[73] The composition of the GI tract content determined by food/feed and the endogenous microflora are of pivotal importance. The immunologic response to intestinal colonization and bacterial exposure was studied in colostrum-deprived piglets that were delivered germ-free by cesarean section and reared in gnotobiotic isolators. Piglets were inoculated with different *Escherichia coli* strains. Colonization with *E. coli* strains resulted in recruitment of B cells in blood and lymphatic organs and increases in antigen-specific IgA in the gut and serum. In addition, the amount of total immunoglobulins of all isotypes increased in both sera and intestinal washings. IgM-, IgA-, and IgG-secreting cells were increased in spleen, mesenteric lymph nodes, and Peyers patches. Thus at the onset of intestinal colonization, nonpathogenic *E. coli* specifically and polyclonally stimulated the mucosal and systemic humoral immunity in pigs.[80] Intranasal administration of a Herpes virus (pseudorabies virus) to germ-free piglets gave rise to numerous double positive (CD4[+] CD8[+]) T cells in the periphery and the spleen.[13]

Very little is known about prenatal programming of the intestinal immune system. In chickens, the response to an intestinal infection was influenced by prenatal feeding.[81] No data are available for the pig; however, several porcine models are available for studies on intestinal function.

LARGE ANIMAL MODELS OF INFECTION AND ALLERGY

Infection models

As described in the section on maternal infections, a number of interesting infection models are available in domestic animals. An example of a very useful infection model is bovine respiratory syncytial virus (BRSV). BRSV has been employed as a model for human respiratory syncytial virus (HuRSV), which causes a disease resulting in significant mortality in newborns. Since the first report of BRSV in the 1970s, the understanding of this agent and its respective disease has increased dramatically. BRSV disease in cattle is similar in clinical, immunologic and virologic aspects to infection in humans.[82] The results of experimental infection point to an important role for local IgA, rather than for serum IgG1, in the protection against BRSV infection. The capacity to mount a local memory IgA response seems especially important. Priming for such a mucosal response was possible even in young animals when the primary immune response was suppressed by the presence of maternal antibodies in circulation.[83]

In cattle a BRSV vaccine from inactivated virus similar to the human RSV vaccine showed the same benefits for disease prevention.[84] Immunization with this formalin-inactivated BRSV mainly primes for a Th2-like inflammatory response, characterized by a significant eosinophilic influx in the bronchial alveolar lung fluid and lung tissues and high levels of serum IgE. While this response can enhance clinical outcome it can also lead to IgE allergic responses to the vaccine similar to the observations in human.[84] These findings emphasize the usefulness of this animal model to unravel questions about preventive and therapeutic antiviral agents.

Because both chickens and pigs are natural hosts for influenza, they provide an excellent model for investigation of new strains. The pig may act as a mixing vessel that is involved in the generation of new reassortant viruses with pandemic properties. New European Union rules for licensing of vaccines require that animal models are used for toxicity and safety studies. The pig is an excellent model species for such studies. Clinical and immunologic features of influenza infections are to a large extent similar to those observed in humans.[85] In addition the strains that pigs harbor show high similarity to those found in humans, such as 'Hongkong flu' which is an H3N2 strain. Systemic and immune responses in the airways to flu have been studied in the pig.[86] The effect of maternal antibody on vaccine effectiveness in offspring has also been evaluated,[87] and modern vaccine techniques, such as DNA vaccination, have been studied in the pig.[88]

Other virus models in pig that can be used to study basic infection mechanisms include Herpes and pseudorabies viruses for initial transmission and invasion of the nerve tissues,[89] and the effects of breastfeeding on rotavirus infections.[90]

A special category of porcine models include neonatal diarrhea. Diarrheal diseases are still a large problem, claiming more than 2 million lives per year among children under 5 years of age in the developing world. In the developed world, diarrheal diseases continue to occur in neonatal and intensive care wards. Furthermore, globalization increases the risk of cholera outbreaks. In the majority of noncholera cases, the causative organisms are rotavirus and enterotoxigenic *E. coli* (ETEC). In pig husbandry, diarrhea caused by ETEC and rotavirus is also a major problem. Thus, both rotavirus- and ETEC-induced diarrhea can be studied in weaning piglets. The small intestinal segment perfusion (SISP) model provides a means to study the disease processes *ex vivo*.

For the latter model, the small intestine from an anesthetized pig is divided into 10 segments, with separate inlet and outlet tubes. These segments are subsequently perfused for 8 hours. Intestinal segments can be separately infected with enteropathogens or enterotoxins, and the effect of different foods and components on the net fluid absorption and electrolyte balance tested simultaneously within one animal. This technique is very useful for testing the functionality of food components, novel foods, pre- and probiotics and food additives. Furthermore, as testing is done in a functional intestine, with intact blood flow and innervation, it also allows for simultaneous testing of different compounds within the same animal. Results obtained in the SISP have a high predictive value for secretory diarrhea *in vivo* in pigs.[91] Within the SISP model, both curative and preventive approaches can be tested. Also, this technique allows for continuous sampling of intestinal tissue for genomic analysis. Using this technique, the influence of prenatal programming on the expression and function of intestinal genes, intestinal immunology, and the defense against pathogens could be tested.

Models for allergic asthma

Epidemiological data reveal that children from allergic mothers are more likely to develop allergies or asthma than are children who have only an allergic father. However, the mechanism behind this differential inheritability is unknown. This is an example of a subject that cannot easily be studied in humans.

Recently, a dog model was established to study maternal influences on allergic sensitivity of offspring.[92] Beagle puppies that were born from allergic parents (sensitized with ragweed) or nonallergic parents were then exposed to ragweed beginning within 1 week after birth. Offspring from sensitized dogs exposed to ragweed developed elevated serum total and ragweed specific IgE and showed an increased pulmonary resistance to histamine and ragweed, and increased numbers of eosinophils in bronchoalveolar lavage. Offspring from nonsensitized parents did not show this immune response. This dog model offers unique possibilities to investigate the role that early events play in the development of atopic disorders.

A number of other animal models of asthma are available, and the most widely used one is probably the guinea pig. Although this model resembles many features seen in human asthma, there are also quite a few differences. A late phase response to allergen has been seen only under certain experimental conditions and the immune response is mainly due to IgG, which is in contrast to the predominant IgE response in humans.[93] Animal models of asthma have also been developed in farm animal species, such as sheep and pigs. Allergic sensitivity in sheep has been induced by *Ascaris suum* and more recently by sensitization to house dust mite.[94–96] Changes in respiratory physiology as well as pulmonary immunology and the development of airway hyperreactivity are similar to those seen in humans. Another advantage is the animal size, which eases the accessibility of the lungs for measurements of respiratory parameters in the conscious animal.

Only a small number of publications refer to the use of a pig model of asthma, but both the early and late phase responses to allergens have been found.[97–100] The studies mainly focused on the airway responses and pharmacological interventions; and so far only limited information on the immunological mechanisms is

available. However, the similarity of the hyperresponsiveness after sensitization with *Ascaris suum* or ovalbumin, and the comparability of pig to human lungs,[101,102] make swine promising for studies on prenatal programming and the immunology of asthma.

FUTURE POSSIBILITIES

Large animals offer excellent opportunities to take the research on the long-term consequences of prenatal conditions a step forward. However, the traditional separation of agricultural and animal husbandry research institutions from biological and medical university departments often poses a barrier to ready exchange of ideas and findings. Integration of knowledge from these fields will enhance the interpretation and the generalizability of results. Porcine and bovine models are valid and predictive, and appear to meet the criteria of clinical relevance.

REFERENCES

1. Birch RA, Padmanabhan V, Foster DL et al. Prenatal programming of reproductive neuroendocrine function: fetal androgen exposure produces progressive disruption of reproductive cycles in sheep. Endocrinology 2003; 144: 1426–34.
2. Bauer R, Walter B, Hoppe A et al. Body weight distribution and organ size in newborn swine (*Sus scrofa domestica*) – a study describing an animal model for asymmetrical intrauterine growth retardation. Exp Toxicol Pathol 1998; 50: 59–65.
3. Kanitz E, Otten W, Tuchscherer M et al. Effects of prenatal stress on corticosteroid receptors and monoamine concentrations in limbic areas of suckling piglets (*Sus scrofa*) at different ages. J Vet Med A Physiol Pathol Clin Med 2003; 50: 132–9.
4. Hein WR, Griebel PJ. A road less travelled: large animal models in immunological research. Nat Rev Immunol 2003; 3: 79–84.
5. Hart SL. Large animal models: bridging the gap. Mol Ther 2003; 8: 528–9.
6. Kirk AD. Crossing the bridge: large animal models in translational transplantation research. Immunol Rev 2003; 196: 176–96.
7. Finch AM, Antipatis C, Pickard AR et al. Patterns of fetal growth within Large White × Landrace and Chinese Meishan gilt litters at three stages of gestation. Reprod Fertil Dev 2002; 14: 419–25.
8. Pere MC. Maternal and fetal blood levels of glucose, lactate, fructose, and insulin in the conscious pig. J Anim Sci 1995; 73: 2994–9.
9. Beglinger R, Becker M, Eggenberger E et al. [The Goettingen miniature swine as an experimental animal. 1. Review of literature, breeding and handling, cardiovascular parameters.] Res Exp Med (Berl) 1975; 165: 251–63.

10. Kvetina J, Svoboda Z, Nobilis M et al. Experimental Goettingen minipig and beagle dog as two species used in bioequivalence studies for clinical pharmacology (5-aminosalicylic acid and atenolol as model drugs). Gen Physiol Biophys 1999; 18 (Spec No): 80–5.

11. Hughes GC, Post MJ, Simons M et al. Translational physiology: porcine models of human coronary artery disease: implications for preclinical trials of therapeutic angiogenesis. J Appl Physiol 2003; 94: 1689–701.

12. Rolandsson O, Haney MF, Hagg E et al. Streptozotocin induced diabetes in minipig: a case report of a possible model for type 1 diabetes? Autoimmunity 2002; 35: 261–4.

13. Sinkora J, Rehakova Z, Sinkora M et al. Early development of immune system in pigs. Vet Immunol Immunopathol 2002; 87: 301–6.

14. Lai L, Kolber-Simonds D, Park KW et al. Production of alpha-1,3-galactosyltransferase knockout pigs by nuclear transfer cloning. Science 2002; 295: 1089–92.

15. Uchida M, Shimatsu Y, Onoe K et al. Production of transgenic miniature pigs by pronuclear microinjection. Transgenic Res 2001; 10: 577–82.

16. Holemans K, Aerts L, Van Assche FA. Fetal growth restriction and consequences for the offspring in animal models. J Soc Gynecol Investig 2003; 10: 392–9.

17. Vuguin P. Animal models for assessing the consequences of intrauterine growth restriction on subsequent glucose metabolism of the offspring: a review. J Matern Fetal Neonatal Med 2002; 11: 254–7.

18. Van der Lende T, Hazeleger W, De Jager D. Weight distribution within litters at the early fetal stage and at birth in relation to embryonic mortality in the pig. Livest Prod Sci 1990; 26: 53–65.

19. Van der Lende T, Soede NM, Kemp B. Embryo mortality and prolificacy in the pig. In: Principles of Pig Science (Cole DJA, Wiseman J, Varley MA, eds). Nottingham: Nottingham University Press, 1994: 297–317.

20. Steven DH. Comparative Placentation. Essays in Structure and Function. London: Academic Press, 1975.

21. Ashworth CJ, Finch AM, Page KR et al. Causes and consequences of fetal growth retardation in pigs. Reprod Suppl 2001; 58: 233–46.

22. Thornbury JC, Sibbons PD, van Velzen D et al. Histological investigations into the relationship between low birth weight and spontaneous bowel damage in the neonatal piglet. Pediatr Pathol 1993; 13: 59–69.

23. Bauer R, Walter B, Ihring W et al. Altered renal function in growth-restricted newborn piglets. Pediatr Nephrol 2000; 14: 735–9.

24. Da Silva-Buttkus P, van den Hurk R, te Velde ER et al. Ovarian development in intrauterine growth-retarded and normally developed piglets originating from the same litter. Reproduction 2003; 126: 249–58.

25. Bauer R, Walter B, Brust P et al. Impact of asymmetric intrauterine growth restriction on organ function in newborn piglets. Eur J Obstet Gynecol Reprod Biol 2003; 110: S40–S49.

26. Dwyer CM, Stickland NC, Fletcher JM. The influence of maternal nutrition on muscle fiber number development in the porcine fetus and on subsequent postnatal growth. J Anim Sci 1994; 72: 911–17.

27. Ezekwe MO, Ezekwe EI, Sen DK et al. Effects of maternal streptozotocin-diabetes on fetal growth, energy reserves and body composition of newborn pigs. J Anim Sci 1984; 59: 974–80.

28. Ren MQ, Kuhn G, Wegner J et al. Feeding daidzein to late pregnant sows influences the estrogen receptor beta and type 1 insulin-like growth factor receptor mRNA expression in newborn piglets. J Endocrinol 2001; 170: 129–35.

29. Tumbleson M. Swine in Biomedical Research. New York: Plenum Press, 1986.

30. Biensen NJ, Wilson ME, Ford SP. The impact of either a Meishan or Yorkshire uterus on Meishan or Yorkshire fetal and placental development to days 70, 90, and 110 of gestation. J Anim Sci 1998; 76: 2169–76.

31. Handel S, Stickland N. Catch-up growth in pigs – a relationship with muscle cellularity. Anim Prod 1988; 47: 291–5.

32. Powell SE, Aberle ED. Skeletal muscle and adipose tissue cellularity in runt and normal birth weight swine. J Anim Sci 1981; 52: 748–56.

33. Poore KR, Fowden AL. Insulin sensitivity in juvenile and adult Large White pigs of low and high birthweight. Diabetologia 2004; 47: 340–8.

34. Braastad B. Effects of prenatal stress on behaviour of offspring of laboratory and farmed mammals. Appl Anim Behav Sci 1998; 61: 159–80.

35. Janssens CJ, Helmond FA, Wiegant VM. Increased cortisol response to exogenous adrenocorticotropic hormone in chronically stressed pigs: influence of housing conditions. J Anim Sci 1994; 72: 1771–7.

36. Loijens L, Schouten W, Wiepkema P et al. Brain opioid receptor density reflects behavioral and heart rate responses in pigs. Physiol Behav 2002; 76: 579–87.

37. Janssens CJ, Helmond FA, Wiegant VM. Chronic stress and pituitary-adrenocortical responses to corticotropin-releasing hormone and vasopressin in female pigs. Eur J Endocrinol 1995; 132: 479–84.

38. Ruis MAW, De Groot J, te Brake JHA et al. Behavioural and physiological consequences of acute social defeat in growing gilts: effects of the social environment. Appl Anim Behav Sci 2001; 70: 201–25.

39. De Jonge FH, Bokkers EA, Schouten WG et al. Rearing piglets in a poor environment: developmental aspects of social stress in pigs. Physiol Behav 1996; 60: 389–96.

40. Olsson I, de Jonge F, Schuurman T et al. Poor rearing conditions and social stress in pigs: repeated social challenge and the effect on behavioural and physiological responses to stressors. Behav Process 1999; 46: 201–15.

41. Otten W, Kanitz E, Tuchscherer M. Prenatal stress in pigs: effects on growth, physiological stress reactions and immune function. Archiv Fur Tierzucht 2000; 43: 159–64.

42. Haussmann MF, Carroll JA, Weesner GD et al. Administration of ACTH to restrained, pregnant sows alters their pigs' hypothalamic-pituitary-adrenal (HPA) axis. J Anim Sci 2000; 78: 2399–411.

43. Kranendonk G, Hopster H, Van Eerdenburg FJ et al. Evaluation of oral administration of cortisol as a model for prenatal stress in pregnant sows. Am J Vet Res 2005; 66: 780–90.

44. Kranendonk G, Hopster H, Fillerup M et al. Effects of increased maternal plasma cortisol levels during gestation on postnatal piglet behaviour and physiology. In: Annual Conference of the International Society for Applied Ethology ; Helsinki, Finland, 2004.

45. De Groot J, Kranendonk G, Hopster H et al. Prenatal cortisol exposure affects sensitivity to LPS in young pigs. In: Annual Conference of the Psychoneuroimmunology Research Society, Titisee, Germany, 2004.

46. Roussel S, Hemsworth P, Boissy A et al. Effects of repeated stress during pregnancy in ewes on the behavioural and physiological responses to stressful events and birth weight of their offspring. Appl Anim Behav Sci 2004; 85: 259–76.

47. Pond WG, Boleman SL, Fiorotto ML et al. Perinatal ontogeny of brain growth in the domestic pig. Proc Soc Exp Biol Med 2000; 223: 102–8.

48. Adams RD, Victor M, Ropper AH. Principles of Neurology, 6th edn. New York: McGraw-Hill, 1997.

49. Wiebers DO, Feigin VL, Brown RD Jr. Handbook of Stroke. Philadelphia: Lippincott-Raven, 1997.

50. Tamura A, Kawai K, Takagi K. Animal models used in cerebral ischemia and stroke research. In: Clinical Pharmacology of Cerebral Ischemia (Ter Horst GJ, Korf J, eds). Totowa NJ: Humana Press, 1997: 265–94.

51. Costa LG. Signal transduction in environmental neurotoxicity. Annu Rev Pharmacol Toxicol 1998; 38: 21–43.

52. Chen WJ, Maier SE, Parnell SE et al. Alcohol and the developing brain: neuroanatomical studies. Alcohol Res Health 2003; 27: 174–80.

53. Foster KA, Colditz PB, Lingwood BE et al. An improved survival model of hypoxia/ischaemia in the piglet suitable for neuroprotection studies. Brain Res 2001; 919: 122–31.

54. Grate LL, Golden JA, Hoopes PJ et al. Traumatic brain injury in piglets of different ages: techniques for lesion analysis using histology and magnetic resonance imaging. J Neurosci Methods 2003; 123: 201–6.

55. Haaland K, Loberg EM, Steen PA et al. Posthypoxic hypothermia in newborn piglets. Pediatr Res 1997; 41 (4 Pt 1): 505–12.

56. Munkeby BH, Lyng K, Froen JF et al. Morphological and hemodynamic magnetic resonance assessment of early neonatal brain injury in a piglet model. J Magn Reson Imaging 2004; 20: 8–15.

57. Ioroi T, Peeters-Scholte C, Post I et al. Changes in cerebral haemodynamics, regional oxygen saturation and amplitude-integrated continuous EEG during hypoxia-ischaemia and reperfusion in newborn piglets. Exp Brain Res 2002; 144: 172–7.

58. Roohey T, Raju TN, Moustogiannis AN. Animal models for the study of perinatal hypoxic-ischemic encephalopathy: a critical analysis. Early Hum Dev 1997; 47: 115–46.

59. Siegrist C. Mechanisms by which maternal antibodies influence infant vaccine responses: review of hypotheses and definition of main determinants. Vaccine 2003; 21: 3406–12.

60. Lyon A. Chronic lung disease of prematurity. The role of intra-uterine infection. Eur J Pediatr 2000; 159: 798–802.

61. Boksa P, El-Khodor B. Birth insult interacts with stress at adulthood to alter dopaminergic function in animal models: possible implications for schizophrenia and other disorders. Neurosci Biobehav Rev 2003; 27: 91–101.

62. Grigsby P, Hirst J, Scheerlinck J et al. Fetal responses to maternal and intra-amniotic lipopolysaccharide administration in sheep. Biol Reprod 2003; 68: 1695–702.

63. Johansen M, Bogh H, Nansen P et al. *Schistosoma japonicum* infection in the pig as a model for human schistosomiasis japonica. Acta Trop 2000; 76: 85–99.

64. Hill D, Dubey J. *Toxoplasma gondii*: transmission, diagnosis and prevention. Clin Microbiol Infect 2002; 8: 634–40.

65. Jungersen G, Bille-Hansen V, Jensen L et al. Transplacental transmission of *Toxoplasma gondii* in minipigs infected with strains of different virulence. J Parasitol 2001; 87: 108–13.

66. Van Oirschot J. Congenital infections with nonarbo togaviruses. Vet Microbiol 1983; 8: 321–61.

67. Narita M, Imada T, Fukusho A. Pathologic changes caused by trans-placental infection with an adenovirus-like agent in pigs. Am J Vet Res 1985; 46: 1126–9.

68. Edington N, Watt R, Plowright W et al. Experimental transplacental transmission of porcine Cytomegalovirus. J Hyg (Camb) 1977; 78: 243–51.

69. Wegener H, Skov Jensen E. A Longitudinal study of *Staphylococcus hyicus* colonization of vagina of gilts and transmission to piglets. Epidemiol Infect 1992; 109: 433–44.

70. Brownlie J, Hooper L, Thompson I et al. Maternal recognition of foetal infection with bovine virus diarrhoea virus (BVDV) – the bovine pestivirus. Clin Diagn Virol 1998; 10: 141–50.

71. Grooms D. Reproductive consequences of infection with bovine viral diarrhea virus. Vet Clin North Am Food Anim Pract 2004; 20: 5–19.

72. Bielefeldt-Ohmann H. The pathologies of bovine viral diarrhea virus infection. A window on the pathogenesis. Vet Clin North Am Food Anim Pract 1995; 11: 447–76.

73. Rothkotter HJ, Sowa E, Pabst R. The pig as a model of developmental immunology. Hum Exp Toxicol 2002; 21: 533–6.

74. Dresser D. The influence of maternal humoral responsiveness on the specific immunocompetence of the progeny in mice. J Reprod Immunol 1990; 18: 293–9.

75. Ogra PL, Dayton DH. Immunology of Breast Milk. New York: Raven Press, 1979.

76. Bianchi A, Scholten J, Leusen B et al. Development of the natural response of immunoglobulin secreting cells in the pig as a function of organ, age and housing. Dev Comp Immunol 1999; 23: 511–20.

77. Bianchi A, Zwart R, Jeurissen S et al. Development of the B-cell and T-cell compartments in porcine lymphoid organs from birth to adult life – an immunohistochemical approach. Vet Immunol Immunopathol 1992; 33: 201–21.

78. Joling P, Bianchi A, Kappe A et al. Distribution of lymphocyte subpopulations in thymus, spleen, and peripheral-blood of specific pathogen-free pigs from 1 to 40 weeks of age. Vet Immunol Immunopathol 1994; 40: 105–17.

79. Butler J, Sun J, Weber P et al. Switch recombination in fetal porcine thymus is uncoupled from somatic mutation. Vet Immunol Immunopathol 2002; 87: 307–19.

80. Cukrowska B, Kozakova H, Rehakova Z et al. Specific antibody and immunoglobulin responses after intestinal colonization of germ-free piglets with non-pathogenic *Escherichia coli* 086. Immunobiology 2001; 204: 425–33.

81. Rebel J, van Dam J, Zekarias B et al. Vitamin and trace mineral content in feed of breeders and their progeny: effects of growth, feed conversion and severity of malabsorption syndrome of broilers. Br Poultry Sci 2004; 45: 201–9.

82. Kimman T, Westenbrink F. Immunity to human and bovine respiratory syncytial virus. Arch Virol 1990; 112: 1–25.

83. Kimman T, Westenbrink F, Schreuder B et al. Local and systemic antibody-response to bovine respiratory syncytial virus-infection and reinfection in calves with and without maternal antibodies. J Clin Microbiol 1987; 25: 1097–106.

84. Antonis A, Schrijver R, Daus F et al. Vaccine-induced immunopathology during bovine respiratory syncytial virus infection: exploring the parameters of pathogenesis. J Virol 2003; 77: 12067–73.

85. Easterday B. Animals in the influenza world. Philos Trans R Soc Lond B Biol Sci 1980; 288: 433–7.

86. Heinen P, de Boer-Luijtze E, Bianchi A. Respiratory and systemic humoral and cellular immune responses of pigs to a heterosubtypic influenza A virus infection. J Gen Virol 2001; 82: 2697–707.

87. Loeffen W, Heinen P, Bianchi A et al. Effect of maternally derived antibodies on the clinical signs and immune response in pigs after primary and secondary infection with an influenza H1N1 virus. Vet Immunol Immunopathol 2003; 92: 23–35.

88. Heinen P, Rijsewijk F, de Boer-Luijtze E et al. Vaccination of pigs with a DNA construct expressing an influenza virus M2-nucleoprotein fusion protein exacerbates disease after challenge with influenza A virus. J Gen Virol 2002; 83: 1851–9.

89. Kritas S, Pensaert M, Nauwynck H et al. Neural invasion of two virulent Suid Herpesvirus 1 strains in neonatal pigs with or without maternal immunity. Vet Microbiol 1999; 69: 143–56.

90. Parreno V, Hodgins D, de Arriba L et al. Serum and intestinal isotype antibody responses to Wa human rotavirus in gnotobiotic pigs are modulated by maternal antibodies. J Gen Virol 1999; 80: 1417–28.

91. Niewold TA, Kerstens HH, van der Meulen J, Smits MA, Hulst MM. Development of a porcine small intestinal cDNA micro-array: characterization and functional analysis of the response to enterotoxigenic E. coli. Vet Immunol Immunopathol 2005; 105: 317–29.

92. Barrett E, Rudolph K, Bowen L et al. Parental allergic status influences the risk of developing allergic sensitization and an asthmatic-like phenotype in canine offspring. Immunology 2003; 110: 493–500.

93. Bice DE, Seagrave J, Green FH. Animal models of asthma: potential usefulness for studying health effects of inhaled particles. Inhal Toxicol 2000; 12: 829–62.

94. Abraham WM, Delehunt JC, Yerger L et al. Characterization of a late phase pulmonary response after antigen challenge in allergic sheep. Am Rev Respir Dis 1983; 128: 839–44.

95. Abraham WM, Laufer S, Tries S. The effects of ML 3000 on antigen-induced responses in sheep. Pulm Pharmacol Ther 1997; 10: 167–73.

96. Bischof RJ, Snibson K, Shaw R et al. Induction of allergic inflammation in the lungs of sensitized sheep after local challenge with house dust mite. Clin Exp Allergy 2003; 33: 367–75.

97. Alving K, Matran R, Fornhem C et al. Late phase bronchial and vascular responses to allergen in actively-sensitized pigs. Acta Physiol Scand 1991; 143: 137–8.

98. Fornhem C, Lundberg JM, Alving K. Allergen-induced late-phase airways obstruction in the pig: the role of endogenous cortisol. Eur Respir J 1995; 8: 928–37.

99. Mitchell HW, Turner DJ, Gray PR et al. Compliance and stability of the bronchial wall in a model of allergen-induced lung inflammation. J Appl Physiol 1999; 86: 932–7.

100. Turner DJ, Gray PR, Taylor SA et al. Physiological responses of the airway wall and lung in hyperresponsive pigs. Eur Respir J 2001; 18: 935–41.

101. Magno M. Comparative anatomy of the tracheobronchial circulation. Eur Respir J Suppl 1990; 12: 557s–562s; discussion 62s–63s.

102. McKay KO, Wiggs BR, Pare PD et al. Zero-stress state of intra- and extraparenchymal airways from human, pig, rabbit, and sheep lung. J Appl Physiol 2002; 92: 1261–6.

103. Sell DR, Lane MA, Johnson WA et al. Longevity and the genetic determination of collagen glycoxidation kinetics in mammalian senescence. Proc Natl Acad Sci USA 1996; 93: 485–90.

Section III – Early life programming of immunity – links to infectious and allergic disorders

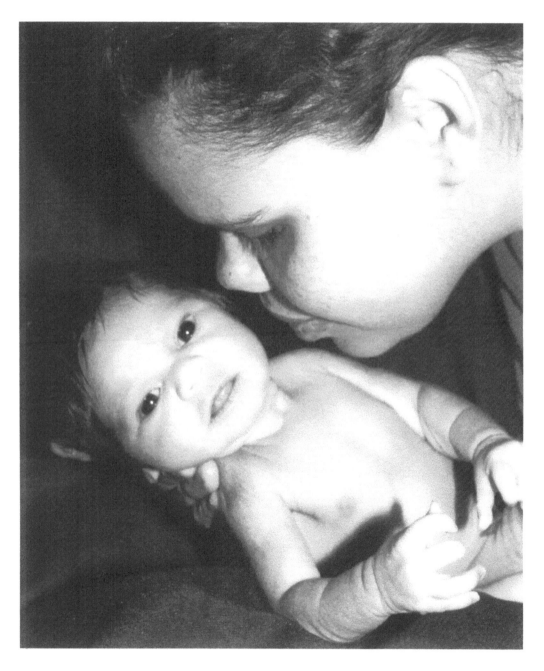

'Every people should be originators of their own destiny'
Martin Delany

10

Prenatal influences on immunity and the developmental trajectory of infant primates

Christopher L Coe and Gabriele R Lubach

INTRODUCTION

During the excitement of observing a child's birth, one is not usually inclined to contemplate the myriad number of complex processes that contributed to the successful outcome. When it involves the birth of an animal, it is also common to have a noninquiring acceptance of this momentous event, because the mother's solicitous care and the infant's responses seem to unfold so naturally that all the antecedent biology, and the remarkable coordination that was required, are not overtly apparent. However, when there are pregnancy or delivery complications, or if the baby develops an illness, then we begin to appreciate the full significance of the many prenatal events that guide and enable normal development. From a research point of view, perturbing the pregnancy and assessing if there is a deleterious change is one of the more effective ways to reveal the important maternal and fetal processes that underlie and ensure a baby's normal behavior and physiology. It is the approach our laboratory has used to investigate how gestational factors influence the development of brain, behavioral, and immune responses in young monkeys.

Our major interest has been focused on the development of the immune system, especially with regard to determining if a period of prenatal stress can compromise an infant's immune competence after birth. However, the immune system does not act autonomously so it was also necessary to study many other aspects of the monkey's physiology in order to identify the critical pathways that could explain any long-term change in immunity. In keeping with the seminal findings that initially heralded the importance of 'fetal programming',[1] we evaluated growth processes both before and after birth. This chapter begins with a short summary of factors that con-tribute to an infant monkey's weight at birth and the potential significance for later development. Next, we discuss several types of disturbances during pregnancy that were found to exert long-term effects on the infant's behavior and physiology after birth.

In addition to periods of maternal stress, administering hormones to increase the adrenal activity of the gravid female caused lasting changes in brain and immune responses. Similarly, injecting drugs, such as dexamethasone (Dex) that cross the placenta and act like adrenal hormones, also impacted the fetus and were found to still have an influence on immune responses when the monkey was 1 year of age. We briefly describe how one assesses the behavioral status of a young monkey in order to ascertain the potential effect of different pregnancy conditions, especially with regard to its maturational and emotional state. Finally, a number of immune alterations caused by perturbations of the maternal/fetal relationship are summarized, along with several mediators that were identified. For example, some hormone and immune changes appear to be associated with a decrease in the size of the hippocampus, a brain area that seems to be particularly sensitive to stress. Across growth, behavior, brain, and immunity, it is clear that important aspects of the infant's developmental trajectory are initiated *in utero*. As evident in many species, from rodents to farm animals and humans, processes that shape and ultimately establish the set points for many of the monkey's physiological systems start during fetal life.

NONHUMAN PRIMATE MODEL

There are over 200 species in the Order Primates, including the prosimians, many different types of monkeys, and the larger great apes. Our studies focused primarily on just one of these primate species, the rhesus monkey (*Macaca mulatta*), which normally lives in the forests of India and southern Asia. This particular monkey is the one used most commonly in biomedical research. Our colony was first established over 50 years ago, in order to conduct learning and developmental studies. Today, the facility houses nearly 500 monkeys, descendants of the founder population originally imported from India. Each year between 50 and 100 new infants are generated from normal and different types of treated pregnancies.

Learning a few facts about the reproduction and development of monkeys will help to better appreciate the findings that we will be discussing. The rhesus monkey gives birth to one infant at a time; in fact, twinning is a very rare event, occurring only 3 times in 1500 births at our facility (as compared to a prevalence of 1:60–80 in humans). The monkey mother's physiology is quite similar to that of women in terms of the hormonal changes across pregnancy. For example, there are comparable increases in important hormones like cortisol by midgestation, which is one reason that we focused on how maternal stress affected the pituitary-adrenal axis. Monkeys also have the same type of hemachorial placenta as humans do, which makes them a good animal model for evaluating changes in placental physiology. In addition, their gestation is relatively long, lasting 5.5 months, which afforded the opportunity in many experiments to compare the impact of disturbance during early and late pregnancy. To create the babies for our research, we used a time-mating protocol, keeping the male and female together for a delimited period around ovulation so that it was possible to designate date of conception and gestational age. Unless there was a clinical need to intervene and assist in the delivery, the monkeys gave birth naturally at night, typically after a labor of 30–240 minutes. In all of the studies we will be describing, the experimental manipulations ended at least 3 weeks prior to parturition, so that postpartum effects on the infant were not due to premature birth or delivery complications.

The rhesus monkey infant typically weighs a little over one pound at birth (490 ± 50 g). However, there is a considerable range of normal variation in size. At the lower end, 330 g is the smallest baby that would usually be viable without human intervention; at the upper end, 790 g was the largest monkey delivered naturally without veterinary assistance. This range corresponds to a comparable variation between 2.3 and 4.6 kg (5–10 pounds) in full-term human infants. We have conducted many analyses to assess predictors of birth weight, because a change in fetal growth rates is one of the more

direct ways through which the mother and the environment can affect the baby's development. Using multivariate regression analyses for 1321 births over 25 years, a number of influential variables emerged, but it was striking that maternal variables far outweighed the influence of any paternal factor (e.g. the female's weight gain across pregnancy was very important).[2] In a second study we turned our attention more specifically to the smallest and largest babies born in the colony.[3] Babies were selected on the basis of being small for gestational age (SGA < 390 g, *n* = 88) or large for gestational age (LGA > 590 g, *n* = 91), and then the birth records were re-analyzed, clustering together relatives on their mother's or father's side (Figure 10.1). A high concordance of birth weight was seen among maternal relatives, especially siblings, but not with relatives on the father's side, highlighting one of the major influences a mother has on the baby developing within her. The significance of birth weight did not end at parturition. Applying the statistical technique of growth curve modeling, it was possible to show that size at birth, whether small or large, was then associated with the slope of growth across the next 3 years of life, and predictive of a female's age at menarche and reproductive maturity.[4]

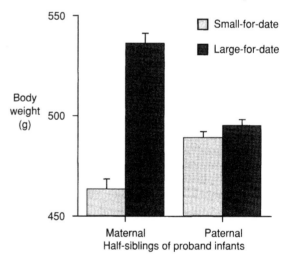

Figure 10.1 Association between birth weights among half-siblings indicating a greater maternal influence on fetal growth. More similarity in birth weights was found for maternal than for paternal relatives of small-for-gestational age (< 390 g, *n* = 88) and large-for-gestational age (> 590 g, *n* = 91) rhesus monkey infants.[3] Female monkeys had been mated with different male sires across successive pregnancies, which enabled this analysis of half-siblings.

One consequence of this awareness about the maternal influence on fetal and infant growth was that we established certain inclusion and exclusion criteria for adult females used as breeders in the following research on prenatal stress. They had to be of optimal reproductive age (5–18 years), multiparous, and without a history of pregnancy complications or SGA babies. In addition, the experimental manipulations were tailored to ensure that they would not alter birth weight. Even the Dex treatments, which can cause a slowing of fetal growth for several days, were ended 3 weeks before term so that they no longer had an effect on infant size by the time of delivery. Thus, the effects on brain and immunity were not mediated either by infant prematurity or a small size at birth. As a consequence, we return to the topic of growth only briefly at the end of the chapter. It turned out to be important for understanding the effect of pregnancy stress on the prenatal transfer and utilization of iron by the baby. The faster-growing babies placed more demands on their iron stores and were at greater risk for developing an iron deficiency anemia (IDA).

DISTURBANCES OF PREGNANCY

The previous descriptions characterized normal births from undisturbed pregnancies, but one can think of experimental or even natural conditions that might challenge the gravid female monkey and perturb the developing fetus. In nature, it could be harsh climatic conditions, such as a drought or extreme temperatures, difficulties in obtaining enough food, or perhaps aggression from other members of the troop. Physical and psychological challenges can also be simulated in a number of different ways for experimental purposes in the laboratory. In one study, we assessed the impact of relocation: moving females into new cages and social groups during their pregnancy.[5] To gain greater control over the timing and level of the disturbance, our studies have more typically employed a stressful condition that could be scheduled at exact times during gestation.[6] It involved a 10-minute period of daily disturbance, evoked for 6 weeks or 25% of the 24-week pregnancy. Specifically, the pregnant female was relocated to another room in the mid-afternoon for 10 minutes, where a 1-second horn was sounded three times randomly by a computer program. This acoustical startle protocol elicited a brief period of agitation and evoked an acute release of the stress hormone cortisol from the adrenal gland. Although brief and delimited, when carried out during early or late pregnancy (days 50–92 postconception or 105–147 postconception), the babies were found to be significantly different from undisturbed ones. These lasting effects were found despite the fact that the disturbance was determined to still be moderate enough that it did not reduce birth weight, which was of concern given the importance ascribed previously to fetal growth.

We were interested in investigating the possible role of pituitary-adrenal hormones in mediating the effects of maternal stress on the fetus, because these hormones have been implicated so often in rodent studies.[7–9] The type of hormone activation that would accompany psychological arousal was induced in other experiments by injecting the gravid female monkey with adrenocorticotropin hormone (ACTH). ACTH is the regulatory hormone released from the pituitary and stimulates the adrenal gland. For 2 weeks during pregnancy (from days 120 to 133 postconception), ACTH was administered daily to raise cortisol secretion for > 4 hours, as if there was a recurrent stressor, and then the females were left undisturbed for the remaining month of pregnancy.[10] In other projects, additional females received 2-day treatments of Dex.[11] Dex is a potent corticosteroid receptor agonist known to cross the placenta, and thus it provided a test of the effect of fetal exposure to unusually high corticosteroid levels. Beyond shedding some light on whether Dex acts in a manner like stress, these assessments were of interest because Dex and betamethasone have been used commonly in clinical practice to stimulate a rapid maturation of lung function when infants are born premature.[12,13] As we will describe, this type of Dex treatment can also have some adverse side effects on other physiological systems, including on the immune responses of infant monkeys.[14]

BEHAVIORAL AND EMOTIONAL EFFECTS OF PRENATAL STRESS

To the casual observer, monkey babies generated from these disturbed or hormone-treated pregnancies look normal at birth. They were full-term and of typical weight. But when evaluated more systematically, it soon became apparent that they were quite different both in their behavior and physiology. For many years, we have employed a modified version of the Brazelton Neonatal Assessment Scale to assess the developmental status and maturity of infant monkeys.[6,15] When they are 2 weeks of age, a prescribed set of motor reflexes is tested, as well as the baby's emotional reactions and capacity to orient and attend to visual and auditory stimuli. As shown in Figure 10.2, one consistent finding has been that disturbed pregnancies result in babies with immature neuromotor reflexes and an

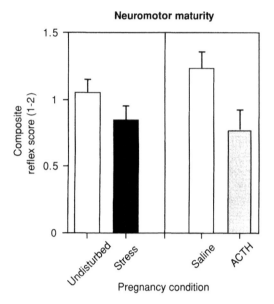

Figure 10.2 Neuromotor maturity ratings in infant monkeys generated from two experiments manipulating pregnancy conditions.[6,16] Prenatally stressed infants were compared to babies from undisturbed control pregnancies (*n* =18 and 12, respectively). Babies were also generated from pregnancies that included a 2-week treatment of the mother with adrenocorticotrophin hormone (ACTH) and compared to controls injected daily with saline for the same period from day 120 to 133 postconception (*n* = 12 and 10, respectively).

impaired capacity to attend and orient. Similar effects also occurred when ACTH was administered to the gravid female.[16] The latter finding seemed to implicate the transfer of maternal cortisol into the fetal compartment, because the exogenous ACTH could not cross the placenta. Because of how high the mother's cortisol became, it may have exceeded the capacity of protective placental enzymes to convert it to less active forms.[17] (See also Chapter 4 by Nyirenda and Seckl.)

The neuromotor effects at 2 weeks of age were not so debilitating that they posed a health risk, but they did presage other behavioral differences that continued to emerge during the first year of life. Monkeys from disturbed pregnancies were found to be more emotionally reactive when tested in novel situations.[18] As a consequence they also did not perform as well in tests of their learning capabilities, showing a greater propensity to become frustrated. Moreover, when observed as juveniles in small social groups, after weaning from the mother, they tended to be more submissive animals.[19] For this evaluation, the behavior of yearling monkeys was scored while they lived in social

groups comprised of four to eight offspring from both the control and manipulated pregnancies. Based on the frequency of assertive and submissive behavior recorded across 12 5-minute sessions per animal, those from disturbed and ACTH-treated pregnancies ranked lower in the social hierarchies.

BRAIN ALTERATIONS FOLLOWING PRENATAL DISTURBANCE

While these behavioral effects have not been directly linked with specific brain regions, we have documented that there were several neurological changes caused by disturbance of the fetus. Perhaps the most remarkable was finding a substantial reduction in the size of the hippocampus.[20] Eight monkeys from pregnancies disturbed early or late were compared to four age- and gender-matched controls, and the comparison revealed that the overall hippocampal volume was reduced approximately 10% by maternal stress (Figure 10.3). The magnitude of this effect is notable because it rivaled the decrease seen after exposure of fetal monkeys to high levels of Dex, when administered at a dose approximately 10 times that used for clinical treatments of premature human babies.[21,22] In addition, using an innovative technique for labeling new neurons, our study showed that juvenile monkeys from

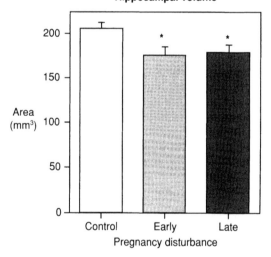

Figure 10.3 Comparison of the hippocampal size in monkeys born after control (*n* = 4) and disturbed pregnancies (*n* = 8).[20] Rhesus monkeys from both early and late disturbance conditions had a significantly smaller hippocampus throughout its length in the temporal lobe (statistical significance indicated by *).

disturbed pregnancies also had a lower level of neurogenesis in the hippocampus. The monkeys were administered bromodeoxyuridine (BrdU), a compound preferentially taken up by new cells, and then the same cells were double-stained with a neuronal marker (anti-neuron specific nuclear protein, NeuN), to verify that they were really neurons. As compared to a typical density of ~650 BrdU-positive cells/mm^3 of granule cell layer in the four control animals, the number of new cells in the eight animals from disturbed pregnancies was reduced by 32%. Because this assessment was done just prior to puberty, when the monkeys were 3 years of age, it suggests that the difference in the rate of cell replacement, and the smaller size of this critical brain area, would persist into adulthood.

In evaluations of additional monkeys, it was found that other brain regions were also changed by disturbances of pregnancy. Using a noninvasive approach, magnetic resonance imaging (MRI) was employed to visualize the corpus callosum of 16 monkeys when they were 7–11 months of age.[23] This change in the size and shape of the corpus callosum was most notable because of a differential effect of prenatal stress on male and female infants. Males showed a decrease in size, whereas females stressed *in utero* actually had a larger splenium or posterior portion of the callosum. The corpus callosum is composed primarily of myelinated nerves connecting the two hemispheres, and thus these differences in the posterior region could indicate an effect on inter-hemispheric communication between the parietal and temporal lobes. Alterations in the size and shape of the corpus callosum in humans have been associated with the degree of hemispheric asymmetry and also learning disabilities that start in fetal life (e.g. the size of the corpus callosum is abnormal in many dyslexic children).[24]

Further insight into how prenatal disturbance in monkeys can influence brain development was obtained through the use of positron emission tomography (PET). This sophisticated assessment was conducted by colleagues at the University of Wisconsin who generated and evaluated rhesus monkeys from similar types of pregnancies at our facility.[25] When the monkeys were young adults, 5–7 years of age, dopamine synthesis and dopamine binding availability (D2 receptor) in the striatal region were estimated by quantification of the uptake of 6-fluoro-m-tyrosine (F-MT) and fallypride (FAL), respectively. The binding levels and ratio of F-MT/FAL suggested that animals from disturbed pregnancies had lower dopamine decarboxylase, a critical enzyme for DA synthesis, accompanied by up-regulation of D2 receptors in two important striatal areas, the caudate and putamen.

Variation in the monkeys' dopamine neurochemistry was also correlated with their fearful and repetitive stereotypic behavior in an arousing test situation, which the researchers interpreted as indicative of a lower capacity for behavioral inhibition.

This sensitivity of monoamine neurons in the brain to prenatal disturbance concurs with studies in rodents, as well as with experiments involving postnatal disturbance in primates. Many investigators have reported that dopamine, serotonin, and norepinephrine levels can be impacted by abnormal rearing conditions in monkeys, even when the infant just experiences a series of repetitive postnatal separations from the mother.[26]

IMMUNE ALTERATIONS AFTER DISTURBED AND HORMONE-TREATED PREGNANCIES

A primary interest of ours was to extend research in rodents which indicated that prenatal disturbance also impacted the immune system.[27,28] It is known that many white blood cells and most lymphoid glands are extremely responsive to stress-related hormones. Thus, it seemed reasonable to expect that certain immune responses would be altered in the infant. Lymphocytes were a likely target, given that the fetal thymus gland is so sensitive to stress and the teratogenic effect of drugs.[29] It can undergo a rapid reduction in size, with many of its immature lymphocytes being directly lysed or self-destructing due to the initiation of cell death programs (apoptosis). However, the magnitude of the possible immune changes was not known, nor for how long they would last after the type of gestational disturbance being tested in our monkeys.

We tailored the assays to the age of the infant at the time of assessment. For example, for the newborn infant an *in vitro* assay was employed that quantified the capacity of its lymphocytes and monocytes to recognize and respond to the presence of nonself antigens.[10,30] This mixed lymphocyte response (MLR) required collecting a small 2 ml blood sample from the baby and incubating its cells with stimulator cells. The stimulators were derived from the infant's mother or father, an unrelated animal, and a virus-transformed cell line. In general, monkeys from disturbed or hormone-treated pregnancies showed reduced MLRs, especially a diminished proliferative response to the more foreign stimulators: cells from the unrelated animal or a monkey B cell line transformed by a Herpes virus (Figure 10.4). One exception to the general conclusion that pregnancy disturbance or hormone treatment always resulted in lower MLRs was seen for infants generated from the early disturbance

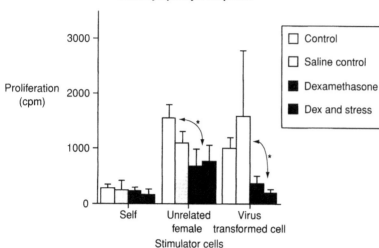

Mixed lymphocyte response

Proliferation (cpm)

- □ Control
- □ Saline control
- ■ Dexamethasone
- ■ Dex and stress

Stimulator cells: Self, Unrelated female, Virus transformed cell

Figure 10.4 Effect of antenatal Dex treatment on the mixed lymphocyte response of the neonate's cells to lymphocytes from an unrelated animal or a Herpes transformed monkey B cell line.[30] Three weeks before term, Dex was given for 2 days to either undisturbed dams or dams that had experienced the 6-week psychological disturbance paradigm ($n = 5$ and 5, respectively). Dex-exposed monkeys were significantly different than both control pregnancy conditions (*).

pregnancy.[10] These babies actually had an exaggerated proliferative response. We hypothesized that disturbance at such an early point in gestation (starting on day 50 postconception) might have affected the positive or negative selection for a unique lymphocyte subset in the thymus, which accounted for the over-reaction in the MLR.

While it might seem that larger immune responses could be preferable, in fact newborn infants have to restrain their reactions, because they are being exposed simultaneously to many thousands of novel antigens and pathogens in the environment. This modulation is accomplished in several ways, including by transferring maternal antibody across the placenta, which obviates the need for the infant to respond (i.e. a process called passive immunity). The neonate also has a distinctive type of T cell that can suppress the response of other lymphocytes. We evaluated how disturbances of pregnancy might affect the functioning of these special suppressor T cells across the first 2 months of life when their action is most evident.[10] The assay involved activating the infant's cells in culture with a mitogen (concanavalin A), and then quantifying the amount of suppressive activity manifest when they were added to proliferating lymphocytes of an adult animal ('responder cells'). At both 2 and 6 weeks of age, infants from disturbed pregnancies showed lower levels of suppressor activity, suggesting that prenatally disturbed infants may also not modulate their own immune responses as well. In fact, they might emerge too quickly from the less reactive immune profile characteristic of the very young infant, or shift too soon from the normal Th2 phenotype of the neonate to the more mature Th1-biased cellular immune responses seen in the older animal.

Beyond assessing different types of immune functions in the young monkey, another important question was the enduring nature of the cellular alterations. When 44 monkeys from various pregnancy conditions were between 1.5 and 2.5 years of age, we evaluated their response to administration of interleukin-1 (IL-1), an important cytokine involved in inflammatory responses.[31] IL-1 is a member of a triad of proinflammatory cytokines, which includes IL-6 and tumor necrosis factor-alpha (TNF-α) that mobilize the body's reaction to bacterial infections. We used the levels of IL-6 in the blood stream and in cerebrospinal fluid as an index of how the monkeys responded to the injections of IL-1. Monkeys generated from the ACTH-treated pregnancies showed significantly lower IL-6 responses at 1 hour after intravenous administration of IL-1, both in the blood and cerebrospinal fluid of the intrathecal compartment. When tested in this way, the monkeys from the psychologically disturbed pregnancies seemed to have a more normal reaction, but we later found that they too had very different cytokine responses.

The suggestion that there might be a long-term effect of prenatal stress on inflammatory responses was confirmed when a different approach was used.[32] Cells from 9 control and 11 prenatally disturbed monkeys were stimulated *in vitro* with lipopolysaccharide (LPS), a protein derived from the bacterial cell wall. LPS is a potent stimulator of monocytes and lymphocytes, and the cells' response was measured by the release of two cytokines. IL-6 and TNF-α levels in the surrounding fluid (the supernatant). The cytokines were quantified by enzyme immunosorbent assay (ELISA) after the blood had been cultured for 1 day with LPS. As illustrated in Figure 10.5, monkeys from

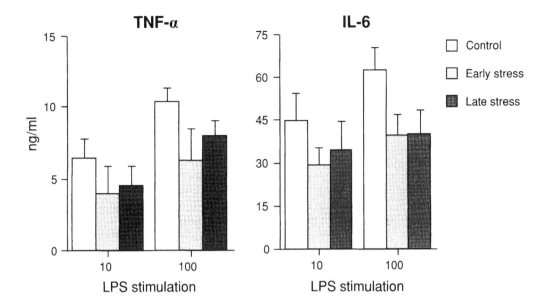

Figure 10.5 Cytokine levels (tumor necrosis factor-alpha, TNF-α, and interleukin-6, IL-6) released after stimulating whole blood cultures with a low or high concentration of lipopolysaccharide (LPS). The trait-like effect of early and late gestational disturbance on these proinflammatory responses was still evident in 2-year old juvenile monkeys.[32]

disturbed pregnancies produced significantly less of both cytokines. This difference was equally evident in monkeys born after early and late pregnancy disturbance, and consistently seen whether cells were stimulated with low or high amounts of LPS. Because these monkeys were already 2.0–2.5 years of age at the time of assessment, it indicated that the pregnancy conditions resulted in a fairly enduring, 'trait-like' alteration in this aspect of their cytokine biology.

MEDIATION OF PRENATAL INFLUENCES ON THE DEVELOPING BABY

We share the prevailing view that hormones from the pituitary-adrenal axis are likely to be involved in mediating some of the effects of gestational stress on the developing monkey baby.[7,8,33] Because ACTH treatment of the gravid females mimicked the psychological disturbance, even though the exogenous ACTH could not cross the placenta, it implicated the transfer of maternal cortisol as one important vector. Further, we and others have found that Dex can recreate some effects of prenatal stress, even when administered for a much shorter time period. Because of its potency, Dex was given for only 2 days in our studies, as compared to 2 weeks for ACTH, and 6 weeks of psychological disturbance;

yet it still had long-term effects. In addition to affecting the HPA activity of the pregnant female, it seems that the prenatal disturbance and hormone treatments may continue to have a lasting effect on the baby's HPA axis postpartum.

To test whether the lingering immune differences might be due to the fact that the disturbed offspring maintain higher cortisol levels in their blood or because they activate cortisol release more frequently, we evaluated how their lymphocytes would respond to exposure to cortisol.[11] Cells were stimulated with mitogen and then incubated with different concentrations of cortisol to assess the lymphocytes' sensitivity to the normal inhibitory actions of cortisol. Monkeys that had been exposed to Dex *in utero* had cells that were quite different in this assay. Their cells proliferated less in culture and also were less sensitive to cortisol feedback *in vitro*. This finding suggested that the cells' cortisol receptors had perhaps been down-regulated endogenously due to higher *in vivo* release of cortisol. Other researchers reached a similar conclusion about the long-term changes in the infants' HPA activity after antenatal Dex treatments. When monkeys were moved to a novel room, the ones from Dex-treated pregnancies had a more protracted cortisol response across several hours, suggesting that they do not recover and return as readily to baseline levels of secretion.[22]

The idea that the relationship between the HPA axis and immune system is not regulated normally in prenatally disturbed infants also concurs with evidence from an evaluation testing how the HPA axis itself responds to negative feedback. When juvenile monkeys were treated with Dex overnight, which should act at the hippocampal and hypothalamic levels to inhibit the release of HPA hormones, the monkeys from disturbed pregnancies did not suppress in the typical way.[32] They were more likely to override the Dex feedback by the following morning.

While these findings suggest that the placental transfer of maternal cortisol is a major mediator of the effects on the fetus, and that altered hippocampal functioning after birth may explain lingering HPA changes in the infant, the etiology of the immune dysregulation proved to be more complex. It is unlikely that any one hormone or pathway entirely accounts for the diverse effects of maternal stress on immunity. For example, it is known that psychological disturbance also changes maternal blood pressure and blood flow to the uterus and placenta.[34] There is further evidence that changes in fetal physiology and development are also elicited by reduced oxygenation and the induction of brief hypoxic episodes. In addition, hormones uniquely released by the placenta during pregnancy, such as corticotrophin-releasing hormone (CRH), have been shown to be associated with some effects of maternal stress, especially with the increased risk for premature labor[33] (see Chapter 3 by Wadwha et al). Our research has demonstrated that there are still other nonendocrine processes that should be considered as important mediators.

In one project, female monkeys were maintained on a diet that had adequate levels of iron for a nonpregnant animal, but not the extra amounts required to fulfill the needs of a gravid female and her growing baby, especially during times of stress. When the effects of maternal disturbance were evaluated under these nutritional conditions, it induced a marked impairment in iron homeostasis in the baby after birth. Monkeys from the early and late disturbance conditions were found to be at high risk for developing an iron deficiency anemia (IDA) as they grew postpartum. Here we also return to the importance of the infant's growth, because infants that doubled their birth weight quickly were at especially high risk for this IDA.

The importance of a high prenatal transfer of iron from mother to baby is not unique to monkeys. Rodents as well as our own children must obtain and then store before birth about 50% of the iron needed to sustain postpartum growth. The additional iron provided by breast milk is important but not sufficient

by itself. As the infant monkeys from the disturbed pregnancies depleted their iron stores and exceeded their dietary intake of iron and started to become anemic by 4–6 months of age, yet another impairment became evident. The compromise in red cell functioning induced by the low iron had a cascading effect on the immune system, providing a second hit to their lymphocytes. In this experiment, we were simultaneously quantifying the ability of the babies' natural killer (NK) cells to lyse virally infected target cells and to kill cancer cells in culture. As soon as the infants from the disturbed pregnancies became iron deficient, the killing capability of their NK cells plummeted.

Perhaps the most novel pathway we have identified as being important for explaining some of the effects of prenatal disturbance on immunity was a change in the infant's gastrointestinal physiology (Figure 10.6).[35] A microbiologist, Dr Michael Bailey, joined our group and his expertise enabled an evaluation of the bacteria that became established as the normal gut flora in baby monkeys. Almost as soon as the baby leaves the sterile environs of the womb, it becomes exposed to bacteria, and within a few days millions of bacteria enter through any orifice in the body's surface. One means of regulating this bacterial influx is to foster a predominance of certain protective types that become the commensal flora residing within us. Our assessment focused on two bacteria, lactobacilli and bifidobacteria, which are known to assist in the defense

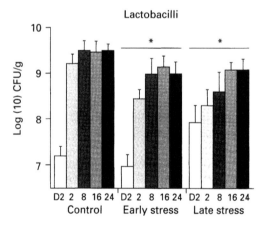

Figure 10.6 Lactobacilli quantified from fecal cultures of 24 infants across the first 6 months of life. Prenatal disturbance resulted in lower levels of protective microflora, which were associated with an increased risk for infection with *Shigella*, a pathogenic bacteria. (*Lactobacilli levels in offspring from both Early and Late Disturbance pregnancies were significantly below normal after 2 weeks of age.) Bifidobacterium levels were also lower in infants from the late disturbance condition.

against enteric pathogens. Fecal swabs were collected from infants across the first 6 months of life, and coprocultures were used to quantify the bacterial concentrations. As can be seen in Figure 10.6, infant monkeys from both early and late disturbance pregnancies had lower levels of lactobacilli; those from the late disturbance condition also had significantly reduced bifidobacteria. The health significance of this effect on the microbiota of the gut became evident when the monkeys were also tested for the presence of an opportunistic pathogen, *Shigella flexneri*. While not seen in the control infants, asymptomatic infections were seen in about 40% of those from disturbed pregnancies. Further, two infants from the late disturbance condition developed clinical infections with diarrheic symptoms, which required antibiotic treatments. This influence of prenatal disturbance on the gut flora concurs with reports in rodents indicating that gestational stress can affect the physiology of the gut wall postpartum and increase the ease with which some pathogenic bacteria can translocate and reach the systemic circulation.[36]

CONCLUSIONS

The overall message from this research on infant monkeys is that there are many important and sustained influences of the fetal stage on later behavioral and physiological responses. Periods of prenatal disturbance or hormone treatments were found to have lasting effects on stress-sensitive brain areas, such as the hippocampus, and also affected several other systems in the body (Figure 10.7). The specific influence on the hippocampus was evident both in terms of its size and the numbers of new neurons being generated in the dentate gyrus. In this region, the brain of the infant monkey appears to show the same vulnerability as the rodent pup to prenatal stress.[37] Because the hippocampus is also an important regulatory center for the HPA axis, where cortisol normally provides a critical negative feedback signal, it may help to explain why prenatally disturbed animals continue to show differences in pituitary-adrenal activity. A more active or a dysregulated HPA axis is a likely explanation for some of the immune alterations found in prenatally disturbed infants. These immune differences in infant monkeys, which involve both proliferative and inflammatory responses, are similar for the most part to those seen in rodents.[27,28]

With regard to the immune system, a primary interest of ours, some responses were already different in the neonate at birth, in terms of how cells proliferated in culture when exposed to nonself antigens. Other alter-

ations, such as the lower production of proinflammatory cytokines, continued to still be evident in animals at 2–3 years of age. In addition to a reduced inflammatory response, we have also discussed an effect on one lymphocyte that plays an important role in innate immunity, the NK cell. This influence of prenatal disturbance on NK activity was most evident in those infants that became anemic as a consequence of the synergistic impact of gestational stress and a maternal diet low in iron. Much more needs to be learned about the possible mediation of stress effects through an influence on the placental transfer of nutrients.

Given the range of brain, immune, and behavioral changes described for the prenatally disturbed monkeys, it is probably important to correct any erroneous impression inadvertently conveyed with respect to the severity or aversive nature of the manipulations. It might seem that the disturbance conditions would have to be extremely stressful. In fact, a more surprising aspect of our research may be the relatively benign and acute nature of the disturbance. The arousal procedure lasted only 10 minutes, and occurred for only 6 weeks or 25% of the pregnancy. It did elicit a stress-related rise in cortisol, but still should be considered a relatively modest provocation when compared to other stressful events that might be experienced by animals in nature or even by women. If gauged against the types of catastrophic accidents that can unfortunately occur, especially in times of famine or war, the stress in our experiments would certainly rank relatively low. Even within the normal realm of experience for animals, considerably less distress was evoked than might occur when a subordinate animal gets into a fight with a more dominant monkey.

Indeed, a question one is led to ask is: what is the magnitude of the challenge or perturbation needed to exert a lasting change on a fetus? It doesn't seem likely that all events would be potent enough to permanently alter the course of infant development, even if the fetus evinces an acute reaction for a few minutes or hours. Moreover, it has been found that the placenta has special enzymes to limit the transfer of stress-responsive hormones like cortisol and presumably thereby to protect the baby. One challenge for future research is to determine how salient and enduring an event must be in order to elicit a protracted effect on the baby. For monkeys, at least, we know that 6 weeks of daily disturbance has sufficient *saliency*.

When considering the issue of fetal vulnerability, it may also be worth reflecting on one other unique aspect of research conducted in the controlled setting of the laboratory. In a way, it could also be argued that the 'undisturbed control' condition was just as distinctive. Food and water were available without effort,

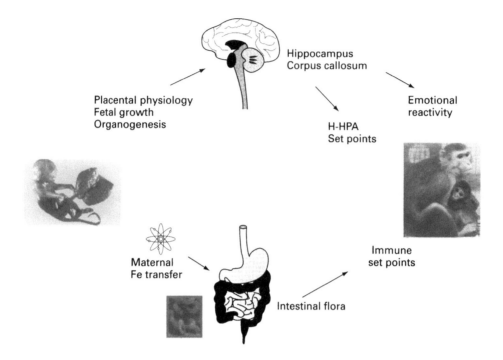

Figure 10.7 Overview of physiological alterations induced by prenatal disturbance and the pathways likely to be involved in mediating immune effects. In addition to the neuroendocrine axis, significant changes in the placental transfer of nutrients and the establishment of microflora in the gut appear to play a role.

temperature and light cycles were invariant, and the social milieu was benign and constant throughout pregnancy. From an experimental point of view, this type of undisturbed pregnancy was essential for generating a reference point against which to compare the effect of disturbance. But it too could be thought of as a distinct type of pregnancy that played some role in shaping and 'programming' the regulatory set points of the baby's physiological systems after birth. Perhaps in a positive way, enhancing the resiliency and health of the infant since the monkeys in our colony do not typically get sick.

One is usually more inclined to highlight the negative impact of prenatal stress, because of the concern that the baby may be pushed out of the tolerable range of normalcy, making it more vulnerable to disease. With regard to this issue of pathology, a few additional comments are warranted. For the most part, the infant monkeys would have appeared healthy and normal to the casual observer. Even the many physiological changes we described might not result in illness, *unless* the young animal experienced an additional challenge or a pathogen. It is then that one sees the potential vulnerability or

risk that had been created. This important lesson was most clearly evident in the association found between the seemingly modest change in the commensal gut bacteria and the increased risk for infection by an enteric pathogen. Similarly, we found greater consequences of prenatal stress when pregnant females were fed a diet containing an adequate but not an optimal amount of iron. Thus, appreciating the significance of stress during pregnancy really requires one to think about the mother and baby from the perspective of a diathesis model. If challenged further from a second insult, a tolerable physiological change caused by the initial stress may cross out of an acceptable range of variation, resulting in pathology or disease.

The full implications for the offspring may also not emerge until much later when adult-onset diseases begin to occur. In the case of the immune system, perhaps not even until old age, with the start of the normal immune decline that takes place at the end of the lifespan. Then, the older host shows a second period of increased susceptibility to infection and more autoimmune and cancerous disease. This type of longitudinal study linking prenatal events and the biology of aging has not yet been conducted in nonhuman primates, but would be a very important endeavor.

ACKNOWLEDGMENTS

This research was supported by grants from the National Institutes of Allergy and Infectious Disease and Child Health and Human Development (AI46521, HD39386). CLC also receives partial salary support from MH61083 and AG20166. Special appreciation is due M. Bailey, H. Crispen, E. Fuchs, M. Kraemer, T. Reyes, M. Schneider, and A. Slukvina for invaluable help with critical aspects of this research.

REFERENCES

1. Barker DJ. Intrauterine programming of adult disease. Mol Med Today 1995; 1: 418–23.

2. Price KC, Hyde JS, Coe CL. Matrilineal transmission of birth weight in the rhesus monkey (*Macaca mulatta*) across several generations. Obstet Gynecol 1999; 94: 128–34.

3. Price KC, Coe CL. Maternal constraint on fetal growth patterns in the rhesus monkey: the intergenerational link between mothers and daughters. Hum Reprod 2000; 15: 452–7.

4. Coe CL, Shirtcliff, EA. Growth trajectory evident at birth affects age of first delivery female monkeys. Pediatr Res 2004; 55: 914–20.

5. Coe CL, Crispen H. Social stress in pregnant monkeys differentially affects placental transfer of maternal antibody to male and female infants. Health Psychol 2000; 19: 1–6.

6. Schneider ML, Coe CL. Repeated stress during pregnancy impairs neuromotor development of the primate infant. J Dev Behav Pediatr 1993; 14: 81–7.

7. Weinstock M. Does prenatal stress impair coping and regulation of hypothalamic-pituitary-adrenal axis? Neurosci Biobehav Rev 1997; 21: 1–10.

8. Takahashi LK. Prenatal stress: consequences of glucocorticoids on hippocampal development and function. Int J Dev Neurosci 1998; 16: 199–207.

9. Rhees RW, Fleming D. Effects of malnutrition, maternal stress or ACTH injections during pregnancy on sexual behavior of male offspring. Physiol Behav 1981; 27: 879–92.

10. Coe CL, Lubach GR, Karaszewski JW, Ershler WB. Prenatal endocrine activation alters postnatal cellular immunity in infant monkeys. Brain Behav Immun 1996; 10: 221–34.

11. Coe CL, Lubach GR. Prenatal influences on neuro-immune set points in infancy. Ann N Y Acad Sci 2000; 917: 468–77.

12. Kay HH, Bird IM, Coe CL, Dudley DJ. Antenatal steroid treatment and adverse fetal effects: what is the evidence? J Soc Gynecol Investig 2000; 7: 269–78.

13. Matthews SG. Antenatal glucocorticoids and programming of the developing CNS. Pediatr Res 2000; 474: 291–300.

14. Coe CL, Lubach, GR. Developmental consequences of antenatal dexamethasone treatments in nonhuman primates. Neurosci BioBehav Rev 2005; 29: 227–35.

15. Roughton EC, Schneider ML, Bromley LJ, Coe CL. Maternal activation during pregnancy alters neurobehavioral state in primate infants. Am J Occup Ther 1998; 52: 90–8.

16. Schneider ML, Coe CL, Lubach GR. Endocrine activation mimics the adverse effects of prenatal stress on the neuromotor development of the primate infant. Devel Psychobiol 1992; 25: 427–39.

17. Seckl JR. Glucocorticoids, feto-placental 11 beta-hydroxysteroid dehydrogenase type 2, and the early life origins of adult disease. Steroids 1997; 62: 89–94.

18. Clarke AS, Wittwer, DJ, Abbott DH, Schneider ML. Long term effects of prenatal stress on HPA axis activity in juvenile rhesus monkeys. Dev Psychobiol 1994; 27: 257–69.

19. Coe CL, Lubach GR, Schneider ML. Neuromotor and socioemotional behavior in the young monkey is presaged by prenatal conditions. In: Soothing and Stress (Lewis M, Ramsay D, eds). Mahwah, NJ: Lawrence Erlbaum Associates, 1999: 19–38.

20. Coe CL, Czeh B, Gould E et al. Prenatal stress diminishes neurogenesis in the dentate gyrus of juvenile rhesus monkeys. Biol Psychiatry 2003; 54: 1025–34.

21. Uno H, Lohmiller L, Thieme C et al. Brain damage induced by prenatal exposure to dexamethasone in fetal rhesus macaques. I. Hippocampus. Dev Brain Res 1990; 53: 157–67.

22. Uno H, Eisele S, Sakai A et al. Neurotoxicity of glucocorticoids in the primate brain. Horm Behav 1994; 28: 236–48.

23. Coe CL, Lubach GR, Schneider M. Prenatal stress alters the size of the corpus callosum in the infant monkey. Dev Psychobiol 2002; 41: 178–85.

24. Geschwind N, Galaburda AM. Cerebral lateralization: Biological mechanisms, associations and pathology III. A hypothesis and a program of research. Arch Neurol 1985; 42: 634–54.

25. Roberts AD, Moore CF, DeJesus OT et al. Prenatal stress, moderate fetal alcohol, and dopamine system function in rhesus monkeys. Neurotoxicol Teratol 2004; 26: 169–78.

26. Kraemer GW, Ebert MH, Schmidt DE, McKinney WT. A longitudinal study of the effect of different social rearing conditions on cerebrospinal fluid norepinephrine and biogenic amine metabolites in rhesus monkeys. Neuro-psychopharmacology 1989; 2: 175–89.

27. Klein SL, Rager DR. Prenatal stress alters immune function in the offspring of rats. Dev Psychobiol 1995; 28: 321–6.

28. Taylor AN, Chiappelli F, Yirmiya R. Fetal alcohol syndrome and immunity. In: Psychoneuroimmunology, 3rd edn (Ader R, Felten DL, Cohen N, eds). San Diego: Academic Press, 2001: 49–71.

29. Sawyer R, Hendrickx A, Osburn B, Terrell T. Abnormal morphology of the fetal monkey (*Macaca mulatta*) thymus exposed to a corticosteroid. J Med Primatol 1977; 6: 145–50.

30. Coe CL, Lubach GR, Karaszewski J. Prenatal stress and immune recognition of self and nonself in the primate neonate. Biol Neonate 1999; 76: 301–10.

31. Reyes TM, Coe CL. Prenatal manipulations reduce the pro-inflammatory response to a cytokine challenge in juvenile monkeys. Brain Res 1997; 769: 29–35.

32. Coe CL, Kramer M, Kirschbaum C et al. Prenatal stress diminishes cytokine production after an endotoxin challenge and induces glucocorticoid resistance in juvenile rhesus monkeys. J Clin Endocrinol Metab 2002; 87: 675–81.

33. Wadhwa PD, Sandman CA, Garite TJ. The neurobiology of stress in human pregnancy: implications for prematurity and development of the fetal central nervous system. Prog Brain Res 2001; 133: 131–42.

34. DiPietro JA, Costigan KA, Gurewitsch ED. Fetal response to induced maternal stress. Early Hum Dev 2003; 74: 125–38.

35. Bailey MT, Lubach GR, Coe CL. Prenatal conditions alter the bacterial colonization of the gut in the infant monkey. J Pediatr Clin Gastroenterol 2004; 17: 1704–8.

36. Wenzl HH, Schimpl G, Feierl G, Steinwender G. Effect of prenatal corticosterone on spontaneous bacterial translocation from gastrointestinal tract in neonatal rat. Dig Dis Sci 2003; 48: 1171–6.

37. Lemaire V, Koehl M, Le Moal M, Abrous DN. Prenatal stress produces learning deficits associated with an inhibition of neurogenesis in the hippocampus. Proc Natl Acad Sci USA 2000; 97: 11032–7.

11

Role of prenatal events in the development of allergic disease

Susan L Prescott and Janet Dunstan

INTRODUCTION

The escalating burden of allergic diseases is anticipated to rise further as 'western' lifestyle changes also begin to impact the developing world. These increasing rates of allergic disease indicate that a high proportion of the population carry some form of genetic predisposition, which is increasingly unmasked by environmental change. There is an urgent need to identify the responsible factors in order to develop safe and effective prevention strategies. As the first signs of allergic disease are often manifest within weeks or months of life, it is logical that factors that influence very early immune development are likely to play a significant role in the mounting propensity for allergy. Growing evidence of presymptomatic differences in the immune function of newborns who later develop allergic disease suggests that events during fetal life are of crucial importance. Both maternal environmental exposures and direct maternal immune responses have the capacity to influence the developing fetal immune system. This chapter will review current concepts of allergy pathogenesis and how events in early life may contribute. It will also explore maternal and environmental factors that may influence immune development in fetal life, including possible avenues for disease prevention during this period.

BACKGROUND

The problem in context

The last 40–50 years have seen an exponential rise in many immune-mediated diseases. This change has been most evident for allergic diseases (including asthma, allergic rhinitis, atopic dermatitis, and food allergies), which have reached epidemic levels. A parallel increase is also apparent for other less common immune-mediated conditions, including type 1 diabetes, Crohn's disease, multiple sclerosis, and other autoimmune disease[1] (Figure 11.1). All of these (autoimmune and allergic) diseases are the result of complex environmental and genetic interactions that lead to inappropriate immune responses to self-antigens or other environmental proteins (allergens) depending on the individual genetic susceptibility. These interactions, shown in the flow diagram in Figure 11.2, are discussed in detail below.

Increasing rates of diseases strongly suggest that changing environmental influences, perhaps related to industrialization and 'western' lifestyle, may be affecting the basic underlying immune regulatory pathways that normally suppress inappropriate immune responses to these tissue or allergen targets. There are concerns that allergic diseases could become pandemic as developing countries become progressively 'westernized'. Adding to this concern, recent genetic studies suggest that nonCaucasian racial groups (particularly in equatorial regions) may be even more predisposed to allergic diseases because of higher frequencies of proinflammatory genetic polymorphisms than found in Caucasians.[2] There is now an urgent need to understand the pathogenesis of these diseases and possible factors (such as changing dietary and infectious exposures) that may be unmasking disease propensities in the genetically predisposed.

Factors which either protect from, or potentiate the development of atopic disease appear to act early in life, during critical stages of immune development. The escalating incidence of atopic disease suggests that genetic factors are readily modified by environmental factors. Emerging evidence that atopic individuals have pre-existing biases in cellular immune

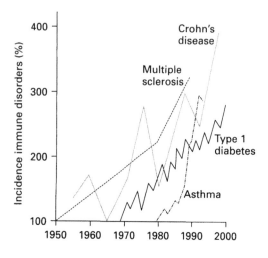

Figure 11.1 The rise in immune-mediated diseases over the last 50 years. Reproduced with permission from Bach JF (2002) The effect of infections on susceptibility to autoimmune and allergic diseases. N Engl J Med 347(12): 911–20.

responses evident at birth raises further interest in the gestational environment.

The basis of the allergic response

Allergic diseases are associated with an increased predisposition to produce allergen-specific IgE antibodies. Although the exact mechanisms are unclear, it is generally accepted that this is mediated by underlying T helper type 2 (Th2) cellular immune responses, characterized by synthesis of cytokines (interleukin [IL]-4, IL-5, IL-9, IL-13) that promote IgE isotype switching and allergic inflammation.[3] This contrasts with the T helper type 1 (Th1) responses (characterized by IL-2 and interferon gamma, IFNγ) seen in nonallergic individuals.

The immunological propensity for Th2 responses can lead to 'atopy' with the production of IgE antibodies. Many (but not all) atopic individuals go on to develop allergic inflammation, generally in tissues that interface with the environment (and hence with allergens) such as the skin, the gastrointestinal tract, and the respiratory tract. In previously sensitized individuals, allergen exposure results in cross-linking of preformed mast cell-bound IgE. This initiates the

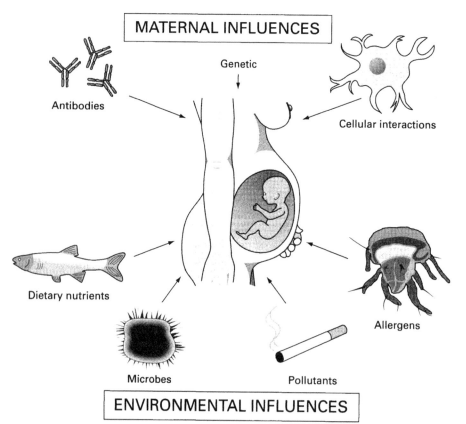

Figure 11.2 Factors influencing early immune development: A flow diagram showing major interactions in fetal life.

release of inflammatory mediators associated with acute allergic inflammation including leukotrienes, histamine, and other mediators. Some of these mediators also serve to attract other inflammatory cells that can lead to the more chronic inflammation seen in asthma, dermatitis, and allergic rhinitis. It is not clear what factors lead to tissue-specific manifestations in some individuals and not in others.

Most research has focused on defining the established allergic immune responses in mature individuals; however, there is now growing recognition that early life events are critical in initiating the fundamental events leading to allergic disease pathogenesis.

The limitations of the Th1/Th2 paradigm in humans

The notion that Th2-mediated allergic disease is the result of a simple 'polarization' of immune responses away from 'normal' Th1 responses has recently been called into question. Although there are clear parallels with the Th1/Th2 paradigm originally described in rodents,[4] the role in development of human disease is less clear. There is certainly a substantial body of evidence implicating various Th2 cytokines in the development and expression of allergy and airways inflammation. However, although 'deficient' Th1 function was initially proposed as an underlying factor, there is no conclusive evidence of impaired Th1 function in either established asthma or atopy,[5–7] suggesting that other possible types of immune dysfunction also have important roles.

New concepts of disease pathogenesis – 'regulatory' dysfunction

At a population level, there has been a parallel rise in both Th1-mediated autoimmune diseases (Figure 11.1) and Th2-mediated allergic diseases,[1] although this has sometimes been debated.[8] At the individual level, there is accumulating evidence that atopy is associated with an increase in both Th1 and Th2 responses.[7] Furthermore, Th1 cells also appear to play a role in allergic inflammation in local tissues, failing to counterbalance Th2 responses in airways inflammation.[9] These observations led to the notion that the atopic response may develop as a result of a more fundamental failure of underlying *immune regulation*, rather than a simple skewing of immune response along a Th1–Th2 continuum as previously thought. It also challenges the notion that modern environmental changes are having a generalized 'Th2 skewing effect' by promoting Th2 responses or inhibiting Th1 responses.

Environmental changes may be having more fundamental effects on common 'regulatory pathways', such that they inadequately prevent over-expression of inappropriate Th1 and Th2 responses in predisposed individuals.[10] There has been intense interest in aspects of the immune network with homeostatic and immunomodulatory functions (particularly cells that produce key regulatory cytokines, such as IL-10 and transforming growth factor, TGF-β) and how these processes might be influenced by environmental factors. Many cells produce these regulatory cytokines, but there has been particular interest in the role of antigen-presenting cells (APCs) and regulatory T cells, which influence both the pattern and magnitude of effector T-cell signaling. Detailed discussion of regulatory pathways can be found elsewhere.[8,11]

THE IMPORTANCE AND RELEVANCE OF EARLY LIFE

It is now generally accepted that events during early life when systems and responses are developing are likely to have more substantive effects.[12] This formative influence also appears to be true of the immune system. Although the etiological factors are still not well defined, presymptomatic immune dysregulation is detectable at birth in individuals who will later develop allergic disease.[13] The first clinical symptoms of allergy can sometimes be detected in the first months of life. These observations strongly suggest that the events which lead to allergic disease begin very early in life, probably even before birth. To be most effective, prevention strategies will ultimately need to be targeted to this period of life before allergic inflammation has become established. Another essential part of this process is developing more accurate ways of identifying individuals who will go on to develop allergic disease, so that prevention strategies can be targeted more effectively. Ultimately, primary prevention is the most logical, cost-effective approach at both the individual and population level, and should be the priority for all areas of medicine.

NORMAL IMMUNE DEVELOPMENT IN FETAL LIFE

Normal events at the materno-fetal interface

Complex immunologic mechanisms have evolved in the placenta to allow the fetal and maternal immune systems to coexist during pregnancy, without harming or rejecting each other. The maternal cellular immune system adapts subtly during pregnancy to a 'Th2 state' in order to down-regulate Th1 cell-mediated allo-immune responses to fetal antigens.[14] This is mediated through constitutive production of Th2 cytokines (including IL-4 and IL-10), hormones (progesterone), and other mediators (such as prostaglandin E2, PGE2) by trophoblastic and decidual cells,[15] which protect the fetus from allograft rejection.[14] However, although excessive Th1 responses are detrimental to later pregnancy, the production of low levels of some cytokines (such as IFNγ) is critical at some stages of gestation (such as implantation).[16] In fact, maternal immune responses in the endometrium of the uterus are critical to the successful implantation of the embryo right after conception.

At the same time, additional cellular mechanisms have evolved to protect the fetus from CD8[+] cytotoxic T cells in the uterus. Placental villous trophoblast cells express high levels of nonpolymorphic HLA G antigens but do not express the usual HLA class I or class II antigens on their surface.[17] These cells do not respond to cytokines which normally increase expression of other HLA antigens. This essentially provides an HLA 'negative' layer, which protects the HLA-positive fetus. In contrast, fetal HLA-positive cells are strongly expressed in the fetal layers of the placenta and serve to protect the fetus from maternal antibodies and infection. They simultaneously inhibit cytotoxic responses by maternal lymphocytes and recruit maternal monocytes to help sculpt the new blood vessels that will nourish the placenta and baby.

Changes in metabolic functions also regulate the activity of maternal lymphocytes during later pregnancy. Enzymes such as adoleamine 2,3-dioxygenase (2,3 IDO; expressed on macrophages and other APCs) appear to play a role in maintaining T-cell tolerance.[18,19] The resulting metabolic products (of tryptophan catabolism) appear to inhibit T-cell function.[19] However, while reduced 2,3 IDO activity has been associated with fetal demise in mice,[18] the role of this enzyme in humans is less clear.

These complex hormonal, metabolic, and immunologic interactions that are required to interact to maintain maternal tolerance for the fetus during pregnancy are still incompletely understood.

Ontogeny of fetal cellular immune responses

Human lymphocytes are derived from the yolk sac and first appear in the fetal liver at 2 weeks, and in the thymus at 10–11 weeks of gestation.[20] These thymocytes show responsiveness to mitogen PHA as early as 10 weeks of gestation.[20,21] Allogeneic 'graft versus host' reactions by human fetal T cells have been demonstrated as early as the 12th week.[22] By week 18, splenic T cells express adult levels of CD3 and CD4, and CD8[23] and MHC class II-positive cells are detected in the skin, gastrointestinal tract, and T-cell area of the thymic medulla,[24] indicating a capacity for an antigen-specific response at this time. Measures of PHA-induced DNA synthesis indicate that there is increasing responsiveness with age, peaking at 19 weeks gestation. Thereafter responsiveness appears to decline. Between 20 and 22 weeks gestation, numbers of antigen-specific binding thymocytes are higher than in neonatal or adult thymic tissue.[25] A number of groups have observed that cord blood T cells are extremely reactive to mitogenic stimulation,[21] and it was initially proposed that high rates of spontaneous transformation may be due to chronic antigen challenge during intrauterine life. In 1978, Toivanen et al.[26] demonstrated that the capacity for developing antigen-specific effector cells is first present in the 28-week preterm infant, and fully developed in the term infant. More recently, one group has demonstrated proliferative responses to environmental allergens as early as 22 weeks gestation.[27] However, others have found that the lymphocyte responses are still immature at birth, due in large part to poor antigen presentation.

The significance of fetal immune responses to allergens

Although neonatal T cells can respond to a range of antigens, these responses are atypical and do not appear to represent classical memory responses. *In vitro* studies have demonstrated allergen-specific responses (to both food and aeroallergens) by cord blood mononuclear cells (CBMCs).[28–35] Microsatellite DNA analysis has confirmed that the allergen-responsive T cells are of fetal rather than maternal origin.[36] However, there has been ongoing speculation about whether allergen-responsive fetal T cells have been primed by allergen exposure *in vivo* or the placental transfer of maternal IgG–antigen complexes. Adding to this uncertainty, in a number of situations CBMC responses to specific stimuli have been observed when there was no previous documented exposure. This includes responses to tetanus[37] and diphtheria toxoid[38] when there was no apparent exposure to these antigens in pregnancy. It has been proposed that these responses may therefore be nonspecific or due to cross-reactivity to other antigens.[39] However, detection of antigen-specific IgE (and IgM) antibodies (which do not generally cross the placenta) specific for parasites,[40] vaccine antigens,[41] and allergens[42] does indicate that the fetus is capable of mounting antigen-specific responses in some situations.

Demonstrating that allergen can reach the fetus has been a logical step in addressing this issue. While transplacental passage of food allergens has been demonstrated in animals,[43] transfer of aeroallergens has been more difficult to prove given the much lower levels of these proteins in the maternal circulation. To address this in humans, Szepfalusi and co-workers[44] used a novel *ex vivo* placenta perfusion model to show that both food and inhaled allergens can pass from the maternal to the fetal circulation. This is dose-dependent, the transfer of aeroallergens is affected by molecular weight (< 500 Da), and occurs more with placentas from earlier pregnancy. Events at mucosal surfaces, known to be important for initiating and informing immune development in the postnatal period, may also be important *in utero*. Allergens have been detected in amniotic fluid[45] and it has been proposed that these may reach the fetus through the amniotic fluid and the fetal gut (and lung).[46] Furthermore, cells capable of presenting antigens have also been detected in the fetal gut.[46] Despite all these observations, it is still not clear whether the fetus is directly exposed to levels of allergens at sufficient levels to induce T-cell priming *in vivo*.

For many reasons, it is inappropriate to assume that neonatal lymphoproliferative responses are equivalent to adult T-cell responses.[47] Only half of the allergen-responsive T cells in cord blood have been shown to have the CD45RO+ 'memory' phenotype and it is not clear why the responses are being observed in 'naïve' cell populations.[48] Although environmental antigens induce MHC class II-dependent cord blood lymphoproliferative responses, this is associated with unusually high levels of apoptosis.[49] Furthermore, the surviving cell populations appear to have 'suppressive' or 'regulatory' properties in culture. These cells also express markers which are common (but not exclusive) to T-regulatory cells, including CD4, CD25, and CTLA4.[49] The significance of these cells and the surface markers is still unclear, and further studies are needed. There is obvious interest given the growing focus on the role of regulatory T cells in early immune development.

Differences in perinatal immune responses in allergic-prone infants

While there is still a great deal of uncertainty surrounding the early immune events that may lead to atopy, there is accumulating evidence of early presymptomatic differences between atopic and nonatopic individuals at birth.[31,32,35,36,50–54] These differences seem to be reflected in a number of different 'read outs' of immune activity at birth, including the magnitude[30,31,33] and pattern on cellular responses *in vitro*,[31,32,35,50–52] circulating neonatal levels of cytokines[53] or cytokine-producing cells,[55] and activity of progenitors that give rise to proallergic inflammatory cells (eosinophil progenitors).[54] Proteins involved in the activation of APC and pro-Th1 signaling (such as sCD14) have also been detected in amniotic fluid and are reduced in those who go on to develop atopic dermatitis.[56] IgE levels have also been reported to be higher in the cord blood of babies from allergic mothers and children who become atopic.

While there is immaturity of Th1 responses in all neonates, the reduced capacity for IFNγ production is more profound in neonates with a family history of atopy.[31,32,35,50–52,57–59] Although this can be overcome by high-level stimulation, these observations suggest early immune dysregulation in this group. It has been proposed that this perinatal Th1 immaturity leads to failure of normal postnatal Th1-driven immune deviation, and to the persistent allergen-specific Th2 responses.[60] Th2 differentiation appears to be the default response in the absence of mature APC signaling.[61] Factors that may affect maturation of these regulatory pathways in the fetus and early postnatal period are therefore of critical interest. Although there is indirect evidence that APC co-stimulation[62] and (IL-12) cytokine production[57] are reduced in neonates at high risk of atopy, the role of these (and regulatory) cells is still unclear.

It is not clear if these early differences are primarily a detectable measure of increased genetic predisposition, or whether they are indicative of early (*in utero*) environmental influences that are already promoting the development of the allergic phenotype. It seems increasingly likely that both are true, particularly as atopic dermatitis and food allergies may be manifest within months of life. It is reasonable to assume that the processes that promote allergic inflammation are initiated in this very early period.

FACTORS WHICH MAY INFLUENCE NORMAL IMMUNE DEVELOPMENT

The effects of events at the materno-fetal interface on fetal immune responses

Maternal (rather than paternal) atopy appears to be associated with a higher risk of allergic disease and with relative immaturity of Th1 function in the perinatal period.[63] This finding suggests that maternal exposures and direct maternal immune interactions can exert important influences on the developing fetal immune system. Fetal responses are clearly sensitive to the ambient cytokine environment of pregnancy, as the fetal responses to allergens reflect the normal Th2 skew of pregnancy.[36] Thus, variations in the cytokine milieu in pregnancy have implications for subsequent immune development. Understanding the regulation of T-cell activity in the feto-placental unit may not only be central to successful pregnancy, but also in the pathogenesis of many disease processes.

While profound cytokine shifts threaten pregnancy and markedly elevated levels of proinflammatory cytokines like TNF are abortifacient, the effects of less marked variation in cytokine production on fetal immune development have yet to be explored. It is possible that mild reactivity between maternal and paternal (fetal) antigens may activate APCs to provide an important stimulus for fetal immune maturation (particularly Th1 responses). Many aspects of immune function are less mature in newborns of atopic parents, and other factors which stimulate Th1 maturation in the early postnatal period may reduce the risk of subsequent Th1 disease.[63,65]

It is not clear if atopic mothers with greater Th2 propensity are more tolerant to paternal antigens. Differences in the cytokine production and HLA reactivity of atopic mothers with a pre-existing Th2 bias (to specific allergens) have not been investigated, although there are reports that maternal atopy has been associated with increased fertility rate.[66] It may be speculated that maternal atopy is more successful in promoting a Th2 milieu during pregnancy, thereby favoring successful feto-placental 'engraftment' and subsequent fetal growth. Of interest, there are several studies linking fetal growth parameters (particularly head circumference) with infant atopic disease.[67] However, these effects seem to occur more in babies with disproportionately large heads relative to body size, and also in large-for-date babies. This further suggests a possible link between placenta viability (fetal nutrition) and atopy. A gestational environment where there is potentially reduced signal for fetal Th1 maturation (as seen at birth in infants of atopic mothers) may contribute atopic risk additional to that conferred by maternal genetic factors alone.

Endogenous maternal influences on fetal immune development

Although the concept of 'fetal origins of adult disease' focused initially on cardiovascular disease,[68] it has now been generalized to include many other processes.

Here we explore the possible gestational influences that could affect the developing fetal immune system and the risk of subsequent allergic disease.

Genetic influences

Familial associations indicate that genetic predisposition is an important factor in the development of allergic disease. Although no 'causal genes' have been identified, more than 11 reported genome screens[69] have identified a growing number of genetic polymorphisms that have been linked with susceptibility to asthma, asthma-associated phenotypes, atopy, elevated IgE levels, and bronchial hyper-responsiveness.[70] This finding suggests that multiple genes are involved. It is also apparent that different genes have a variable role, in different populations.[71] This genetic (and phenotypic) heterogeneity has made the search for causal pathways extremely challenging.

The most studied and most reproducible linkage has been with chromosome 5q, which contains many genes that have been linked with development and progression of allergic disease and asthma (including IL-4, IL-5, IL-9, IL-13, IL-12, and granulocyte macrophage-colony-stimulating factor, GM-CSF).[69] Chromosome 13 also contains a major atopy locus, with linkage between total IgE and the locus 13q14.[69] Other regions of linkage relevant to asthma determined by studying candidate loci include chromosome 14q and T-cell receptor genes, regions on chromosome 12 encoding for IFNγ and STAT6 (a gene important in the IL-4 and IL-13 Th2 signal transduction pathway),[72] chromosome 6, coding for the MHC region,[69] and chromosome 20p encoding for ADAM33 (which plays a role in airway remodeling). Other genes expressed on the epidermal surfaces, such as CD14 and TLR-4,[73] may also play a role in the susceptibility to disease but more studies are required in this area.[69,70]

The influence of maternal IgE and IgG antibodies on fetal immune responses to allergens

IgE antibodies

The association of elevated serum IgE levels and the expression of atopic disease has been recognized since the 1960s. Levels of IgE in umbilical cord blood have been investigated, as a potential predictor for atopic risk in later childhood. Although IgE secretion by the fetus has been documented in the fetal lungs and liver as early as the eleventh week of gestation,[74] the origin of cord IgE remains debatable. There has been some conjecture that this IgE may be of maternal origin; the result of either contamination during delivery, or transplacental passage. There is evidence that neonates with particularly high cord blood IgE levels are likely to develop atopic disease, particularly with respiratory symptoms, and have higher serum IgE later in childhood.[75,76] However, this is not strongly predictive and is quite insensitive for use as a single screening test, with inconsistencies in the literature.

In the absence of transplacental transfer of IgE, it has been proposed that small amounts of antigen bound to maternal IgE could cross into amniotic fluid surrounding the fetus *in utero*.[77] Fetal swallowing of amniotic fluid would expose the fetus to allergen (bound to maternal IgE) via the gastrointestinal tract. In support of this idea, low affinity IgE receptors (CD23) are expressed in the fetal gut from 16 weeks gestation, providing a mechanism for IgE-mediated antigen focusing.[77]

IgG antibodies

Differences in the passage of allergen-specific IgG from mother to fetus could be a potential mechanism of maternal influence on the development of fetal allergen-specific immunity. The transplacental passage of antigenic peptides bound to maternal IgG has been proposed as a potential mechanism of allergen transfer into the fetal circulation. These antibodies may bind via Fc receptors on the placenta and after passage into the fetal compartment affect maturing B cells, NK cells, neutrophils, dendritic cells, and monocytes. Antibody of the G class is the primary type to be transferred, mostly during the last month of pregnancy, and by term the IgG levels in the baby reach 100–200% of the mother's level.

Maternal antibodies have long been associated with the developing infant's health and with the process of 'passive' immunity,[78] but the evidence is conflicting about whether maternal allergen-specific IgG antibodies protect[79,80] or contribute to atopy.[81] Although human cord blood allergen-specific IgG levels have been associated with neonatal immune responses, they did not appear to predict or protect from infantile atopy.[63] Thus, there is currently no convincing evidence that maternal allergen-specific IgG antibodies in cord blood are the mediators of later disease.

The influence of maternal cellular immune responses

A key factor controlling the activity of the maternal immune system in pregnancy is responsiveness to paternal HLA antigens. Maternal reactivity to paternal/fetal antigens varies widely within the normal population, without overtly compromising the fetus.[82] HLA mismatching between maternal and paternal

(fetal) antigens may be a source of Th1 stimulation during pregnancy, and may alter the cytokine balance in the placenta.[83] Excessive Th1 responses do not occur in all cases of significant HLA mismatch, indicating that additional poorly understood maternal factors regulate the magnitude of reactivity. It is postulated that an established predisposition for altered immune responses (i.e. a propensity for Th2 responses in atopic women) may alter the cytokine patterns generated towards paternal antigens. While the effect of 'Th2 tendency' has not been investigated in this capacity, it is known that some women are predisposed to strong Th1 responses to paternal antigens which affect placental function and may result in fetal loss, pre-eclampsia, and poor fetal growth.[14,83]

There also appears to be variability in the capacity of women to develop tolerance to paternal antigens with successive pregnancies. The well-known example of 'Rh factor' is one that demonstrates increasing maternal responsiveness across pregnancies. On the other hand, it has been observed that, at least in some situations, successive pregnancies have 'more successful Th2 skewing' and lower incidence of Th1-mediated complications.[84] In other situations, where Th1 responses are adaptive (i.e. in the protection from placental malaria) higher Th1 (IFNγ) responses are seen with successive pregnancies and protect the fetus.[85] Thus it appears that while all pregnancies have to cope with a degree of maternal/fetal incompatibility, immune responses in pregnancy vary as a result of a complex interplay between maternal immune programming and adaptation to environmental factors. The effects of variations in the magnitude and Th1/Th2 polarity on the fetal immune system have not been explored. The capacity of fetal responses to affect maternal reactivity is also not well studied, although early reports suggested that fetal T cells can modify maternal responses *in vitro*.[86]

Other endogenous maternal factors

Maternal cytokines may also enter the amniotic fluid[87] and can be absorbed via the fetal gastrointestinal tract.[88] Breast milk continues to be a source of cytokines after birth in a similar manner. Although *ex vivo* studies have demonstrated transplacental transfer of cytokines as well as allergens,[44,89] the significance of this transfer is not known.

Influence of exogenous environmental exposures during pregnancy

There is also strong evidence that environmental exposures during early life can have more profound effects during critical periods of immune development. Many studies now indicate that events during perinatal life (beginning *in utero*) may be associated with increased risk of subsequent allergic disease.[90] Environmental influences are likely to be complex and multifactorial. The most logical candidates to investigate initially are those exposures with immunomodulatory properties that have shown changes over the last 50 years.

Maternal smoking in pregnancy

The adverse effects of maternal smoking on infant lung development are well recognized.[91–93] Parental smoking has also been associated with an increased risk of atopy[94,95] and with immunological markers of atopy in children,[96–98] although this effect has not been seen in all studies.[99,100] Increased levels of cord IgE[101] and other immunological parameters[102] in infants of smoking mothers also suggests antenatal effects on immune development.

Bacterial exposures in utero

Intrauterine infection is associated with increased capacity for neonatal Th1 responses,[103] confirming that antenatal exposures have the potential to influence maturation of Th1 function. Thus, it is possible that 'cleaner' environments could be having an effect even before birth. There is speculation that even normal microbial exposures such as through maternal fecal flora might have effects during this antenatal period, but this is unconfirmed. One recent report also observed that giving microbial (probiotic) supplements in pregnancy was associated with reduced atopic dermatitis in infancy and early childhood,[104] but the supplementation was also given in the postnatal period and thus cannot be attributed to an antenatal effect. Although the expression of bacterial recognition receptors (such as CD14) are reduced in the neonate compared with the adult, soluble CD14 has been reported to be at lower levels in amniotic fluid of infants that go on to develop early manifestations of allergic disease (atopic dermatitis).[56] This suggests that the defects in bacterial recognition pathways might also be implicated in the development of allergic responses during this early period of life. The role of bacterial products (given in fetal and early postnatal life) in allergy prevention is being actively explored.

Maternal dietary exposures

Maternal diet in pregnancy represents an important source of antigen exposure, and a pathway to affect fetal growth and well-being. Good maternal nutrition before and during pregnancy is associated with bigger babies,[105,106] and it is of note that fetal growth parameters (particularly head circumference) have also been associated with atopy.[67]

Modern diets differ in many respects from more traditional diets with more complex, processed, and synthetic foods and less fresh fish, fruits, and vegetables. As a result, there have been many changes in the intake of various dietary components (such as dietary polyunsaturated fatty acids [PUFAs] and antioxidants) that have known immunomodulatory effects.[107] It is also likely that effects of dietary factors (such as PUFAs) may be greater during critical stages of early immune development before allergic responses are established.

There are few studies to assess the relationship between specific maternal dietary nutrients in pregnancy and fetal immune development. To address the role of maternal dietary antioxidants Devereux et al.[108] examined the association between maternal dietary intake of vitamins C and E and neonatal immune function. In this study, the magnitude of cord blood mononuclear proliferative response to allergens was significantly lower in infants with the highest intake of vitamin E (determined from a food frequency questionnaire).[108] Vitamin C was not associated with these *in vitro* lymphocyte responses. This study suggested that the amount of dietary intake of antioxidants (vitamin E) during pregnancy may influence the immune system in a way that might affect the development of atopy, but more studies are needed.

To our knowledge there has only been one intervention study to examine the effect of modifying specific maternal nutrient intakes on fetal immune responses to allergens and other factors.[109,110] This study by our group examined the effects of maternal dietary fatty acid intake on neonatal immune responses. In a randomized, double-blind, placebo-controlled design, we confirmed that maternal fish oil supplementation in pregnancy resulted in significantly higher neonatal n-3 PUFA levels compared with the control group. Infant cytokine responses were negatively correlated with n-3 PUFA levels and positively correlated to n-6 PUFA levels. These observations suggest that n-3 PUFAs have immunomodulatory properties during early immune development. Although this study was designed to assess immune rather than clinical outcomes, preliminary data showed a consistent trend for less allergic symptoms and sensitization in the supplementation group.[110]

These observations clearly warrant further studies to confirm these effects, and to assess the mechanisms of action, because at this stage there are insufficient data to support any dietary recommendations.

THE FUTURE: EARLY PREDICTIVE MEASURES AND TARGETED DISEASE PREVENTION

With the development of allergy prevention strategies there is a growing need to more accurately predict children at the highest risk for both atopy and related airways disease. Although there are a number of associations between early patterns of immune responses and either genetic risk of allergic disease (family or parental allergy) or subsequent allergic disease (as discussed above) these measures do not currently have any clear predictive value. It is therefore possible that future technologies may offer the potential to assess the propensity of an individual to a particular pattern of response. Ideally this will allow more targeted prevention when more effective, more definitive strategies become available.

SUMMARY

- The dramatic increase in allergic disease highlights the need to further identify the processes that underlie Th2 differentiation in early life.
- Both maternal environmental exposures and direct maternal–fetal interactions appear to influence the developing fetal immune system, with implications for subsequent immune responses and disease susceptibility.
- These influences are most relevant during early development when immune responses are first developing. Understanding these events may lead to future strategies for disease prevention.

ACKNOWLEDGMENT

We wish to acknowledge Dr Peter Smith for his contribution to the graphics in Figure 11.2.

REFERENCES

1. Bach JF. The effect of infections on susceptibility to autoimmune and allergic diseases. N Engl J Med 2002; 347: 911–20.
2. Le Souef PN, Goldblatt J, Lynch NR. Evolutionary adaptation of inflammatory immune responses in human beings. Lancet 2000; 356: 242–4.
3. Romagnani S. Cytokines and chemoattractants in allergic inflammation. Mol Immunol 2002; 38: 881–5.
4. Romagnani S. Human Th1 and Th2 subsets: doubt no more. Immunol Today 1991; 12: 256–7.
5. Kimura M, Yamaide A, Tsuruta S, Okafuji I, Yoshida T. Development of the capacity of peripheral blood mononuclear cells to produce IL-4, IL-5 and IFN-gamma upon stimulation with house dust mite in children with atopic dermatitis. Int Arch Allergy Immunol 2002; 127: 191–7.
6. Ng TW, Holt PG, Prescott SL. Cellular immune responses to ovalbumin and house dust mite in egg-allergic children. Allergy 2002; 57: 207–14.
7. Smart JM, Kemp AS. Increased Th1 and Th2 allergen-induced cytokine responses in children with atopic disease. Clin Exp Allergy 2002; 32: 796–802.
8. Romagnani S, Romagnani P, Lasagni L et al. The increased prevalence of allergy and the hygiene hypothesis: missing immune deviation, reduced immune suppression, or both? Immunology 2004; 112: 352–63.
9. Hansen G, Berry G, DeKruyff RH, Umetsu DT. Allergen-specific Th1 cells fail to counterbalance Th2 cell-induced airway hyperreactivity but cause severe airway inflammation. J Clin Invest 1999; 103: 175–83.
10. Wills-Karp M, Santeliz J, Karp CL. The germless theory of allergic disease: revisiting the hygiene hypothesis. Nat Rev Immunol 2001; 1: 69–75.
11. Robinson DS. Regulation: the art of control? Regulatory T cells and asthma and allergy. Thorax 2004; 59: 640–3.
12. Barker DJ. Fetal origins of cardiovascular disease. Ann Med 1999; 31 (Suppl 1): 3–6.
13. Prescott S, Macaubas C, Smallacombe T et al. Development of allergen-specific T-cell memory in atopic and normal children. Lancet 1999; 353: 196–200.
14. Wegmann TG, Lin H, Guilbert L, Mosmann TR. Bidirectional cytokine interactions in the maternal-fetal relationship: is successful pregnancy a Th2 phenomenon? Immunol Today 1993; 14: 353–6.
15. Romagnani S. The role of lymphocytes in allergic disease. J Allergy Clin Immunol 2000; 105: 399–408.
16. Jones CA, Williams KA, Finlay-Jones JJ, Hart PH. Interleukin 4 production by human amnion epithelial cells and regulation of its activity by glycosaminoglycan binding. Biol Reprod 1995; 52: 839–47.
17. Schmidt C, Orr H. Maternal-fetal interactions: the role of the MHC class I molecule HLA-G. Crit Rev Immunol 1993; 13: 207–24.
18. Munn DH, Shafizadeh E, Attwood JT et al. Inhibition of T cell proliferation by macrophage tryptophan catabolism. J Exp Med 1999; 189: 1363–72.
19. Terness P, Bauer TM, Rose L et al. Inhibition of allogeneic T cell proliferation by indoleamine 2,3-dioxygenase-expressing dendritic cells: mediation of suppression by tryptophan metabolites. J Exp Med 2002; 196: 447–57.
20. Stites D, Pavia C. Ontogeny of human T cells. Pediatrics 1979; 64 (Suppl): 795–802.
21. August CS, Izzet-Berkel A, Driscoll S, Merler E. Onset of lymphocyte function in developing human fetus. Pediatr Res 1971; 5: 539–47.
22. Asantila T, Sorvani T, Hirvonen T, Toivanen P. Xenogeneic reactivity of human fetal lymphocytes. J Immunol 1973; 111: 984–7.
23. von Hoegen P, Sarin S, Krowka JF. Deficiency in T cell responses of human fetal lymph node cells: a lack of accessory cells. Immunol Cell Biol 1995; 73: 353–61.
24. Janossy G, Bofill M, Poulter LW et al. Separate ontogeny of two macrophage-like accessory cell populations in the human fetus. J Immunol 1986; 136: 4354–61.

25. Dwyer JM, MacKay IR. Antigen binding lymphocytes in human fetal thymus. Lancet 1970; 1: 1119–212.

26. Toivanen P, Asantila T, Grauberg C, Leino A, Hirvonen T. Development of T cell repertoire in the human and sheep fetus. Immunol Rev 1978; 42: 185–201.

27. Jones A, Miles E, Warner J et al. Fetal peripheral blood mononuclear cell proliferative responses to mitogenic and allergenic stimuli during gestation. Pediatr Allergy Immunol 1996; 7: 109–116.

28. Kondo N, Kobayashi Y, Shinoda S et al. Cord blood lymphocyte responses to food antigens for the prediction of allergic disorders. Arch Dis Child 1992; 67: 1003–7.

29. Piccinni MP, Mecacci F, Sampognaro S et al. Aeroallergen sensitization can occur during fetal life. Int Arch Allergy Immunol 1993; 102: 301–3.

30. Piastra M, Stabile A, Fioravanti G et al. Cord blood mononuclear cell responsiveness to beta-lactoglobulin: T-cell acitivity in 'atopy-prone' and 'non-atopy-prone' newborns. Int Arch Allergy Immunol 1994; 104: 358–65.

31. Warner JA, Miles EA, Jones AC et al. Is deficiency of interferon gamma production by allergen triggered cord blood cells a predictor of atopic eczema? Clin Exp Allergy 1994; 24: 423–30.

32. Rinas U, Horneff G, Wahn V. Interferon gamma production by cord blood mononuclear cells is reduced in newborns with a family history of atopic disease and is independent from cord blood IgE levels. Pediatr Allergy Immunol 1993; 4: 60–4.

33. Miles EA, Warner JA, Jones AC et al. Peripheral blood mononuclear cell proliferative responses in the first year of life in babies born to atopic parents. Clin Exp Allergy 1996; 26: 780–88.

34. Van Duren-Schmidt K, Pichler J, Ebner C et al. Prenatal contact with inhalant allergens. Pediatr Res 1997; 41: 128–31.

35. Prescott SL, Macaubas C, Smallacombe T et al. Reciprocal age-related patterns of allergen-specific T-cell immunity in normal vs. atopic infants. Clin Exp Allergy 1998; 28 (Suppl 5): 39–44; discussion 50–1.

36. Prescott S, Macaubas C, Holt B, et al. Transplacental priming of the human immune system to environmental allergens: universal skewing of initial T-cell responses towards Th-2 cytokine profile. J Immunol 1998; 160: 4730–7.

37. Smillie FI, Elderfield AJ, Patel F et al. Lymphoproliferative responses in cord blood and at one year: no evidence for the effect of in utero exposure to dust mite allergens. Clin Exp Allergy 2001; 31: 1194–204.

38. Prescott SL. The significance of immune responses to allergens in early life. Clin Exp Allergy 2001; 31: 1167–9.

39. Platts-Mills TA, Woodfolk JA. Cord blood proliferative responses to inhaled allergens: is there a phenomenon? J Allergy Clin Immunol 2000; 106: 441–3.

40. Weil GJ, Hussain R, Kumaraswami V et al. Prenatal allergic sensitization to helminth antigens in offspring of parasite-infected mothers. J Clin Invest 1983; 71: 1124–9.

41. Gill TJ 3rd, Repetti CF, Metlay LA et al. Transplacental immunization of the human fetus to tetanus by immunization of the mother. J Clin Invest 1983; 72: 987–96.

42. Johnson CC, Ownby DR, Peterson EL. Parental history of atopic disease and concentration of cord blood IgE [comment]. Clin Exp Allergy 1996; 26: 624–9.

43. Dahl GM, Telemo E, Westrom BR, Jacobsson I, Karlson BW. The passage of orally fed proteins from mother to foetus in the rat. Comp Biochem Physiol 1984; 77A: 199–201.

44. Szepfalusi Z, Loibichler C, Pichler J et al. Direct evidence for transplacental allergen transfer. Pediatr Res 2000; 48: 404–7.

45. Holloway JA, Warner JO, Vance GH et al. Detection of house-dust-mite allergen in amniotic fluid and umbilical cord blood. Lancet 2000; 356: 1900–2.

46. Jones CA, Vance GH, Power LL et al. Costimulatory molecules in the developing human gastrointestinal tract: a pathway for fetal allergen priming. J Allergy Clin Immunol 2001; 108: 235–41.

47. Prescott SL, Jones CA. Cord blood memory responses: are we being naive? Clin Exp Allergy 2001; 31: 1653–6.

48. Devereux G, Seaton A, Barker RN. In utero priming of allergen-specific helper T cells. Clin Exp Allergy 2001; 31: 1686–95.

49. Thornton CA, Upham JW, Wikstrom ME et al. Functional maturation of CD4+CD25+CTLA4+CD45RA+ T regulatory cells in human neonatal T cell responses to environmental antigens/allergens. J Immunol 2004; 173: 3084–92.

50. Tang MLK, Kemp AS, Thorburn J, Hill D. Reduced interferon gamma secretion in neonates and subsequent atopy. Lancet 1994; 344: 983–5.

51. Liao S, Liao T, Chiang B et al. Decreased production of IFNγ and decreased production of IL-6 by cord blood mononuclear cells of newborns with a high risk of allergy. Clin Exp Allergy 1996; 26: 397–405.

52. Martinez F, Stern D, Wright A et al. Association of interleukin-2 and interferon-γ production by blood mononuclear cells in infancy with parental allergy skin tests and with subsequent development of atopy. J Allergy Clin Immunol 1995; 96: 652–60.

53. Macaubas C, de Klerk NH, Holt BJ et al. Association between antenatal cytokine production and the development of atopy and asthma at age 6 years. Lancet 2003; 362: 1192–7.

54. Upham JW, Hayes LM, Lundahl J, Sehmi R, Denburg JA. Reduced expression of hemopoietic cytokine receptors on cord blood progenitor cells in neonates at risk for atopy. J Allergy Clin Immunol 1999; 104 (2 Pt 1): 370–5.

55. Spinozzi F, Agea E, Russano A et al. CD4+IL13+ T lymphocytes at birth and the development of wheezing and/or asthma during the 1st year of life. Int Arch Allergy Immunol 2001; 124: 497–501.

56. Jones CA, Holloway JA, Popplewell EJ et al. Reduced soluble CD14 levels in amniotic fluid and breast milk are associated with the subsequent development of atopy, eczema, or both. J Allergy Clin Immunol 2002; 109: 858–66.

57. Gabrielsson S, Soderlund A, Nilsson C et al. Influence of atopic heredity on IL-4-, IL-12- and IFN-gamma-producing cells in in vitro activated cord blood mononuclear cells. Clin Exp Immunol 2001; 126: 390–6.

58. Szepfalusi Z, Nentwich I, Gerstmayr M, Jost E, Toloran L. Prenatal allergen contact with milk proteins. Clin Exp Allergy 1997; 27: 28–35.

59. Lehmann I, Thoelke A, Weiss M et al. T cell reactivity in neonates from an East and a West German city – results of the LISA study. Allergy 2002; 57: 129–36.

60. Holt PG. Development of sensitization versus tolerance to inhalant allergens during early life. Pediatr Pulmonol Suppl 1997; 16: 6–7.

61. Ridge J, Fuchs E, Matzinger P. Neonatal tolerance revisited: turning on newborn T cells with dendritic cells. Science 1996; 271: 1723–6.

62. Pohl D, Bockelmann C, Forster K, Reiger C, Schauer U. Neonates at risk of atopy show impaired production of interferon-gamma after stimulation with bacterial products (LPS and SEE). Allergy 1997; 52: 732–8.

63. Prescott S, Jenmalm M, Bjorksten B, Holt P. Effects of maternal allergen-specific IgG in cordblood on early post-

natal development of allergen-specific T-cell immunity. Allergy 2000; 55: 470–5.

64. Aaby P, Shaheen SO, Heyes CB et al. Early BCG vaccination and reduction in atopy in Guinea-Bissau. Clin Exp Allergy 2000; 30: 644–50.

65. Shirakawa T, Enomoto T, Shimazu S, Hopkin J. Inverse association between tuberculin responses and atopic disorder. Science 1997; 272: 77–9.

66. Nilsson L, Kjellman NI, Lofman O, Bjorksten B. Parity among atopic and non-atopic mothers. Pediatr Allergy Immunol 1997; 8: 134–6.

67. Oryszczyn MP, Annesi-Maesano I, Campagna D et al. Head circumference at birth and maternal factors related to cord blood total IgE. Clin Exp Allergy 1999; 29: 334–41.

68. Barker D, Godfrey K, Fall C et al. Relation of birthweight and childhood respiratory infection to adult lung function and death from chronic obstructive airways disease. BMJ 1991; 303: 671–5.

69. Cookson W. Genetics and genomics of asthma and allergic diseases. Immunol Rev 2002; 190: 195–206.

70. Hakonarson H, Halapi E. Genetic analyses in asthma: current concepts and future directions. Am J Pharmacogenomics 2002; 2: 155–66.

71. Tattersfield AE, Knox AJ, Britton JR, Hall IP. Asthma. Lancet 2002; 360: 1313–22.

72. Barnes KC. Atopy and asthma genes – where do we stand? Allergy 2000; 55: 803–17.

73. Song PI, Park YM, Abraham T et al. Human keratinocytes express functional CD14 and toll-like receptor 4. J Invest Dermatol 2002; 119: 424–32.

74. Miller D, Hiravonen T, Gitlin D. Synthesis of IgE by the human conceptus. J Allergy Clin Immunol 1973; 52: 182–8.

75. Croner S, Kjellman NIM. Development of atopic disease in relation to family history and cord blood IgE levels. Eleven year follow-up in 1654 children. Pediatr Allergy Immunol 1990; 1: 14–20.

76. Hansen LG, Halken S, Host A, Møller K, Østerballe O. Prediction of allergy from family history and cord blood IgE levels. Pediatr Allergy Immunol 1993; 4: 34–40.

77. Thornton CA, Holloway JA, Popplewell EJ et al. Fetal exposure to intact immunoglobulin E occurs via the gastrointestinal tract. Clin Exp Allergy 2003; 33: 306–11.

78. Jarrett EEE. Perinatal influences on IgE responses. Lancet 1984; 2: 797.

79. Dannaeus A, Inganäs N. A followup study of children with food allergy: clinical course in relation to serum IgE and IgG antibodies to milk, egg and fish. Clin Allergy 1981; 11: 533–9.

80. Casimir G, Duchateau J, Cuvelier P, Vis H. Maternal immune status against beta-lactoglobulin and cow's milk allergy in the infant. Ann Allergy 1989; 63: 517–19.

81. Iikura Y, Akimoto K, Odajima Y, Akazawa A, Nagakura T. How to prevent allergic disease. I. Study of specific IgE, IgG, and IgG4 antibodies in serum of pregnant mothers, cord blood, and infants. Int Arch Allergy Appl Immunology 1989; 88: 250–2.

82. Manyonda IT, Pereira RS, Pearce JM, Sharrock CE. Limiting dilution analysis of the allo-MHC anti-paternal cytotoxic T cell response. I: Normal primigravid and multiparous pregnancies. Clin Exp Immunol 1993; 93: 126–31.

83. Saito S, Umekage H, Sakamoto Y et al. Increased T-helper-1-type immunity and decreased T-helper-2-type immunity in patients with preeclampsia. Am J Reprod Immunol 1999; 41: 297–306.

84. Barrat F, Lesourd B, Boulouis HJ et al. Sex and parity modulate cytokine production during murine ageing. Clin Exp Immunol 1997; 109: 562–8.

85. Moore JM, Nahlen BL, Misore A, Lal AA, Udhayakumar V. Immunity to placental malaria. I. Elevated production of interferon-gamma by placental blood mononuclear cells is associated with protection in an area with high transmission of malaria. J Infect Dis 1999; 179: 1218–25.

86. Saji F, Tanaka F, Fumita Y, Nakamuro K, Tanizawa O. Immunoregulatory effects of human cord blood T lymphocytes on mixed lymphocyte reaction. Nippon Sanka Fujinka Gakkai Zasshi 1986; 38: 1115–9.

87. Kent AS, Sullivan MH, Elder MG. Transfer of cytokines through human fetal membranes. J Reprod Fertil 1994; 100: 81–4.

88. Jones CA, Kilburn SA, Warner JA, Warner JO. Intrauterine environment and fetal allergic sensitization [editorial; comment]. Clin Exp Allergy 1998; 28: 655–9.

89. Reisenberger K, Egarter C, Vogl S et al. The transfer of interleukin-8 across the human placenta perfused in vitro. Obstet Gynecol 1996; 87: 613–16.

90. Prescott SL. Early origins of allergic disease: a review of processes and influences during early immune development. Curr Opin Allergy Clin Immunol 2003; 3: 125–32.

91. Stick SM, Burton PR, Gurrin L, Sly PD, LeSouef PN. Effects of maternal smoking during pregnancy and a family history of asthma on respiratory function in newborn infants. Lancet 1996; 348: 1060–4.

92. Brown RW, Hanrahan JP, Castille RG, Tager IB. Effect of maternal smoking during pregnancy on passive respiratory mechanics in early infancy. Pediatr Pulmonol 1995; 19: 23–8.

93. Hoo A, Matthias H, Dezateux C, Costeloe K, Stocks J. Respiratory function among preterm infants whose mothers smoked during pregnancy. Am J Respir Crit Care Med 1998; 158: 700–5.

94. Weiss ST, Tager IB, Munoz A, Speizer FE. The relationship of respiratory infections in early childhood to the occurrence of increased levels of bronchial responsiveness and atopy. Am Rev Respir Dis 1985; 131: 573–8.

95. Martinez FD, Antognoni G, Macri F et al. Parental smoking enhances bronchial responsiveness in nine-year-old children. Am Rev Respir Dis 1988; 138: 518–23.

96. Kulig M, Luck W, Lau S et al. Effect of pre- and postnatal tobacco smoke exposure on specific sensitization to food and inhalant allergens during the first 3 years of life. Multicenter Allergy Study Group, Germany [In Process Citation]. Allergy 1999; 54: 220–8.

97. Ronchetti R, Macri F, Ciofetta G et al. Increased serum IgE and increased prevalence of eosinophilia in 9-year-old children of smoking parents. J Allergy Clin Immunol 1990; 86 (3 Pt 1): 400–7.

98. Wjst M, Heinrich J, Liu P et al. Indoor factors and IgE levels in children. Allergy 1994; 49: 766–71.

99. Soyseth V, Kongerud J, Boe J. Postnatal maternal smoking increases the prevalence of asthma but not of bronchial hyperresponsiveness or atopy in their children. Chest 1995; 107: 389–94.

100. Ownby DR, McCullough J. Passive exposure to cigarette smoke does not increase allergic sensitization in children. J Allergy Clin Immunol 1988; 82: 634–8.

101. Magnusson C. Maternal smoking influences cord serum IgE and IgD levels and increases the risk for subsequent infant allergy. J Allergy Clin Immunol 1986; 78: 898–904.

102. Noakes PS, Holt PG, Prescott SL. Maternal smoking in pregnancy alters neonatal cytokine responses. Allergy 2003; 58: 1053–8.

103. Matsuoka T, Matsubara T, Katayama K et al. Increase of cord blood cytokine-producing T cells in intrauterine infection. Pediatr Int 2001; 43: 453–7.

104. Kalliomaki M, Salminen S, Poussa T, Arvilommi H, Isolauri E. Probiotics and prevention of atopic disease: 4-year follow-up of a randomised placebo-controlled trial. Lancet 2003; 361: 1869–71.

105. Luke B. Maternal-fetal nutrition. Clin Obst Gynecol 1994; 37: 93–109.

106. Brown E. Improving pregnancy outcomes in the United States: the importance of preventative nutrition services. J Am Diet Assoc 1989; 89: 631–3.

107. Weiss S. Diet as a risk factor for asthma. In: CIBA Foundation Symposium (Holgate S, ed). New York: Wiley, 1997: 244–57.

108. Devereux G, Barker RN, Seaton A. Antenatal determinants of neonatal immune responses to allergens. Clin Exp Allergy 2002; 32: 43–50.

109. Dunstan JA, Mori TA, Barden A et al. Maternal fish oil supplementation in pregnancy reduces interleukin-13 levels in cord blood of infants at high risk of atopy. Clin Exp Allergy 2003; 33: 442–8.

110. Dunstan J, Mori TA, Barden A et al. Fish oil supplementation in pregnancy modifies neonatal allergen-specific immune responses and clinical outcomes in infants at high risk of atopy: a randomised controlled trial. J Allergy Clin Immunol 2003; 112: 1178–84.

12

Perinatal characteristics and asthma and allergies in offspring

Sami T Remes and Juha Pekkanen

INTRODUCTION

The hypothesis that pre- and perinatal factors may contribute to the risk of childhood asthma was proposed in 1974 by Salk and colleagues.[1] At that time, psychological factors and stress were believed to have an important role in the pathogenesis of asthma. Salk et al. concluded that 'complications during the pregnancy and birth experience may well be predictive of a predisposition to manifest respiratory symptoms of asthma'.[1] Since that time, there has been considerable expansion of the literature on asthma and allergy.

It has been suggested that during pregnancy and the first year of life, the Th1/Th2 balance of the immune system is determined, possibly for life.[2] In some subjects, the initial postnatal Th2 skew of the immune system may persist, which may lead to increased occurrence of persistent asthma and allergic diseases in later life.[2] Microbial exposure before and after birth may have an important effect on this development trajectory. The mother's immune status during pregnancy may also affect the immune development of the child. This idea that early life events program the immune development of the child links closely with the fetal programming hypothesis, which is very popular in the literature on cardiovascular diseases and diabetes.[3,4] Repeated studies have shown that low birth weight predicts development of these diseases in adulthood and several older studies have linked prematurity with asthma and respiratory problems.

On the other hand, the fetal programming hypothesis has been criticized for its focus on only a limited time period early in life as a cause of chronic diseases later in life. A book edited by Kuh and Ben-Shlomo[5] provides a broader perspective: early life events form only part of a continuum in the developmental process lasting throughout the human lifespan, and modifying the disease risk of an individual.[5]

Asthma is a complex disorder, in which several factors play a role, especially lung function and immune development. Childhood asthma also has several phenotypes,[6] like transient wheezing, which is more related with low lung function, and persistent wheezing, which is more related with immune processes. The factors operating during fetal and early postnatal life may influence both of these outcomes.[7–9] There is evidence that the same surrogate markers of fetal growth (such as birth weight or gestational age) may have opposite associations with the different outcomes, either lung growth or altered immune response. Therefore, in this chapter, we try to disentangle the effects of perinatal factors on these different components of asthma, which ultimately may lead to clinical expression of asthma. We focus on epidemiological studies that assessed markers of fetal growth (such as gestational age and anthropometric measurements at birth) and other perinatal factors (such as pregnancy complications and early life infections) and consider their association with the subsequent development of asthma, atopic sensitization, and allergic disease.

EPIDEMIOLOGICAL TOOLS IN STUDYING PERINATAL FACTORS IN ASTHMA AND ATOPY

Anthropometric measures at birth, such as weight, length, head circumference, or gestational age, have been utilized by a number of historical cohort studies, because such data have been recorded in many countries. Research on such epidemiological data, perhaps in combination with a cross-sectional follow-up, can be carried out with low cost and in a relatively short time.

Most of the analyses, however, have been based on pre-existing studies that were not originally designed to address these issues. Since many studies were based on retrospective, historical birth cohorts, the completeness of information on perinatal and other factors depends on which variables were originally ascertained. Many studies also lack information on important confounding factors. In addition, the definition of outcome, especially that of asthma, varies between the studies due to incomplete data. They may be subject to recall bias when information has been provided by memory from the parents. Some were carried out only in selected subpopulations; for example, in low birth weight infants, making it difficult to generalize their results.

It is clear, therefore, that prospective studies would be preferable in terms of quality of the data. However, since prospective birth cohort studies are extremely expensive and time-consuming, the literature on asthma and allergy based on prospective cohorts has been scanty until recent years. The first large, population-based birth cohort study on asthma and allergy was initiated in the 1980s.[10] This study, the Tucson Children's Respiratory Study (TCRS), is a birth cohort of 1246 children born in 1980–84 in Tucson, Arizona. The study subjects have been repeatedly evaluated from birth until adolescence. Since the initiation of that study, many other birth cohort studies have been started. In the meantime, the results from the cross-sectional and retrospective cohort studies provide an important basis for formulating hypotheses that can later be tested in prospective birth cohort studies. The ultimate goal of these studies would be to provide tools for effective population-based prevention strategies, and thus curtail the current 'allergy epidemic' in the westernized world. The studies with a sample size of over 1000 subjects are presented in Table 12.1.[11–29]

DEFINITIONS OF ASTHMA, ALLERGIC DISEASES, AND ATOPY

Asthma is a sum of several factors leading to its clinical presentation. The manifestation of asthmatic symptoms depends on the total level of variable airway obstruction, which is dependent on at least two factors. A primary factor is the airway size. The second factor is the level of airway inflammation and the subsequent airway hyper-responsiveness (i.e. reactivity to inhaled airway stimulants, such as allergens or tobacco smoke).[30] Both of these factors need to be considered when studying asthma.

Developmental anatomy and physiology of the respiratory tract

When discussing abnormal airway size, it is necessary to understand normal physiology and development. Post-mortem studies have shown that bronchial structures and branches develop before the 16th week of gestation, followed by growth of airway size and complexity. There is a rapid increase in the number of alveoli during the first 2 years of life and very little or no increase thereafter. After the age of 2–3 years, alveolar volume increases by age until adolescence.[31] Stable tracking of lung function from the first year of life up to school age has been suggested.[32] Similarly, the results from the TCRS[10] showed that lung function in infancy (before any respiratory illnesses) is the most important determinant of lung function at the age of 6 years.[33] The progressive tracking of lung function seems to continue until early adulthood.[34] These studies suggest that the level of lung function in early life is a significant determinant of lung function throughout life, highlighting the potential importance of factors operating during pregnancy and in early life.

Two phenotypes of asthma

Both the outcome and risk factors of childhood asthma vary between the different phenotypes.[6,10] The first phenotype consists of children who experience transient wheezing in early life. These 'transient wheezers' seem to be born with low lung function, and they are probably no more bronchial hyper-responsive than nonwheezing children.[6,35] This proposal is supported by the results of a large, prospective cohort study that found an association between low birth weight and early transient wheezing.[17] No association between low birth weight was found with continued wheezing until the age of 16 years. It is tempting to speculate that persistently lower lung function among the transient wheezers may have been caused by factors related to impaired fetal or early postnatal growth, leading to structural alterations and disturbance in lung growth. If this hypothesis is true, we should see an association between measures of fetal growth and lung function soon after birth. To our knowledge, this issue has been directly assessed in only one recent study, which supported the hypothesis.[36] In that study, reduced airway function was observed among the children with low birth weight for gestation age, the latter indicating impaired fetal growth. The importance of that study was that the authors measured lung function very early in infancy (before 12 weeks of age), before the child had experienced any overt respiratory illnesses.

Table 12.1 Studies on association between gestational age or anthropometry at birth and the risk of respiratory disease or atopy (only studies with a sample size of 1000 or more have been included)

Study	Design	n	Age (years)	Main exposure	Main outcome	Main result	Definitions/comments
Bager et al. 2003[11]	Retrospective cohort	9722	20–28	Mode of delivery, BW, GE	Asthma, allergic rhinitis	GE inversely associated with allergic rhinitis, cesarean section positively with asthma	Self-reported allergic rhinitis, asthma ever, current asthma
Barker et al. 1991[12]	Retrospective cohort	6543	59–70	BW	LF	BW positively associated with FEV_1	Substantial loss to follow-up
Bråbäck & Hedberg 1998[13]	Retrospective cohort (conscripts)	149 398	18	BW, GE	Asthma, allergic rhinitis	Allergic rhinitis positively associated with GE, asthma inversely related to BW	MD asthma or rhinitis; 12 months period prevalence
Bolte et al. 2004[14]	Cross-sectional	1138	5–7	BW, BL, HC, GE	Asthma, eczema, hay fever, IgE, SPT	BW & GE positively associated with SPT & IgE, no association with diseases	Number of children in extreme BW and GE categories small
Butland et al. 1997[15]	Prospective birth cohorts	n_1: 11 195 n_2: 9387	16	Birth weight	Hay fever, eczema	No associations	Parental report of eczema, hay fever or allergic rhinitis; 12 months period prevalence
Fergusson et al. 1997[16]	Prospective birth cohort	1265	16	BW, BL, HC, GE	Asthma, eczema, 'other allergies'	Large HC associated with increased risk of asthma	'Medical consultation' for asthma, eczema, or other allergies; cumulative incidence since birth
Lewis et al. 1995[17]	Birth cohort	15 712	16	BW, GE	Wheeze, persistent wheeze	BW inversely related to wheeze by 5 years of age, and to persistent wheeze by 16 years (borderline significance)	Parental report at 5 and 16 years of age

Table 12.1 (*continued*)

Study	Design	n	Age (years)	Main exposure	Main outcome	Main result	Definitions/comments
Von Mutius et al. 1993[18]	Cross-sectional	7445	9–11	BW, GE, mechanical ventilation after birth	Asthma, wheeze, lung function, BHR, SPT	Premature girls had elevated risk of asthma, recurrent wheeze, and low lung function	MD asthma; 12 months period prevalence
Olesen et al. 1997[19]	Retrospective cohort	n₁: 7862 n₂: 985	5–10	BW, GE	Atopic dermatitis	Atopic dermatitis associated with high GE, and with high BW in one study	MD atopic dermatitis; cumulative incidence
Pekkanen et al. 2001[20]	Birth cohort	5192	31	BW, BL, GE	Asthma, SPT	GE positively associated with SPT	MD asthma ever
Rona et al. 1993[21]	Retrospective cohort	5573	5–11	BW, GE	Asthma, wheeze, LF	BW positively associated with LF, wheeze inversely related to GE	Wheezing ever/most days; cumulative incidence
Rusconi et al. 1999[22]	Cross-sectional	16 333	6–7	BW	Wheeze	LBW associated with transient wheeze	
Schwartz et al. 1990[23]	Retrospective cohort	4661	6 months–11 years	BW, premature birth	Asthma, wheeze	BW inversely associated with asthma, LBW associated with asthma and wheeze, prematurity associated with wheeze	MD asthma; point prevalence. Frequent wheeze; 12 months period prevalence
Sears et al. 1996[24]	Prospective birth cohort	1037	18	BW	Asthma, wheeze, SPT, BHR	No association with asthma, wheeze, or BHR, atopy most prevalent in the median BW group	MD asthma, wheeze: cumulative incidence (to 9 and 18 years).
Seidman et al. 1991[23]	Retrospective cohort (conscripts)	20 312	17	BW	Asthma	LBW (< 2500 g) associated with asthma	MD asthma; cumulative incidence

Table 12.1 (continued)

Study	Design	n	Age (years)	Main exposure	Main outcome	Main result	Definitions/comments
Shaheen et al. 1999[26]	Prospective cohort	8960	26	BW	Asthma, hay fever, eczema	Inverse association between BW and asthma	Self-report of asthma, hay fever, eczema: 12 months period prevalence
Sin et al. 2004[27]	Retrospective cohort	83 595	10	BW	Asthma	High BW associated with asthma	Emergency visit for asthma up to 10 years of age
Steffensen et al. 2000[28]	Retrospective cohort (conscripts)	4795	18	BW, GE	Asthma, atopic eczema	LBW nonsignificantly associated with asthma and eczema	MD asthma or atopic eczema, current
Yuan et al. 2002[29]	Retrospective cohort	10 440	12	BW, BL, GE	Asthma	High BW associated with asthma	Hospitalization with asthma

BW, birth weight; BL, birth length; GE, gestational age; HC, head circumference at birth; LF, lung function; MD, doctor-diagnosed; BHR, bronchial hyperresponsiveness; LBW, low birth weight; SPT, skin prick test; LRI, lower respiratory illness.

The second phenotype of childhood asthma includes children who suffer from wheezing in early life and then continue to wheeze through childhood.[6,10] Persistent wheezing is often associated with IgE-mediated allergy (see below) and eosinophil recruitment into the airways. This group, often called 'persistent wheezers', represents a group of children with chronic childhood asthma. There may be a critical period during childhood when chronic inflammatory airway disease may permanently deteriorate lung function among susceptible individuals. Children who developed persistent wheezing had only marginally (but not significantly) lower lung function in infancy before any respiratory illnesses than children who had never wheezed.[6] However, by the age of 6 years, the lung function of the children with persistent wheezing had significantly decreased. In other words, the children who developed persistent asthma had a progressive decline in lung function during the first 6 years of life. A longitudinal study from Australia showed that asthmatic children with different severity of the disease had parallel lung function growth curves from 7–10 years up to the age of 35 years, those with most severe disease initially ending up with the lowest lung function.[37] These studies suggest that the deterioration of lung function among chronic asthmatics occurs mostly (if not entirely) during early childhood. Therefore, understanding the immune process leading to inflammatory airway disease will be crucial when looking for strategies to prevent childhood asthma.

Atopy and allergic diseases

Atopy is generally defined as the presence of circulating IgE antibodies against common environmental allergens in an individual.[38] Sensitization in an individual, i.e. the presence of IgE antibodies, is usually measured by determination of allergen-specific serum IgE antibodies or by skin prick testing. Due to low cost, skin prick testing is generally used in epidemiological surveys. In these studies, atopy is usually defined as having one or more positive (≥ 3 mm mean weal size) skin prick reactions against the tested allergens.[39]

Allergic diseases consist of hay fever, atopic eczema, and asthma. However, atopy is not synonymous with allergic diseases, and the association between allergic diseases and atopic sensitization varies. For example, there is a strong association of hay fever with atopic sensitization.[40] On the contrary, the association is weaker for asthma, and it has been estimated that at the population level, less than 50% of asthma can be attributed to atopy.[41] The association is even weaker in early childhood asthma, which often includes children

with transient early wheezing. This variation is often seen in clinical practice; there are many sensitized children who do not have any signs of atopic disease, and some children with typical allergic symptoms who do not show evidence of sensitization.[38]

STUDIES ON BIRTH WEIGHT

Birth weight is probably a rather imprecise marker of fetal growth. For example, some children who are tiny at birth may be normal, being small because they have genetically small parents or because of other reasons not related to an adverse fetal environment. Another newborn with the same birth weight may have suffered from maternal undernutrition or from other adverse conditions *in utero*. This mix of causal factors is especially evident in the middle of the birth weight distribution. It may also explain why the associations between birth weight and asthma, or lung function and asthma, have been seen primarily at the extreme ends of the birth weight distribution (i.e. low and high birth weight).

Low birth weight and asthma

Several studies, mainly based on historical birth cohorts, found that children born at a low weight had decreased lung function in later life.[12,21,42–44] On the other hand, some studies have observed no relation between birth weight and lung function.[26] There is also rather consistent evidence for an association between low birth weight and asthma,[13,23,25,26,45,46] although some studies have found no association[12,13,16,24,25] (Figure 12.1, Table 12.1).

The simplest explanation for the association between low birth weight and asthma,[18,47,48] wheezing,[21] or decreased lung function[18] would be that there are lung complications related to prematurity. However, the findings that the association between birth weight and asthma remain significant after adjustment for gestational age[13,26] argue against this interpretation. Moreover, the inverse association was observed within the normal range of birth weight in one study.[49] In fact, the inverse association of birth weight and asthma remained even after children with low birth weight or prematurity were excluded.

Recent studies have shown that the association of low birth weight and asthma is strongest for nonatopic asthma[50] and for transient wheezing.[22,50,51] A similar but weaker association has been observed with regard to persistent wheeze, a marker of chronic asthma.[22,50] It seems, therefore, that the association between low birth weight and asthma may be

(a)

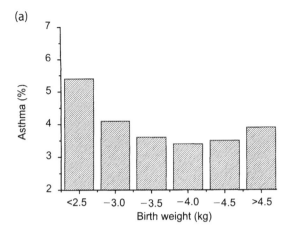

(b)

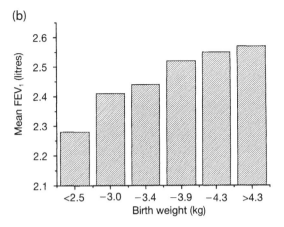

(c)

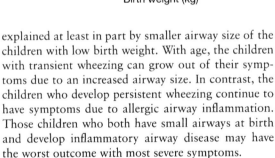

Figure 12.1 The associations of birth weight with (a) asthma, (b) lung function, and (c) allergic rhinitis. The relationship between birth weight and asthma seems to be U-shaped, the highest risk being among those with either low or high birth weight (a). Risk among those with low birth weight may be explained by reduced lung function (b), whereas the risk in high birth weight infants may be due to a higher frequency of atopy (c) or factors related to the development of obesity. Data presented in the figure are derived from Seidman et al. 1991[25] (a), Barker et al. 1991[12] (b), and Braback et al. 1998[13] (c). Forced expiratory volume in 1 second (FEV₁) values in (b) have been standardized for age and height.

explained at least in part by smaller airway size of the children with low birth weight. With age, the children with transient wheezing can grow out of their symptoms due to an increased airway size. In contrast, the children who develop persistent wheezing continue to have symptoms due to allergic airway inflammation. Those children who both have small airways at birth and develop inflammatory airway disease may have the worst outcome with most severe symptoms.

Low birth weight may also be considered as a surrogate marker of multiple factors that can have adverse effects on the fetus and impair lung growth. Such factors may include maternal asthma, smoking, hypertension, undernutrition, poor maternal health, or adverse environmental conditions during pregnancy.[36,42,43,52–55] On the other hand, low birth weight babies may be more likely to experience other postnatal risk factors, like infections (see below), that can have a harmful effect on lung function. This view is also supported by several recent studies that have shown an association between various complications during pregnancy and asthma.[56,57] Therefore, the asso-

ciations between pregnancy complications, low birth weight and asthma are likely mediated through an effect on the lungs. One recent study also reported an association between uterus-related complications and allergic rhinitis linking pregnancy complications with the development of atopy in addition to asthma.[58]

High birth weight and asthma

In addition to the association between low birth weight and asthma, two recent studies observed an increased risk of asthma among the children born with a high birth weight[27,29] (Table 12.1). Both studies were large and registry-based, providing enough subjects to examine extreme categories of birth weight. The definition of asthma was based on cumulative incidence of either asthma hospitalization[29] or emergency visits for asthma[27] by adolescence, and the results did not significantly change when the occurrence of these events in early childhood was excluded. Using a smooth interpolation method, Sin et al. fitted a probability curve of developing asthma by birth weight. Interestingly, the probability of asthma remained stable until the birth weight of 4.5 kg, thereafter increasing progressively in a linear manner.[27] A similar trend was observed in the other study.[29]

Two potential hypotheses have been offered to explain the association between high birth weight and asthma.[27] The first explanation relates to lung mechanics, such as the disadvantage of respiratory muscle function due to obesity. In addition, obesity may influence the development of certain immune responses, altering the risk of developing chronic asthma (Figure 12.1). The latter explanation is of special interest, since obesity has been suggested to be an important factor for incident asthma at adolescence.[59] On the other hand, there may be other factors associated with fetal macrosomy (such as maternal diabetes) and their role in mediating the association of asthma and high birth weight is unknown. However, it is tempting to speculate that the association of asthma and obesity may start much earlier than previously suggested, although the evidence to date supporting this hypothesis is still weak. This linkage would concur with the proposal that enhanced fetal growth may increase the risk of asthma and atopy.[14,60,61] These findings raise the interesting speculation that the recent increase in childhood asthma and atopy may be partially attributed to obesity and overnutrition in the westernized countries. The results also suggest that the association of birth weight and asthma may have changed over time. In other words, the associations found in one cohort may not be seen in others due to secular changes in the time of exposure (cohort effect).[62,63]

INFECTIONS

Infections in early life have been suggested to be both harmful or beneficial with regard to asthma. Respiratory viral infections are common triggers of asthmatic symptoms among children who already have asthma. The impact of infections on the initiation of asthma is less clear. Many studies have shown that severe infections of the lower respiratory tract may damage lung structure and lead to permanently decreased lung function. On the other hand, the hygiene hypothesis suggests that some types of infections may actually have a beneficial effect on immune maturation and protect against the development of childhood asthma and allergy.[64] As the impact of microbial exposure on immune development is covered in detail in Chapter 11, our focus below is on clinical infections and their treatment.

Respiratory infections – the bad?

The influence of infections during early life on lung growth is controversial. Many studies have shown that severe infections of the lower respiratory tract may damage lung structure and lead to permanently decreased lung function.[3,42] However, interpretation of the historical birth cohort studies is hampered by substantial selection bias, selective loss to follow-up, and misclassification of early infections because of diagnostic inaccuracy.[52] In addition, the reversibility of the deficits in lung function has not been assessed,[65] making it difficult to distinguish between reversible obstruction and irreversible tissue damage. However, these findings suggest that the developing lung may be more vulnerable to the adverse effects of infections during the first year of life than later. It is even possible that prenatal infections, such as chorioamnionitis, may adversely influence the lung development.[65] In a study from Netherlands, there was a tendency for increased obstructive airway disease among those exposed to famine during early or mid-gestation. These results are in keeping with the proposal that suboptimal lung growth and early childhood insults reduce the lung capacity and may leave these children with an increased risk of chronic obstructive pulmonary disease (COPD) in adulthood.[65,66]

It would be important to know whether lower respiratory tract infections early in life contribute to or modify the potential effect of other prenatal factors on lung growth. For example, one could argue that the association between birth weight and lung function is explained by a higher susceptibility of low birth weight infants to lower respiratory tract infections, decreasing lung function by infection-associated lung damage. However, a recent study from Britain did not find evidence to support this hypothesis. In their study the association between birth weight and lung function in later life (see Figure 12.1) was independent of the postnatal infection history.[12] Unfortunately, many studies analyzing the association between perinatal factors and subsequent respiratory health have no information on respiratory or other infections during the first year of life. The follow-up of the cohort of Dezateux et al.[36] could provide answers to the question whether there are differential effects of lower airway infections on lung growth in children with small or appropriate birth weight for gestational age.

Respiratory infections – the good?

The possible preventive effect of infections on the risk of asthma has gained popularity and is often described as the 'hygiene hypothesis'.[64] However, it should be noted that clinical infections are a poor marker of microbial exposure and the epidemiological evidence for the protective effect of infections has been quite conflicting.[67] Moreover, the evidence for a protective effect of microbes is stronger for atopy than for asthma.[68] This finding fits with the theory that microbes affect primarily the Th1/Th2 balance[2] and thereby atopy, but may have less of an effect on asthma.[41]

Another possible explanation for the controversial findings on infections and the risk of childhood asthma is the variance in immune response between the children.[69–72] Asthmatics, or children who will later develop asthma, are likely to have more frequent severe respiratory symptoms. As a result, respiratory infections would appear to be associated with an increased risk of asthma. However, this risk may not be caused by the infection *per se*, but rather by underlying defects in the immune responses of the symptomatic subjects. Factors determining the phenotype and competence of immune responses in children are still incompletely understood, but are known to have strong genetic determinants.[73]

A corollary of this discussion is the idea that antibiotics could increase the risk of asthma by reducing the possible protective effect of childhood infections. There is, again, the possibility that children with asthma are more prone to have lower respiratory symptoms when infected with a pathogen,[69] leading to an increased use of antibiotics by asthmatics. This 'reverse causation' is potentially a concern in those studies reporting on an association between antibiotic use and the risk for asthma. In fact, two recent cohort studies have found that the association between antibiotic use in early life and asthma appeared to be due to 'reverse causation'.[74,75] On the other hand, the large birth cohort study by McKeever et al.,[76] indicated that maternal use of antibiotics during pregnancy was associated with asthma, suggesting that drug use was an antecedent factor. The association was clearly weaker for hay fever in this study. If this finding indicates causality, it is likely to be due to 'hygiene hypotheses', as infections and other complications during pregnancy have been associated with increased risk of asthma.[76,77] Possibly there is some common and non-specific mechanism, like increased maternal stress,[78] that explains these associations. However, in the future it will probably be more fruitful to focus on microbial exposure and less on symptomatic infections and their treatment, when searching for the etiology of atopy and asthma.

OTHER FACTORS

Head circumference

When the discussion on the impact of fetal growth on risk of atopy started in 1994, Godfrey et al. reported that babies who were born with disproportionately large heads relative to body size had elevated IgE levels as adults.[79] These results were later supported by another study.[80] In addition, positive correlations between head circumference and cord blood IgE[81] and IgE at the age of 11 years[61] have been reported. Having a disproportionately large head may indicate that the fetus sustained brain growth, while utilizing less resource for growing other parts of the body. Godfrey et al. hypothesized that fetal undernutrition in late gestation may impair thymic maturation, leading to permanently altered immune function and increased IgE concentrations in adult age.

Assuming that the babies who were exposed to an adverse fetal environment really do have a higher risk of becoming atopic, as suggested by Godfrey et al.,[79] one would expect there to be many atopic children in developing countries where poor maternal health is the rule rather than an exception. In fact, the opposite is true, atopic diseases are less common in the poorest countries of the third world.[82] In support of this conclusion, no influence of undernutrition was found on markers of atopy in the Dutch famine study, when looking for a long-term effect on lung function and serum IgE in adulthood.[83]

Godfrey's theory[79] may be further challenged by a Scandinavian study in which the relationship between head circumference and thymic size was assessed by sonography soon after birth.[84,85] In contrast to Godfrey's hypothesis, there was a positive association between head circumference at birth and sonography-estimated thymus size, and between birth weight and thymus size, the latter being the strongest determinant of thymus size. In the same study, the correlation between thymus size and development of allergic disease by 5 years of age was examined, and no association was found. However, the latter results cannot be regarded as conclusive, because the 'allergy' group included children with early childhood wheezing, making the group heterogeneous. No markers of atopy, such as skin prick tests or serum IgE, were studied.

Head circumference at birth has been reported to be positively associated with childhood asthma in some[16] but not all studies.[14] In the other studies, head circumference has been inversely associated with wheezing during the first year of life,[51] and positively associated with lung function later in life.[44] The latter findings suggest that small head circumference, like low birth weight, may be an indicator of adverse lung growth, leading to susceptibility to transient wheezing.

Gestational age

No consistent associations have been reported between gestational age and the risk of asthma[11,13,16,20] (Table 12.1). The impact of gestational age on lung growth seems to be variable as well (apart from the complication of bronchopulmonary dysplasia among very preterm babies). Some authors found an association between low birth weight and poor lung function independent of gestational age,[21,36] whereas others have found an association only among babies born at term.[86]

In contrast to asthma, the associations between gestational age and atopy have been more consistent. Large epidemiological studies have reported positive associations between gestational age and hay fever[11,13] (Table 12.1). In accordance with these results, a study from Finland showed a strong positive association between gestational age and atopy (measured by skin prick tests) at the age of 30 years.[20] In contrast, no association was observed between gestational age and atopy in adulthood in a British cohort,[87] but the article presented only the data on mean gestational age and atopy.

The positive association of gestational age and atopy could be due to the longer period of time spent by the fetus in the uterus, where the baby is exposed to the Th2 skewed immune responses of the mother. This greater duration of exposure might skew the developing immune responses of the infant toward a Th2 direction.[88] Some authors have challenged this

explanation, however, by arguing that normal human pregnancy may not be dominated by the Th2 profile, proposing that the placental cytokine milieu of humans may be in a more balanced state than seen in mice.[89,90] Another possible explanation could be an earlier postnatal exposure to microbial products, leading to the earlier maturation of the antigen-presenting cells (APCs) in the neonate and establishment of the Th1 responses.[9] This hypothesis is supported by a Finnish study,[20] in which the association of gestational age and atopy was found to be stronger among farmers' children who presumably were more exposed to microbes postnatally than were those living in a more hygienic environment. The importance of postnatal exposures is suggested further by the fact that all infants typically show a rapid decrease in thymic size after birth[91] and yet there is no association between gestational age and thymus size at the time of birth.[85]

Cesarean section

It has been suggested that the microbial gut flora can affect the balance between Th1/Th2 lymphocytes in early childhood.[92] The colonization of microbial flora varies between babies born through cesarean section and through normal, vaginal delivery.[93] Therefore, it is tempting to speculate that babies born by cesarean section might have higher risk of atopic disease, as their gut is not as rapidly colonized with bacteria from the mother's reproductive tract.

In a birth cohort born in 1966, a strong association between cesarean section and doctor-diagnosed asthma was observed at the age of 31 years (adjusted OR 3.23, 95% CI 1.53, 6.80) (Table 12.2).[11,57,58,76,94–96]

Table 12.2 Odds ratios (OR) for the association between ceserean section and asthma, atopy or hay fever in birth cohort studies (sorted by decade of birth)

Reference	n	Decade of birth	Frequency of sections (%)	Asthma (OR)	Atopy or hay fever (OR)
Xu et al. 2001[94]	1953	1960s	5	3.2*	1.3
Bager et al. 2003[11]	9722	1970s	12	1.3*	1.2
Xu et al. 2000[57]	8086	1980s	14	1.4*	NA
Kero et al. 2002[95]	59 927	1980s	17	1.2*	NA
Håkansson 2003[96]	863 846	1980–90	7	1.3	NA
Nafstad et al. 2000[58]	2531	1990s	10	1.1	1.2
McKeever et al. 2002[76]	24 690	1990s	20	1.1	1.0

NA, not available. *$p < 0.05$.

However, no significant association was observed with atopy, hay fever, or eczema.[94] The frequency of cesarean sections was only 5%, in contrast to the prevalence in more recent studies. Weaker associations between cesarean section and asthma have been observed subsequently in four other birth cohorts born during the 1970s and 1980s, with odds ratios ranging between 1.2 and 1.4 (Table 12.2). In addition, no associations were observed in two birth cohorts from the 1990s, either with asthma or atopy or hay fever. However, a small birth cohort of 219 children has also recently suggested increased risk of atopy, as measured by skin prick test and specific IgE, among those delivered by cesarean section.[95]

Based on these findings, it is unlikely that association between cesarean section and asthma is mediated by atopy, while there is still the intriguing possibility of an effect on microbial flora and thereby on Th1/Th2 balance. Based solely on the hygiene hypothesis, one might have expected a stronger association between cesarean section and atopy than with asthma, but it was not observed.

On the other hand, cesarean section often occurs in the context of other obstetrical complications, which could be the cause of respiratory problems in the newborn.[56,57]

In the earlier studies one might expect that emergency cesarean sections constituted a larger proportion of the deliveries. However, Håkansson and Källén[96] reported no difference in asthma risk among those born after acute or elective cesarean section. Another potential confounding factor is that maternal asthma is associated with an increased risk of obstetric complications,[47] but the study by Xu et al.[94] adjusted for maternal asthma. It could be hypothesized that fetuses that will later develop asthma also are at risk for obstetrical complications and thus cesarean section delivery. However, taken together, the most likely explanation for the associations observed in the older studies is obstetric complications or other factors associated with cesarean section.

CONCLUSIONS

In summary, we can draw four major conclusions, as follows. I) Low birth weight is associated with decreased lung function in adult life. This association is possibly explained by an adverse perinatal environment altering lung growth, leading to persistently lower lung function and to an increased susceptibility to COPD in later life. II) Low birth weight seems to be associated with a greater risk for asthma. This finding is less readily explained, although it might be partially

due to lower lung function among low birth weight infants more readily provoking asthmatic symptoms than in children with larger airways.[26,97] III) Enhanced or extended fetal growth seems to be associated with an increased risk of asthma, especially in children with the highest birth weight. This finding may be related to the likelihood of later obesity, but the predisposition is already evident at birth. IV) Gestational age is positively associated with the development of atopy. The mechanisms for this association are still debated, but may be related to the age of the neonate at the initial postnatal exposure to environmental microbes.[20]

When using anthropometric measures to study the early origins of asthma, several etiological factors may be linked with a single marker. This is clearly seen in birth weight: low birth weight is associated with impaired lung growth and decreased lung function, whereas high birth weight is associated with an increased risk of asthma, possibly due to atopy or obesity.

It is also important to view asthma as a heterogeneous disorder consisting of several phenotypes, each with different etiological factors. It is imperative to consider atopy, lung function, and asthma separately, when evaluating the role of perinatal risk factors in the development of these outcomes. Therefore, more comprehensive studies with specific markers, like airway inflammation, are needed to expand our understanding of the complex association between perinatal factors and respiratory health in later life.

REFERENCES

1. Salk L, Grellong BA, Strauss W, Dietrich J. Perinatal complications in the history of asthmatic children. Am J Dis Child 1974; 127: 30–3.
2. Holt PG, Macaubas C, Stumbles PA et al. The role of allergy in the development of asthma. Nature 1999; 402: B12–B17.
3. Barker DJP, Robinson RJ. Fetal and Infant Origins of Adult Disease. London: British Medical Journal, 1993.
4. Marmot MG. Early life and adult disorder: research themes. Br Med Bull 1997; 53: 3–9.
5. Kuh D, Ben-Shlomo Y. A Life Course Approach to Chronic Disease Epidemiology. New York: Oxford University Press, 1997.
6. Martinez FD, Wright AL, Taussig LM et al. Asthma and wheezing in the first 6 years of life. N Engl J Med 1995; 332: 133–8.
7. Bjorksten B. The intrauterine and postnatal environments. J Allergy Clin Immunol 1999; 104: 1119–27.
8. Jones CA, Holloway JA, Warner JO. Does atopic disease start in foetal life? Allergy 2000; 55: 2–10.
9. Martinez FD. Maturation of immune responses at the beginning of asthma. J Allergy Clin Immunol 1999; 103: 355–61.

10. Taussig LM, Wright AL, Holberg CJ et al. Tucson Children's Respiratory Study: 1980 to present. J Allergy Clin Immunol 2003; 111: 661–75.

11. Bager P, Melbye M, Rostgaard K et al. Mode of delivery and risk of allergic rhinitis and asthma. J Allergy Clin Immunol 2003; 111: 51–6.

12. Barker DJP, Godfrey KM, Fall C et al. Relation of birth-weight and childhood respiratory infection to adult lung-function and death from chronic obstructive airways disease. Br Med J 1991; 303: 671–5.

13. Braback L, Hedberg A. Perinatal risk factors for atopic disease in conscripts. Clin Exp Allergy 1998; 28: 936–42.

14. Bolte G, Schmidt M, Maziak W et al. The relation of markers of fetal growth with asthma, allergies and serum immunoglobulin E levels in children at age 5–7 years. Clin Exp Allergy 2004; 34: 381–8.

15. Butland BK, Strachan DP, Lewis S et al. Investigation into the increase in hay fever and eczema at age 16 observed between the 1958 and 1970 British birth cohorts. Br Med J 1997; 315: 717–21.

16. Fergusson DM, Crane J, Beasley R et al. Perinatal factors and atopic disease in childhood. Clin Exp Allergy 1997; 27: 1394–401.

17. Lewis S, Richards D, Bynner J et al. Prospective study of risk factors for early and persistent wheezing in childhood. Eur Respir J 1995; 8: 349–56.

18. von Mutius E, Nicolai T, Martinez FD. Prematurity as a risk factor for asthma in preadolescent children. J Pediatr 1993; 123: 223–9.

19. Olesen AB, Ellingsen AR, Olesen H et al. Atopic dermatitis and birth factors: historical follow up by record linkage. Br Med J 1997; 314: 1003–8.

20. Pekkanen J, Xu B, Jarvelin MR. Gestational age and occurrence of atopy at age 31 – a prospective birth cohort study in Finland. Clin Exp Allergy 2001; 31: 95–102.

21. Rona RJ, Gulliford MC, Chinn S. Effects of prematurity and intrauterine growth on respiratory health and lung-function in childhood. BMJ 1993; 306: 817–20.

22. Rusconi F, Galassi C, Corbo GM et al. Risk factors for early, persistent, and late-onset wheezing in young children. Am J Respir Crit Care Med 1999; 160: 1617–22.

23. Schwartz J, Gold D, Dockery DW et al. Predictors of asthma and persistent wheeze in a national sample of children in the United States – Association with social-class, perinatal events, and race. Am Rev Respir Dis 1990; 142: 555–62.

24. Sears MR, Holdaway MD, Flannery EM et al. Parental and neonatal risk factors for atopy, airway hyper-responsiveness, and asthma. Arch Dis Child 1996; 75: 392–8.

25. Seidman DS, Laor A, Gale R et al. Is low-birth-weight a risk factor for asthma during adolescence. Arch Dis Child 1991; 66: 584–7.

26. Shaheen SO, Sterne JAC, Montgomery SM et al. Birth weight, body mass index and asthma in young adults. Thorax 1999; 54: 396–402.

27. Sin DD, Spier S, Svenson LW et al. The relationship between birth weight and childhood asthma – a population-based cohort study. Arch Pediatr Adolesc Med 2004; 158: 60–4.

28. Steffensen FH, Sorensen HT, Gillman MW et al. Low birth weight and preterm delivery as risk factors for asthma and atopic dermatitis in young adult males. Epidemiology 2000; 11: 185–8.

29. Yuan W, Basso O, Sorensen HT et al. Fetal growth and hospitalization with asthma during early childhood: a follow-up study in Denmark. Int J Epidemiol 2002; 31: 1240–5.

30. Masoli M, Fabian D, Holt S et al. The global burden of asthma: executive summary of the GINA Dissemination Committee Report. Allergy 2004; 59: 469–78.

31. Thurlbec WM. Postnatal human lung growth. Thorax 1982; 37: 564–71.

32. Dezateux C, Stocks J. Lung development and early origins of childhood respiratory illness. Br Med Bull 1997; 53: 40–57.

33. Marotti F, Holberg CJ, Wright AL et al. Predictors of lung function at 6 years of age. Am J Respir Crit Care Med 1999; 159: A147.

34. Lebowitz MD, Sherrill DL. The assessment and interpretation of spirometry during the transition from childhood to adulthood. Pediatr Pulmonol 1995; 19: 143–9.

35. Martinez FD. The relationship between impaired lung growth and onset of bronchial asthma in early life. Pediatr Pulmonol 1997; 16: 84–5.

36. Dezateux C, Lum S, Hoo AF et al. Low birth weight for gestation and airway function in infancy: exploring the fetal origins hypothesis. Thorax 2004; 59: 60–6.

37. Oswald H, Phelan PD, Lanigan A et al. Childhood asthma and lung function in mid-adult life. Pediatr Pulmonol 1997; 23: 14–20.

38. von Mutius E. Epidemiology of allergic diseases. In: Pediatric Allergy: Principles and Practice. (Leung DYM, Sampson HA, Geha RS, Szefler SJ, eds). Missouri: Mosby, 2003: 1–9.

39. Haahtela T. Skin tests used for epidemiologic studies. Allergy 1993; 48 (Suppl 14): 76–80.

40. Braun-Fahrlander C, Wuthrich B, Gassner M et al. Validation of a rhinitis symptom questionnaire (ISAAC core questions) in a population of Swiss school children visiting the school health services. SCARPOL-team. Swiss Study on Childhood Allergy and Respiratory Symptom with respect to Air Pollution and Climate. International Study of Asthma and Allergies in Childhood. Pediatr Allergy Immunol 1997; 8: 75–82.

41. Pearce N, Pekkanen J, Beasley R. How much asthma is really attributable to atopy? Thorax 1999; 54: 268–72.

42. Shaheen S. The beginnings of chronic airflow obstruction. Br Med Bull 1997; 53: 58–70.

43. Shaheen SO, Sterne JAC, Tucker JS et al. Birth weight, childhood lower respiratory tract infection, and adult lung function. Thorax 1998; 53: 549–53.

44. Stein RT, Holberg CJ, Morgan WJ et al. Peak flow variability, methacholine responsiveness and atopy as markers for detecting different wheezing phenotypes in childhood. Thorax 1997; 52: 946–52.

45. Chan KN, Elliman A, Bryan E et al. Respiratory symptoms in children of low birth-weight. Arch Dis Child 1989; 64: 1294–304.

46. Oliveti JF, Kercsmar CM, Redline S. Pre- and perinatal risk factors for asthma in inner city African-American children. Am J Epidemiol 1996; 143: 570–7.

47. Kelly YJ, Brabin BJ, Milligan P et al. Maternal asthma, premature birth, and the risk of respiratory morbidity in schoolchildren in Merseyside. Thorax 1995; 50: 525–30.

48. Schaubel D, Johansen H, Dutta M et al. Neonatal characteristics as risk factors for preschool asthma. J Asthma 1996; 33: 255–64.

49. Svanes C, Omenaas E, Heuch JM et al. Birth characteristics and asthma symptoms in young adults: results from a population-based cohort study in Norway. Eur Respir J 1998; 12: 1366–70.

50. Tariq SM, Matthews SM, Hakim EA et al. The prevalence of and risk factors for atopy in early childhood: a whole

population birth cohort study. J Allergy Clin Immunol 1998; 101: 593.

51. Gold DR, Burge HA, Carey V et al. Predictors of repeated wheeze in the first year of life – the relative roles of cockroach, birth weight, acute lower respiratory illness, and maternal smoking. Am J Respir Crit Care Med 1999; 160: 227–36.

52. Britton J, Martinez FD. The relationship of childhood respiratory infection to growth and decline in lung function. Am J Respir Crit Care Med 1996; 154: S240–S245.

53. Goldenberg RL, Davis RO, Cliver SP et al. Maternal risk-factors and their influence on fetal anthropometric measurements. Am J Obstet Gynecol 1993; 168: 1197–205.

54. Morgan WJ, Martinez FD. Maternal smoking and infant lung function – further evidence for an in utero effect. Am J Respir Crit Care Med 1998; 158: 689–90.

55. Murphy VE, Gibson PG, Giles WB et al. Maternal asthma is associated with reduced female fetal growth. Am J Respir Crit Care Med 2003; 168: 1317–23.

56. Nafstad P, Samuelsen SO, Irgens LM et al. Pregnancy complications and the risk of asthma among Norwegians born between 1967 and 1993. Eur J Epidemiol 2003; 18: 755–61.

57. Xu BZ, Pekkanen J, Jarvelin MR. Obstetric complications and asthma in childhood. J Asthma 2000; 37: 589–94.

58. Nafstad P, Magnus P, Jaakkola JJK. Risk of childhood asthma and allergic rhinitis in relation to pregnancy complications. J Allergy Clin Immunol 2000; 106: 867–73.

59. Castro-Rodriguez LA, Holberg CJ, Morgan WJ et al. Increased incidence of asthmalike symptoms in girls who become overweight or obese during the school years. Am J Respir Crit Care Med 2001; 163: 1344–9.

60. Beasley R, Leadbitter P, Pearce N et al. Is enhanced fetal growth a risk factor for the development of atopy or asthma? Int Arch Allergy Immunol 1999; 118: 408–10.

61. Leadbitter P, Pearce N, Cheng S et al. Relationship between fetal growth and the development of asthma and atopy in childhood. Thorax 1999; 54: 905–10.

62. Collins JW, Wu SY, David RJ. Differing intergenerational birth weights among the descendants of US-born and foreign-born whites and African Americans in Illinois. Am J Epidemiol 2002; 155: 210–16.

63. Vagero D, Koupilova I, Leon DA et al. Social determinants of birthweight, ponderal index and gestational age in Sweden in the 1920s and the 1980s. Acta Paediatr 1999; 88: 445–53.

64. Liu AH, Murphy JR. Hygiene hypothesis: fact or fiction? J Allergy Clin Immunol 2003; 111: 471–8.

65. Merkus PJFM. Effects of childhood respiratory diseases on the anatomical and functional development of the respiratory system. Paediatr Respir Rev 2003; 4: 28–39.

66. Sethi S. Bacterial infection and the pathogenesis of COPD. Chest 2000; 117: 286S–291S.

67. Strachan DP. Family size, infection and atopy; the first decade of the 'Hygiene hypothesis'. Thorax 2000; 55 (Suppl 1): S2–S10.

68. von Hertzen LC, Haahtela T. Asthma and atopy – the price of affluence? Allergy 2004; 59: 124–37.

69. Corne JM, Marshall C, Smith S et al. Frequency, severity, and duration of rhinovirus infections in asthmatic and non-asthmatic individuals: a longitudinal cohort study. Lancet 2002; 359: 831–4.

70. Martinez FD, Stern DA, Wright AL et al. Differential immune responses to acute lower respiratory illness in early life and subsequent development of persistent wheezing and asthma. J Allergy Clin Immunol 1998; 102: 915–20.

71. Papadopoulos NG, Stanciu LA, Papi A et al. Rhinovirus-induced alterations on peripheral blood mononuclear cell phenotype and costimulatory molecule expression in normal and atopic asthmatic subjects. Clin Exp Allergy 2002; 32: 537–42.

72. Parry DE, Busse WW, Sukow KA et al. Rhinovirus-induced PBMC responses and outcome of experimental infection in allergic subjects. J Allergy Clin Immunol 2000; 105: 692–8.

73. Nagy A, Kozma GT, Keszei M et al. The development of asthma in children infected with *Chlamydia pneumoniae* is dependent on the modifying effect of mannose-binding lectin. J Allergy Clin Immunol 2003; 112: 729–34.

74. Celedon JC, Litonjua AA, Ryan L et al. Lack of association between antibiotic use in the first year of life and asthma, allergic rhinitis, or eczema at age 5 years. Am J Respir Crit Care Med 2002; 166: 72–5.

75. Cullinan P, Harris J, Mills P et al. Early prescriptions of antibiotics and the risk of allergic disease in adults: a cohort study. Thorax 2004; 59: 11–15.

76. McKeever TM, Lewis SA, Smith C et al. The importance of prenatal exposures on the development of allergic disease – A birth cohort study using the West Midlands General Practice Database. Am J Respir Crit Care Med 2002; 166: 827–32.

77. Xu BZ, Pekkanen J, Jarvelin MR et al. Maternal infections in pregnancy and the development of asthma among offspring. Int J Epidemiol 1999; 28: 723–7.

78. von Hertzen LC. Maternal stress and T-cell differentiation of the developing immune system: possible implications for the development of asthma and atopy. J Allergy Clin Immunol 2002; 109: 923–8.

79. Godfrey KM, Barker DJP, Osmond C. Disproportionate fetal growth and raised IgE concentration in adult life. Clin Exp Allergy 1994; 24: 641–8.

80. Gregory A, Doull I, Pearce N et al. The relationship between anthropometric measurements at birth: asthma and atopy in childhood. Clin Exp Allergy 1999; 29: 330–3.

81. Oryszczyn MP, Annesi-Maesano I, Campagna D et al. Head circumference at birth and maternal factors related to cord blood total IgE. Clin Exp Allergy 1999; 29: 334–41.

82. The International Study of Asthma and Allergies in Childhood (ISAAC) steering committee. Worldwide variation in prevalence of symptoms of asthma, allergic rhinoconjunctivitis, and atopic eczema: ISAAC. Lancet 2004; 351: 1225–32.

83. Lopuhaa CE, Roseboom TJ, Osmond C et al. Atopy, lung function, and obstructive airways disease after prenatal exposure to famine. Thorax 2000; 55: 555–61.

84. Benn CS, Jeppesen DL, Hasselbalch H et al. Thymus size and head circumference at birth and the development of allergic diseases. Clin Exp Allergy 2001; 31: 1862–6.

85. Hasselbalch H, Jeppesen DL, Ersboll AK et al. Sonographic measurement of thymic size in healthy neonates – relation to clinical variables. Acta Radiol 1997; 38: 95–8.

86. Wjst M, Popescu M, Trepka MJ et al. Pulmonary function in children with initial low birth weight. Pediatr Allergy Immunol 1998; 9: 80–90.

87. Strachan DP, Harkins LS, Johnston IDA et al. Childhood antecedents of allergic sensitization in young British adults. J Allergy Clin Immunol 1997; 99: 6–12.

88. Bergmann RL, Bergmann KE, Wahn U. Can we predict atopic disease using perinatal risk factors? Clin Exp Allergy 1998; 28: 905–7.

89. Jones CA, FinlayJones JJ, Hart PH. Type-1 and type-2 cytokines in human late-gestation decidual tissue. Biol Reprod 1997; 57: 303–11.

90. Brown MA, Chun A, Lohman IC et al. Human decidual cells produce both Th1-like and Th2-like cytokines in vitro (abstract). ALA/ATS International Conference, 1998.

91. Dominguez-Gerpe L, Rey-Mendez M. Evolution of the thymus size in response to physical and random events throughout life. Microsc Res Tech 2003; 62: 464–76.

92. Bjorksten B, Naaber P, Sepp E et al. The intestinal microflora in allergic Estonian and Swedish 2-year-old children. Clin Exp Allergy 1999; 29: 342–6.

93. Gronlund MM, Lehtonen OP, Eerola E et al. Fecal microflora in healthy infants born by different methods of delivery: permanent changes in intestinal flora after cesarean delivery. J Pediatr Gastroenterol Nutr 1999; 28: 19–25.

94. Xu B, Pekkanen J, Hartikainen AL et al. Caesarean section and risk of asthma and allergy in adulthood. J Allergy Clin Immunol 2001; 107: 732–3.

95. Kero J, Gissler M, Gronlund MM et al. Mode of delivery and asthma – is there a connection? Pediatr Res 2002; 52: 6–11.

96. Hakansson S, Kallen K. Caesarean section increases the risk of hospital care in childhood for asthma and gastroenteritis. Clin Exp Allergy 2003; 33: 757–64.

97. Liu AH. Consider the child: how early should we treat? J Allergy Clin Immunol 2004; 113: S19–S24.

98. Martinez FD, Wright AL, Taussig LM et al. Asthma and wheezing in the first 6 years of life. N Engl J Med 1995; 332: 133–8.

99. Haahtela T, Laitinen A, Laitinen LA. Using biopsies in the monitoring of inflammation in asthmatic-patients. Allergy 1993; 48: 65–9.

100. Prescott SL, Macaubas C, Smallacombe T et al. Development of allergen-specific T-cell memory in atopic and normal children. Lancet 1999; 353: 196–200.

13

Maternal alcohol consumption and neuroendocrine-immune interactions in the offspring

Anna N Taylor, Francesco Chiappelli, Susan H Tritt, and Raz Yirmiya

INTRODUCTION

Fetal alcohol exposure: overview

Exposure of the human fetus to alcohol *in utero* leads to pleiotropic, teratogenic effects referred to as the fetal alcohol syndrome (FAS). The characteristic features of FAS include cranio-facial dysmorphologies, growth retardation, and central nervous system (CNS) dysfunction that manifests as mental retardation, cognitive and behavioral problems, and impaired motor performance and communication skills. As reviewed previously,[1] frequently associated features include dysregulation of T-cell-mediated immune surveillance reminiscent of DiGeorge syndrome, and impairment of neuroendocrine feedback and the allostatic response to stressors. FAS patients present with a characteristic lack of coordination, hyperactivity, diminished or distorted sense of danger, lack of ability to function as independent adults, and a more frequent incidence of a constellation of medical symptoms. For example, when assessed with the FAS checklist,[2] they often manifest attention deficit hyperactivity disorder (40%), mental retardation (15–20%), learning disorders (25%), speech and language disorders (30%), sensory impairment (30%), cerebral palsy (4%) and epilepsy (8–10%). The hallmarks of FAS are thus multi-system, and encompass the cardiac, skeletal, and muscular systems, as well as the CNS, neuroendocrine and immune systems, which are the focus of this chapter.

FAS represents one end of a continuum of effects of prenatal alcohol exposure that encompass alcohol-related birth defects (ARBD), i.e. one or more congenital defects, including malformations and dysplasias of the heart, bone, kidney, visual or auditory systems, and alcohol-related neurodevelopmental disorder (ARND), i.e. CNS neurodevelopmental abnormalities and/or complex patterns of behavioral or cognitive deficits.[3] Among the factors that affect the risk and severity of fetal alcohol damage are the timing of the alcohol exposure, the occurrence of binge drinking that produces high blood alcohol concentrations, polydrug use, and genetic vulnerability. Prenatal alcohol exposure, particularly during the first trimester, predicts deficits in learning, short- and long-term memory, specifically in the verbal domain of word-pairs, with or without the complete manifestation of FAS.[4] The deficits suggest alcohol-induced damage to the prefrontal cortex and related brain areas, such as hippocampus and caudate nucleus, that process meaning, memory, and language.[4] Preclinical and clinical studies have demonstrated that these brain structures are vulnerable to the effects of prenatal alcohol exposure.[5–9]

The fundamental mechanisms for FAS (as well as ARBD and ARND) at the cellular and molecular biology levels include increased oxidative stress, damage to the mitochondria, interference with the activity of growth factors, effects on glial cells, impaired development and function of chemical messenger systems involved in neuronal communication, changes in the transport and uptake of glucose, effects on cell adhesion, and changes in the regulation of gene activity during development. This multitude of mechanisms may act simultaneously or consecutively and differ among cell types. Many of these mechanisms result in cell death by necrosis or apoptosis and appear to involve inhibition of protein and DNA synthesis, and alteration in the uptake of critical nutrients such as glucose and amino acids, with consequential impairment in several kinase-mediated signal transduction pathways that regulate a variety of developmental processes.[10]

Rodent models of FAS (including ARBD and ARND, *vide infra*) have been used extensively to investigate the significant effects on the body's physiological systems, including the neuroendocrine and immune systems. These studies have also established that there are alterations in the neuroendocrine-immune interactions in response to experimental stress (i.e. allostatic response) in animals exposed prenatally to ethanol. Following a brief discussion of the organization of the neuroendocrine-immune axis, this chapter will review the experimental evidence for effects of alcohol exposure on the prenatal programming of neuroendocrine-immune regulation and integration.

The neuroendocrine-immune axis: overview

The immune system and the CNS communicate in a bidirectional manner: on the one hand, the brain regulates immunity via the autonomic nervous system and the neuroendocrine system, and on the other hand, the immune system can signal the brain to initiate physiological and behavioral processes that promote recovery following infection.[11,12] Infection characteristically elicits fever and a variety of physiological, neuroendocrine and behavioral responses mediated by the CNS, including hypothalamic-pituitary-adrenal (HPA) axis activation, anorexia, hypoactivity and altered sleep patterns. Collectively the changes have been termed 'sickness behaviors' and represent a primary host defense response to infection.[13–16] Cytokines, such as interleukin (IL)-1β, tumor necrosis factor (TNF)-α, and IL-6, released from antigen-activated immune cells, are the chief messengers of afferent signals to the brain and play a key role as regulators of host defense. Cytokines can gain access to the CNS via both humoral and neural routes, including through areas with a poorly developed blood-brain barrier (BBB), such as the circumventricular organs. They may also reach the brain via active transport, by induction of mediators that can cross the BBB, or by stimulation of cytokine production within the CNS. In addition, peripheral cytokines act on neural pathways, such as the vagus or the glossopharyngeal nerves.[11,12,17,18] The CNS, in turn, regulates and provides feedback to the immune system via the HPA hormones and the autonomic and peripheral nervous systems (Figure 13.1).

The central and peripheral components of the neural-endocrine-immune interactions outlined above provide loci for the actions of maternal alcohol consumption on the developing fetus. Indeed, impairment of the reciprocal communication between the immune

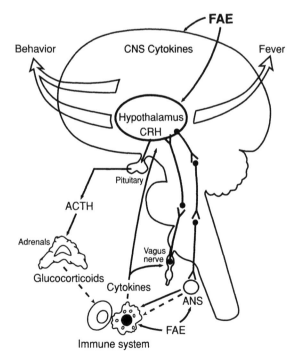

Figure 13.1 Fetal alcohol exposure (FAE) and neuroendocrine-immune interactions. Schematic representation of the communication amongst the immune system, the central nervous system (CNS), and the hypothalamo-pituitary-adrenal axis, and the potential intervention of FAE in this circuitry. ANS, autonomic nervous system; CRH, corticotropin releasing hormone; ACTH, adrenocorticotropic hormone. Solid lines indicate stimulatory effects and broken lines indicate inhibitory effects. (Adapted from refs 17 and 85.)

and nervous systems may be an important risk factor for the increased susceptibility to infection and altered immune competence of children exposed to alcohol *in utero*. The discussion that follows aims to relate the neuroendocrine-immune outcome effects of maternal alcohol consumption to the ontogeny of these interactive feedback loops. In a previous publication[1] we described in considerable detail the experimental evidence from our own studies, as well as those of other investigators for the relationship between fetal alcohol exposure (FAE) and immunity. In this chapter we aim to bring the description of this experimental evidence up to date within the context of perinatal programming.

FETAL ALCOHOL EXPOSURE (FAE) AND THE NEUROENDOCRINE-IMMUNE AXIS IN THE OFFSPRING

Immune system: FAE and cell-mediated immunity

Children exposed to alcohol *in utero* can exhibit serious impairments in both cellular and humoral immunity, e.g. decreased counts of eosinophils, neutrophils and T cells, lower immunoglobulin (Ig) levels, reduced thymus size, and mitogen-induced proliferative responses of T and B lymphocytes. As reviewed previously[1], children with FAE also have increased incidence of infections and malignancies (particularly of embryonic origin), which may be associated with their immune suppression. Although the propensity to infection may not persist, teens with FAE appear to have an increased rate of atopic hypersensitivity reactions such as allergic rhinitis and persistent skin rashes, and asthma.[19]

Rodent models of the effects of prenatal alcohol exposure also show profound alterations in cellular immune outcomes. FAE markedly reduced the number of T-helper and T-suppressor/cytotoxic cells in fetal and neonatal mice,[20] reduced the number of B cells and suppressed the mitogen-induced proliferative response of splenic T and B cells in weanling mice[21] and in adult male rats.[22–24] These deficits in cell-mediated immunity may be due to FAE-induced alterations in sympathetic nervous system (SNS) regulation of lymphoid tissues.[25] The mitogen-induced response to IL-2 was also suppressed in FAE rats.[22,25] The alterations in mitogen-induced proliferation of thymocytes that result from FAE are age-dependent because thymocyte proliferation was reduced in near-term fetal mice[20] and in 21-day-old male rats,[23] but this cellular immune response was increased in 30–44-day-old rats

after FAE, and returned to normal levels by 72 days of age.[26] The effects of FAE on cellular immune responses in rodents have also been found in the progeny of nonhuman primates exposed to ethanol *in utero*;[27] however, neither the rodent nor the monkey model of FAE has demonstrated deleterious effects on natural killer cells[28] or humoral immunity.[24,27,29] We have extended these studies by *in vivo* priming of the peripheral myeloid populations with lipopolysaccharide (LPS), using a low dose (5 µg/kg) that is considered to be suboptimal from the perspective of eliciting increases in proinflammatory cytokines.[30] One hour and a half after priming, when we stimulated the peripheral blood mononuclear cells *in vitro* with LPS (2.5 µg/ml), we found that TNF-α production was significantly blunted in male but not female FAE rats, as compared with control animals. These results provided another demonstration of the frequent observation that fetal alcohol-induced alterations in cellular immune responses are more often detected in male than in female rats.[24,31]

In vivo immune responses, such as hypersensitivity to the contact-sensitizing trinitrochlorobenzene, and the graft vs host response, are also impaired following FAE.[25] In addition, FAE has been found to reduce serum levels of IL-2 as well as IgM and IgG responses in weanling rats challenged with the intestinal parasite, *Trichinella spiralis*.[32] The development of immunity to an antigenic challenge reflects the integrated actions of antigen processing by macrophages and T/B-cell interactions leading to B-cell activation, as well as Ig production and isotype switching.[33] Antibody secretion and isotype switching depend upon certain cytokines produced by T helper type 1 (Th1) cells (e.g. IL-2, IFN) and Th2 cells (e.g. IL-4, IL-5, and IL-10).[34] It has been shown that the shift from IgM to IgG production represents a genetic switch in B cells mediated by Th1 and Th2 cells.[34] While Th1 cells appear to be primarily involved in the development of cellular immune responses, Th2 cells are more implicated in the regulation of B-cell growth, differentiation and maturation.[34] The generation and interaction of Th1 and Th2 cells and T-cell cytokine production that occur in response to an antigenic challenge are modulated by the regulatory influences exerted by many hormones including glucocorticoids and androgens.[35,36] Thus, it is reasonable to expect that stress or ethanol, which can increase the output of glucocorticoids, would have an inhibitory effect on immune responses that depend upon IL-2 or IFN for optimal expression, while perhaps augmenting those driven by IL-4, IL-5, and IL-10.

We determined the effects of FAE on the *in vivo* antibody response to a primary challenge with the

T-cell-dependent antigen, keyhole limpet hemocyanin (KLH). In this study, we assessed antibody levels at 7, 14, and 21 days after KLH in the adult offspring of dams that had consumed an ethanol-containing liquid diet *ad libitum* or been pair-fed just the isocaloric liquid diet without ethanol during the last 2 weeks of gestation (this is our standard protocol for the FAE rat model). IgM and IgG levels were quantified by an enzyme-linked immunosorbent assay (ELISA). We found no effects of FAE on peak IgM production in either males or females, i.e. on day 7, after administration of either 10 or 250 μg/kg KLH. However, at the low KLH dose, normal (N) males showed a strong trend for higher IgG, as compared to the pair-fed (PF) and FAE (E) males. In keeping with the previously discussed sex differences, N females showed significant delays in IgG production. Animals were also evaluated from pregnancies in which the dams were adrenalec-

tomized (ADX) or given a sham surgery. When tested at the higher dose, N male offspring of sham-operated dams had significantly higher IgG compared to E and PF males (Figure 13.2A). Removal of maternal adrenal hormones during pregnancy by ADX brought the IgG levels in N males down to those of the PF and E males (Figure 13.2A), but left the levels of N females unaltered (Figure 13.2B). The implications of this prenatal treatment will be discussed later in this chapter. Given that IgM production was unaffected by FAE, it appears that FAE may influence the switch from IgM to IgG production in response to KLH, which occurs maximally at about 21 days after KLH administration.[37] The steps involved in isotype switching from IgM to IgG may have been altered by prenatal ethanol exposure of males but not females, explaining why the effects on IgG are seen between 7 and 21 days following the antigen challenge. A previous study reported a lack of

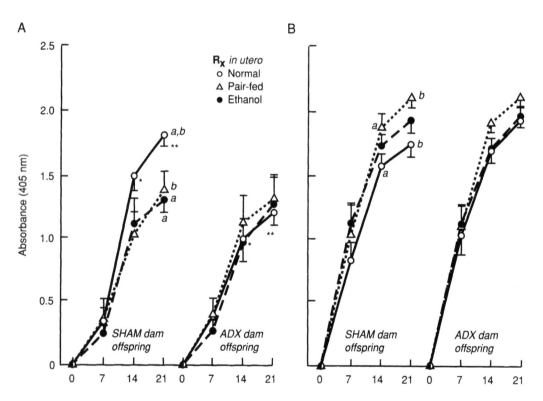

Figure 13.2 IgG antibody production (absorbance at 405 nm) before and at 7, 14, and 21 days after administration of KLH (250 μg/kg, i.p.) to adult males (A) and females (B). The rats were the offspring of sham-operated (SHAM) or adrenalectomized (ADX) dams that were fed ethanol-containing or pair-fed liquid or normal chow and water diets during the last 2 weeks of gestation. Values are means ± SEM for 3–8 rats/group. Letters (a, b) indicate where prenatal diets induced significant ($p < 0.05$) differences in male (A) and female (B) offspring of SHAM-treated dams on days 14 and 21; maternal ADX abolished these differences. Asterisks (* or **) indicate where maternal treatment (SHAM or ADX) produced significant ($p < 0.05$) differences for the same prenatal diet conditions in males (A); females (B) were unaffected by maternal ADX.

effect of FAE and pair-feeding on IgM and IgG production following immunization of rats with sheep red blood cells (SRBCs) at 25–33 days of age.[29] The difference with our results may be due to the fact that the effects of FAE on humoral immune responses are age-dependent, as we have found previously for cellular immune responses.[22]

The finding of opposite effects of the pair-feeding (PF) in males and females (Figure 13.2) indicates that the stress of maternal food restriction that invariably occurs when matching food intake of pair-fed control dams with alcohol-exposed dams may also impact the humoral immunity. Maternal restraint stress during the last week of gestation has also been reported to increase anti-KLH antibody response (IgM and IgG) in adult rat offspring of both sexes, albeit in response to a several fold higher dose of KLH than we used.[38] The gender differences that we observed may reflect the differential action of gonadal hormones on lymphokine production by T cells.[39,40] Additionally, the gender-related dose-response effects may also represent a switch in the influence on Th1 to Th2 cells with increasing antigen dose, insofar as moderate doses of antigen appear to stimulate Th1 cells, preferentially, while high doses stimulate Th2 cells.[34] On the other hand, the enhanced IgG response of PF females (Figure 13.2B) may represent stimulation of both Th1 and Th2 cells, due to estrogen.[39] Thus, these prenatal manipulations of ethanol and feeding may act via a number of hormones that affect different components of the immune system.

CNS: FAE and the acute phase response

Infectious agents can elicit fever, a component of the acute phase response that serves to enhance host defense. In fact, an elevated body temperature reduces the morbidity and mortality caused by a variety of pathogens.[15,41] The interactions of pyrogenic cytokines, such as IL-1β, IL-6, and TNF-α, with their receptors, particularly within the hypothalamus, produce an increase in body temperature by raising the thermoregulatory set point.[15,42] Simultaneously, these cytokines exert potent effects on the hypothalamic-pituitary axis, activating the adrenal gland depending upon the species, and a number of other neuroendocrine axes.[11] During infections, these cytokines also facilitate behavioral patterns that promote conservation of body resources, while inhibiting goal-directed behavior.[12,43,44] This sickness behavior syndrome induced by IL-1β includes a reduction of motor activity, suppression of food ingestion, exploratory behavior, social activity, and sexual behavior, as well as increased slow wave sleep.

Among the first demonstrations that FAE affected neuroimmune function in adult offspring was our finding[45] of an impaired febrile response to systemic (i.p.) administration of the endotoxin LPS in FAE male rats. The FAE rats required a higher dose of LPS to show any hyperthermia (50 μg/kg vs 10 μg/kg), and even with the higher dose, they manifested a smaller and shorter hyperthermic response than control animals. LPS induces fever by stimulating the endogenous release of the proinflammatory cytokines IL-1β, TNF-α, and IL-6, peripherally and/or centrally (Figure 13.1). Thus, it was not surprising to find that the fever induced by IL-1β (2 μg/kg, i.p.) was also attenuated in adult FAE males, as shown in Figure 13.3.[46] Furthermore, FAE also attenuated the anorexic and adypsic, but not the immobilizing responses to IL-1β.[46] In females, FAE also produced a blunting of the IL-1β-induced febrile response (Figure 13.3);[47] however, this effect was not associated with a differential effect on anorexia in control and FAE females. Together, these findings indicate that FAE impairs the expression of the febrile and sickness behavioral components of the acute phase response to an infection agent, such as endotoxin and a proinflammatory cytokine. In view of the adaptive functions of the acute phase response in infection,[13–16] these impairments may contribute to the decreased resistance to infections observed in animals and humans following FAE.[1]

In order to determine whether the FAE-related impairments of the febrile and anorexic responses occurred centrally or peripherally, we examined the effects of FAE on LPS-induced secretion of several cytokines in blood and brain.[48,49] There was no effect of FAE on the amount of TNF-α, IL-1β, IL-6, and IL-10 secretion after LPS in the blood of males. There was also no effect of FAE on LPS-induced blood levels of TNF-α in females; however, ovariectomized FAE rats responded to LPS with significantly lower TNF-α secretion than their controls.[48] In view of another observation that ovariectomy reverses the blunting effect of FAE on the females' febrile response during the light phase,[50] the TNF-α finding suggests that it may be acting as a cryogen in this model.[15] This interpretation is supported by the elevated levels of hypothalamic TNF-α that were observed at 2 hours after peripheral injection of LPS in prenatal FAE males (Figure 13.4). Moreover, at the 2-hour time point, hypothalamic levels of IL-1β were significantly lower in E males compared with those of normal males[49] (Figure 13.4).

An alteration in the kinetics of IL-1β production could reflect impairments in a number of immune-to-brain communication pathways (e.g. decreased effects of circulating IL-1β at the circumventricular organs, less active transport or diminished IL-1β-induced

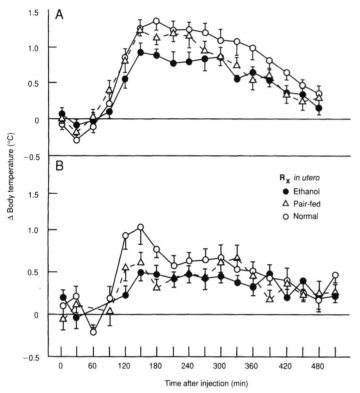

Figure 13.3 Febrile responses to IL-1β in adult male (A) and female (B) rats. Body temperature was recorded biotelemetrically in adult rats exposed to ethanol-containing (E) or pair-fed (PF) liquid or normal (N) rat chow and water diets *in utero*. The rats (n = 8–9/group) were injected intraperitoneally with either IL-1β (2 μg/kg) or saline early in the light period and body temperature was recorded continuously for 510 min. The results are presented as the mean ± SEM difference between temperature recorded at comparable time points after injection of IL-1β and saline on the day prior to the injection of IL-1β (the zero line). The febrile responses of both E males (A) and females (B) were significantly lower than the respective N responses, while PF responses were intermediate. (Adapted from ref. 47.)

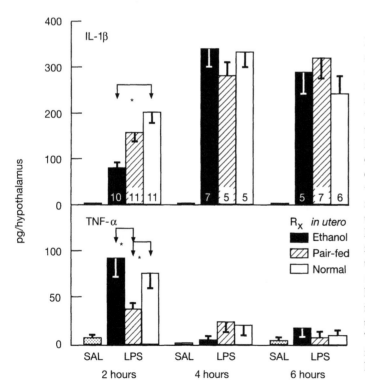

Figure 13.4 Hypothalamic levels of IL-1β and TNF-α after administration of LPS (500 μg/kg, i.p.) or saline (SAL) to adult male rats. Mean ± SEM content of IL-1β and TNF-α in each hypothalamic block was determined by ELISA in rats exposed to ethanol-containing (E) or pair-fed (PF) liquid or normal (N) rat chow and water diets *in utero*. LPS or SAL was injected early in the light period and hypothalami were obtained 2, 4, and 6 h later. The numbers in each LPS histogram indicate the number of animals sampled. SAL histograms represent the combined data from two E and two PF animals at each time point. IL-1β was significantly (p < 0.05) lower in the E than in the N hypothalami at 2-hours after LPS, as indicated by the asterisk (*) connecting the arrows between these groups, while TNF-α was significantly (p < 0.05) lower in the PF than in either the E or N hypothalami. (Adapted from ref. 49.)

vagal afferent activation) as well as disturbed thermoregulatory processes either peripherally or centrally. To begin to address these possibilities, we determined whether intracerebroventricular (i.c.v.) administration of IL-1β could bypass this FAE-related impairment and produce a normal febrile response. Infusion of IL-1β (20 ng/rat, i.c.v.) resulted in characteristic febrile responses in the control adult males; however, the febrile response of the FAE rats was still significantly attenuated.[49] These results indicate that FAE has a direct effect on central mechanisms that mediate the pyrogenic effects of IL-1β. In contrast, there were no differential effects of FAE on the reduction of food and water consumption and body weight loss that occurred in the 24 hour period after i.c.v. IL-1β.

Having found that the febrile response to i.c.v. IL-1 was blunted in FAE rats,[49] it was of interest to ascertain whether this was indicative of a general impairment of thermoregulatory effector mechanisms that mediate the febrile response. Prostaglandin E_2 (PGE), administered i.c.v., can bypass the IL-1β signal and produce fever by acting directly on temperature-sensitive neurons in the hypothalamus.[1] Indeed, FAE rats had a normal febrile response to exogenous administration of PGE.[49] Taken together, these results suggest that FAE impairs one or more of the neurochemical signaling mechanisms for the febrile response without affecting central thermoregulatory processes that permit the generation of fever subsequent to prostaglandin release.

Gender differences in the effects of FAE on the acute phase response have already been noted. With respect to the IL-1β-induced hyperthermia, we have found that FAE blunts the response of both male and female rats when IL-1β is administered in the light phase[46,47] (Figure 13.3). In contrast, in the dark phase, IL-1β (10 µg/kg, i.p.) reveals gender-specific effects of FAE on febrile responses, i.e. IL-1β-induced hyperthermia was significantly attenuated in E females while not differentially affected in E males.[46] Additionally, in both males[46] and females, IL-1β-induced hyperthermia is preceded by an initial hypothermia that during the dark phase is significantly greater in E males, but not E females, when compared with their respective controls. Moreover, the attenuated dark phase hyperthermia of E females was unaffected by prepubertal ovariectomy in contrast to its normalizing effect in the light phase.[50] Collectively, our findings in males and females indicate long-lasting gender-specific effects of FAE on the acute phase responses.

Neuroendocrine system: FAE and the HPA axis

We and others have repeatedly shown that FAE alters the stress responsiveness of the offspring: during the preweaning period, FAE offspring exhibit lower pituitary-adrenal and β-endorphin responses to a wide range of stressors. Beyond the weaning age and persisting through adult life, FAE animals often show increased responsiveness to stressors, such as footshock, ether, restraint, cold, neurogenic stressors, and acute challenges with ethanol or morphine. The altered responsiveness of the HPA axis to stressors in FAE rats is also reflected by changes in the hormone response to immune activation. Thus, FAE blunts IL-1-induced ACTH and β-endorphin secretion in immature rats and augments IL-1 and LPS-induced secretion of ACTH in mature rats.[51] These findings also generalize to monkey FAE models.[52] For example, rhesus monkeys (*Macaca mulatta*) exposed prenatally to alcohol or alcohol and stress characteristically show poorer behavioral adaptations to stress postnatally which are correlated with both baseline and stress-induced ACTH levels.

Glucocorticoids can be potent inhibitors of many IL-1β actions. This inhibition may be achieved directly via effects on IL-1 transcription or mRNA stability,[53] as well as on post-transcriptional synthesis[54] or release.[55] In addition, glucocorticoids can act secondarily to block IL-1 actions on tissue and physiology, e.g. on fever and thermogenesis. IL-1β-induced fever was almost completely prevented by preadministration of the synthetic glucocorticoid agonist, dexamethasone.[56] This effect of glucocorticoids is at least partly mediated by the release of lipocortin-1, which acts as an endogenous inhibitor of the pyrogenic and thermogenic responses to IL-1β, interfering in part with the thermogenic effects of corticotrophin releasing hormone (CRH). Consistent with these findings, we found that male PF rats, which showed significantly lower levels of IL-1β-induced corticosterone secretion, also showed significantly elevated IL-1β-induced fever compared to FAE rats when IL-1β was administered at the onset of the dark period.[46] Although IL-1β-induced corticosterone secretion was not differentially affected by FAE in male rats,[46,48] glucocorticoid receptor expression in the hypothalamus has been shown to be increased in FAE adults.[31] The resulting augmented sensitivity to normal corticosterone levels could contribute to the decreased febrile response.

CRH has been shown to be involved in several components of the febrile response, including stimulation of sympathetic outflow, thermogenesis, and activity of brown adipose tissue (BAT).[42] These effects are probably independent of the role of CRH in activation of the HPA axis, which inhibits the IL-1β-induced fever. Administration of exogenous IL-1β induces the release of hypothalamic CRH, which contributes to the effects of IL-1β on thermogenesis and fever. For example, i.c.v. administration of a CRH receptor antagonist or neutralizing antibody to CRH inhibits the febrile and thermogenic responses to IL-1β.[56] FAE has been shown to alter hypothalamic CRH levels, although the results of such studies are not always consistent. Some reported an increase,[31,57] while others found no change[58] in CRH mRNA levels. Lee and Rivier also showed that CRH content in the median eminence is decreased in FAE rats.[59] If the latter finding represents a decrease of CRH content in nerve terminals of FAE rats, particularly during the light period of the day/night cycle, a reduced thermogenic response to IL-1β could be expected following FAE, consistent with the results reported above.

FAE AFFECTS PRENATAL PROGRAMMING OF THE NEUROENDOCRINE-IMMUNE AXIS

There is ample opportunity for FAE to affect prenatal programming of a variety of biological systems. As summarized earlier, maternal drinking during pregnancy adversely influences the developing organism with effects ranging from mild cognitive impairment to full-blown FAS, characterized by growth deficiency and CNS disorders. Thus, the effect of alcohol on fetal programming will depend not only upon level of consumption, but also on the temporal association of alcohol consumption with the developmental sequence of each system. For example, as the formation of facial cartilage and bone occurs early in fetal development, exposure to alcohol during the first week of fetal life in the rodent may produce the facial anomalies associated with FAS, while the cognitive deficits are produced by coincidental exposure during the third week of gestation extending into the first week postnatally.[10,60]

The studies reviewed above lead to the conclusion that maternal alcohol consumption during the second and third weeks of the rodent's fetal life affects the developmental programming of the neuroendocrine-immune axis. Among the multiple actions of alcohol exposure in utero on growth, behavior, and immune function of the offspring, a recurrent finding was an effect on maternal glucocorticoids. FAE has been shown to increase corticosterone levels in pregnant rats[61,62] and it is well known that corticosterone can readily cross the placenta from the mother to the fetus and vice versa.[63] Indeed, this transfer of maternal hormone during periods of FAE or prenatal stress may affect the development of the fetal HPA axis.[64] Additional evidence for this conclusion is derived from studies that eliminated the influence of maternal glucocorticoids by ADX. Maternal ADX is known to produce some compensatory increases in corticosterone levels of fetuses near term. Nevertheless, the corticosterone increases were found to be lower in fetuses of FAE dams after ADX than in fetuses of ADX dams maintained on a pair-fed diet,[65] suggesting an additional effect of ethanol directly on the fetal pituitary-adrenal axis.

As indicated above, maternal ADX brought the IgG responses to KLH in N males down to those of PF and E males (Figure 13.2A), but did not modify the antibody response levels of N females (Figure 13.2B). Maternal ADX has also been shown to prevent several postnatal effects of FAE, including growth retardation,[62] hyperresponsiveness to stress,[57,65] increased proopiomelanocortin mRNA in the anterior pituitary, and suppression of mitogen-stimulated lymphocyte proliferation.[31] We have also investigated the effects of maternal ADX on the blunted febrile response of male and female FAE offspring.[47] Pregnant rats were ADX or sham-operated on gestation day (GD) 7, or remained intact (without any surgery), and were fed E-containing liquid diets, pair-fed (PF) or ate normal (N) rat chow and water from GD 8 to GD 21. As adults, all male and female offspring were injected with IL-1β (2 µg/kg, i.p.) at 0900 and body temperature was recorded biotelemetrically for 8.5 hours. FAE significantly attenuated the IL-1β-induced febrile response in both male and female offspring of intact dams. In males, FAE also attenuated the febrile response in the offspring of the sham-operated dams, and this effect was completely reversed by maternal ADX (Figure 13.5). In females, both sham surgery and maternal ADX reversed the effect of FAE on the febrile response (Figure 13.5). Thus, these findings suggest that maternal adrenal hormones are essential for the long-term effect of FAE on the febrile response in male offspring.

FAE also affects developmental programming of other components of the neuro-endocrine-immune system.[1] For example, fetal male rats exposed to alcohol in utero do not exhibit the normal testosterone surge right before parturition and their testosterone levels are significantly depressed below normal on the day of birth. Consistent with these effects, FAE was found to feminize physiological and behavioral systems in male rats, as well as to affect the size of a sexually dimorphic nucleus of the preoptic hypothalamus. It was also demonstrated that maternal ADX exacerbates this ethanol-induced suppression of the fetal testosterone surge in males and similarly abolishes the surge of the adrenal androgen,

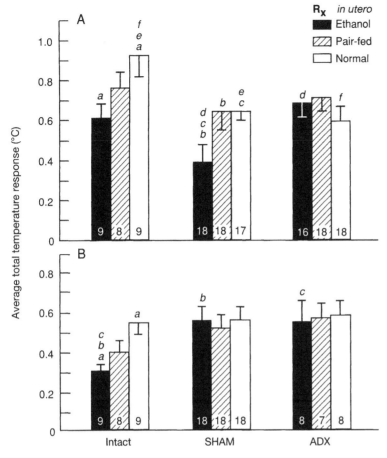

Figure 13.5 Effect of maternal adrenalectomy (ADX), sham operation (SHAM) or no surgery (Intact) on the febrile response to IL-1β in adult male (A) and female (B) rats. Body temperature was recorded biotelemetrically in adult offspring of dams fed ethanol-containing (E) or pair-fed (PF) liquid or normal (N) rat chow and water diets during the last 2 weeks of gestation. Shown are the mean ± SEM sums of the half-hourly body temperature responses to IL-1β (2 μg/kg, i.p.) averaged over the hyperthermic response period (90–480 min; cf. Figure 13.3). The numbers in each histogram indicate the number of animals in each group; the bar is one SEM. Similar letters above the histograms in each panel indicate significant ($p < 0.05$) differences between the designated groups. Thus, in addition to differential effects of maternal treatment on the febrile responses of males (A) and females (B) in the same diet groups, the febrile responses of both male and female E offspring of intact dams were significantly lower than those of the N rats. Differential diet effects on the febrile responses in the offspring of SHAM dams persisted for E males but not for E females, while maternal ADX abolished the differential effects of E exposure in males. (Adapted from ref. 47.)

dehydroepiandrosterone (DHEA), typically seen in maternal plasma on GD 19.[66] Interestingly, administration of DHEA to pregnant rats has been reported to reduce the proliferative response of splenic lymphocytes of male, but not female offspring during the prepubertal period.[67] These data suggest that the disruptive effects of FAE on cellular immunity in males may be related to a combined effect on fetal T and maternal corticosterone, and possibly also DHEA.[66,67] However, it is also possible that the passage of alcohol across the placenta may directly affect fetal testicular capacity to synthesize steroids, and not act via the hypothalamic-pituitary axis, as suggested by Westney et al.[68] These investigators reported that at

birth 4-androstenedione, testosterone, and estradiol are significantly decreased in the amniotic fluid of male children from alcohol users as compared with control neonates. Their levels of DHEA sulfate were in the normal range, as were the pituitary hormones that regulate the gonads (follicle stimulating hormone, FSH, and luteinizing hormone, LH).

SNS innervation of BAT may be involved in the reduced febrile response in FAE animals. The febrile response to IL-1β depends to a large extent on SNS activation, which induces nonshivering thermogenesis in BAT.[42] FAE has been found to markedly alter the development of the SNS innervation of BAT.[69] Norepinephrine concentration in BAT was significantly lower in 5-day-old FAE rats and significantly higher in 20-day-old FAE rats compared with control rats, suggesting a delay in the development of innervation, followed by a compensatory overactivation.[69] The number of β1-adrenoreceptor binding sites in BAT was also increased in FAE rats.[69] To what extent the altered LPS-induced febrile responses of adults reflect the influence of FAE on thermoregulation, as has been demonstrated in neonates[69] and adults,[69,70] remains to be determined.

CLINICAL IMPLICATIONS

We have reviewed the mechanisms by which prenatal exposure to ethanol produces long-term effects on the neuroendocrine-immune axis in the rat. While some effects may be produced directly by the toxic effect of ethanol, the finding that maternal ADX can protect the fetus suggests that activation of the maternal HPA axis may play a role. In other words, ethanol may affect the fetus in part because of the stress response it induces in the pregnant female. It is estimated that in the US about 4000 children per year are affected by FAS and another 7000 suffer some effects of prenatal alcohol exposure.[71] These numbers are unfortunate, but still infrequent enough that the average obstetrician or pediatrician might not often care for an alcoholic woman and her baby. If activation of the maternal stress response plays a significant role, our results may have a much wider clinical application with regard to the effects of prenatal stress. For example, it has also been estimated that 10% of pregnant women suffer domestic violence that begins or is exacerbated during pregnancy (ACOG Educational Bulletin, No. 255, Nov. 1999). Community-based studies report[72] that 9–20% of pregnant women meet criteria for a depressive disorder and 10–20% have substance use or dependence during gestation. In a large population-based cohort analysis of birth records,[72] maternal psychiatric and substance use diagnoses were independently associated with low birth weight and preterm delivery.

Previous clinical studies[73,74] have related maternal anxiety, as assessed on psychological questionnaires and interviews, to adverse pregnancy outcomes such as decreased birth weight, early delivery, and fetal movements. Elevated maternal anxiety scores were correlated with an increased uterine artery resistance assessed by Doppler ultrasound.[74] The increased resistance to blood flow in the uterine circulation results in decreased placental perfusion and may be part of the explanation of the association between maternal stress and low birth weight in humans. Whether the decrease in uterine flow is secondary to elevation of glucocorticoids or catecholamines in the mother has not been determined.

In human pregnancy the placenta is an important link between the HPA axes of the mother and the fetus because it produces CRH.[75–77] *In vitro* studies have shown that trophoblasts increase production of CRH in response to stress-related hormones, such as cortisol and catecholamines, as well as to cytokines. Elevated levels of maternal CRH in plasma have been found to be associated with preterm labor, and there is a significant correlation between CRH levels in maternal and fetal circulation. Elevated CRH may have at least two effects on the fetus. First, it may activate the fetal pituitary-adrenal axis and promote organ maturation that would be associated with early delivery. Second, it acts as a vasodilator in the placental circulation to maintain umbilical blood flow.[75] Maternal stress would be associated with increased blood levels of cortisol and catecholamines that are known to stimulate release of placental CRH. This would be an adaptive short-term response to help maintain blood flow to the placenta when the uterine blood flow decreases. However, chronic stress that elevates CRH in the placental circulation appears to have adverse effects on fetal growth because umbilical cord blood CRH is higher in neonates with intrauterine growth retardation (IUGR).[78]

Altered cytokine expression at the feto-placental interface may potentially be an additional mechanism for the development of neuroendocrine-immune dysfunction in children with FAS. Indeed, trophoblasts may be an important source of fetal cytokines, as suggested by the finding[79] that human first trimester trophoblasts express high levels of granulocyte colony-stimulating factor (G-CSF) and IL-6 when exposed *in vitro* to 0.5% ethanol. It has also been shown that chronic alcohol use during pregnancy induces significantly more release of pro-inflammatory cytokines, including IL-1β, IL-6, and TNF-α, in response to LPS stimulation *in vitro* of cord blood mono-nuclear cells as compared to cells obtained from control children.[80] Clinical evidence indicates that the human placenta releases TNF-α when there is fetal growth restriction secondary to placental insufficiency.[81] Moreover, human neonates exposed to the stress of infection or IUGR are more at risk for sepsis, pneumonia, respiratory distress syndrome and necrotizing enterocolitis[82,83] and for the development of brain white matter lesions.[84] Thus, altered cytokine levels consequential to the passage of alcohol through the placenta could have an adverse effect on the development of the immune system.

In summary, the FAS rodent model has allowed us to examine some aspects of how this prenatal teratogen affects the development and subsequent postnatal functioning of the HPA axis and immune system. Clinical studies suggest that similar maternal–fetal interactions may account for the effects of stress on the fetus in human pregnancy. A better understanding of how ethanol acts to alter development in the fetal rat may give us insight into the way that this teratogen as well as other stressors affect normal maternal–fetal physiology. This insight may help us to develop psychological, social and medical therapies to reduce the impact on the mother and her developing baby. It may also improve our evaluation and long-term care of children at risk because of prenatal exposure to alcohol.

ACKNOWLEDGMENTS

We are grateful to Delia L. Tio for her expert assistance in our studies. Our work reported herein was supported by grants from the Department of Veterans Affairs Medical Research Service, the NIAAA-NIH, and the United States-Israel Binational Science Foundation.

REFERENCES

1. Taylor AN, Chiappelli F, Yirmiya R. Fetal alcohol syndrome and immunity. In: Psychoneuroimmunology, 3rd edn, Vol. 2 (Ader R, Felten DL, Cohen N, eds). San Diego: Academic Press, 2001: 49–71.

2. Burd L, Martsolf JT, Klug MG et al. Diagnosis of FAS: a comparison of the Fetal Alcohol Syndrome Diagnostic Checklist and the Institute of Medicine Criteria for Fetal Alcohol Syndrome. Neurotoxicol Teratol 2003; 25: 719–24.

3. Warren KR, Foudin LL. Alcohol-related birth defects – the past, present, and future. Alcohol Res Health 2001; 25: 153–8.

4. Willford JA, Richardson GA, Leech SL et al. Verbal and visuospatial learning and memory function in children with moderate prenatal alcohol exposure. Alcohol Clin Exp Res 2004; 28: 497–507.

5. Bookstein FL, Sampson PD, Streissguth AP et al. Geometric morphometrics of corpus callosum and subcortical structures in the fetal-alcohol-affected brain. Teratology 2001; 64: 4–32.

6. Clark CM, Li D, Conry J et al. Structural and functional brain integrity of fetal alcohol syndrome in non-retarded cases. Pediatrics 2000; 105: 1096–9.

7. Maier SE, West JR. Regional differences in cell loss associated with binge-like alcohol exposure during the first two trimesters equivalent in the rat. Alcohol 2001; 23: 49–57.

8. Mattson SN, Riley EP, Sowell ER et al. A decrease in the size of the basal ganglia in children with fetal alcohol syndrome. Alcohol Clin Exp Res 1996; 20: 1088–93.

9. Savage DD, Becher M, de la Torre A et al. Dose-dependent effects of prenatal ethanol exposure on synaptic plasticity and learning in mature offspring. Alcohol Clin Exp Res 2002; 26: 1752–8.

10. Goodlett CR, Horn KH. Mechanisms of alcohol-induced damage to the developing nervous system. Alcohol Res Health 2001; 25: 175–84.

11. Besedovsky HO, Del Rey A. Cytokines as mediators of central and peripheral immune-neuroendocrine interactions. In: Psychoneuroimmunology, 3rd edn, Vol. 1 (Ader R, Felten DL, Cohen N, eds). San Diego: Academic Press, 2001: 1–17.

12. Maier SF, Watkins LR. Cytokines for psychologists: implications of bi-directional immune-to-brain communication for understanding behavior, mood, and cognition. Psychol Rev 1998; 105: 83–107.

13. Hart BL. Biological basis of the behavior of sick animals. Neurosci Biobehav Rev 1988; 12: 123–37.

14. Blatteis CM. Neural mechanisms in the pyrogenic and acute-phase responses to interleukin-1. Int J Neurosci 1988; 38: 223–32.

15. Kluger MJ. Fever: role of pyrogens and cryogens. Physiol Rev 1991; 72: 93–127.

16. Kent S, Bluthe R, Kelley KW et al. Sickness behavior as a new target for drug development. Trends Pharmacol Sci l992; 13: 24–8.

17. Sternberg EM. Neural-immune interactions in health and disease. J Clin Invest 1997; 11: 2641–7.

18. Romeo HE, Tio DL, Rahman SU et al. The glossopharyngeal nerve as a new pathway in immune-to-brain interactions: relevance to neuroimmune surveillance of the oral cavity. J Neuroimmunol 2001; 115: 91–100.

19. Oleson DR, Magee RM, Donahoe RM et al. Immunity and prenatal alcohol exposure. A pilot study in human adolescents. Adv Exp Med Biol 1998; 437: 255–64.

20. Ewald SJ. Fetal alcohol exposure and immunity. In: Alcohol, Immunity, and Cancer (Yirmiya R, Taylor AN, eds). Boca Raton: CRC Press, 1993: 123–132.

21. Moscatello KM, Biber KL, Jennings SR et al. Effects of in utero alcohol exposure on B cell development in neonatal spleen and bone marrow. Cell Immunol 1999; 191: 124–30.

22. Norman DC, Chang M-P, Wong CM et al. Changes with age in the proliferative response of splenic T cells from rats exposed to ethanol in utero. Alcohol Clin Exp Res 1991; 15: 428–32.

23. Redei E, Clark W, McGivern RF. Alterations in immune responsiveness, ACTH and CRF content of brains in animals exposed to alcohol during the last week of gestation. Alcohol Clin Exp Res 1989; 13: 439–43.

24. Weinberg J, Jerrells TR. Suppression of immune responsiveness: sex differences in prenatal ethanol effects. Alcohol Clin Exp Res 1991; 15: 525–31.

25. Gottesfeld Z, Christie R, Felten DL et al. Prenatal ethanol exposure alters immune capacity and noradrenergic synaptic transmission in lymphoid organs of the adult mouse. Neuroscience 1990; 35: 85–94.

26. Wong CM, Chiappelli F, Norman DC et al. Prenatal exposure to alcohol enhances thymocyte mitogenic responses postnatally. Int J Immunopharmacol 1992; 14: 303–9.

27. Grossman A, Astley SJ, Liggitt HD et al. Immune function in offspring of non-human primates (*Macaca memestrina*) exposed weekly to 1.8 g/kg ethanol during pregnancy: preliminary observations. Alcohol Clin Exp Res 1993; 17: 822–7.

28. Wolcott RM, Jennings SR, Chervenak R. In utero exposure to ethanol affects postnatal development of T- and B-lymphocytes, but not natural killer cells. Alcohol Clin Exp Res 1995; 19: 170–6.

29. Gottesfeld Z, Ulrich SE. Prenatal alcohol exposure selectively suppresses cell-mediated but not humoral immune responsiveness. Int J Immunopharmacol 1995; 17: 247–54.

30. Chiappelli F, Kung MA, Tio DL et al. Fetal alcohol exposure augments the blunting of tumor necrosis factor production in vitro resulting from in vivo priming with lipopolysaccharide

in young adult male but not female rats. Alcohol Clin Exp Res 1997; 21: 1542–6.

31. Redei E, Halasz I, Li L et al. Maternal adrenalectomy alters the immune and endocrine functions of fetal alcohol-exposed male offspring. Endocrinology 1993; 133: 452–60.

32. Seelig LL Jr, Steven WM, Steward GL. Effects of maternal ethanol consumption on the subsequent development of immunity to *Trichinella spiralis* in rat neonates. Alcohol Clin Exp Res 1996; 20: 514–22.

33. Stenzel-Poore M, Rittenberg MG. Clonal diversity, somatic mutation and immune memory to phosphocholine-keyhole limpet hemocyanin. J Immunol 1989; 143: 4123–30.

34. Mossmann TR, Sad S. The expanding universe of T-cell subsets: Th1, Th2 and more. Immunol Today 1996; 17: 138–46.

35. Daynes RA, Meikle AW, Araneo BA. Locally active steroid hormones may facilitate compartmentalization of immunity by regulating the types of lymphokines produced by helper T cells. Res Immunol 1991; 142: 40–5.

36. Chiappelli F, Manfrini E, Franceschi C et al. Steroid regulation of cytokines: relevance for Th1 to Th2 shift? Ann N Y Acad Sci 1994; 746: 204–16.

37. Fleshner M, Brennan FX, Nguyen K et al. RU-486 blocks differentially suppressive effect of stress on in vivo anti-KLH immunoglobulin response. Am J Physiol 1996; 271: R1344–52.

38. Klein SL, Rager DR. Prenatal stress alters immune function in the offspring of rats. Devel Psychobiol 1995; 28: 321–6.

39. Grossman CJ. Regulation of the immune system by sex steroids. Endocr Rev 1984; 5: 435–55.

40. Araneo BA, Dowell T, Diegel M et al. Dihydrotestosterone exerts a depressive influence on the production of interleukin-4 (IL-4), IL-5 and gamma-interferon, but not IL-2 by activated murine T cells. Blood 1991; 78: 688–99.

41. Moltz H. Fever: causes and consequences. Neurosci Biobehav Rev 1993; 17: 237–69.

42. Rothwell NJ. Cytokines and thermogenesis. Int J Obes 1993; 17: S98–S101.

43. Yirmiya R. Endotoxin produces a depressive-like episode in rats. Brain Res 1996; 711: 163–74.

44. Yirmiya R. Behavioral and psychological effects of immune activation: implication for 'depression due to a general medical condition.' Curr Opin Psychiatry 1997; 10: 470–6.

45. Yirmiya R, Pilati ML, Chiappelli F et al. Fetal-alcohol exposure attenuates LPS-induced fever in rats. Alcohol Exp Clin Res 1993; 17: 906–10.

46. Yirmiya R, Tio DL, Taylor AN. Effects of fetal alcohol exposure on fever, sickness behavior, and pituitary-adrenal activation induced by interleukin-1 beta in young adult rats. Brain Behav Immunol 1996; 10: 205–20.

47. Taylor AN, Tritt SH, Tio DL et al. Maternal adrenalectomy abrogates the effect of fetal alcohol exposure on the interleukin-1β-induced febrile response: gender differences. Neuroendocrinology 2002; 76: 185–92.

48. Yirmiya R, Chiappelli F, Tio DL et al. Effect of fetal alcohol exposure and pair feeding on lipopolysaccharide-induced secretion of TNFalpha and corticosterone. Alcohol 1998; 15: 327–35.

49. Taylor AN, Tio DL, Yirmiya R. Fetal alcohol exposure attenuates interleukin-1β-induced fever: neuroimmune mechanisms. J Neuroimmunol 1999; 99: 44–52.

50. Taylor AN, Tio DL, Yirmiya R. Fetal alcohol exposure (FAE) and ovariectomy interact to affect febrile and hypothermic responses to interleukin-1β (IL-1). Alcohol Clin Exp Res 1998; 22: 27A.

51. Lee S, Rivier C. Gender differences in the effect of prenatal alcohol exposure on the hypothalamic-pituitary-adrenal

axis response to immune signals. Psychoneuroendocrinology 1996; 21: 145–55.

52. Schneider ML, Moore CF, Kraemer GW. Moderate level alcohol during pregnancy, prenatal stress, or both and limbic-hypothalamic-pituitary-adrenocortical axis response to stress in rhesus monkeys. Child Dev 2004; 75: 96–109.

53. Amano Y, Lee SW, Allison AC. Inhibition by glucocorticoids of the formation of interleukin-1 alpha, interleukin-1 beta, and interleukin-6: mediation by decreased mRNA stability. Mol Pharmacol 1993; 43: 176–82.

54. Knudsen PJ, Dinarello CA, Strom TB. Glucocorticoids inhibit transcriptional and post-transcriptional expression of interleukin-1 in U937 cells. J Immunol 1987; 139: 4129–34.

55. Kern JA, Lamb RJ, Reed JC et al. Dexamethasone inhibition of interleukin-1 beta production by human monocytes. Posttranscriptional mechanisms. J Clin Invest 1988; 81: 237–44.

56. Strijbos PJ, Hardwick AJ, Relton JK et al. Inhibition of central actions of cytokines on fever and thermogenesis by lipocortin-1 involves CRF. Am J Physiol 1992; 263: E632–6.

57. Lee SY, Imaki T, Vale W et al. Effects of prenatal exposure to alcohol on the activity of hypothalamic-pituitary-adrenal axis of the offspring: importance of the time of exposure to ethanol and possible modulating mechanisms. Mol Cell Neurosci 1990; 1: 168–77.

58. Lee S, Rivier C. Prenatal alcohol exposure blunts interleukin-1-induced ACTH and β-endorphin secretion by immature rats. Alcohol Clin Exp Res 1993; 17: 940–5.

59. Lee S, Rivier C. Prenatal alcohol exposure alters the hypothalamic-pituitary-adrenal axis response of immature offspring to interleukin-1: is nitric oxide involved? Alcohol Clin Exp Res 1994; 18: 1242–7.

60. Chen W-JA, Maier SE, Parnell SE et al. Alcohol and the developing brain: neuroanatomical studies. Alcohol Res Health 2003; 27: 174–80.

61. Weinberg J, Bezio S. Alcohol-induced changes in pituitary-adrenal activity during pregnancy. Alcohol Clin Exp Res 1987; 11: 274–80.

62. Tritt SH, Tio DL, Brammer G et al. Adrenalectomy but not adrenal demedullation during pregnancy prevents the growth retarding effects of fetal alcohol exposure. Alcohol Clin Exp Res 1993; 17: 1281–9.

63. Chatelain A, Dupuoy JP, Allaume P. Fetal-maternal adrenocorticotrophin and corticosterone relationship in the rat: effects of maternal adrenalectomy. Endocrinology 1980; 106: 1297–303.

64. Barbazanges A, Piazza PV, Le Moel M et al. Maternal glucocorticoid secretion mediates long-term effects of prenatal stress. J Neurosci 1996; 16: 3943–9.

65. Slone JL, Redei EE. Maternal alcohol and adrenalectomy: asynchrony of stress response and forced swim behavior. Neurotoxicol Teratol 2002; 24: 173–8.

66. Sinha P, Halasz I, Choi JF et al. Maternal adrenalectomy eliminates a surge of plasma dehydroepiandrosterone in the mother and attenuates the prenatal testosterone surge in the male fetus. Endocrinology 1997; 138: 4792–7.

67. Shelat SG, Aird F, Redei E. Exposure to dehydroepiandrosterone in utero affects T-cell function in males only. Neuroimmunomodulation 1997; 4: 154–62.

68. Westney L, Bruney R, Ross B et al. Evidence that gonadal hormone levels in amniotic fluid are decreased in males born to alcohol users in humans. Alcohol Alcohol 1991; 26: 403–7.

69. Zimmerberg B. Brown adipose tissue: a model system to investigate fetal alcohol effects on thermoregulation. In:

Fetal Alcohol Syndrome: From Mechanisms to Prevention. (Abel E, ed). Boca Raton: CRC Press, 1996: 285–316.

70. Taylor AN, Branch BJ, Liu S et al. Fetal exposure to ethanol enhances pituitary-adrenal and temperature responses to ethanol in adult rats. Alcohol Clin Exp Res 1981; 5: 237–46.

71. Shibley IA Jr, Pennington SN. Metabolic and mitotic changes associated with the fetal alcohol syndrome. Alcohol Alcohol 1997; 32: 423–34.

72. Kelly RH, Russo J, Holt VL et al. Psychiatric and substance use disorders as risk factors for low birth weight and preterm delivery. Obstet Gynecol 2002; 100: 297–304.

73. Herrenkohl LR. The impact of prenatal stress on the developing fetus and child. In: Psychiatric Consultation in Childbirth Settings (Cohen RL, ed). New York: Plenum, 1988: 21–35.

74. Teixeira JMA, Fisk NM, Glover V. Association between maternal anxiety in pregnancy and increased uterine artery resistance index: cohort based study. BMJ 1999; 318: 153–7.

75. Giles WB, McLean M, Davies JJ et al. Abnormal umbilical artery Doppler waveforms and cord blood corticotropin-releasing hormone. Obstet Gynecol 1996; 87: 107–11.

76. Holzman C, Jetton J, Siler-Khodr T et al. Second trimester corticotropin-releasing hormone levels in relation to preterm delivery and ethnicity. Obstet Gynecol 2001; 97: 657–63.

77. Hobel CJ, Arora CP, Korst LM. Corticotrophin-releasing hormone and CRH-binding protein. Differences between patients at risk for preterm birth and hypertension. Ann N Y Acad Sci 1999; 897: 54–65.

78. Goland RS, Jozak S, Warren WB et al. Elevated levels of umbilical cord plasma corticotropin-releasing hormone in growth-retarded fetuses. J Clin Endocrinol Metab 1993; 77: 1174–9.

79. Svinarich DM, DiCerbo JA, Zaher FM et al. Ethanol-induced expression of cytokines in a first-trimester trophoblast cell line. Am J Obstet Gynecol 1998; 179: 470–5.

80. Ahluwalia B, Wesley B, Adeyiga O et al. Alcohol modulates cytokine secretion and synthesis in human fetus: an in vivo and in vitro study. Alcohol 2000; 21: 207–13.

81. Bartha JL, Romero-Carmona R, Comino-Delgado R. Inflammatory cytokines in intrauterine growth retardation. Acta Obstet Gynecol Scand 2003; 82: 1099–102.

82. Weeks JW, Reynolds L, Taylor D et al. Umbilical cord blood interleukin-6 levels and neonatal morbidity. Obstet Gynecol 1997; 90: 815–18.

83. Hitti J, Tarczy-Hornoch P, Murphy J et al. Amniotic fluid infection, cytokines, and adverse outcome among infants at 34 weeks' gestation or less. Obstet Gynecol 2001; 98: 1080–8.

84. Yoon H, Jun JK, Romero R et al. Amniotic fluid inflammatory cytokines interleukin-6, interleukin-1β, and tumor necrosis factor-α, neonatal brain white matter lesions, and cerebral palsy. Am J Obstet Gynecol 1997; 177: 19–26.

85. Pavlov VA, Tracey KJ. Neural regulators of innate immune responses and inflammation. Cell Mol Life Sci 2004; 61: 2322–31.

14

The 'Old Friends' hypothesis; how early contact with certain microorganisms may influence immunoregulatory circuits

Graham AW Rook, Roberta Martinelli, and Laura Rosa Brunet

INTRODUCTION

In general, the populations of industrialized and affluent countries are healthier than those of developing countries. However, for a number of diseases the reverse is true. Since the late 19th century, there has been a paradoxical increase in the incidences of at least three groups of disease in developed countries that are rare in developing ones. These include the allergies (eczema, food allergy, asthma, hay fever),[1,2] the inflammatory bowel diseases (IBD; Crohn's disease, CD; and ulcerative colitis),[3,4] and some autoimmune diseases (type 1 diabetes and multiple sclerosis; MS).[2] There is also a North–South gradient in the prevalence of these diseases, all of which tend to be more common in Northern Europe.[2] In this chapter we review evidence that these increases are due to fundamental changes in our lifestyle that have deprived our immune system of inputs without which its regulatory mechanisms may respond inappropriately. In the absence of these inputs, the immune system mounts unwanted and destructive immune responses to self (resulting in autoimmunity), gut contents (leading to IBD) or benign allergens in the air (which may cause allergies). This failure of immunoregulation is most likely to occur in those individuals with genetic polymorphisms that further diminish the efficiency of their immunoregulatory mechanisms, so these are classic 'gene/environment' interactions.[5] This theme is relevant to this book, because epidemiological studies indicate that the perinatal period is particularly important for the relevant inputs into the immune system. We suggest that important inputs come from our physiological interactions with relatively harmless microorganisms that, as a consequence of their presence throughout mammalian evolutionary history, affect immunoregulatory circuits. These organisms are now significantly reduced in our environment, and we need to understand how to replace them, or mimic their effects in other ways.

THE INCREASE IN ALLERGIC DISORDERS, AND THE BIRTH OF THE HYGIENE HYPOTHESIS

In developed countries the incidence of allergic disorders has been increasing since the 19th century. The greatest increases seem to have occurred in the 1960s and 1970s.[6,7] This upward trend may have now stopped, and reached a plateau in some parts of Europe.[8,9] This increase in developed countries has resulted in enormous variations in the occurrence of allergic disorders in different parts of the world. For instance, in different centers the prevalence of rhinoconjunctivitis varied from 0.8% to 14.9% in children aged 6–7 years, and from 1.4% to 39.7% in those aged 13–14 years.[1] In 1989 it was suggested that modern hygiene might be in some way responsible for the epidemic of allergies, and the term 'hygiene hypothesis' was born.[10] At this time, no detailed mechanism was proposed, but it was rapidly assumed that hygiene was altering the balance of lymphocyte subsets within the immune system. There are many types of lymphocytes, but the most crucial distinction is between the T helper 1 lymphocytes (Th1) and T helper 2 lymphocytes (Th2). Th1 cells preferentially release interferon gamma (IFNγ) and interleukin (IL)-2 and mediate cell-mediated immunity, which combats many infections and cancers. Th2 lymphocytes are more prone to release IL-4, IL-5 and IL-13, which are involved in humoral immunity and also the immune reactions to some parasites. It was thought, therefore, that hygiene might be leading to reduced contact with pathogens that prime Th1 responses. It was generally believed that decreased Th1 activity would result in a compensatory increase in the Th2 activity. This concept, requiring Th1-inducing infections to control Th2-mediated allergic conditions (the Th1/Th2 see-saw), arose because there is some experimental evidence for regulation of Th2 responses by Th1.[11] However, for reasons detailed in the next few paragraphs, this concept has been discarded.

Do Th1 and Th2 effector cells have mutual regulatory effects?

First, it is often forgotten that IFNγ is in fact a major cytokine in human asthma, despite the major Th2 component.[12] Secondly, recent evidence suggests that Th1 effector responses may *not* be physiological regulators of Th2 activity in humans *in vivo*. The earlier view that Th1 cells can down-regulate Th2 responses was the result of attempts to interpret data while ignorant of the presence of distinct subsets of regulatory T cells (T_{reg}) that control both Th1 and Th2 effector cells.[13] For instance when the presence of T_{reg} is rigorously excluded, cloned polarized Th1 cells transferred into allergic mice may even exacerbate ongoing Th2-mediated inflammation.[14] This conclusion is not contradicted by the recent observation that mice that lack T-bet, a transcription factor needed for development of Th1 cells, have dominantly Th2 responses and develop some asthma-like pathology.[15] This is a default mechanism restoring T-cell numbers with the only subsets available. However, individuals with congenitally defective IFNγ receptors do not have increased Th2 activity, suggesting that IFNγ is not involved in control of Th2 activity in humans.[16]

Simultaneous increases in allergies, autoimmunity, and IBD

The interpretation of a Th1/Th2 imbalance was further weakened by the realization that Th2-mediated and Th1-mediated immunoregulatory disorders were increasing simultaneously and in the same countries. Indeed, there is a striking correlation between the prevalence of type 1 diabetes (Th1-mediated destruction of beta cells in the pancreas) and allergies, both within Europe and outside.[17] Similarly, IBD (CD and ulcerative colitis) are increasing in the same regions.[3,4] CD is unquestionably mediated by Th1 cells, and is

beginning to occur in young children in whom its effects are devastating. Clearly, the explanation for the increased prevalence of allergic disorders cannot be a lack of stimuli for Th1 activity if Th1-mediated diseases such as CD, type 1 diabetes, and multiple sclerosis (MS) are also increasing. It is just as clear that increasing Th1-mediated disorders (CD, MS, type 1 diabetes) cannot be attributable to decreased Th2 activity, when there is a simultaneous rapid rise in the prevalence of allergies.

The role of regulatory T cells

The failure of the Th1/Th2 imbalance hypothesis suggests a role for the T_{reg} mentioned in the previous section. We propose that a relative lack of T_{reg} is permitting a simultaneous increase in immune responses against targets that should be tolerated, irrespective of whether the pathology is mediated by Th1 or Th2 effector cells. These pathological targets include allergens, self antigens, and the contents of the gut (resulting in allergies, autoimmunity, and IBD, respectively). So rather than Th1/Th2 balance, the crucial factor in maintaining a state of health might be $T_{effector}/T_{reg}$ balance (Figure 14.1). In the absence of optimal levels of immunoregulation, the individual may develop a Th1- or a Th2-mediated inflammatory disorder, depending on his/her own particular Th1/Th2 bias, immunological history, and genetic background (discussed later). The argument that a similar lack of T_{reg} activity could underlie the increases in such diverse disorders as allergies, IBD,

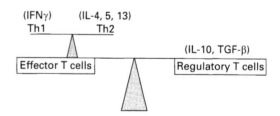

Figure 14.1 The rising incidence of immunoregulatory disorders, such as allergies, IBD, and autoimmunity, is at least partly attributable to an imbalance between effector T cells and regulatory T cells. Diseases mediated by Th1 or Th2 cells are rising in parallel in developed countries. An individual with inadequate regulatory cell activity will have a greater chance of developing these diseases, but their own immunological history and genetic background will determine whether it is a Th1 disease (much autoimmunity, and Crohn's disease) or a Th2 disease (allergies).

and autoimmunity is given added weight by the observation that mice or humans who have genetic defects of the transcription factor Foxp3, which is required for some T_{reg} functions, have a syndrome that includes components of all three of these immunoregulatory disorders.[18]

T_{reg} defects in chronic immunoregulatory disorders

If this re-interpretation of the hygiene hypothesis is correct, the increase in human immunoregulatory disorders is at least partly attributable to defective T_{reg} activity. Therefore, there should be evidence of failed immunoregulation in modern patients with these disorders. Evidence to confirm this hypothesis has come from studies of allergic disorders,[19] MS,[20] autoimmune polyglandular syndromes,[21] and cow's milk intolerance.[22] It is likely to be true for IBD too, though more difficult to prove. The intestine is always in a state of controlled inflammation, and T cells of regulatory phenotype are present in the guts of patients with IBD.[23] Nevertheless, the data from animal models of IBD suggest that the problem is likely to be an immunoregulatory one.[24] IBD occurs rapidly in animals with defective immunoregulation, whether because they lack T_{reg}, or because T_{reg} function is compromised by a lack of an immunoregulatory cytokine such as IL-10. There is also evidence that there is defective induction of oral tolerance in IBD patients.[25] Moreover, they have exaggerated responses to bowel flora,[26] which appear to be the disease-triggering antigens in the animal models.[24]

Microbial exposure and immunoregulation

How does this T_{reg}-orientated concept relate to the original hygiene hypothesis? Why would microbial exposure affect maturation of regulatory pathways? To answer these questions we must first establish what we mean by hygiene.

One interpretation of the word 'hygiene' in this context, mostly promoted by the media, assumes that the critical factor is domestic hygiene (bathing, soaps, detergents, antibacterial kitchen cutting boards, etc.). However, a comprehensive recent report has shown that the development of these practices in the home does not correlate with the observed changes in the occurrence of immunoregulatory disorders.[27]

A second view is that the critical change resulting from modern hygiene is the decreased frequency of infections due to *pathogenic* organisms. When the data available from the Centers for Disease Control

and Prevention for the prevalance of some infections are plotted against time, the graphs suggest that some of the falls did occur during the critical period 1960–1985 when some chronic inflammatory immunoregulatory disorders were doubling every decade.[2] However, more detailed analysis of European data reveals that most of the changes in exposure to pathogens took place long before this crucial period.[27] In addition, there is strong epidemiologic evidence to suggest that certain pathogens, such as childhood viruses and respiratory infections, cause an *increase* rather than a decrease in the incidence of allergic disorders.[28] Interestingly, despite the detrimental effect of infections, this study still identified protective effects of being sent to daycare, keeping pets, and living on a farm.[28] The latter has been a consistently robust observation, and the protective effect of exposing children to cowsheds is well documented.[29] So childhood infections do not protect, and home hygiene does not correlate, but there is still something protective associated with pets, farms, and day-care centers. What might this be?

THE 'OLD FRIENDS' HYPOTHESIS

The answer might lie in exposure to certain relatively harmless microorganisms (including helminths, saprophytic mycobacteria and lactobacilli) that have been present throughout mammalian evolution. We have called this the 'Old Friends' hypothesis.[30] Contact with 'Old Friends' is greatly diminished in rich countries, but still occurs on farms, in cowsheds, and through contact with pets.

Helminths were present throughout mammalian evolution, and are common in developing countries, but rare in developed ones. Indeed, the critical fall in the presence of some harmless helminths, such as *Enterobius vermicularis,* is recent and coincides with the timing of the greatest increases in immunoregulatory disorders.[31] Moreover, allergic disorders are less frequent in individuals with helminth infections, and atopic sensitization increases after treatment of intestinal helminths.[32] Clinical trials using living ova of *Trichuris suis* in patients with IBD are providing encouraging results.[33]

Lactobacilli were very abundant in the human diet during human evolution, because of the use of vegetable foods stored underground, malo-lactic fermentation of alcoholic drinks, and the unavoidable rapid lactic fermentation of milk products. Interestingly, there are fewer lactobacilli in the intestinal flora in people living in developed countries, and more specifically, fewer lactobacilli in the guts of children with allergies.[34] A preliminary clinical study suggests that high doses of lactobacilli may inhibit development of atopic eczema in genetically high-risk children.[35]

Finally, almost everyone in developing countries has skin test positivity to multiple environmental saprophytic mycobacteria. There are at least 80 species, and they are probably the most abundant bacteria in untreated water and mud. Untreated water can contain 10^9 mycobacteria/liter. The saprophytic mycobacterium *M. vaccae,* originally isolated, as its name suggests, from the environment of cows, potently drives maturation of T_{reg} that will treat pre-existing allergy in a mouse model,[36] and has given encouraging results in clinical trials in allergic disorders.[37,38]

The mechanism behind the Old Friends hypothesis

We suggest that because of our long evolutionary association with these organisms, they are recognized by the innate immune system as harmless, or in the case of some helminths, treated as 'guests' because a response might lead to immunopathology. So rather than eliciting aggressive immune responses, these organisms prime immunoregulation.[30] They do it by inducing an unusual pattern of maturation of dendritic cells (DCs) such that they become DC_{reg}, which retain the ability to drive T_{reg}, and often secrete IL-10 rather than IL-12 (Figure 14.2). The previous dogma, based on *in vitro* experiments, stated that DCs drive immunoregulation when immature, but effector responses when mature. This interpretation made sense to the extent that in the absence of 'danger signals', the DC remains immature, and no response is required. However, each of the three groups of Old Friends highlighted here can still have important effects. Certain components of schistosomes will drive T_{reg} maturation in human peripheral blood cell populations.[39] Similarly, when allergic animals are treated with *M. vaccae*, a DC population appears that expresses TGF-β, IL-10 and IFNα, all of which are involved in the driving and maintenance of T_{reg}.[40] Finally, those lactobacilli that are therapeutically active in models of Th1-mediated immunoregulatory disorders tend to suppress IL-12 and Th1 cytokines while preserving the release of TGF-β.[41] These also are likely to be operating via induction of T_{reg}.

The role of the innate immune system in T_{reg} induction

In order to drive maturation of T_{reg}, the Old Friends need to trigger cells of the innate immune system. Innate immunity is involved in early recognition of potential pathogens. It also provides temporary non-specific defense mechanisms, while information about the nature of the threat is assessed and a decision about the appropriate immunologic response mechanism is made. The innate immune system operates via a multitude of pattern recognition receptors (PRR). When PRR recognize the organism as an Old Friend, they divert the response towards immunoregulation rather than attack. Children exposed to a farming way of life that protects from allergies[29] had higher levels of mRNA encoding the PRR, CD14, and TLR2.[42] The farming environment, particularly the cowshed, is likely to be rich in lactobacilli and saprophytic mycobacteria (such as *M. vaccae*) and also in helminth species that can perhaps undergo partial life cycles in man. These observations make TLR2 of particular interest, because it is prominent in the recognition of both mycobacteria and helminths by the innate immune system[39,43] (Figure 14.2). A dysfunctional polymorphism of TLR2 increases susceptibility to lepromatous leprosy,[44] and in an *in vitro* system, materials derived from *Schistosoma mansoni* (i.e. one of the postulated Old Friends) that cause DCs to drive IL-10-secreting T_{reg}, failed to do so if TLR2 was blocked.[39] Therefore it is of great interest that the protective effect of the farming environment was dependent upon the polymorphisms of TLR2 present.[45]

Another example is seen in experimental models using lactobacilli to prevent or treat colitis. The protective effect of the lactobacilli depended upon TLR9, which binds CpG motifs.[46] However, there is nothing special about the DNA of the lactobacilli. Rather they seem to present their DNA in a 'package', or in the context of other signals to the innate immune system, that permit recognition of the lactobacilli as Old Friends.

Several studies indicated that levels of endotoxin (a component of the cell wall of gram-negative bacteria) in childrens' bedding were inversely related to the occurrence of hay fever, atopic asthma, and atopic sensitization.[47] Since mutations of TLR4 are associated with hyporesponsiveness to endotoxin in humans,[48] it was logical to seek a relationship between polymorphisms in this gene, and susceptibility to asthma. Surprisingly, no such relationship was found.[49] This finding may imply that endotoxin is a robust marker of bacterial contamination rather than directly relevant in its own right. The endotoxin might be a surrogate marker for other microbial components that are ligands for TLR-2 or NOD2, but less easily measured in environmental samples.

NOD2, also known as CARD15, is an important intracellular PRR that recognizes fragments of the peptidoglycan of bacterial cell walls (Figure 14.2). Polymorphisms of this molecule are linked to

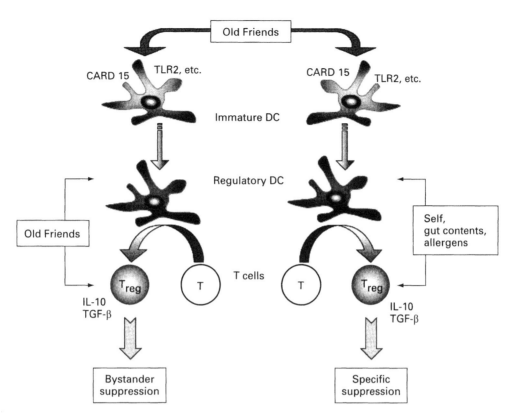

Figure 14.2 Two types of regulatory activity triggered by the microorganisms considered to be Old Friends. Pattern recognition receptors (PRR) of the innate immune system, such as CARD15 or TLR2, recognize them as harmless. Consequently, the antigen-presenting cells (dendritic cells, DC) become DC_{reg}, and drive T_{reg} rather than effector T cells. On the left, the Treg recognize the Old Friend itself and so exert bystander suppression whenever it is present. On the right, the DC_{reg} have picked up and processed self proteins, gut contents, and allergens, and so drive T_{reg} specific for these 'forbidden' targets. The T_{reg} are probably not active when the PRR detect genuine danger signals, so the immune system can initiate the appropriate protective response.

increased susceptibility to both CD[50] and asthma.[51] Although NOD2 has not yet been implicated in driving T_{reg}, we predict that it will prove to be so. This would provide an explanation for its relevance to these two entirely different immunoregulatory disorders.

Gene/environment interactions

The identification of genes within the innate immune system relevant to susceptibility to immunoregulatory disorders allows certain predictions. Thus, an extension of the Old Friends hypothesis suggests that in an environment that less actively primes T_{reg} activity, immunoregulatory disorders will occur first in those individuals whose innate immune systems are least efficient at driving T_{reg}.[5] In other words, disease will occur in those individuals who have certain polymor-

phisms of the important PRR such as NOD2, TLR2 or TLR9. This is a classic 'gene by environment' effect.

Other sets of genes may explain the fact that although Th1-mediated and Th2-mediated inflammatory disorders are increasing in parallel within populations,[2,17] there does seem to be some segregation of Th1 and Th2 at the level of the individual. Thus, in some communities, people suffering from the Th1-mediated autoimmune diseases, type 1 diabetes or MS, are less likely to be allergic .[52,53] It is beyond the scope of this review to go into the detail of the genes that lead to disease-specific susceptibilities, although there is a large literature on each disorder.

Two functions of immunoregulation driven by Old Friends

The increased DC_{reg} and T_{reg} induced by Old Friends lead to two immunoregulatory mechanisms mediated in part by release of IL-10 and TGF-β (Figure 14.2). First, continuing exposure to the Old Friends will cause continuous background activation of T_{reg} specific for the Old Friends themselves, resulting in a constant background release of IL-10 and TGF-β, and bystander suppression. This mechanism has been elegantly demonstrated in a model of colitis.[54] Clearly, for this mechanism to work, exposure to the triggering organism must be frequent or constant. Such continuous exposure was an inevitable feature of infection with helminths, consumption of untreated water rich in saprophytic mycobacteria, and a diet rich in products fermented, deliberately or by accident, with lactobacilli. Secondly, the DC_{reg} will inevitably sample self, gut contents and allergens, and so induce T_{reg} specific for the target antigens of the three major groups of chronic inflammatory disorder. Effects of this type might not require ongoing exposure to the Old Friends, because once established, T_{reg} activity will be maintained by continuing exposure to the target antigens. It is important to point out that these two mechanisms do not result in the immune system being brought to a standstill. T_{reg} seem to be most efficient at damping down the inappropriate immune responses characteristic of the immunoregulatory disorders. These mechanisms may be aborted when there are legitimate 'danger' signals. For example, T_{reg} function can be turned off by appropriate 'danger signals' *in vitro*.[55] Infections of pathogens will still trigger effective immune responses.

WHAT OTHER DISEASES MIGHT ALSO BE INCREASING BECAUSE OF DIMINISHED EXPOSURE TO OLD FRIENDS? SOME SPECULATIONS

What other diseases, in addition to the three groups of inflammatory disorders already discussed, might be changing in incidence or presentation as a result of the altered cytokine patterns that result from a different microbial environment, and diminished T_{reg} activity? Premature speculation could be misleading, but the striking increases in the metabolic syndrome and in atherosclerosis deserve comment. The metabolic syndrome, which involves abdominal obesity, hypertriglyceridemia, low high-density lipoprotein cholesterol, and insulin resistance, now affects 20–25% of the US population.[56] It has been observed recently that whereas women with uncomplicated obesity have increased serum levels of IL-10, those with the metabolic syndrome do not.[57] Could this imply less regulatory T-cell activity? The hypothesis is strengthened by considering atherosclerosis, which is a T-cell-mediated inflammatory lesion in blood vessel walls, considerably more common in patients with the metabolic syndrome. Atherosclerosis is exaggerated in IL-10-deficient mice, particularly if they are kept in a conventional environment.[58] Mice with transgenic T cells overexpressing IL-10 are protected from atherosclerosis.[59] There is similar evidence that IL-10 has a beneficial role in human atherosclerotic plaques,[60–62] and serum levels of IL-10 are reduced in patients with unstable angina.[63] There is a relationship between obesity and asthma.[64] But does asthma occur more commonly in those obese individuals who have the metabolic syndrome and/or atherosclerosis and reduced serum IL-10?

THE OLD FRIENDS HYPOTHESIS AND THE PERINATAL PERIOD

In the previous sections we set out the current understanding of the Old Friends hypothesis, and of the organisms, genes, and mechanisms involved. Most of the work has come from studies of older children and adults. Here we outline information that suggests a particular importance of the perinatal period. The immune system resembles the brain in that we are born with the hardware, and a limited amount of software and data, but correct function depends heavily on the information received *in utero* and in the postnatal period. This developmental sequence should not deviate too far from that which our evolutionary history has set up the system to expect. The information passed on by the mother (and father) includes genetically encoded information that can be considered as knowledge of how to set up an effective immune system. This knowledge has accumulated during the evolution of our species. Parents also pass on genetic variations in disease susceptibility. Childhood asthma is associated with maternal asthma, and to a slightly lower extent, with paternal asthma.[65] Most of this increased risk is likely to be genetic, but the greater importance of the mother points to the possibility of other immunologically relevant influences. For instance, the mother also passes on additional information based on her own immunological experience and history. The proteins and cells that convey this information are antibodies, anti-idiotypes, agalactosyl IgG, and possibly some T cells. At birth, the mother also transfers some of her commensal flora to her child. In some species, such as whales and dolphins, the nipple is close to the anus and the mother may defecate while the infant suckles to ensure intake of the bowel flora. Perhaps human births are also intended to be fecally contaminated so that gut colonization can occur rapidly. Finally, the way in which the mother cares for the child, and the environment in which she does it, will affect exposure to other organisms from the environment that colonize intermittently, or interact with the immune system without colonization, perhaps by being taken up by the tonsils, and by M cells on Peyer's patches throughout the gut.

Sensitization to allergens *in utero*

Sensitization to allergens can occur *in utero*. For example, cord blood lymphocytes may respond to allergens present in the mother's environment. One study sought to determine at what gestational age these responses appear. Blood samples were obtained from fetuses and premature babies. Their cells were stimulated with the allergens, house dust mite, cat fur, birch tree pollen, β-lactoglobulin, ovalbumin, and bee venom. The responses became significant from around 22 weeks gestation.[66] How does this sensitization occur? An allergen from house dust mite was detectable in 24 of 43 amniotic fluid samples. It was also present in maternal blood, and in 15 of 24 cord-plasma samples at significantly higher concentrations than in the maternal plasma. The presence of allergen in the fetal circulation suggests passage of allergen across the placenta. Moreover, allergen in the amniotic fluid will be swallowed by the fetus, and absorbed via the gut.[67]

So what is the relationship between *in utero* sensitization and subsequent allergic disorder? In a study seeking to address this issue, data from immunologic assessments performed at birth, 1 and 2 years of age were compared with subsequent clinical outcome. Surprisingly, neonatal responses to allergen did not predict the allergic status of the child at 6 years.[68] This finding casts doubt on the hypothesis that following allergen sensitization *in utero*, postnatal high dose allergen exposure localizes inflammation to the airways, leading to the clinical manifestations of allergy.[69] In fact, further analysis suggests that the neonatal responses are complex, involving both unusual, presumably immature effector cells, and T_{reg}. Some of the previously recorded responses might have been manifestations of T_{reg} rather than of effector cells.[70] Therefore, once again, before we can understand what is happening, we need to distinguish between $T_{effector}$ and T_{reg}. There is no doubt, however, that immunization can occur *in utero*. (This is leading to the useful possibility that the baby can be indirectly

vaccinated against infections by immunizing the mother.) Below we consider factors in the maternal environment that may influence the outcome in terms of the type of response generated by deliberately administered vaccines, or accidentally encountered allergens or food antigens.

Family size, birth order, and allergic disorders

One observation that supported the hygiene hypothesis was the lower risk of allergies found in children from large families. This protective effect was most striking in children with multiple older siblings, especially if they were boys.[71] Since children from large families are exposed to more childhood infections, it seemed to support the hygiene hypothesis. The observation appears to be reliable, but interpretation is now less clear. As discussed earlier, most childhood infections do *not* protect from allergies; they increase them.[28] Meanwhile, it has emerged that cord blood IgE levels fall with increasing number of live births.[72] It is not clear whether the level of IgE transferred to the fetus has a major influence on the subsequent development of allergic disorders. Nevertheless others have shown that the cord blood mononuclear cell proliferative responses to allergens also decreased significantly with increasing birth order,[73] and so did the risk of subsequent allergic rhinitis.[74] Therefore, the protective effect of birth order might not have anything to do with increased exposure to infections passed on by older siblings, but rather be a consequence of a physiological change in the mother. The sibling effect might be initiated *in utero*.

The effect of maternal diet, smoking, and helminth infections

The magnitude of the cord blood mononuclear cell proliferative responses to allergens increased significantly in association with maternal smoking, and decreased significantly with greater maternal dietary intake of vitamin E.[73] Similarly, fish oil supplementation (n-3 polyunsaturated fatty acids, n-3 PUFAs) of the maternal diet resulted in a trend towards lower neonatal cytokine responses to allergens, and fewer positive skin prick tests.[75] As discussed above, the significance of the cord blood lymphoproliferative response is unclear, but nevertheless maternal dietary factors have an influence on the level of proliferation.

Another example, which brings us back to the Old Friends hypothesis, is provided by co-infection with helminths. The vaccine currently used for tuberculosis (bacillus Calmette-Guérin; BCG) induced an abnormal response in babies that had been sensitized *in utero* to antigens of *Wuchereria bancrofti* or *Schistosoma haematobium* because their mothers were suffering from these infections.[76] At 10–14 months after neonatal BCG vaccination, peripheral blood mononuclear cells from the helminth-sensitized children cultured with antigen from *M. tuberculosis* released strikingly less IFNγ, and more IL-5 than did cells from nonsensitized controls. Therefore, exposure to helminth antigens *in utero*, or to factors derived from a mother suffering from a helminth infection, was able to exert a long-term effect on the balance of the immune response to subsequently encountered antigens. Helminths are potent inducers of T_{reg}, and epidemiological studies show that helminth infections limit allergies.[32] It seems possible that some of this effect is exerted *in utero*.

Antibiotics

Several studies have suggested that early use of antibiotics is associated with increased risk of subsequent atopic disease, particularly if the antibiotic was used during the first year or two of life.[77,78] It is not clear whether the antibiotics increase the risk, or whether children with allergies are more likely to wheeze, and so are prescribed more antibiotics. However, it has been noted that when animals are given antibiotics during 'infancy', the immune system is diverted towards Th2, so the effects seen in human children may represent a real example of the Old Friends hypothesis at work.[79] The effect is presumably mediated by changes in the bowel flora.

The farming environment

One of the most conclusively demonstrated protective effects of lifestyle is seen when infants spend time in cowsheds while the mother milks the cows. If this occurs during the first year of life, the level of protection from allergic disorders is very significant.[29] The study could not identify the protective agent, though it must either be in the cowshed environment, or in the unpasteurized milk that many of the infants were given.[29] Dust samples from this environment are undergoing intensive study, and will certainly contain mycobacteria, helminth ova, and lactobacilli in addition to a vast range of other factors.

Persistent effects in older children

Interestingly, immunologic effects that are likely to be due to diminished microbial exposure in early life are also evident in older children. Peripheral blood lymphocytes from children living in Munich and Dresden (which is less economically developed because it was within the old East Germany) were stimulated *in vitro* with phorbol myristate acetate (PMA) and ionomycin, and the cytokines released were then measured. Stimulating lymphocytes in this way drives memory cells to secrete cytokines they are primed to make, giving a glimpse of the consequences of the child's past immunologic history. If there had been less immunologic activity, there will be a smaller response. The findings were extraordinary. Many of the 5–7-year-old children from Munich had no response, while others were strongly biased towards Th2.[80] Indeed, the incidence of allergic disorders is higher in Munich than in Dresden. By contrast, almost all children from Dresden were responders, and the pattern of cytokines released was mixed (i.e. both Th1 and Th2 cytokines were found) suggesting a diverse and perhaps more balanced immunologic experience.[80] In fact, the poor responses of the lymphocytes from the children brought up in Munich were more reminiscent of the responses seen with cells from naïve specific pathogen-free (SPF) laboratory mice that have been reared in isolators. That such differences were evident when two German cities were compared in the 21st century is remarkable, but it illustrates the powerful immunologic consequences of apparently small differences in lifestyle.

THE POTENTIAL FOR HEALTH-CARE INTERVENTIONS BASED ON THE PRINCIPLES OF THE OLD FRIENDS HYPOTHESIS

Lifestyle

There has been pressure from journalists and the public to suggest safe changes in lifestyle that might increase exposure to the organisms that promote our immunoregulatory circuits. However, it is not clear that we can give sensible advice. Many aspects of domestic hygiene, particularly food hygiene, are clearly beneficial, and protect us from *Salmonella*, *Campylobacter* and pathogenic *E. coli*. In fact, hygiene along with antibiotics and vaccines, is certainly the most valuable and cost-effective achievement of modern medicine. On the other hand, exposures to pet dogs and farm animals seem to protect against allergic disorders. So perhaps home hygiene needs to be applied sensibly rather than excessively. There may be no need for obsessive hand-washing every time a child encounters animals, earth or untreated water in ponds and streams. Similarly, farm produce purchased in markets, perhaps still coated with earth and harmless Old Friends, might be better at driving the regulatory circuits than the clean, sterilized cling-wrapped supermarket produce. However, the truth is that we should not abandon hygiene, and it is not practical to advocate 'selective' hygiene. So the future lies in identifying the Old Friends, and devising novel types of vaccines that can selectively put the Old Friends back into the environment.

Novel vaccines

So can such vaccines be devised? This would constitute a novel vaccine strategy (Figure 14.3). Current vaccines routinely given to children are designed to elicit potent effector responses targeting specific pathogens. They are designed *not* to evoke a dominant regulatory response. So although the vaccines cannot, in our opinions, be blamed for the increases in immunoregulatory disorders, it probably is true to suggest that they do not help to combat the rise. So we may need to develop additional vaccines that do not target a specific infection, but can interact with the innate immune system in a way that primes regulatory circuits. As discussed earlier, clinical trials are taking place using saprophytic mycobacteria,[37,38] lactobacilli,[35] and helminths[33] in allergic disorders and IBD. It is interesting to note that the lactobacilli and helminths were given by the oral route, and it has been found recently that the mycobacteria are also most active by this route. The gut is a major site for the induction of T_{reg}. This is exciting because the oral

route of administration is more acceptable to the public, which is growing wary of injected vaccines. If the Old Friends used individually as oral treatments (or prophylactics) are clinically effective, then the objective may be achieved. If they are not sufficiently potent, or work only in discrete subsets of patients with appropriate polymorphisms of the innate immune system, then capsules that incorporate multiple Old Friends could be developed. Taken daily, these would evoke both bystander and specific mechanisms of immunoregulation. Taken intermittently they would preferentially evoke immunoregulation by specific T_{reg}. We suspect that the public would welcome this approach, which might come from the food industry rather than the pharmaceutical one.

Probiotics

Probiotics are living microorganisms given orally to benefit health. Prebiotics are materials given orally to influence the nature and balance of the bowel flora; effectively an attempt to cultivate them. Prebiotics and probiotics are often given together. For many years, these concepts lurked on the fringes of medicine, but recently there has been a lot of excellent research that has identified a variety of mechanisms and molecular pathways. These mechanisms include competition for ecological niches within the gut, inhibition of signaling via NFκB, direct antimicrobial effects of secreted components, modulation of apoptosis, and activation of macrophages that take part in driving epithelial repair (partly reviewed in ref. 81). In addition it has emerged recently that some probiotics induce T_{reg}.

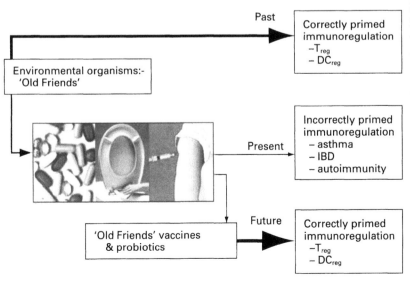

Figure 14.3 The changing pattern of exposure to organisms that can prime immunoregulatory mechanisms. In the past they were encountered in diets and the environment. In the modern world we use vaccines that are not intended to prime immunoregulation, and antibiotics and hygiene that diminish our exposure to microorganisms and parasites. The future might include supplementing the missing Old Friends in other ways, including vaccines or probiotics, probably by the oral route.

Orally administered *Lactobacillus casei* reduced skin inflammation due to contact sensitivity in animals sensitized to dinitrofluorobenzene.[82] This finding cannot be attributed to local gut-specific effects of *L. casei*, but rather appears to require CD4+ T cells, and is likely to have been mediated by T_{reg}. Moreover, some strains of lactobacilli stimulate the maturation of DC so that they release little TNF-α or IL-12, but maintain their ability to release IL-10. This might facilitate the induction of T_{reg}.[83] In IL-10 knockout mice, probiotics that attenuate the colitis to which these animals are susceptible, down-regulate Th1 cytokines while maintaining TGF-β.[41] Both oral and subcutaneous administration promote this effect.[84] This activity of lactobacilli via the subcutaneous route protects not only against colitis in IL-10 knockout mice, but also against collagen arthritis, a mainly Th1-mediated model of autoimmunity.[84]

These results all suggest that some probiotics are acting via T_{reg}. Others may act by entirely different mechanisms, and this confusion needs to be resolved. Those probiotic strains that do drive DC_{reg} and T_{reg} are excellent candidates for early administration to infants in developed countries, with the objective of reducing the incidences of chronic immunoregulatory disorders. Therefore, this new interpretation of the actions of probiotics needs to be integrated within the Old Friends hypothesis (Figure 14.3). In addition to the studies in allergic disorders, where a probiotic *Lactobacillus* strain was given orally to pregnant women and to the neonate,[35] there have been several preliminary studies of the efficacy of bacterial probiotics, usually derived from *Lactobacillus* strains, for inducing or maintaining remission in IBD (reviewed in ref. 85).

CONCLUSIONS

1. Allergies, autoimmunity and IBD have been increasing in parallel in rich countries. There is evidence that this is partly attributable to a failure of immunoregulatory mechanisms (T_{reg} and DC_{reg}) that should block inappropriate responses to allergens, self antigens, and gut contents, respectively.
2. Evidence from epidemiology, animal models, and clinical studies suggests that the failure of immunoregulation is attributable at least in part to diminished exposure to certain groups of relatively harmless microorganisms that are tolerated by the innate immune system, and can prime regulatory mechanisms.
3. There have been encouraging clinical trials using these types of microorganisms and appropriately selected probiotics may prove to be particularly important in the neonatal period.

REFERENCES

1. Strachan D, Sibbald B, Weiland S et al. Worldwide variations in prevalence of symptoms of allergic rhinoconjunctivitis in children: the International Study of Asthma and Allergies in Childhood (ISAAC). Pediatr Allergy Immunol 1997; 8: 161–76.
2. Bach JF. The effect of infections on susceptibility to autoimmune and allergic diseases. N Engl J Med 2002; 347: 911–20.
3. Sawczenko A, Sandhu BK, Logan RF et al. Prospective survey of childhood inflammatory bowel disease in the British Isles. Lancet 2001; 357: 1093–1094.
4. Lindberg E, Lindquist B, Holmquist L, Hildebrand H. Inflammatory bowel disease in children and adolescents in Sweden, 1984–1995. J Pediatr Gastroenterol Nutr 2000; 30: 259–64.
5. Rook GA, Martinelli R, Brunet LR. Innate immune responses to mycobacteria and the downregulation of atopic responses. Curr Opin Allergy Clin Immunol 2003; 3: 337–42.
6. Warner JO. Worldwide variations in the prevalence of atopic symptoms: what does it all mean? Thorax 1999; 54 (Suppl 2): S46–S51.
7. Platts-Mills TA, Carter MC, Heymann PW. Specific and nonspecific obstructive lung disease in childhood: causes of changes in the prevalence of asthma. Environ Health Perspect 2000; 108 (Suppl 4): 725–31.
8. Fleming DM, Sunderland R, Cross KW, Ross AM. Declining incidence of episodes of asthma: a study of trends in new episodes presenting to general practitioners in the period 1989–98. Thorax 2000; 55: 657–61.
9. Ronchetti R, Villa MP, Barreto M et al. Is the increase in childhood asthma coming to an end? Findings from three surveys of schoolchildren in Rome, Italy. Eur Respir J 2001; 17: 881–6.
10. Strachan DP. Hay fever, hygiene, and household size. BMJ 1989; 299: 1259–60.
11. Romagnani S. Regulation of the development of type 2 T-helper cells in allergy. Curr Opin Immunol 1994; 6: 838–46.
12. Krug N, Madden J, Redington AE et al. T-cell cytokine profile evaluated at the single cell level in BAL and blood in allergic asthma. Am J Respir Cell Mol Biol 1996; 14: 319–26.
13. Jiang H, Chess L. An integrated model of immunoregulation mediated by regulatory T cell subsets. Adv Immunol 2004; 83: 253–88.
14. Hansen G, Berry G, DeKruyff RH, Umetsu DT. Allergen-specific Th1 cells fail to counterbalance Th2 cell-induced airway hyperreactivity but cause severe airway inflammation. J Clin Invest 1999; 103: 175–83.
15. Finotto S, Neurath MF, Glickman JN et al. Development of spontaneous airway changes consistent with human asthma in mice lacking T-bet. Science 2002; 295: 336–8.
16. Lammas DA, Casanova JL, Kumararatne DS. Clinical consequences of defects in the IL-12-dependent interferon-gamma (IFN-gamma) pathway. Clin Exp Immunol 2000; 121: 417–25.
17. Stene LC, Nafstad P. Relation between occurrence of type 1 diabetes and asthma. Lancet 2001; 357: 607.

18. Wildin RS, Smyk-Pearson S, Filipovich AH. Clinical and molecular features of the immunodysregulation, polyendocrinopathy, enteropathy, X linked (IPEX) syndrome. J Med Genet 2002; 39: 537–45.

19. Akdis M, Verhagen J, Taylor A et al. Immune responses in healthy and allergic individuals are characterized by a fine balance between allergen-specific T regulatory 1 and T helper 2 cells. J Exp Med 2004; 199: 1567–75.

20. Viglietta V, Baecher-Allan C, Weiner HL, Hafler DA. Loss of functional suppression by CD4+CD25+ regulatory T cells in patients with multiple sclerosis. J Exp Med 2004; 199: 971–9.

21. Kriegel MA, Lohmann T, Gabler C et al. Defective suppressor function of human CD4+ CD25+ regulatory T cells in autoimmune polyglandular syndrome type II. J Exp Med 2004; 199: 1285–91.

22. Karlsson MR, Rugtveit J, Brandtzaeg P. Allergen-responsive CD4+CD25+ regulatory T cells in children who have outgrown cow's milk allergy. J Exp Med 2004; 199: 1679–88.

23. Makita S, Kanai T, Oshima S et al. CD4+CD25bright T cells in human intestinal lamina propria as regulatory cells. J Immunol 2004; 173: 3119–30.

24. Powrie F, Read S, Mottet C, Uhlig H, Maloy K. Control of immune pathology by regulatory T cells. Novartis Found Symp 2003; 252: 92–8; discussion 98–105, 106–14.

25. Kraus TA, Toy L, Chan L, Childs J, Mayer L. Failure to induce oral tolerance to a soluble protein in patients with inflammatory bowel disease. Gastroenterology 2004; 126: 1771–8.

26. Duchmann R, Kaiser I, Hermann E et al. Tolerance exists towards resident intestinal flora but is broken in active inflammatory bowel disease (IBD). Clin Exp Immunol 1995; 102: 448–55.

27. Stanwell-Smith R, Bloomfield S. The hygiene hypothesis and its implications for home hygiene. Milan: NextHealth Srl, 2004.

28. Benn CS, Melbye M, Wohlfahrt J, Bjorksten B, Aaby P. Cohort study of sibling effect, infectious diseases, and risk of atopic dermatitis during first 18 months of life. BMJ 2004; 328: 1223.

29. Riedler J, Braun-Fahrlander C, Eder W et al. Exposure to farming in early life and development of asthma and allergy: a cross-sectional survey. Lancet 2001; 358: 1129–33.

30. Rook GA, Adams V, Hunt J et al. Mycobacteria and other environmental organisms as immunomodulators for immunoregulatory disorders. Springer Semin Immunopathol 2004; 25: 237–55.

31. Gale EA. A missing link in the hygiene hypothesis? Diabetologia 2002; 45: 588–94.

32. Yazdanbakhsh M, Matricardi PM. Parasites and the hygiene hypothesis: regulating the immune system? Clin Rev Allergy Immunol 2004; 26: 15–24.

33. Weinstock JV, Summers R, Elliott DE. Helminths and harmony. Gut 2004; 53: 7–9.

34. Bjorksten B, Naaber P, Sepp E, Mikelsaar M. The intestinal microflora in allergic Estonian and Swedish 2-year-old children. Clin Exp Allergy 1999; 29: 342–6.

35. Kalliomaki M, Salminen S, Arvilommi H et al. Probiotics in primary prevention of atopic disease: a randomised placebo-controlled trial. Lancet 2001; 357: 1076–9.

36. Zuany-Amorim C, Sawicka E, Manlius C et al. Suppression of airway eosinophilia by killed Mycobacterium vaccae-induced allergen-specific regulatory T-cells. Nat Med 2002; 8: 625–9.

37. Arkwright PD, David TJ. Intradermal administration of a killed Mycobacterium vaccae suspension (SRL 172) is associated with improvement in atopic dermatitis in children with moderate-to-severe disease. J Allergy Clin Immunol 2001; 107: 531–4.

38. Camporota L, Corkhill A, Long H et al. The effects of Mycobacterium vaccae on allergen-induced airway responses in atopic asthma. Eur Respir J 2003; 21: 287–93.

39. van der Kleij D, Latz E, Brouwers JF et al. A novel host-parasite lipid cross-talk. Schistosomal lyso-phosphatidylserine activates Toll-like receptor 2 and affects immune polarization. J Biol Chem 2002; 277: 48122–9.

40. Adams VC, Hunt J, Martinelli R et al. Mycobacterium vaccae induces a population of pulmonary antigen presenting cells that have regulatory potential in allergic mice. Eur J Immunol 2004; 34: 631–8.

41. McCarthy J, O'Mahony L, O'Callaghan L et al. Double blind, placebo controlled trial of two probiotic strains in interleukin 10 knockout mice and mechanistic link with cytokine balance. Gut 2003; 52: 975–80.

42. Lauener RP, Birchler T, Adamski J et al. Expression of CD14 and Toll-like receptor 2 in farmers' and non-farmers' children. Lancet 2002; 360: 465–6.

43. Heldwein KA, Fenton MJ. The role of Toll-like receptors in immunity against mycobacterial infection. Microbes Infect 2002; 4: 937–44.

44. Kang TJ, Lee SB, Chae GT. A polymorphism in the toll-like receptor 2 is associated with IL-12 production from monocyte in lepromatous leprosy. Cytokine 2002; 20: 56–62.

45. Eder W, Klimecki W, Yu L et al. Toll-like receptor 2 as a major gene for asthma in children of European farmers. J Allergy Clin Immunol 2004; 113: 482–8.

46. Rachmilewitz D, Katakura K, Karmeli F et al. Toll-like receptor 9 signaling mediates the anti-inflammatory effects of probiotics in murine experimental colitis. Gastroenterology 2004; 126: 520–8.

47. Braun-Fahrlander C, Riedler J, Herz U et al. Environmental exposure to endotoxin and its relation to asthma in school-age children. N Engl J Med 2002; 347: 869–77.

48. Arbour NC, Lorenz E, Schutte BC et al. TLR4 mutations are associated with endotoxin hyporesponsiveness in humans. Nat Genet 2000; 25: 187–91.

49. Raby BA, Klimecki WT, Laprise C et al. Polymorphisms in toll-like receptor 4 are not associated with asthma or atopy-related phenotypes. Am J Respir Crit Care Med 2002; 166: 1449–56.

50. Ogura Y, Bonen DK, Inohara N et al. A frameshift mutation in NOD2 associated with susceptibility to Crohn's disease. Nature 2001; 411: 603–6.

51. Kabesch M, Peters W, Carr D et al. Association between polymorphisms in caspase recruitment domain containing protein 15 and allergy in two German populations. J Allergy Clin Immunol 2003; 111: 813–17.

52. Douek IF, Leech NJ, Gillmor HA, Bingley PJ, Gale EA. Children with type-1 diabetes and their unaffected siblings have fewer symptoms of asthma. Lancet 1999; 353: 1850.

53. Tremlett HL, Evans J, Wiles CM, Luscombe DK. Asthma and multiple sclerosis: an inverse association in a case-control general practice population. Q J Med 2002; 95: 753–6.

54. Groux H, O'Garra A, Bigler M et al. A CD4+ subset inhibits antigen-specific T cell responses and prevents colitis. Nature 1997; 389: 737–42.

55. Pasare C, Medzhitov R. Toll pathway-dependent blockade of CD4+CD25+ T cell-mediated suppression by dendritic cells. Science 2003; 299: 1033–6.

56. Ford ES, Giles WH, Dietz WH. Prevalence of the metabolic syndrome among US adults: findings from the third

National Health and Nutrition Examination Survey. JAMA 2002; 287: 356–9.

57. Esposito K, Pontillo A, Giugliano F et al. Association of low interleukin-10 levels with the metabolic syndrome in obese women. J Clin Endocrinol Metab 2003; 88: 1055–8.

58. Mallat Z, Besnard S, Duriez M et al. Protective role of interleukin-10 in atherosclerosis. Circ Res 1999; 85: e17–24.

59. Pinderski LJ, Fischbein MP, Subbanagounder G et al. Overexpression of interleukin-10 by activated T lymphocytes inhibits atherosclerosis in LDL receptor-deficient mice by altering lymphocyte and macrophage phenotypes. Circ Res 2002; 90: 1064–71.

60. Uyemura K, Demer LL, Castle SC et al. Cross-regulatory roles of interleukin (IL)-12 and IL-10 in atherosclerosis. J Clin Invest 1996; 97: 2130–8.

61. Mallat Z, Heymes C, Ohan J et al. Expression of interleukin-10 in advanced human atherosclerotic plaques: relation to inducible nitric oxide synthase expression and cell death. Arterioscler Thromb Vasc Biol 1999; 19: 611–16.

62. Pinderski Oslund LJ, Hedrick CC et al. Interleukin-10 blocks atherosclerotic events in vitro and in vivo. Arterioscler Thromb Vasc Biol 1999; 19: 2847–53.

63. Smith DA, Irving SD, Sheldon J, Cole D, Kaski JC. Serum levels of the antiinflammatory cytokine interleukin-10 are decreased in patients with unstable angina. Circulation 2001; 104: 746–9.

64. O'Brien PE, Dixon JB. The extent of the problem of obesity. Am J Surg 2002; 184(6B): 4S–8S.

65. Litonjua AA, Carey VJ, Burge HA, Weiss ST, Gold DR. Parental history and the risk for childhood asthma. Does mother confer more risk than father? Am J Respir Crit Care Med 1998; 158: 176–81.

66. Kondo N, Kobayashi Y, Shinoda S et al. Cord blood lymphocyte responses to food antigens for the prediction of allergic disorders. Arch Dis Child 1992; 67: 1003–7.

67. Holloway JA, Warner JO, Vance GH et al. Detection of house-dust-mite allergen in amniotic fluid and umbilical-cord blood. Lancet 2000; 356: 1900–2.

68. Prescott SL, King B, Strong TL, Holt PG. The value of perinatal immune responses in predicting allergic disease at 6 years of age. Allergy 2003; 58: 1187–94.

69. Warner JO, Pohunek P, Marguet C, Clough JB, Roche WR. Progression from allergic sensitization to asthma. Pediatr Allergy Immunol 2000; 11 (Suppl 13): 12–14.

70. Thornton CA, Upham JW, Wikstrom ME et al. Functional maturation of CD4+CD25+CTLA4+CD45RA+ T regulatory cells in human neonatal T cell responses to environmental antigens/allergens. J Immunol 2004; 173: 3084–92.

71. Strachan DP, Harkins LS, Golding J. Sibship size and self-reported inhalant allergy among adult women. ALSPAC Study Team. Clin Exp Allergy 1997; 27: 151–5.

72. Karmaus W, Arshad SH, Sadeghnejad A, Twiselton R. Does maternal immunoglobulin E decrease with increasing order of live offspring? Investigation into maternal immune tolerance. Clin Exp Allergy 2004; 34: 853–9.

73. Devereux G, Barker RN, Seaton A. Antenatal determinants of neonatal immune responses to allergens. Clin Exp Allergy 2002; 32: 43–50.

74. Braback L, Hedberg A. Perinatal risk factors for atopic disease in conscripts. Clin Exp Allergy 1998; 28: 936–42.

75. Dunstan JA, Mori TA, Barden A et al. Fish oil supplementation in pregnancy modifies neonatal allergen-specific immune responses and clinical outcomes in infants at high risk of atopy: a randomized, controlled trial. J Allergy Clin Immunol 2003; 112: 1178–84.

76. Malhotra I, Mungai P, Wamachi A et al. Helminth- and Bacillus Calmette-Guerin-induced immunity in children sensitized in utero to filariasis and schistosomiasis. J Immunol 1999; 162: 6843–8.

77. Farooqi IS, Hopkin JM. Early childhood infection and atopic disorder. Thorax 1998; 53: 927–32.

78. Droste JH, Wieringa MH, Weyler JJ et al. Does the use of antibiotics in early childhood increase the risk of asthma and allergic disease? Clin Exp Allergy 2000; 30: 1548–53.

79. Oyama N, Sudo N, Sogawa H, Kubo C. Antibiotic use during infancy promotes a shift in the T(H)1/T(H)2 balance toward T(H)2-dominant immunity in mice. J Allergy Clin Immunol 2001; 107: 153–9.

80. Renz H, Mutius E, Illi S, Wolkers F, Hirsch T, Weiland SK. T(H)1/T(H)2 immune response profiles differ between atopic children in eastern and western Germany. J Allergy Clin Immunol 2002; 109: 338–42.

81. Ghosh S, van Heel D, Playford RJ. Probiotics in inflammatory bowel disease: is it all gut flora modulation? Gut 2004; 53: 620–2.

82. Chapat L, Chemin K, Dubois B, Bourdet-Sicard R, Kaiserlian D. *Lactobacillus casei* reduces CD8(+) T cell-mediated skin inflammation. Eur J Immunol 2004; 34: 2520–8.

83. Asseman C, Powrie F. Interleukin 10 is a growth factor for a population of regulatory T cells. Gut 1998; 42: 157–8.

84. Sheil B, McCarthy J, O'Mahony L et al. Is the mucosal route of administration essential for probiotic function? Subcutaneous administration is associated with attenuation of murine colitis and arthritis. Gut 2004; 53: 694–700.

85. Sartor RB. Therapeutic manipulation of the enteric microflora in inflammatory bowel diseases: antibiotics, probiotics, and prebiotics. Gastroenterology 2004; 126: 1620–33.

Section IV – Early life programming of pain responsiveness

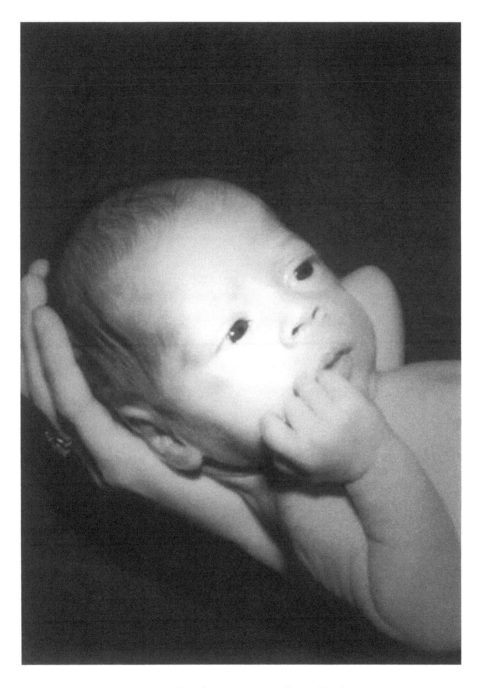

'Tomorrow lurks in us, the latency to be all that was not achieved before' Loren Eiseley

15

Long-term effects of repetitive pain in the neonatal period: neuronal vulnerability, imprinting, and plasticity

Kanwaljeet Singh Anand, Adnan T Bhutta, Richard W Hall, Cynthia R Rovnaghi, and Elie D Al-Chaer

Pain is an inseparable part of everyday life. It is universal, protective, and crucial for survival.
Pain can have profound deleterious and disruptive effects on the quality of life.

Menon, Anand, McIntosh, 1998[1]

INTRODUCTION

Each year, 300 000 neonates are admitted to neonatal intensive care units (NICUs) in the United States,[2] often subjected to hundreds of diagnostic and therapeutic procedures that are necessary for an improved survival.[3] The repetitive acute pain caused by invasive procedures, established pain resulting from neonatal surgery, and prolonged pain due to neonatal diseases or chronic conditions may contribute to the clinical complications or adverse neurological outcomes.[4-6] Follow-up studies of ex-preterm children and adolescents have reported major developmental deficits with lifetime needs for special assistance and increased health-care costs for early intervention and special education.[7] Persistent changes in pain processing, neuroendocrine function, and neurologic development may follow early repetitive pain and maternal separation, both routine occurrences in the NICU.[6,8] This chapter reviews the widespread effects of repetitive or prolonged pain on developmental changes in the brain during the prenatal, postnatal, infantile, or childhood periods in human infants and animal models, and speculates on their implications for adult behavior and health.

PAIN PROCESSING IN THE FETUS AND NEONATE: A BRIEF PRÉCIS

Following exposure to acute painful stimuli, newborn infants show changes in various physiological and behavioral parameters including stress hormone levels,[9-11] behavioral state,[11] cry features,[12] facial expressions,[13] altered sleep states, disorganized behavior, and decreased responses to developmentally supportive care.[14,15] These changes indicate a multi-layered response to pain, graded according to the intensity of the painful stimulus, and modulated by factors such as gestational immaturity, postnatal age, concurrent medications, and previous exposures to pain in preterm and term neonates.

The newborn rat as a model for human pain experience

Similarities in the pain system of newborn rodents and humans provide an animal model for characterizing the exaggerated dorsal cutaneous flexor reflexes,[16] properties of functional nociceptors,[17] sensitization caused by repeated noxious stimulation,[18] relatively large receptive fields of dorsal horn cells,[19] and immaturity of the descending inhibitory systems.[20-22] The expression of pain-related neurotransmitters in the spinal cord – e.g. substance P, calcitonin gene-related peptide (CGRP), vasoactive intestinal polypeptide (VIP) – follows a similar developmental blueprint in newborn rats and human neonates[23,24] and the patterns of supraspinal processing following acute pain also appear to be comparable.[25,26]

Behavioral responses

Behaviors associated with pain in neonates include facial expression, crying, gross motor movement, and changes in behavioral state and bodily functions (such as sleeping or eating patterns). The subjective state of the newborn before a pain stimulus occurs, their severity of illness, time since the previous painful procedure, and their cumulative exposure to pain are important determinants of the pattern of pain behavior, particularly in preterm neonates.[12,27,28] Determining if these behaviors are specific to pain versus other states such as fear, fatigue or hunger presents a challenge to researchers and clinicians.[29] Most methods of behavioral pain assessment in infants have focused on acute noxious events and the indicators tend to reflect the psycho-physiologic activation resulting from the event. Facial expressions, crying, and gross body movements all appear to be at peak amplitude in the immediate period following pain, thus easily incorporated into measurement schemes.

Facial activity is less variable and more consistent in infants than crying or body movements[30–32] and specific facial actions, including brow bulge, eye squeeze, nasolabial furrow and open lips are consistently associated with pain in preterm, full-term, and older infants.[13,27,33] Facial activity is the most reliable and consistent indicator of pain across all situations and populations.[29,34] Crying is an indicator that signals distress to care providers, mostly described in terms of its presence or absence, or in terms of its duration (cry latency, duration of expiratory or inspiratory cries, pause between cries, or rhythm of the crying), amplitude and/or pitch (the variability, melody pattern, harmonic structure, jitter, formants, bi-phonation, and spectral energy of its fundamental frequency).[13,35,36] Body movements are used as indicators of pain in older infants and toddlers using the Infant Body Coding System, but very preterm or sick infants may become limp and flaccid in response to noxious stimuli.[37–39] The flexion withdrawal reflex (FWR) is the distinct withdrawal of a limb evoked by pain (or elicited by Von Frey filaments). In adults, the threshold and amplitude of this reflex are linearly correlated with pain perception,[40] whereas in preterm and full-term neonates, the latency, amplitude, and duration of the FWR are correlated with the intensity of stimuli.[41,42] The FWR, evoked by stimuli of much lower intensity in neonates than in the adult, may serve as an indicator of somatic or visceral hyperalgesia (lower pain threshold) or allodynia (pain caused by non-noxious stimuli).[41–44]

Similarly, neonatal rat behavior mimics the typical responses observed in adult animals[45] in classical tests of nociception, such as the formalin test,[46] hot plate[47] and tail withdrawal tests,[48] or following stimulation with von Frey filaments.[49] Formalin injection into the hindlimb was followed by paw-lifting, paw-licking, and other recuperative behaviors in rats at P3, P7, and P10.[46,50,51] All studies have noted uniphasic response to formalin in neonatal rats (P0–P14), which lasts up to 60 minutes in the younger rats and 30 minutes in older rats.[50,51] The combination of paw flexion, shaking, and licking as well as kicking movements were specifically related to increases in formalin concentration,[52] whereas nonspecific behaviors decrease with advancing neonatal age.[51]

Cardiovascular changes

Autonomic responses in the human neonate lead to increased blood pressure, heart rate, respiratory rate, palmar sweating, desaturation episodes, and changes in intracranial pressure.[4,53] Blood pressure, heart rate, and respiratory rate changes have been documented during minor procedures such as heel lance, venipuncture and circumcisions, as well as during major surgery, and numerous studies documented an amelioration of these changes after local/topical anesthesia, sucrose or other interventions.[8,11,15,53,54] Correlation of cardiovascular changes with pain behavior in immature animals may give some insight into the development of autonomic responses in rat pups.[55] For example, neonatal rats subjected to the formalin test at postnatal (P) days 7, 14, and 21 showed significant increases in heart rate, as compared to saline-injected controls, but did not develop the typical biphasic response noted in adult rats until P35.[50]

Cellular responses

Until recently, it was difficult to study the cellular activation of supraspinal areas associated with pain processing in the human newborn, particularly if premature. Near-infrared spectroscopy (NIRS) and other neuroimaging techniques may define the neonatal patterns of supraspinal pain processing. NIRS monitoring in 40 preterm neonates (28–36 weeks) showed that regional cerebral blood flow (Hb O_2) increased bilaterally in the somatosensory cortex following unilateral tactile or painful stimuli (venipuncture), but not in other cortical areas such as the occipital cortex.[25] Pain-related cortical activation was more pronounced in male neonates, inversely correlated with gestational age (consistent with greater pain sensitivity at earlier gestational ages[56]) and directly correlated with postnatal age (suggesting greater hypersensitivity with continued exposure to painful procedures in the NICU[57]). Greater cortical responses were reported in awake neonates undergoing a heelstick procedure, as compared with neonates who were sleeping at the time of the heelstick procedure.[58] Accumulating data provide the first evidence that preterm neonates may be consciously aware of the painful experiences resulting from invasive procedures, laying to rest the controversy regarding conscious sensory perception in the neonate.[59]

In experimental animal models, the expression of Fos-like immunoreactivity in neurons has been used as an anatomical and functional measure. Mechanical (pinch), thermal (hot water immersion), or inflammatory stimuli (formalin injection) applied to the hindpaw of newborn rats on the day of birth, elicited Fos expression in dorsal horn cells, indicating the functioning of nociceptive primary afferents.[19] Cellular Fos expression increased linearly with the intensity of stimulation at an early age in the neonatal rat (P0, P1, P2, P3) and was greater than in P14 rats.[19] Similar data for supraspinal Fos expression, reported from our laboratory,[60] found specific patterns of neuronal activation at different postnatal ages. Nuclear Fos expression mostly occurred in the subcortical areas (thalamus, hypothalamus, amygdalar nuclei, and piriform cortex) in the rat pups at P1 and P7, with a shift to cortical activation in P14 rats. Following a unilateral stimulus, a bilateral cellular response was noted at all ages in the neonatal period. In the P14 rats, robust neuronal activation occurred in areas/nuclei associated with emotional regulation (amygdaloid complex, hippocampus, piriform cortex), sensory processing (somatosensory cortex, other cortical areas), and neuroendocrine regulation (hypothalamus, hippocampus). These data described the ontogeny of the cellular responses to pain in neonatal and infant rats.[26]

Increased pain sensitivity in neonates

The traditional view that neonates are relatively insensitive to pain was refuted more than a decade ago.[61] Comparative studies of human infants and rat pups found that thresholds for the dorsal cutaneous withdrawal reflex increase progressively in preterm neonates and postnatal rat pups, suggesting lower pain thresholds during early development.[16,56] Multiple other studies demonstrated that the intensity and duration of pain responses are developmentally regulated in the neonatal period, across different types of stimuli: foot-shock,[62] inflammatory,[50–52,62] mechanical[41] or thermal[48,63] stimuli, showing lower pain thresholds in the younger rats.

EPIDEMIOLOGY OF PAIN IN EARLY LIFE

Despite the current knowledge that preterm and full-term infants are capable of experiencing pain, many invasive procedures are still performed without the use of pharmacological or nonpharmacological analgesic therapy.[3] Table 15.1 shows some of the recent epidemiological data, indicating that large numbers of

Table 15.1 Studies investigating the number of invasive procedures performed in the neonatal intensive care unit (NICU)

References	Duration of study	Sample size	Total number of procedures	Average number of procedures	Most frequent procedures
Barker & Rutter, 1995[64]	Total NICU stay	54	3283	60.8 per patient	Heelstick (56%)
Johnston et al., 1997[65]	7 days of NICU stay	239	2134	2–10 per patient per day	Heelstick (61%)
Porter & Anand, 1998[66]	Total NICU stay	144	7672	53.3 per patient	Heelstick (87%)
Benis & Suresh, 2001[67]	Total NICU stay	15	5663	6 per patient per day	Suctioning (51%)
Simons et al., 2003[3]	First 14 days in NICU	151	19 674	14 per patient per day	Suctioning (64%)

invasive procedures are performed on newborns admitted to NICUs in several different countries.[3,64-67]

Many neonates are exposed to 6–14 painful procedures per day and it is remarkable that most of these procedures are performed without appropriate analgesic therapy.[3,65] Simons et al. reported a higher number of painful procedures compared with previous studies, because they recorded a more extensive list of procedures. They also accounted for failed procedures, and studied infants during their first 14 days in the NICU, which is likely to be the period of critical illness.[3] Barker and Rutter first reported a higher number of procedures in preterm neonates born at less than 31 weeks of gestation as compared with older infants,[64] whereas Simons et al. alluded that an increased frequency of procedures per day was probably related to their severity of illness rather than the gestational age.[3]

As described below, the risk and severity of long-term changes increases with the duration of admission to the NICU in these neonates, which may be a consequence of the degree of prematurity, or severity of illness, or the cumulative exposure to acute pain resulting from invasive procedures, prolonged postoperative pain or inflammatory pain, or the pain/discomfort related to their disease states.

LONG-TERM EFFECTS OF REPETITIVE PAIN

Subsequent pain processing in the human

Multiple lines of evidence indicate that the long-term effects of tissue injury or inflammation in the neonatal period[68] are associated with *hyperalgesia* (increased perception of noxious stimuli) and *allodynia* (pain caused by a stimulus not normally associated with pain), which result from peripheral sensitization of nociceptors, wind-up and central sensitization in spinal areas,[69] and altered processing in supraspinal areas.[70,71] For example, thresholds for the cutaneous flexor reflex in preterm neonates were 50% lower in the heel exposed to heelsticks than in the undamaged contralateral heel.[16]

Neuronal activity results in the maturation, proliferation, and stabilization of various cortical processes, whereas inactivity may lead to developmentally regulated apoptosis in the immature brain. These developmental patterns are refined by activity-dependent mechanisms leading to the differentiation and specialization of neurons, matching axonal processes with target cells, and other maturational events.[18,72,73] *Plasticity* is the process of fine-tuning brain development via activity-dependent mechanisms.[72] The combination of increased sensitivity to pain and greater plasticity of the developing brain make it vulnerable to long-term alterations resulting from repetitive pain in early life and this vulnerability appears to be greatest in the postnatal period.[74] For example, healthy, term neonates exposed to gastric suctioning at birth were three times more likely to develop functional gastrointestinal symptoms like irritable bowel syndrome than their matched siblings.[74]

Increasing degrees of tissue damage cause acute pain, which is followed by primary and secondary hyperalgesia that decrease pain thresholds in the injured area and areas surrounding the damaged tissue.[4,18,73,75] Repeated sub-threshold (or even innocuous) stimuli in neonates may elicit a 'wind-up' phenomenon with an increased excitability of the neurons within the dermatomes supplied by spinal cord segments above and below the area of stimulation or tissue damage.[69] Significantly, preterm neonates before 34 weeks gestation lack the ability to modulate pain, progressively lowering their thresholds to pain occurring with repeated stimulation.[42,76]

Repeated heelsticks, one of the most common procedures performed in the NICU, results in hyperalgesic responses to subsequent stimuli, possibly mediated by the peripheral sensitization, exuberant outgrowth of nerve fibers supplying the injured area, increased expression of afferent nociceptors, and increased excitability of afferent nerve fibers. The ensuing inflammation may cause central sensitization as a result of increased excitability of the spinal cord neurons. Topical anesthesia may alleviate some, but not all, of the adverse effects of repetitive heel sticks, which has worrisome clinical implications.[18] Hyperalgesia was also noted in infants of diabetic mothers who were exposed to repeated heelsticks as compared with uninjured controls.[77] Later in infancy, Taddio et al. showed that term neonates exposed to unanesthetized circumcision at birth had exaggerated responses to immunization pain at 4–6 months of age versus their treated controls.[78]

As noted above, long-term memory appears to be functioning even in preterm neonates. Long-term memory is only possible with the functional integrity of the hippocampus, limbic system, and other parts of the diencephalon. At a cellular level, the glutamatergic and opioidergic receptors and neurotransmitters, as well as long-term potentiation and depression of cellular responses to environmental stimuli, must be in place for long-term memory. All these systems are active in preterm neonates as early as 25–26 weeks gestation.[4] Noxious stimuli are probably retained in the subconscious rather than the conscious memory. Nevertheless, it is clear that human neonates exposed to early postnatal pain show altered behavioral responses to subsequent pain.

Beyond infancy, clinical evidence for altered pain systems is somewhat indirect. Parent reports, however, indicated that 18-month old ex-preterm toddlers with birth weights between 480 and 1000 grams were less reactive to commonplace, everyday pain than matched groups of toddlers born either later in gestation or at full term.[79] Ex-preterm children at 4–5 years of age also seemed to have a higher incidence of unexplained somatic complaints (somatization) compared to term-born controls,[80] and this was clinically abnormal in approximately 25% of ex-preterm children. Additional research showed that ex-preterm children at 8–10 years of age rated the pictures of painful events, such as a child being hit with a baseball, as higher in intensity than their term born counterparts.[81] The increases in pain intensity ratings and increased affective responses were directly proportional to the duration of their NICU stay.[81] Thus, pain in the neonatal period may lead to alterations in neuronal pathways, leading to changes in pain processing during infancy and childhood.

Subsequent pain processing in animal models

Tissue injury or inflammation in the early neonatal period causes profound and long-lasting changes in the pain thresholds and subsequent patterns of pain processing.[5] Although there are some discrepancies in the long-term consequences of pain, produced by using different animal models of neonatal pain,[82] the consensus is that early periods of development are especially vulnerable to the long-term effects of brief or repetitive pain exposures.

When neonatal rat pups were stimulated four times each day from P0 to P7 with either needle pricks or tactile stimuli, decreased pain latencies were noted at P16 and P22 in the rats exposed to acute pain in the neonatal period, indicating effects of repetitive neonatal pain on subsequent development of the pain system, although no significant differences occurred in the adult rats.[47] Surgical injury, with removal of small piece of skin, was followed by robust sprouting of the local sensory nerve terminals resulting in cutaneous hyperinnervation that lasted into adulthood.[83] This response was more pronounced when it occurred at birth in newborn rats as compared with older ages and continued to mediate a heightened sensitivity to pain even into adulthood.[83] Another study showed that, in infant rats exposed to a brief period of inflammation just after birth, the receptive field (areas of skin) supplied by individual dorsal horn neurons was

decreased by >30% in adulthood,[84] implying permanent alterations in the spinal pain processing for these areas.

A model using repetitive inflammatory pain in neonatal rats on P1–P7, showed a significant hypoalgesia in adult rats exposed to neonatal inflammatory pain.[85] Using a similar paradigm, Lidow et al. reported that a short-lasting inflammation of the neonatal rat hind paw was associated with baseline hypoalgesia and exacerbated hyperalgesia after reinflammation of that hind paw in the adult.[86] Subsequent experiments tested the effects of neonatal hind paw inflammation at P3 or P14 on the visceral and somatic pain sensitivity in adult rats. In P3-treated rats, a greater degree of inhibitory processing of somatic and visceral stimuli during adulthood but no long-term consequences were noted in the P14-treated rats.[87] However, inflammation in the adult rat in previously uninjured tissue reversed the relative hypoalgesia resulting from neonatal inflammation and evoked the normal hyperexcitability associated with tissue injury.[87]

In a rat model of short-lasting local inflammation (produced by injection of 0.25% carageenan), the long-term hypoalgesia at baseline occurred equally in the previously injured and uninjured paws,[88] which suggested centrally mediated mechanisms.[71,84] Long-term hyperalgesia occurred in the neonatally-injured paw after re-inflammation, indicating a significant segmental involvement in the spinal processing of pain.[88] The critical window for generation of both these long-term effects (global hypoalgesia and segmental hyperalgesia) occurred within the first postnatal week in newborn rats and they were also detectable in 120–125-day-old rats.[88] A clinically relevant model employed a laparotomy under cold anesthesia on the day of birth, followed by morphine analgesia postoperatively (or a saline control) in mouse pups. Laparotomy produced increased distress ultrasonic vocalizations, but did not change maternal care for these pups. In adulthood, various tests for nociceptive sensitivity showed that neonatal surgery decreased pain behavior relative to the control groups, and this effect was reversed by postoperative morphine treatment in the neonatal period.[89]

Accumulating clinical and experimental data, therefore, point to a global, centrally mediated, hypoalgesia that is noted during adulthood following exposure to prolonged or repetitive neonatal pain. It is likely that these effects may be associated with long-term changes in stress responsiveness and autonomic regulation.

Biobehavioral stress responses

Other chapters in this volume have described the long-term alterations in stress response systems following exposure to maternal separation or other adverse conditions before or just after birth. Repeated exposures to painful stimuli in the NICU have also been implicated in altered biobehavioral responses of preterm neonates to acute heelstick pain at 32 weeks of gestation.

Preterm infants who had spent gestational weeks 28 through 32 in the NICU were less mature in their pain responses to heelsticks than preterm infants born at 32 weeks gestation: the earlier-born infants had less behavioral manifestations of acute pain than the later-born infants. The number of invasive procedures was the primary factor that explained these behavioral differences, whereas physiological differences were explained by the perinatal factors of gestational age at birth and birth weight.[90] In another study, the most significant factors associated with altered behavioral and autonomic pain reactivity at 32 weeks of postconceptional age were a greater number of previous invasive procedures since birth and the gestational age at birth, both of which were correlated with a dampened response to heelstick pain (lower behavioral and sympathetic reactivity).[91] After controlling for severity of illness and other perinatal factors, previous exposure to morphine analgesia was associated with 'normalized' (i.e. increased) rather than diminished autonomic and behavioral responses to heelstick pain.[91]

Alterations in physiologic and behavioral response to acute pain were also reported by Oberlander et al., who found that 4-month-old infants with birth weights <801 grams seemed to have a less intense parasympathetic withdrawal in the lance period and a more sustained sympathetic response during recovery than the control group.[92] During the recovery period, two behavioral patterns associated with early recovery and late recovery emerged among the ex-preterm infants at 4 months,[92] but were not apparent at 8 months of age.[93] The same investigators reported that preterm infants (<28 weeks gestational age) have a higher basal and sustained cortisol levels after visual stimulation with novel toys at 8 months of age in comparison with less premature (28–32 weeks gestation) and term infants.[94] After controlling for early illness severity and the duration of supplemental oxygen, the higher baseline cortisol levels were associated with a higher number of neonatal skin breaking procedures (e.g. heel lancing).[94] Thus, it is likely that exposure to repetitive pain in preterm infants alters the regulation of their pain/stress processing mechanisms during later infancy. This finding has enormous implications for hippocampal development as well as their vulnerability to stress-related disorders during later childhood, adolescence, and adult life.[95,96]

Exposure to repetitive acute pain in neonatal rats, however, did not alter subsequent stress responses mediated via the hypothalamic-pituitary-adrenal (HPA) axis.[47] Subsequent experiments by Walker et al. showed that exposure to repeated pain in newborn rat pups was associated with increased maternal pup grooming on day 6 of life. Thus, increased maternal grooming might act as a buffer against the cumulative effect of pain on stress responsiveness, preventing the long-term changes in HPA axis regulation, as measured by ACTH and corticosterone responses under basal or stimulated conditions.[97] It remains to be seen whether kangaroo care or skin-to-skin contact with the mother, which prevents the biobehavioral responses to acute pain in preterm and term neonates,[98,99] would similarly prevent the long-term changes in stress responsiveness of the HPA axis or the autonomic system in humans.[94,100]

Other behavioral changes

Repetitive pain leaves a legacy of widespread changes in the neonatal brain that are accentuated in preterm neonates. Infants exposed to repetitive pain exhibit sleeplessness and sudden or maladaptive behavioral state changes. In addition, they spend less time in the quiet alert state when they are able to absorb more information from their environment or interact with their caregivers.[13,101,102] Too much stimulation, which occurs with repetitive pain in the NICU, also results in increased excitotoxicity leading to neuronal cell death and can cause permanent alterations in brain development.[5] Thus, cortical development is vulnerable to aberrations in postnatal activity and can be permanently affected by acute, chronic, or repetitive pain and stress.

Many children born prematurely are noted to have 'minor' deficits in cognition, learning disorders, attentional disorders, behavioral problems, and motor abnormalities. Deficits commonly seen in children born preterm include impulsivity, inability to cope with novel situations, poor adaptive behavior, and specific learning deficits.[7,103] When neonates weighing <1000 grams with normal intelligence are compared to term-born normal weight controls, they show major differences in higher order executive functions of attention, planning, and problem solving.[104] Sociodemographic factors may often modify some, but not all, of these factors. For example, language, depressive tendencies, and IQ testing are more related to maternal factors while visual-spatial abilities and anxiety are more related to neonatal factors.[105] The acute changes in cerebral blood flow in preterm infants with impaired autoregulation predispose neonates to intraventricular hemorrhage (IVH) as well as neuronal cell loss and white matter injury. These aberrations are likely responsible for a wide range of subclinical brain alterations including the learning and behavioral problems associated with extreme prematurity.[106]

There is a growing body of literature which establishes the role of repetitive neonatal pain as a cause of change in adult behavior in animal models. These behavioral changes may be attributable to long-term effects on the supraspinal processing of pain or altered stress responses. Adult rats exhibit increased preference to alcohol, greater anxiety and defensive withdrawal behavior, prolonged chemosensory memory, and diminished activation of the somatosensory cortex by thermal pain following exposure to repeated needlesticks in the neonatal period.[47] These changes suggested a change in the supraspinal processing of pain as a result of the neonatal pain experience. Although a growing body of literature establishes the role of supraspinal processing of painful stimuli, the long-term effects of pain on the development of these brain regions are less well understood. Pain in adult rats induced by intraspinal injection of quisqualic acid (an AMPA/mGluR1 agonist) resulted in increased regional cerebral blood flow (rCBF) measured 24–41 days after injection in several forebrain regions, the limbic system, the thalamus and the somatosensory cortex.[107] Similar changes during critical windows in development would be expected to cause major changes in brain development.

In an animal model looking at the effects of inflammatory pain, neonatal rat pups were exposed to repeated formalin injections from P1 to P7. The rats exhibited decreased alcohol preference and reduced locomotor activity, suggesting that plasticity of the neonatal brain may be causing permanent changes in spinal cord or brain development leading to these behavioral changes.[85] Other investigators have used complete Freund's adjuvant (CFA), which produces intense inflammation and lasts for a relatively prolonged period. Using this model, Ruda et al. showed that, as adults, these animals exhibited spinal neuronal circuits with increased input and segmental changes in nociceptive primary afferent axons and altered responses to sensory stimulation.[108] This group also showed that the dorsal horn neurons in rats treated with CFA in the neonatal period showed increased activity in response to both innocuous and noxious stimuli and that the receptive field was significantly larger in the treated group as compared with the controls.[109] Other investigators have used carrageenan as an inflammatory agent which induces less

inflammation than CFA, and for a shorter duration. These investigators have demonstrated that adult animals injected with carrageenan as neonates show decreased sensitivity to thermal and mechanical stimuli.[86]

Widespread changes in behavioral and neuromotor functions imply that the long-term effects of repetitive or prolonged neonatal pain may be pervasive to all parts of the brain. A greater vulnerability to neuronal cell death occurs in the hippocampal and other areas associated with memory, learning, and cognitive processing;[75] therefore, the study of cognitive and executive functions following neonatal pain/stress is particularly important.

Cognitive functions

The long-term cognitive effects of early pain remain unclear because of the difficulty of differentiating long-term effects of acute and chronic pain on a child from other neonatal stressors such as sepsis, hypoglycemia, hypoxia, poor nutrition, and immature brain at birth. We know that preterm infants (<37 weeks) are at risk for lower cognitive scores (10.9 IQ points lower) compared with full-term controls at school age even in the absence of gross mental retardation.[7] The lower cognitive scores are directly proportional to the gestational age and birth weight (i.e. the lower the gestational age and birth weight, the lower the mean IQ score) even after controlling for demographic and socio-economic factors. These children are also at increased risk for behavioral problems including an almost three-fold risk of being diagnosed with attention deficit hyperactivity disorder (ADHD). Kilbride et al. compared preschool cognitive outcomes of extremely low birthweight (ELBW) (<800 grams) children with their term siblings and found them to have a 10 point lower mean score on tests of cognition, lower academic achievement test scores, and decreased language and motor skills.[109] This study suggests that even if the environment remains similar after birth, the biological events occurring in the perinatal period are major determinants of long-term complications.

The etiology of this cognitive decline and behavioral problems is hypothesized to be related to neonatal stressors leading to neuronal injury and death via excitotoxic and apoptotic mechanisms.[103] Cell death may in turn lead to magnetic resonance imaging (MRI) findings, such as loss of cortical gray and white matter volume, and this loss of brain volume correlates with decreased cognitive assessment scores and altered behaviors.[111,112] In addition to these structural abnormalities, there is also evidence to suggest that there is a long-term abnormality in brain function.

Peterson et al. compared brain activity in preterm and term children, associated with the phonologic and semantic processing of language, using functional MRI and found that preterm children with the poorest language skills did not engage normal semantic processing pathways in a language comprehension task. Instead these children engaged pathways that normal term children used to process meaningless phonologic sounds.[113] This abnormal language processing may explain the lower verbal IQ and learning disabilities commonly noted in school-aged children who were born preterm.

Visceral pain

The accumulating clinical and experimental evidence indicates that repetitive exposures to painful stimuli in the early postnatal period can alter the physiological and behavioral profile of the adult and may lead to intractable chronic disorders. To study the effect of neonatal peripheral irritation on structural and functional outcomes in adults, we exposed newborn rat pups to nociceptive or inflammatory treatments and followed their development. Working with this animal model, our group provided for the first time physical evidence that pain and inflammation in newborns alters the development of sensory pathways circuitry, causing a stronger response to pain in adulthood. We found that adult rats exposed to neonatal colon pain exhibit a hypersensitivity to colon and somatic stimuli, central and peripheral neural sensitization in addition to other functional changes in colon motility, sensory pathways, exploratory activity, and responses to stress. In a study on adult rats that received high intensity colorectal distention (CRD) or colon inflammation during pre-adolescence, residual visceral and somatic hypersensitivity were documented beyond the age of 4 months – long after the initial injury had resolved.[114] This hypersensitivity was associated with central and peripheral neural sensitization[115] and functional changes in pain processing pathways;[116] for example, changes in the role of the dorsal column (DC) of the spinal cord.[117] In addition, a shift in the role of the thalamus was observed between rats with neonatal colon pain and controls. The ventrobasal nuclear complex (VBC) of the thalamus is a major sensory relay for somatic and visceral pain. Thalamic stimulation in the region of the VBC is known to cause inhibition of nociceptive neuronal responses in the dorsal horn under normal conditions;[118] however, in adult rats exposed to neonatal colon pain, thalamic stimulation had largely a facilitatory effect.[118] In addition to viscerosomatic hypersensitivity and neurophysiological plasticity, adult rats exposed to neonatal colon pain showed changes in metabolic outcomes characterized mainly by disturbances in colon motility and changes in fecal output.[114] These symptoms were observed in the absence of colon inflammation. When combined, these observations mimic to a large extent the symptoms commonly seen in patients with irritable bowel syndrome (IBS). In fact, a recent study concluded that noxious stimulation caused by gastric suction at birth may promote the development of long-term visceral hypersensitivity and cognitive hypervigilance, leading to an increased prevalence of functional intestinal disorders in later life.[74]

On the other hand, a decrease in exploratory activity was also seen in adults rats exposed to neonatal colon pain. These rats confined themselves to a limited area of an open field. The decrease in exploratory activity was aggravated by stress.[119] In general, voluntary exploratory behavior of animals in a new environment may be used as a measure of discomfort that may be associated with ongoing pain,[120] distress and anxiety,[121] socio-sexual behavior,[122] or adaptation to or fear of leaving a familiar place, clinically known as agoraphobia, often a symptom comorbid with IBS. These symptoms were studied in male and female rats at different stages of the estrus cycle and early results indicate a differential outcome in males and females with female rats showing more sensitivity to nociceptive stimuli, particularly when their circulating levels of estrogen are elevated.

Other groups have also looked at the effect of subjecting rat neonates to somatic pain or the stress of maternal separation and found that as adults, these animals exhibited increased input and segmental changes in nociceptive primary afferent axons and spinal neural circuits as well as altered responses to sensory stimulation.[86,107,123] Such investigations substantiate a long-lasting belief in the impact of postnatal events on the neural processing of sensory information. This effect includes alterations in the afferent pathways, hyperexcitability or sensitization of the receptive neurons, and possibly a shift in the dynamics of sensory channels and descending controls, which in turn determines the visceral sensitivity of the adult organism and predisposes to chronic visceral pain.

CLINICAL IMPLICATIONS

Confounding variables

Interpreting human data from the NICU is fraught with difficulty because life in the NICU is supported by a thread of artificial technology that is accompanied by pain, stressors, and many other events. Life-saving procedures such as mechanical ventilation, intravenous hyperalimentation, and monitors come with a price of chronic and acute repetitive pain, noise, light, inadequate nutrition, and maternal anxiety and separation.[124]

There are three problems with conducting pain research in human neonates. First, there is an understandable reluctance due to ethical and humane concerns to have a pure placebo group when dealing with neonatal pain. In the recently completed NEOPAIN trial, 242 of 444 patients (55%) randomized to the placebo arm of the study received additional analgesia, which made interpretation difficult.[125]

Next, it is almost impossible to separate pain from other stressors in the NICU. Patients who are subjected to the most pain are the most immature and have the highest acuity, subjecting them to more stress in other areas. Noise has been difficult to control in the NICU environment and frequently reaches levels up to 105 decibels.[126] Like pain, noise causes marked changes in autonomic response[127] as well as EEG changes[128] that are different in preterm versus term infants (see Figure 15.1). Light causes changes in mela-

tonin and it can elicit changes in oxygen saturation.[129] Inadequate nutrition is a common cause for stress in the NICU and like pain can affect brain growth and cell death in the preterm infant.[130–132] Maternal separation increases glucocorticoid activity and subsequent excitatory cell death and is all too common in the NICU environment.[75,133,134] Finally, hypothyroxinemia of prematurity affects axon and dendrite formation, which is also found in animal models for pain.[135]

Finally, the long-term effects of repetitive pain are most likely to manifest in neurological aberrations or behavioral disorders that have variable and unique effects during the different phases of childhood development. Some conditions, such as attention deficit disorder,[104] may remain throughout the period of development and into adulthood. Most long-term consequences of neonatal pain during adulthood are not as easily testable and would require long-term follow-up studies. Further, atypical behaviors and other outcomes are likely to be affected by numerous factors such as gender, race, parenting styles, peer pressure, cultural milieu, and socioeconomic factors that must be adjusted in statistical modeling to determine the effects of pain without contamination from other

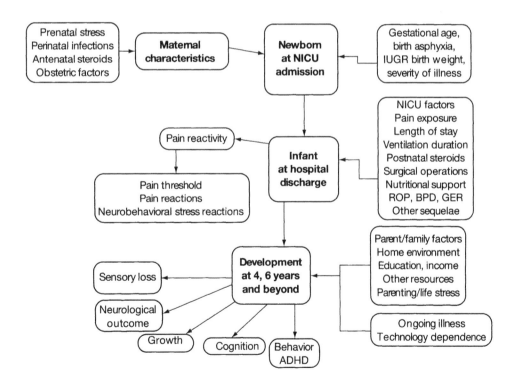

Figure 15.1 A simple model proposed to explain the sequential effects of perinatal and postnatal factors on the development of ex-preterm children. IUGR, intrauterine growth retardation; NICU, neonatal intensive care unit; ROP, retinopathy of prematurity; BPD, bronchopulmonary dysplasia; GER, gastroesophageal reflux.

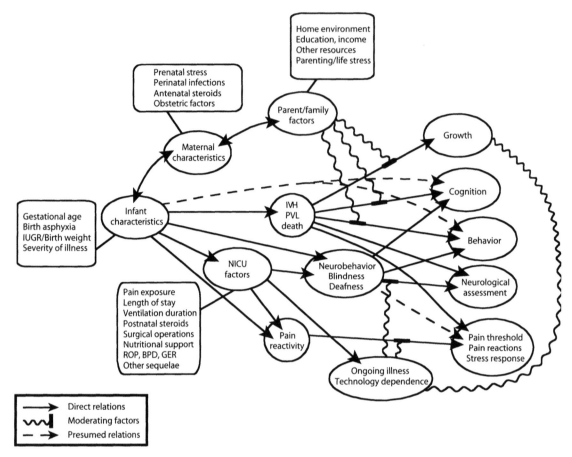

Figure 15.2 Hierarchical model showing the sequential impact of clinical, familial, and environmental factors on the developmental outcomes measured in this project. IUGR, intrauterine growth retardation; NICU, neonatal intensive care unit; IVH, intraventricular hemorrhage; PVL, periventricular leukomalacia, ROP, retinopathy of prematurity; BPD, bronchopulmonary dysplasia; GER, gastroesophageal reflux.

moderating variables. The ability to solve these problems requires long-term follow-up, which is time-consuming, expensive, and requires high follow-up rates that are difficult to achieve in the United States. Nevertheless, the potential difficulties associated with untreated repetitive pain mandate a firm research commitment.

For this research to be successful, some conceptual models are required for a starting point, based on well-established covariates and statistical correlations from early infancy data. Some of these preliminary and hypothetical models are described in the next section as an exemplary framework for further research.

Hypothetical models

Children do not develop in a vacuum, therefore, the long-term effects of repetitive neonatal pain or stress

need to be investigated in a comprehensive manner, where long-term testing will include an assessment of the home environment, quality of parenting, and other confounding or mediating factors. Studies focused on cognitive or behavioral outcomes should include detailed assessments of (a) executive functions, (b) academic skills, (c) intellectual abilities, and (d) visual-motor integration, as well as information from parents/caregivers about functional independence (self-care, mobility, and cognition), everyday behaviors related to executive functions, and a broad screening of other behaviors. Data collection must also include mediating variables such as anthropometric measurements, clinical history, and neurological examination, in addition to the relevant perinatal and postnatal data. Definition of confounding factors may be obtained by a detailed interim history, home screening, parent intelligence, an assessment of life stressors and the social resources available to parents. Despite the critical importance of early development in ex-preterm children, there is a paucity of published data on the evaluation of ex-preterm children using these innovative methods. Hierarchical models must be developed to link the individual factors at various developmental stages (fetus, neonate, infant) to the long-term outcomes.

Another example of a relatively complex model is presented in Figure 15.2, which shows the sequential interplay of proximal clinical and environmental factors leading to intermediate and distal outcomes, while accounting for the distinct effects of direct correlations, moderating factors, and confounding variables.

SUMMARY

Neonates definitely respond to pain both acutely and chronically. Preterm infants are more vulnerable than their term-born counterparts because 1) pain is 'developmentally unexpected' in this population, 2) there is greater brain plasticity associated with epochal changes occurring in brain development in this developmental period, and 3) their life support and illnesses may require multiple exposures to pain and stress. Animal and human data unequivocally indicate a significant long-term impact of acute and repetitive neonatal pain. The mechanisms of these long-term changes may be defined using animal models,[82,136] but ascertaining their wide-ranging impact on behaviors, cognitive or executive functions, or later disease vulnerability will require the design and careful analysis of epidemiological and prospective follow-up studies in humans.[137–140]

REFERENCES

1. Menon G, Anand KJS, McIntosh N. Practical approach to analgesia and sedation in the neonatal intensive care unit. Semin Perinatol 1998; 22: 417–24.
2. Hoyert DL, Freedman MA, Strobino DM, Guyer B. Annual summary of vital statistics: 2000. Pediatrics 2001; 108: 1241–55.
3. Simons SHP, van Dijk M, Anand KJS et al. Do we still hurt newborn babies? A prospective study of procedural pain and analgesia in neonates. Arch Pediatr Adolesc Med 2003; 157: 1058–64.
4. Anand KJS, Hickey PR. Special Article: Pain and its effects in the human neonate and fetus. N Engl J Med 1987; 317: 1321–9.
5. Anand KJS. Pain, plasticity, and premature birth: a prescription for permanent suffering? Nat Med 2000; 6: 971–3.
6. Bhutta AT, Cleves MA, Casey PH, Cradock MM, Anand KJS. Cognitive and behavioral outcomes of school-aged children who were born preterm: a meta-analysis. JAMA 2002; 288: 728–37.
7. Bhutta AT, Anand KJS. Vulnerability of the developing brain: neuronal mechanisms. Clin Perinatol 2002; 29: 357–72.
8. Simons SHP, van Dijk M, van Lingen RA et al. Routine morphine infusion in preterm newborns who received ventilatory support: a randomized controlled trial. JAMA 2003; 290: 2419–27.
9. Anand KJS, Brown MJ, Causon RC et al. Can the human neonate mount an endocrine and metabolic response to surgery? J Pediatr Surg 1985; 20: 41–8.
10. Anand KJS, Hansen DD, Hickey PR. Hormonal-metabolic stress responses in neonates undergoing cardiac surgery. Anesthesiology 1990; 73: 661–70.
11. Guinsburg R, Kopelman BI, Anand KJS et al. Physiological, hormonal, and behavioral responses to a single fentanyl dose in intubated and ventilated preterm neonates. J Pediatr 1998; 132: 954–9.
12. Johnston CC, Stevens BJ, Franck LS et al. Factors explaining lack of response to heel stick in preterm newborns. J Obstet Gynecol Neonatal Nurs 1999; 28: 587–94.
13. Grunau RV, Johnston CC, Craig KD. Neonatal facial and cry responses to invasive and non-invasive procedures. Pain 1990; 42: 295–305.
14. Holsti L, Grunau RE, Oberlander TF, Whitfield MF. Specific Newborn Individualized Developmental Care and Assessment Program movements are associated with acute pain in preterm infants in the neonatal intensive care unit. Pediatrics 2004; 114: 65–72.
15. Whitfield MF, Grunau RE. Behavior, pain perception, and the extremely low-birth weight survivor. Clin Perinatol 2000; 27: 363–79.
16. Fitzgerald M, Shaw A, MacIntosh N. The postnatal development of the cutaneous flexor reflex: a comparative study in premature infants and newborn rat pups. Dev Med Child Neurol 1988; 30: 520–6.
17. Fitzgerald M. Spontaneous and evoked activity of foetal primary afferents 'in vivo'. Nature 1987; 326: 603–5.
18. Fitzgerald M, Millard C, McIntosh N. Cutaneous hypersensitivity following peripheral tissue damage in newborn infants and its reversal with topical anaesthesia. Pain 1989; 39: 31–6.
19. Yi DK, Barr GA. The induction of fos-like immunoreactivity by noxious thermal, mechanical and chemical stimuli in the lumbar spinal cord of infant rats. Pain 1995; 60: 257–65.
20. Boucher T, Jennings E, Fitzgerald M. The onset of diffuse noxious inhibitory controls in postnatal rat pups: a C-Fos study. Neurosci Lett 1998; 257: 9–12.
21. Ren K, Blass EM, Zhou Q, Dubner R. Suckling and sucrose ingestion suppress persistent hyperalgesia and spinal Fos expression after forepaw inflammation in infant rats. Proc Natl Acad Sci USA 1997; 94: 1471–5.
22. Fitzgerald M, Koltzenburg M. The functional development of descending inhibitory pathways in the dorsolateral funiculus of the newborn rat spinal cord. Brain Res 1986; 389: 261–70.
23. Anand KJS. Physiology of pain in infants and children. Annales Nestle 1999; 57: 7–18.
24. Marti E, Gibson SJ, Polak JM et al. Ontogeny of peptide- and amine-containing neurones in motor, sensory and autonomic regions of rat and human spinal cord, dorsal root ganglia and rat skin. J Comp Neurol 1987; 266: 332–59.
25. Bartocci M, Bergqvist LL, Lagercrantz H, Anand KJS. Pain activates cortical areas in the preterm newborn brain. Pain 2005 (under review).
26. Narsinghani U, Anand KJS. Developmental neurobiology of pain in neonatal rats. Lab Anim 2000; 29: 27–39.

27. Johnston CC, Stevens B, Craig KD, Grunau RV. Developmental changes in pain expression in premature, full-term, two- and four-month-old infants. Pain 1993; 52: 201–8.

28. Hadjistavropoulos HD, Craig KD, Grunau RV, Johnston CC. Judging pain in newborns: facial and cry determinants. J Pediatr Psychol 1994; 19: 485–91.

29. Craig KD, Whitfield MF, Grunau RV, Linton J, Hadjistavropoulos HD. Pain in the preterm neonate: behavioural and physiological indices. Pain 1993; 52: 287–99.

30. Johnston CC, Strada ME. Acute pain response in infants: a multidimensional description. Pain 1986; 24: 373–82.

31. Guinsburg R, Kopelman BI, Anand KJS et al. Physiological, hormonal, and behavioral responses to a single fentanyl dose in intubated and ventilated preterm neonates. J Pediatr 1998; 132: 954–9.

32. Pereira AL, Guinsburg R, de Almeida MF et al. Validity of behavioral and physiologic parameters for acute pain assessment of term newborn infants. Rev Paul Med 1999; 117: 72–80.

33. Rushforth JA, Levene MI. Behavioural response to pain in healthy neonates. Arch Dis Child Fetal Neonatal Ed 1994; 70: F174–6.

34. Grunau RV, Craig KD. Pain expression in neonates: facial action and cry. Pain 1987; 28: 395–410.

35. Porter FL, Miller RH, Marshall RE. Neonatal pain cries: effect of circumcision on acoustic features and perceived urgency. Child Dev 1986; 57: 790–802.

36. Fuller BF, Conner DA. The effect of pain on infant behaviors. Clin Nurs Res 1995; 4: 253–73.

37. Hadjistavropoulos HD, Craig KD, Grunau RE, Whitfield MF. Judging pain in infants: behavioural, contextual, and developmental determinants. Pain 1997; 73: 319–24.

38. Grunau RE, Holsti L, Whitfield MF, Ling E. Are twitches, startles, and body movements pain indicators in extremely low birth weight infants? Clin J Pain 2000; 16: 37–45.

39. Morison SJ, Holsti L, Grunau RE et al. Are there developmentally distinct motor indicators of pain in preterm infants? Early Hum Dev 2003; 72: 131–46.

40. Willer JC, Bergeret S, Gaudy JH. Epidural morphine strongly depresses nociceptive flexion reflexes in patients with postoperative pain. Anesthesiology 1985; 63: 675–80.

41. Andrews K, Fitzgerald M. The cutaneous withdrawal reflex in human neonates: sensitisation, receptive fields and the effects of contralateral stimulation. Pain 1994; 56: 95–101.

42. Andrews K, Fitzgerald M. Cutaneous flexion reflex in human neonates: a quantitative study of threshold and stimulus-response characteristics after single and repeated stimuli. Dev Med Child Neurol 1999; 41: 696–703.

43. Andrews K, Fitzgerald M. Wound sensitivity as a measure of analgesic effects following surgery in human neonates and infants. Pain 2002; 99: 185–95.

44. Andrews KA, Desai D, Dhillon HK, Wilcox DT, Fitzgerald M. Abdominal sensitivity in the first year of life: comparison of infants with and without prenatally diagnosed unilateral hydronephrosis. Pain 2002; 100: 35–46.

45. Abbott FV, Franklin KB, Westbrook RF. The formalin test: scoring properties of the first and second phases of the pain response in rats. Pain 1995; 60: 91–102.

46. McLaughlin CR, Lichtman AH, Fanselow MS, Cramer CP. Tonic nociception in neonatal rats. Pharmacol Biochem Behav 1990; 36: 859–62.

47. Anand KJS, Coskun V, Thrivikraman KV, Nemeroff CB, Plotsky PM. Long-term behavioral effects of repetitive pain in neonatal rat pups. Physiol Behav 1999; 66: 627–37.

48. Falcon M, Guendellman D, Stolberg A, Frenk H, Urca G. Development of thermal nociception in rats. Pain 1996; 67: 203–8.

49. Fitzgerald M. The postnatal development of cutaneous afferent fibre input and receptive field organization in the rat dorsal horn. J Physiol 1985; 364: 1–18.

50. Barr GA. Maturation of the biphasic behavioral and heart rate response in the formalin test. Pharmacol Biochem Behav 1998; 60: 329–35.

51. Guy ER, Abbott FV. The behavioral response to formalin in preweanling rats. Pain 1992; 51: 81–90.

52. Teng CJ, Abbott FV. The formalin test: a dose-response analysis at three development stages. Pain 1998; 76: 337–47.

53. Stevens B, Taddio A, Ohlsson A, Einarson T. The efficacy of sucrose for relieving procedural pain in neonates – a systematic review and meta-analysis. Acta Paediatr 1997; 86: 837–42.

54. Hall RW, Kronsberg SS, Barton BA, Kaiser JR, Anand KJS. Morphine, hypotension and adverse outcomes in preterm neonates: who's to blame? Secondary results from the NEOPAIN trial. Pediatrics 2005; 115: 1351–9.

55. Quigley KS, Shair HN, Myers MM. Parasympathetic control of heart period during early postnatal development in the rat. J Auton Nerv Syst 1996; 59: 75–82.

56. Fitzgerald M, Shaw A, MacIntosh N. Postnatal development of the cutaneous flexor reflex: comparative study of preterm infants and newborn rat pups. Dev Med Child Neurol 1988; 30: 520–6.

57. Taddio A, Ohlsson A, Einarson TR, Stevens B, Koren G. A systematic review of lidocaine-prilocaine cream (EMLA) in the treatment of acute pain in neonates. Pediatrics 1998; 101: E1.

58. Cantarella A, Slater R, Gallella S et al. Haemodynamic response to noxious stimuli is larger in awake neonates than in sleeping neonates. Proceedings of the 2nd International Conference on Infant Development in Neonatal Intensive Care, Vol. 1. London, UK, March 3–4, 2005.

59. Anand KJS, Rovnaghi C, Walden M, Churchill J. Consciousness, behavior, and clinical impact of the definition of pain. Pain Forum 1999; 8: 64–73.

60. Newton BW, Rovnaghi CR, Golzar Y, Anand KJS. Supraspinal Fos expression in neonatal rat pups following graded inflammatory pain. Soc Neurosci Abstr 1999; 25: 1044.

61. Anand KJS, Hickey PR. Pain and its effects in the human neonate and fetus. N Engl J Med 1987; 317: 1321–9.

62. Collier AC, Bolles RC. The ontogenesis of defensive reactions to shock in preweanling rats. Dev Psychobiol 1980; 13: 141–50.

63. Hu D, Hu R, Berde CB. Neurologic evaluation of infant and adult rats before and after sciatic nerve blockade. Anesthesiology 1997; 86: 957–65.

64. Barker DP, Rutter N. Exposure to invasive procedures in neonatal intensive care unit admissions. Arch Dis Child Fetal Neonatal Ed 1995; 72: F47–8.

65. Johnston CC, Collinge JM, Henderson SJ, Anand KJS. A cross-sectional survey of pain and pharmacological analgesia in Canadian neonatal intensive care units. Clin J Pain 1997; 13: 308–12.

66. Porter FL, Anand KJS. Epidemiology of pain in neonates. Res Clin Forums 1998; 20: 9–16.

67. Benis MM, Suresh GK. Frequency of invasive procedures in very low birth weight (VLBW) infants in the neonatal intensive care unit. Pediatr Res 2001; 49: 392A (abstract 2253).

68. Alvares D, Fitzgerald M. Building blocks of pain: the regulation of key molecules in spinal sensory neurones during

development and following peripheral axotomy. Pain 1999; Suppl 6: S71–S85.

69. Woolf CJ, Salter MW. Neuronal plasticity: increasing the gain in pain. Science 2000; 288: 1765–8.

70. Price DD. Psychological and neural mechanisms of the affective dimension of pain. Science 2000; 288: 1769–72.

71. Liu JG, Rovnaghi CR, Garg S, Anand KJS. Hyperalgesia in young rats associated with opioid receptor desensitization in the forebrain. Eur J Pharmacol 2004; 491: 127–36.

72. Anand KJS. Effects of perinatal pain. In: The Biological Basis for Mind-Body Interactions, Vol. 122 (Mayer EA, Saper CB, eds). New York: Elsevier Science, 2000: 117–29.

73. Fitzgerald M, McIntosh N. Pain and analgesia in the newborn. Arch Dis Child 1989; 64: 441–3.

74. Anand KJS, Runeson B, Jacobson B. Gastric suction at birth associated with long-term risk for functional intestinal disorders in later life. J Pediatr 2004; 144: 449–54.

75. Anand KJS, Scalzo FM. Can adverse neonatal experiences alter brain development and subsequent behavior? Biol Neonate 2000; 77: 69–82.

76. Porter FL, Grunau RVE, Anand KJS. Long-term effects of neonatal pain. J Behav Dev Pediatr 1999; 20: 253–61.

77. Taddio A, Shah V, Gilbert-MacLeod C, Katz J. Conditioning and hyperalgesia in newborns exposed to repeated heel lances. JAMA 2002; 288: 857–61.

78. Taddio A, Katz J, Ilersich AL, Koren G. Effect of neonatal circumcision on pain response during subsequent routine vaccination. Lancet 1997; 349: 599–603.

79. Grunau RV, Whitfield MF, Petrie JH. Pain sensitivity and temperament in extremely low-birth-weight premature toddlers and preterm and full-term controls. Pain 1994; 58: 341–6.

80. Grunau RV, Whitfield MF, Petrie JH, Fryer EL. Early pain experience, child and family factors, as precursors of somatization: a prospective study of extremely premature and fullterm children. Pain 1994; 56: 353–9.

81. Grunau RE, Whitfield MF, Petrie J. Children's judgements about pain at age 8–10 years: do extremely low birthweight (< or = 1000 g) children differ from full birthweight peers? J Child Psychol Psychiatry 1998; 39: 587–94.

82. Lidow MS. Long-term effects of neonatal pain on nociceptive systems. Pain 2002; 99: 377–83.

83. Reynolds ML, Fitzgerald M. Long-term sensory hyperinnervation following neonatal skin wounds. J Comp Neurol 1995; 358: 487–98.

84. Rahman W, Fitzgerald M, Aynsley-Green A, Dickenson AH. The effects of neonatal exposure to inflammation and/or morphine on neuronal responses and morphine analgesia in adult rats. In: Proceedings of the 8th World Congress on Pain, Vol. 8 (Jensen TS, Turner JA, Wiesenfeld-Hallin Z, eds). Seattle: IASP Press, 1997: 783–94.

85. Bhutta AT, Rovnaghi CR, Simpson PM et al. Interactions of inflammatory pain and morphine treatment in infant rats: long-term behavioral effects. Physiol Behav 2001; 73: 51–8.

86. Lidow MS, Song Z-M, Ren K. Long-term effects of short-lasting early local inflammatory insult. Neuroreport 2001; 12: 399–403.

87. Wang G, Ji Y, Lidow MS, Traub RJ. Neonatal hind paw injury alters processing of visceral and somatic nociceptive stimuli in the adult rat. J Pain 2004; 5: 440–9.

88. Ren K, Anseloni V, Zou SP et al. Characterization of basal and re-inflammation-associated long-term alteration in pain responsivity following short-lasting neonatal local inflammatory insult. Pain 2004; 110: 588–96.

89. Sternberg WF, Scorr L, Smith LD, Ridgway CG, Stout M. Long-term effects of neonatal surgery on adulthood pain behavior. Pain 2005; 113: 347–53.

90. Johnston CC, Stevens BJ. Experience in a neonatal intensive care unit affects pain response. Pediatrics 1996; 98: 925–30.

91. Grunau RE, Oberlander TF, Whitfield MF, Fitzgerald C, Lee SK. Demographic and therapeutic determinants of pain reactivity in very low birth neonates at 32 weeks' postconceptional age. Pediatrics 2001; 107: 105–12.

92. Oberlander TF, Grunau RE, Whitfield MF et al. Biobehavioral pain responses in former extremely low birth weight infants at four months' corrected age. Pediatrics 2000; 105: e6.

93. Grunau RE, Oberlander TF, Whitfield MF et al. Pain reactivity in former extremely low birth weight infant at corrected age 8 months compared with term born controls. Infant Behav Dev 2001; 24: 41–55.

94. Grunau RE, Weinberg J, Whitfield MF. Neonatal procedural pain and preterm infant cortisol response to novelty at 8 months. Pediatrics 2004; 114: e77–84.

95. Liu D, Diorio J, Tannenbaum B et al. Maternal care, hippocampal glucocorticoid receptors, and hypothalamic-pituitary-adrenal reponses to stress. Science 1997; 277: 1659–62.

96. Ladd CO, Huot RL, Thrivikraman KV et al. Long-term behavioral and neuroendocrine adaptations to adverse early experience. Prog Brain Res 2000; 122: 81–103.

97. Walker CD, Kudreikis K, Sherrard A, Johnston CC. Repeated neonatal pain influences maternal behavior, but not stress responsiveness in rat offspring. Brain Res Dev Brain Res 2003; 140: 253–61.

98. Gray L, Watt L, Blass EM. Skin-to-skin contact is analgesic in healthy newborns. Pediatrics 2000; 105: e14.

99. Johnston CC, Stevens B, Pinelli J et al. Kangaroo care is effective in diminishing pain response in preterm neonates. Arch Pediatr Adolesc Med 2003; 157: 1084–8.

100. Liu D, Diorio J, Day JC, Francis DD, Meaney MJ. Maternal care, hippocampal synaptogenesis and cognitive development in rats. Nature Neurosci 2000; 3: 799–806.

101. Grunau RE, Linhares MB, Holsti L, Oberlander TF, Whitfield MF. Does prone or supine position influence pain responses in preterm infants at 32 weeks gestational age? Clin J Pain 2004; 20: 76–82.

102. Beacham PS. Behavioral and physiological indicators of procedural and postoperative pain in high-risk infants. J Obstet Gynecol Neonatal Nurs 2004; 33: 246–55.

103. Bhutta AT, Cleves M, Casey PH, Anand KJS. Prematurity and later cognitive outcomes. JAMA 2002; 288: 2542–3.

104. Botting N, Powls A, Cooke RW. Attention deficit hyperactivity disorders and other psychiatric outcomes in very low birthweight children at 12 years. J Child Psychol Psychiatry 1997; 38: 931–41.

105. Botting N, Powls A, Cooke RWI, Marlow N. Attention deficit hyperactivity disorders and other psychiatric outcomes in very low birth weight children at 12 years. J Child Psychol Psychiatry 1997; 38: 931–41.

106. Volpe JJ. Brain injury in the premature infant. Neuropathology, clinical aspects, pathogenesis, and prevention. Clin Perinatol 1997; 24: 567–87.

107. Morrow TJ, Paulson PE, Brewer KL et al. Chronic, selective forebrain responses to excitotoxic dorsal horn injury. Exp Neurol 2000; 161: 220–6.

108. Ruda MA, Ling QD, Hohmann AG, Peng YB, Tachibana T. Altered nociceptive neuronal circuits after neonatal peripheral inflammation. Science 2000; 289: 628–31.

109. Peng YB, Ling QD, Ruda MA, Kenshalo DR. Electrophysiological changes in adult rat dorsal horn neurons after neonatal peripheral inflammation. J Neurophysiol 2003; 90: 73–80.

110. Kilbride HW, Thorstad K, Daily DK. Preschool outcome of less than 801-gram preterm infants compared with full-term siblings. Pediatrics 2004; 113: 742–7.

111. Peterson B, Vohr B, Staib L et al. Regional brain volume abnormalities and long-term cognitive outcome in preterm infants. JAMA 2000; 284: 1939–47.

112. Peterson BS, Anderson AW, Ehrenkranz R et al. Regional brain volumes and their later neurodevelopmental correlates in term and preterm infants. Pediatrics 2003; 111: 939–48.

113. Peterson BS, Vohr B, Kane MJ et al. A functional magnetic resonance imaging study of language processing and its cognitive correlates in prematurely born children. Pediatrics 2002; 110: 1153–62.

114. Al-Chaer ED, Kawasaki M, Pasricha PJ. A new model of chronic visceral hypersensitivity in adult rats induced by colon irritation during postnatal development. Gastroenterology 2000; 119: 1276–85.

115. Lin C, Al-Chaer ED. Long-term sensitization of primary afferents in adult rats exposed to neonatal colon pain. Brain Res 2003; 971: 73–82.

116. Park Y, Al-Chaer ED. Thoracolumbar neuronal sensitization to colon stimuli in Al-Chaer's animal model of chronic visceral pain. J Pain 2002; 3: 27 (abstract no. 708).

117. Al-Chaer ED, Lin C. Sex-related differences in exploratory activity in adult rats exposed to neonatal colon pain. Society for Neuroscience Annual Meeting, Washington, DC, 2003, Vol. 2.

118. Saab CY, Arai Y-CP, Al-Chaer ED. Modulation of visceral nociceptive processing in the lumbar spinal cord following thalamic stimulation or inactivation and after dorsal column lesion in rats with neonatal colon irritation. Brain Res 2004; 1008: 186–92.

119. Hinze CL, Lin C, Al-Chaer ED. Estrous cycle and stress related variations in open field activity in adult female rats with neonatal colon irritation (CI). Society for Neuroscience Annual Meeting, Washington, DC, 2002, Vol. 1.

120. Palecek J, Paleckova V, Willis WD. The roles of pathways in the spinal cord lateral and dorsal funiculi in signaling nociceptive somatic and visceral stimuli in rats. Pain 2002; 96: 297–307.

121. Griebel G, Perrault G, Sanger DJ. Limited anxiolytic-like effects of non-benzodiazepine hypnotics in rodents. J Psychopharmacol 1998; 12: 356–65.

122. Randolph AG, Gonzales CA, Cortellini L, Yeh TS. Growth of pediatric intensive care units in the United States from 1995 to 2001. J Pediatr 2004; 144: 792–8.

123. Mayer EA, Naliboff BD, Chang L, Coutinho SV. Stress and irritable bowel syndrome. Am J Physiol – Gastrointest & Liver Physiol 2001; 280: G519–G524.

124. Perlman JM. Neurobehavioral deficits in premature graduates of intensive care – potential medical and neonatal environmental risk factors. Pediatrics 2001; 108: 1339–48.

125. Anand KJS, Hall RW, Desai NS et al. Effects of pre-emptive morphine analgesia in ventilated preterm neonates: primary outcomes from the NEOPAIN trial. Lancet. 2004; 363: 1673–82.

126. Bremmer P, Byers JF, Kiehl E. Noise and the premature infant: physiological effects and practice implications. J Obstet Gynecol Neonatal Nurs 2003; 32: 447–54.

127. Morris R, Paxinos G, Petrides M. Architectonic analysis of the human retrosplenial cortex. J Comp Neurol 2000; 421: 14–28.

128. Trinder J, Newman NM, Le Grande M et al. Behavioural and EEG responses to auditory stimuli during sleep in newborn infants and in infants aged 3 months. Biol Psychol 1990; 31: 213–27.

129. Shogan MG, Schumann LL. The effect of environmental lighting on the oxygen saturation of preterm infants in the NICU. Neonatal Netw 1993; 12: 7–13.

130. Uauy R, Mena P, Rojas C. Essential fatty acid metabolism in the micropremie. Clin Perinatol 2000; 27: 71–93.

131. Birch EE, Garfield S, Hoffman DR, Uauy R, Birch DG. A randomized controlled trial of early dietary supply of long-chain polyunsaturated fatty acids and mental development in term infants. Dev Med Child Neurol 2000; 42: 174–81.

132. Uauy R, Mena P, Rojas C. Essential fatty acids in early life: structural and functional role. [Review] [109 refs]. Proceedings of the Nutrition Society 2000; 59: 3–15.

133. Goldman RD, Koren G. Biologic markers of pain in the vulnerable infant. Clin Perinatol 2002; 29: 415–25.

134. Meaney MJ. The sexual differentiation of social play. Psychiatr Dev 1989; 7: 247–61.

135. Porterfield SP, Hendrich CE. The role of thyroid hormones in prenatal and neonatal neurological development – current perspectives. Endocr Rev 1993; 14: 94–106.

136. Johnston CC, Walker CD, Boyer K. Animal models of long-term consequences of early exposure to repetitive pain. Clin Perinatol 2002; 29: 395–414.

137. Anand KJS, Runeson B, Jacobson B. Gastric suction at birth associated with long-term risk for functional intestinal disorders in later life. J Pediatr 2004; 144: 449–54.

138. Jacobson B, Eklund G, Hamberger L et al. Perinatal origin of adult self-destructive behavior. Acta Psychiatr Scand 1987; 76: 364–71.

139. Jacobson B, Bygdeman M. Obstetric care and proneness of offspring to suicides as adults: case-control study. BMJ 1998; 317: 1346–9.

140. Nyberg K, Allebeck P, Eklund G, Jacobson B. Socioeconomic versus obstetric risk factors for drug addiction in offspring. Br J Addict 1992; 87: 1669–76.

16

Pain sensitivity during ontogeny and long-term effects of prenatal noxious events

Irina P Butkevich, Viktor A Mikhailenko, Ludmila I Khozhai, and Vladimir A Otellin

INTRODUCTION

The nociceptive (pain) system serves important protective functions in reducing and preventing trauma and promoting the organization of adequate responses to external and internal stimuli. Despite a long history of pain research and considerable progress in this scientific field, including new research in molecular biology, many pain mechanisms are still not well understood. It is known that two types of pain exist: acute, phasic pain and tonic, prolonged pain. These two types are distinguished by distinctive anatomical, physiological, and neurochemical characteristics.[1-4] Experimentally, the mechanisms of phasic pain and its alleviation are better investigated than those of tonic pain.[1,2,5,6] Investigations of the nociceptive tonic system, and the underlying mechanisms of how it functions, are not only of fundamental importance, but are of practical clinical significance since pain produced by inflammation or tissue injury is more common and problematic in patients. Clinicians need more effective agents for pharmacological treatment and amelioration of tonic pain, especially agents that do not predispose to addiction.

Most of the work on experimental nociception has been done in adult animals. Obviously, age-specific functioning of the nociceptive system must be taken into account.[7-11] Investigations of the developmental dynamics of pain can help us to better understand the regulation of pain. Our experience in the study of ontogenetic aspects of pain sensitivity indicates that individuals vary in the rate of maturation and that there are important gender differences. There are also critical periods during the development of pain systems with different sensitivities to noxious events.[7,11-13] The prenatal period is the most vulnerable to environmental influences and experimental treatments. It has been demonstrated, for example, that prenatal stress can induce irreversible morphological changes in the developing brain,[14-18] and create imbalances in neuroendocrine[19-24] and neurotransmitter systems,[19,25-29] impair behavior,[18,26,27,30-32] and even modify expression of the genetic program.[33] Morphological and functional abnormalities in brain development that result from prenatal stress can lead to neuropsychological and somatic pathology persisting throughout life.[29,30,32,34] One consequence induced by prenatal stress is a change in behavioral responses to nociceptive stimuli.[35-38] Prior to our studies, the effects of prenatal stress were investigated only with respect to acute pain.[35-38] Our current research is dedicated to the study of tonic nociceptive responses.

Analysis of the literature on the ontogeny of pain allows one to focus on a practically unexplored area: the maturation of the descending inhibitory system and the supraspinal pathways.[39] Recent findings emphasize the significance of the descending supraspinal serotonergic system in the modulation of dorsal horn neurons involved in prolonged, tonic pain[40-43] and suggest new insights into the mechanisms underlying modulation of these two types of pain.[44,45] Many contributions have been made by experimental use of the widely accepted formalin test,[46-48] which allows one to quantify pain behavior in a reliable and reproducible manner and to study the function of the descending systems modulating pain processing at the spinal level.[40,41]

Recent data emphasizes the significance of the supraspinal descending serotonergic systems in the modulation of formalin-induced pain in dorsal horn neurons.[40-43] We hypothesized that among the prenatal factors underlying stress-induced changes in pain sensitivity observed in female and male rats is alterations in the descending serotonergic system.[49,50] It could also be involved in the sexual dimorphism in tonic pain described in the literature[51] and by us.[52]

We begin our chapter with the consideration of ontogenetic features of the biphasic behavioral pain response to formalin, a noxious chemical irritant, in female and male rats, that developed under normal conditions. In the next section we focus our attention on the effects of prenatal stress on pain behavior. To test our hypothesis about the importance of serotonergic pathways, we assessed behavioral responses in rats that developed prenatally under conditions of 5HT (5-hydroxytryptamine) deficiency.[53,54] Morphological analyses of the neocortex, hippocampus, and dorsal raphe nuclei, brain structures involved in the biphasic behavioral response in the formalin test, were also performed.

BEHAVIORAL INDICES OF PAIN SENSITIVITY IN THE FORMALIN PAIN TEST DURING RAT ONTOGENY

Ontogenetic characteristics of pain sensitivity in the formalin test were previously investigated in rats only during the first 21–25 days of life.[55–57] We pioneered the more systematic testing of pain sensitivity during critical development periods, prepubertal (25-day-old pups), pubertal (40-day-old rats), and in adults. Injection of formalin (2.5%, 10–50 µl) into the plantar pad of a hind limb of a Wistar rat produces a specific and biphasic behavioral response. The first, early phase is short (1–5 minutes) and considered to be the acute pain behavior induced by chemical irritant. The second, prolonged phase (20–45 minutes) is considered to result partly from the development of inflammation induced by the formalin and may reflect sensitization of primary afferents and spinal cord dorsal horn neurons. Between the first and second phases, there is a more nonresponsive phase (the interphase) lasting 5–20 minutes during which specific reactions (flexing, shaking, and licking) indicative of pain are lacking. Maturation of the descending supraspinal pathways that occurs by the third week of life[58] determines the division of two response phases and appearance of the interphase.[56–58]

We evaluated pain sensitivity by indices of this biphasic response: duration of the injected paw licking (in seconds), the number of flexes + shakes, and the duration of the first and second phases, and the interphase (in minutes). It was found that as the central nervous system (CNS) developed, the pain sensitivity underwent significant changes. In the tonic phase, pain sensitivity assessed by response patterns organized at the spinal level (the number of flexes + shakes) increased in males (Figure 16.1A), and by response patterns organized at the supraspinal level increased in

females (increased licking duration) (Figure 16.1B). The duration of the tonic phase increased progressively during the course of development in both sexes (Figure 16.2A,B).

In the first acute phase, pain sensitivity reflecting patterns of response organized at the supraspinal level decreased significantly with age in both females and males (Figure 16.3B, 16.4B). This finding supports the conclusion that reactions to a novel environment, which is more distinct in adult rats as compared with the younger ones, suppresses pain sensitivity during the acute phase of the formalin test.[47] These age-related differences in the first and second phases of the pain response are consistent with the assumption that different physiological mechanisms underlie two phases of response in the formalin test.[59–61] More age-related differences in pain sensitivity were also found in females in responses organized at the supraspinal level (Figures 16.1B, 16.3B, 16.4B). In addition, the magnitude of pain behavior revealed a fundamental reorganization in hormonal and neurotransmitter systems during the pubertal period in 40-day-old female and male rats (Figures 16.1B, 16.3B, 16.4B). The prepubertal and pubertal periods are known to be characterized by increased activity of catecholaminergic and serotonergic systems, and elevated secretion of gonadal and adrenal steroids. It is noteworthy that neurotransmitter and hormonal systems in 40-day-old rats are not yet at adult values but differ from those in 25-day-old rats.[62,63]

The duration of the interphase was found to be a very informative index of developmental change. It increased with age, presumably reflecting organizational changes at the spinal level (Figure 16.4A). In addition, marked sex differences in this index were found in adulthood. The increasing interphase duration with age indicated a strengthening of inhibitory processes in the central nervous system (CNS). The absence of behavioral responses during the interphase was considered previously as a quiescent period. However, current data show that the interphase in the formalin test is due to active inhibition.[64,65] The increased duration of the interphase with age enables us to propose that the inhibitory activity of the descending bulbospinal systems increases progressively during the first 3 months of life and this occurs to a greater extent in females. These data extend knowledge about the developmental functions of the descending monoaminergic systems involved in tonic pain modulation at the spinal level beyond the first 2–3 weeks of postnatal life.[39]

Thus, comparative analysis showed that pain sensitivity in the classic formalin test is age- and sex-related, varies across the acute and tonic phase of the

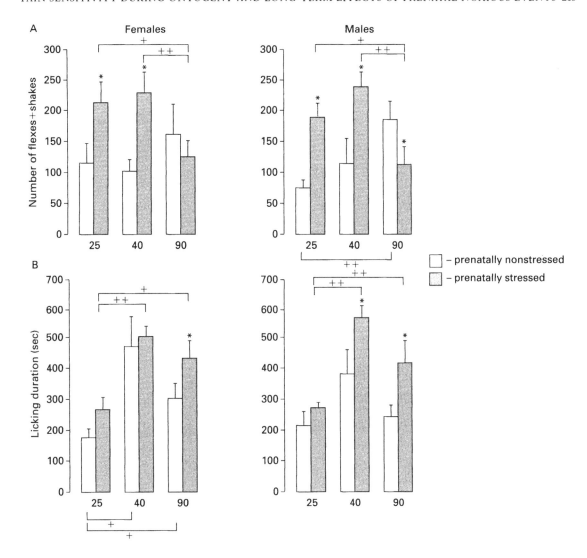

Figure 16.1 Formalin-induced responses (numbers of flexes + shakes and licking duration) during the second phase in control and prenatally stressed rats at different ages. (A) Number of flexes + shakes, (B) licking duration. Numerals under the bars represent age in days. Data are means ± SEM. $p < 0.05$ was considered as statistically significant; *$p < 0.05$, prenatally stressed vs control; + $p < 0.05$; + + $p < 0.001$, age differences.

response, and is dependent on the level of organization in the CNS of behavioral patterns indicative of pain.

LONG-TERM EFFECTS OF PRENATAL STRESS ON PAIN SENSITIVITY AND BRAIN STRUCTURES INVOLVED IN THE BEHAVIORAL RESPONSE TO PAIN

One important realization in developmental biology and pediatrics is the potential significance of prenatal

stress on fetal behavioral development.[18,26,27,30–32] In our study we used 30-minute restraint stress (twice a day) of pregnant rats during the last week of gestation,[49,50] which is a critical developmental period for the nociceptive system.[39] We evaluated pain sensitivity with the formalin test in prenatally stressed rats (25-, 40-, and 90-day-old) and compared them to rats from nonstressed pregnancies.

Tonic pain proved to be more vulnerable to the effects of prenatal stress than acute pain, which serves a protective function. This stress effect was evident from the increased duration of the tonic phase (Figure

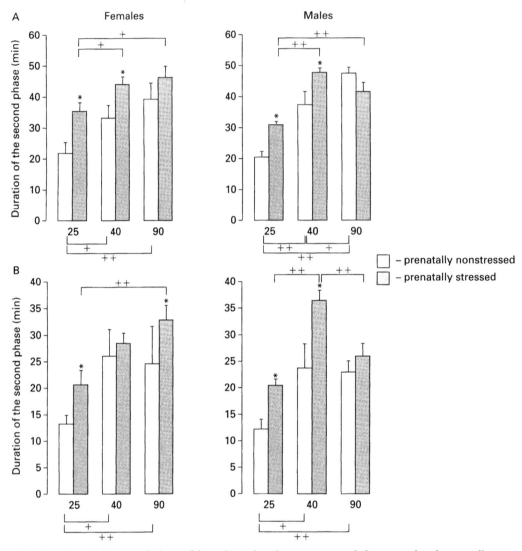

Figure 16.2 Duration of the second phase of formalin-induced response recorded in control and prenatally stressed rats of different ages. (A) Flexes + shakes responses, (B) licking responses. Numerals under the bars represent age in days. Data are means ± SEM. $p < 0.05$ was considered as statistically significant; *$p < 0.05$, prenatally stressed vs controls; + $p < 0.05$; ++ $p < 0.001$, age differences.

16.2A) and from the profound exacerbation of flexing + shaking behaviors in both 25- and 40-day-old female and male rats (Figure 16.1A). In contrast, the number of flexes + shakes in 90-day-old males significantly decreased and was not affected by the prenatal stress at all in females. These findings suggest that at the spinal level, the consequences of prenatal stress were manifested by activation of the descending excitatory processes and suppression of inhibitory processes in 25- and 40-day-old rats, but on the contrary, as activation of the descending inhibitory and suppression of excitatory systems in 90-day-old rats.

At the supraspinal level, the developmental trend of licking behavior (the index of tonic pain) did not change in prenatally stressed rats. However, tonic pain in the 90-day-olds was significantly enhanced in both sexes (Figure 16.1B).

In the adult females, prenatal stress reversed the developmental trends seen in the acute phase responses. Pain sensitivity in prenatally stressed adult females was exacerbated dramatically in comparison to the intact adults (Figure 16.3B). This prenatal effect reflecting supraspinal processes was not seen in adult males. Effects of prenatal stress were also found in

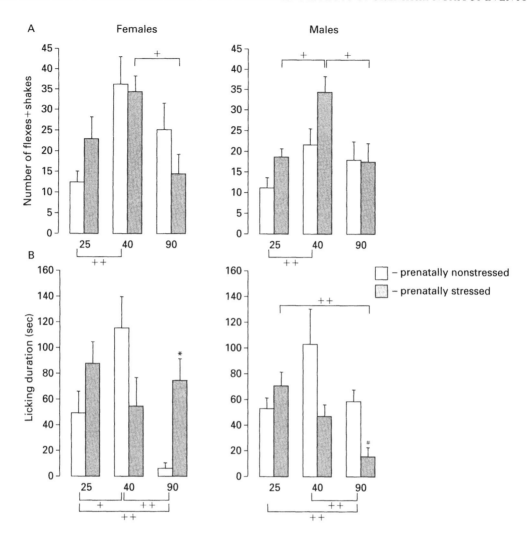

Figure 16.3 Formalin-induced responses (numbers of flexes + shakes and licking duration) during the first phase in control and prenatally stressed rats of different ages. (A) Numbers of flexes + shakes, (B) licking duration. Numerals under the bars represent age in days. Data are means ± SEM. $p < 0.05$ was considered as statistically significant; $*p < 0.05$, prenatally stressed vs controls; $+ p < 0.05$; $++ p < 0.001$, age differences; # $p < 0.01$, prenatally stressed females vs prenatally stressed males.

the measures of acute pain duration (Figure 16.4B). However, here prenatal stress eliminated all age-related differences that had been found in prenatally nonstressed females.

These data support the prevailing view that the first and second phases of formalin-induced pain are different in nature.[59–61] Because the tonic phase is more associated with inflammation, and is influenced by the hypothalamo-pituitary-adrenal (HPA) and sympatho-adrenomedullary systems, this may provide different

explanations for the mediation of prenatal stress effects.[20–24] We believe that the effect of prenatal stress on acute and tonic pain may be realized through different neural circuits.

The duration of the interphase confirmed its informative value for developmental studies. In the 25-day-old rat, prenatal stress resulted in a disinhibition of flexing and shaking behaviors during the interphase. This finding indicated alterations in the descending inhibitory systems modulating pain signals in the spinal dorsal

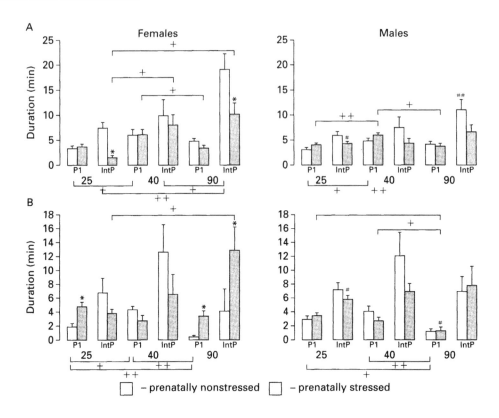

Figure 16.4 Duration of the first phase and the interphase of formalin-induced response in prenatally stressed and control rats of different ages. (A) Flexes + shakes responses, (B) licking responses. P1, the first phase; IntP, the interphase. Numerals under the bars represent age in days. Data are means ± SEM. $p < 0.05$ was considered as statistically significant; *$p < 0.05$, prenatally stressed vs control; + $p < 0.05$; ++ $p < 0.001$; age differences; # $p < 0.01$, prenatally stressed females vs prenatally stressed males; ## $p < 0.05$, control females vs control males.

horns neurons of the prenatally stressed rats. Similar effects on the interphase were observed in prenatally nonstressed adult rats after intrathecal injection of serotonin or adrenaline antagonists.[40] The disinhibition of flexing and shaking behaviors was more pronounced in prenatally stressed, prepubertal females, but not in males (Figure 16.4A). Significant reductions in the interphase duration in females, and a reduced trend in males, suggested that the central inhibition processes were altered more in females. Our results in 25-day-old rats provided additional evidence to support the interpretations about the inhibitory nature of the interphase.[64,65]

Prenatal stress effects at the spinal and supraspinal levels occurred mainly in the opposite direction: 1) decreased tonic pain in flexing + shaking and

increased licking duration in 90-day-old rats; 2) reduced interphase duration in flexing + shaking, but increased licking in 90-day-old females; 3) profound exacerbation of pain as measured by increased flexing + shaking, and the absence of change in licking in 25-day-old rats. This pattern of results indicates that prenatal stress during the last week of gestation produced reorganization of CNS functional morphology. At days 17–19 GA, switching from excitatory to the inhibitory activity occurs in GABA-ergic and glycerinergic synaptic transmission.[66] Thus, the prenatal stress at this critical window may differentially impact the biphasic pain response organized at the different levels of the CNS.

Of further interest are the data demonstrating in 40-day-old prenatally stressed rats, the pronounced tendency for a marked decrease in the large fluctuations in the pain indices typically seen in 40-day-old offspring of nonstressed dams. In prenatally stressed males of this age, licking patterns were more prevalent than in males from the other two age groups (Figure 16.1B, 16.2B). This may be a reflection of a second reorganization in hormonal and neurotransmitter systems during the pubertal period of development.[62,63] It is only during the pubertal period that males demonstrate a greater change in pain sensitivity than females. It is pertinent to mention that the onset of puberty period is different in females (33rd day of age) and males (40th day).[67] An influence of gonadal hormones on nociceptive processing is one of the possible factors determining this sexual dimorphism in pain sensitivity.[68]

Other indices of the biphasic pain responses reflecting inhibitory processes in 25-day-old rats were also sexually dimorphic. Sex differences were seen in the duration of the tonic phase in 40-day-old rats, as well as in duration of the first and second phases in 90-day-old animals. With regard to the intensity of pain response, sex differences were revealed only in the first phase of licking in 90-day-old rats.

Morphological analysis of the brain structures involved in pain responses showed prenatally stressed animals had diffuse loss of chromatosis-like neurons in all layers of neocortex (especially often in the layer V). Cortical layers were thinner, cellular nuclei were rounded, and these cells had less cytoplasm than did the cells of control animals. Cells with foaming cytoplasm and large vacuoles were also observed. Cell loss in the hippocampus was found in the CA_1 and CA_3 areas. In the dorsal raphe nuclei, hyperchromatosis and chromatolysis-like cell death were seen. Because the changes in brain regions associated with formalin-induced pain were more pronounced in rats with more profound alterations in pain behaviors, we concluded that morphological abnormalities led to the altered dynamics of pain sensitivity. The altered brain morphology may have resulted from high levels of glucocorticoids in dams and their fetuses,[15,17] induced by the restraint stress in the last week of pregnancy as well as changes in other hormonal and neurotransmitter systems[19,25–29] that affect regulatory nociceptive systems.

The consequences of prenatal stress depended on age and sex, and were manifest in a wider range of indices in females than males at the age of 25 and 90 days. However, during the pubertal period, the effects were more evident in males. Prenatal stress also altered the maturational changes in pain behavior, and differentially affected responses organized at the spinal and supraspinal levels of the CNS. The tonic phase was found to be more vulnerable to prenatal stress than the acute phase. Finally, our results provide strong evidence to support the conclusion that the interphase in the formalin test[64,65] reflects inhibitory processes.

LONG-TERM EFFECTS OF PRENATAL ALTERING 5HT SYNTHESIS ON THE BEHAVIORAL INDICES OF PAIN AND ON BRAIN STRUCTURES INVOLVED IN PAIN RESPONSE

Our assumption that one cause of exacerbated pain sensitivity in prenatally stressed animals is altered serotonergic modulation at the spinal level is supported by the following facts. First, 5HT along with the HPA axis, is known to be involved in the mediation of the effects of prenatal stress.[25] Second, 5HT has a regulatory influence on development of the nervous system and of brain organization during fetal stages[69–71] and then later functions as a critical neurotransmitter pathway involved in nociception. Changes in 5HT levels during early fetal development (by drugs or 5HT deficiency diets) can result in abnormal development of the brain and alter many functions postnatally.[29,34] It has been shown that inflammatory processes evoked by injection of formalin increase the activity of descending serotonergic systems from the supraspinal areas, which by acting through 5HT1A receptors[40,41,43] cause inhibition of nociceptive signals and by acting through 5HT3 receptors facilitate the response of spinal nociceptive neurons to peripheral stimuli. Finally, this question is of interest because serotonergic receptors are a target of widely used psychotropic drugs for treatment of psychopathic states like anxiety, depression, and schizophrenia.[29,34]

To investigate fetal development under conditions of low levels of 5HT, we followed the method of prenatal 5HT depletion using injection of a water suspension of para-chlorophenylalanine (pCPA; 400 mg/kg/2 ml, i.p.; ICN, USA), an inhibitor of 5HT synthesis injected on day 9 of pregnancy. Control pregnant rats were injected with saline. The level of 5HT content was decreased more than 50% in fetal brains as compared with the controls, and was maximal at 2–3 days after injection, i.e. in the 11–12-day-old fetuses.[53,72] These days are critical for development of the serotonergic system, as cells in the raphe nucleus start to differentiate.[53,73]

Pain sensitivity was assessed in 25- and 90-day-old rats, following these prenatal conditions of 5HT deficiency. Pain sensitivity was differentially affected in prepubertal and adult rats. In young female and male rats, prenatal 5HT depletion caused a large decrease

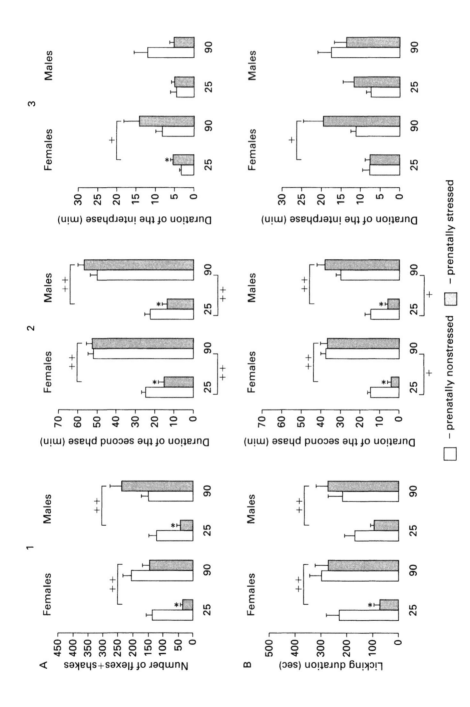

Figure 16.5 Formalin-induced responses in 25- and 90-day-old rats after prenatal injection of pCPA (para-chlorophenylalanine) or saline (controls). (A) Flexes + shakes patterns, (B) licking patterns, (1) intensity of the response, (2) duration of the second phase, (3) duration of the interphase. Numerals under the bars represent age in days. Data are mean ± SEM. $p < 0.05$ was considered statistically significant; *$p < 0.05$, prenatal 5HT depletion vs prenatal saline; + $p < 0.05$; ++ $p < 0.001$, age differences.

A   B

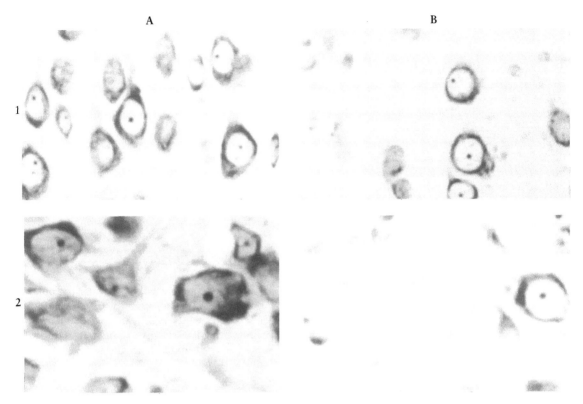

Figure 16.6 Typical morphology and distribution of cells in the neocortex and dorsal raphe nucleus in 25-day-old rats. Morphological alterations after prenatal 5HT depletion: (A) saline-treated (control); (B) pCPA-treated rats. (1) The neocortex (the fifth layer), (2) the dorsal raphe-nucleus. Note the evident cell loss and morphological alterations of neurons, which have large round and very light nuclei with a thin rim of cytoplasm with little Nissl substance in the prenatally pCPA-treated rat as compared with controls. (Nissl staining; magnification ×400.)

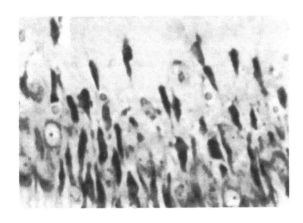

Figure 16.7 The hippocampus (CA3 area) in 90-day-old rat with prenatal 5HT depletion; dying hyperchromic neurons. (Nissl staining; ocular × 7, objective × 40.)

in pain sensitivity in the second, prolonged phase of behavioral response (up to its complete suppression) (Figure 16.5, A1, B1). In addition, the duration of the second phase was also decreased (Figure 16.5, A2, B2). Females displayed an increase in the duration of the interphase (Figure 16.5, A3).

In 6 of the 25 adult rats that had experienced the prenatal 5HT depletion, a suppression of pain responses occurred in one of the phases. The remaining rats did not show significant changes in the response to formalin. However, the duration of the interphase, in both flexing + shaking and licking behaviors, tended to increase in females and decrease in males (Figure 16.5, A3).

Less pronounced changes in the second phase in adults, as compared to 25-day-old rats, suggest that in the course of postnatal development there may be some adaptation to the consequences of prenatal 5HT deficit in the tonic pain transmission system.

Morphological study of brain sections obtained from the rats subjected to prenatal 5HT depletion revealed significant alterations in development of cortical structures, the hippocampus, raphe nuclei, and in the differentiation of neural cells in these structures. In 25-day-old rats, all the cortical layers were thinned and had fewer cells than controls. The cells were distinguished by hyperchromic cytoplasm and nonstained apical dendrites. Cell chromatolysis was observed in the upper cortical layers (Figure 16.6, 1A, B). The raphe nuclei had fewer cells than the control and debris of degenerated neurons and ghost cells were observed (Figure 16.6, 2A, B). Chromatosis-like loss of both single neurons and neuron clusters was revealed in all the brain structures studied in 25-day-old rats. In 90-day-old rats the cell loss was found in the hippocampus, especially in the CA3 zone (Figure 16.7). Analysis of the raphe nuclei demonstrated that they were smaller in size and had fewer cells in comparison with controls. A positive correlation between morphological and behavioral data was found; with more altered behavior in rats manifesting more abnormal development of brain structures. Abnormalities in these brain structures can affect the functional activity of the descending serotonergic systems, which modulate formalin-induced pain at the spinal level, mediating facilitatory effects through 5HT3 receptors and inhibitory effects through 5HT1 receptors. In animals with prenatal 5HT depletion, the inhibitory functions were probably increased, while facilitatory functions decreased, which resulted in an alleviation of tonic pain in the formalin test. Moreover, prenatal 5HT deficiency could impair the development of 5HT1A receptors which take part in regulating prenatal development of the ascending pathways and of 5HT3 receptors that are involved in the descending serotonergic systems.[74,75]

CONCLUSIONS

1. Pain sensitivity to formalin, a prolonged nociceptive irritant, depends on age and sex; the character of age and sex differences is determined by the CNS level of organization of behavioral patterns used as indices of pain sensitivity.
2. Prenatal stress exerted the following influences on pain sensitivity. Long-term, specific changes occurred in females and males, and in each age group (25-, 40- and, 90-day-old). The developmental dynamics of pain response to formalin were altered in stressed animals. Changes in pain sensitivity reflected by patterns of the response were determined by the level of organization of the patterns in the CNS, and the tonic phase was impacted to a greater extent than the acute phase. Finally, prenatal stress impaired inhibitory processes involved in the descending modulatory systems at the level of spinal dorsal horn.
3. Consequences of prenatal 5HT depletion in a critical period of development of the serotonergic system were manifest as an alleviation of prolonged pain, evident to a greater extent in the 25-day-old than in 90-day-old rats.
4. There was a positive correlation between the morphological and behavioral data: greater abnormalities in brain structures after prenatal stress and 5HT depletion were associated with more profound alterations in behavioral responses.

ACKNOWLEDGMENTS

The study was supported by the Russian Foundation for Basic Research (projects N 02-04-48338, 05-04-48677 and N 04-04-48227) and by the Grant of the Leading Scientific Schools of Russia (N 1163.2003.4). We are grateful to our colleague senior staff scientist Galina V. Makukhina for help in the translation of the manuscript.

REFERENCES

1. Kassil GN. Science about Pain. Moscow: Nauka, 1965: 373 (in Russian).
2. Dennis SG, Melzack R. Comparison of phasic and tonic pain in animals. Advances in Pain Research Therapy. New York: Raven Press, 1979: 747–60.
3. Abbott FV, Melzack R, Samuel C. Morphine analgesia in the tail-test and formalin pain tests is mediated by different neural systems. Exp Neurol 1982; 75: 644–51.
4. Basbaum AI. Distinct neurochemical features of acute and persistent pain. Proc Natl Acad Sci USA 1999; 96: 7739–43.
5. Wall PD. Mechanism of acute and chronic pain. In: Advances in Pain Research and Therapy (Kruger L, Liebeskind J, eds). New York: Raven Press, 1984: 95–103.
6. Melzack R. From the gate to the neuromatrix. Pain 1999; 6: 121–6.
7. Butkevich IP, Kassil VG. Antinociceptive effects of brain rewarding system in the developing rabbit: behavioral and electrophysiological analysis. Brain Res 1999; 834: 13–24.
8. Gagliese L, Melzack R. Age differences in the response to the formalin test in rats. Neurobiol Aging 1999; 20: 699–707.
9. McIntosh N. Management of chronic pain in the newborn. In: Pain 1999 – An Updated Review: Refresher Course Syllabus (Max M, ed.). Seattle: IASP Press, 1999: 233–5.
10. Fitzgerald M, Beggs S. The neurobiology of pain: developmental aspects. Neuroscientist 2001; 7: 246–57.
11. Butkevich IP, Vershinina EA. Nociceptive sensitivity to prolonged irritant in formalin test in female and male rats during postnatal ontogeny. Zhurn Evol Biochim Fiziol 2005; 41: 76–81 (in Russian).

12. Butkevich IP, Mikhailenko VA, Leont'eva MN. Consequences of prenatal depletion of serotonin and stress on behavioral indices of pain sensitivity in the formalin test in adult rats. Russian J Physiol 2004; 90: 1246–54 (in Russian).

13. Butkevich IP, Mikhailenko VA, Khozhai LI et al. Influence of prenatal 5-HT depletion and stress on nociceptive sensitivity during prepubertal period of rat development. Zhurn Evol Biochim Fiziol 2005; 41; 168–75 (in Russian).

14. Anderson RH, Fleming DE, Rheess RW et al. Relationships between sexual activity, plasma testosterone, and the volume of the sexually dimorphic nucleus of the preoptic area in prenatally stressed and non-stressed rats. Brain Res 1986; 370: 1–10.

15. Takahashi LK. Prenatal stress: consequences of glucocorticoids on hippocampal development and function. Int J Dev Neurosci 1998; 16: 199–207.

16. Wadhwa PD, Sandman CA, Garite TJ. The neurobiology of stress in human pregnancy: implications for prematurity and development of the fetal nervous system. Prog Brain Res 2001; 133: 131–42.

17. Weinstock M. Alterations induced by gestational stress in brain morphology and behaviour of the offspring. Prog Neurobiol 2001; 65: 427–51.

18. Kofman O. The role of prenatal stress in the etiology of developmental behavioural disorders. Neurosci Biobehav Rev 2002; 26: 457–70.

19. Naumenko EV, Vigash M, Polenov AL. Ontogenetic and Genetico-evolutional Aspects of Neuroendocrine Regulation of Stress. Novosibirsk: Nauka, 1990: 230 (in Russian).

20. Weinstock M, Poltyrev T, Schorer-Apelbaum D et al. Effect of prenatal stress on plasma corticosterone and catecholamines in response to footshock in rats. Physiol Behav 1998; 64: 439–44.

21. Welberg LAM, Seckl JR. Prenatal stress, glucocorticoids and the programming of the brain. J Neuroendocrinol 2001; 13: 113–28.

22. Shaljapina WG, Zaichenko IN, Ordjan NE et al. Changes of neuroendocrinal regulation of adaptive behavior in rats after stress during late prenatal ontogeny. Russian J Physiol 2001; 87: 1193–201 (in Russian).

23. Avishai-Eliner S, Brunson KL, Sandman CA et al. Stressed-out, or in (utero). Trends Neurosci 2002; 25: 518–24.

24. Maccari S, Darnaudery M, Morley-Fletcher S et al. Prenatal stress and long-term consequences: implications of glucocorticoid hormones. Neurosci Biobehav Rev 2003; 27: 119–27.

25. Peters DA. Effects of maternal stress during different gestational periods on the serotonergic system in adult rat offspring. Pharmacol Biochem Behav 1988; 31: 839–43.

26. Takahashi LK, Turner JG, Kalin NH. Prenatal stress alters brain catecholaminergic activity and potentiates stress-induced behavior in adult rats. Brain Res 1992; 574: 131–7.

27. Hayashi A, Nagaoka M, Yamada K et al. Maternal stress induces synaptic loss and developmental disabilities of offspring. Int J Dev Neurosci 1998; 16: 209–16.

28. Reznikov AG, Nosenko ND, Tarasenko LV et al. Early and long-term neuroendocrine effects of prenatal stress in male and female rats. Neurosci Behav Physiol 2001; 31: 1–5.

29. Huizink AC, Mulder EJ, Buitelaar JK. Prenatal stress and risk for psychopathology: specific effects or induction of general susceptibility. Psychol Bull 2004; 130: 115–42.

30. Ward AJ. Prenatal stress and childhood psychopathology. Child Psychiatry Hum Dev 1991; 22: 97–110.

31. Weinstock M. Can the behaviour abnormalities induced by gestational stress in rats be prevented or reversed. Stress 2002; 5: 167–76.

32. O'Connor TG, Heron J, Golding J et al. ALSPAC Study Team. Maternal antenatal anxiety and behavioural/emotional problems in children: a test of a programming hypothesis. J Child Psychol Psychiatry 2003; 44: 1025–36.

33. Kinnunen AK, Koenig JI, Bilbe G. Repeated variable prenatal stress alters pre- and postsynaptic gene expression in the rat frontal pole. J Neurochem 2003; 86: 736–48.

34. Boksa P. Animal model of obstetric complications in relation to schizophrenia. Brain Res Rev 2004; 45: 1–17.

35. Kinsley CH, Mann PE, Bridges RS. Prenatal stress alters morphine- and stress-induced analgesia in male and female rats. Pharmacol Biochem Behav 1988; 30: 123–8.

36. Sternberg WF. Sex differences in the effects of prenatal stress on stress-induced analgesia. Physiol Behav 1999; 68: 63–72.

37. Sternberg WF. Effects of gestational stress and neonatal handling on pain, analgesia, and stress behavior of adult mice. Physiol Behav 2003; 78: 375–83.

38. Szuran T, Zimmerman E, Pliska V et al. Prenatal stress effects on exploratory activity and stress induced analgesia in rats. Dev Psychobiol 1991; 24: 361–72.

39. Narsinghani U, Anand KJS. Developmental neurobiology of pain in neonatal rats. Lab Anim 2000; 29: 27–39.

40. Omote K, Kawamata T, Kawamata M et al. Formalin-induced nociception activates a monoaminergic descending inhibitory system. Brain Res 1998; 814: 194–8.

41. Green GN, Scarth J, Dickenson A. An excitatory role for 5-HT in spinal inflammatory nociceptive transmission; state-dependent actions via dorsal horn 5-HT$_3$ receptors in the anaesthetized rat. Pain 2000; 89: 81–8.

42. Ren K, Dubner R. Descending modulation in persistent pain: an update. Pain 2002; 100: 1–6.

43. Zeit KP, Guy N, Malmberg AB et al. The 5-HT3 subtype of serotonin receptor contributes to nociceptive processing via a novel subset of myelinated and unmyelinated nociceptors. J Neurosci 2002; 22: 1010–19.

44. Basbaum AI, Fields HL. Endogenous pain control systems: brainstem spinal pathways and endorphin circuitry. Annu Rev Neurosci 1984; 7: 309–38.

45. Gebhart FG. Descending modulation of pain. Neurosci Biobehav Rev 2004; 27: 729–37.

46. Dubuisson D, Dennis SG. The formalin test: a quantitative study of the analgesic effects of morphine, meperidine, and brain stem stimulation in rats and cats. Pain 1977; 4: 161–74.

47. Tjölsen A, Berge OG, Hunskaar S et al. The formalin test: an evaluation of the method. Pain 1992; 51: 5–17.

48. Abbott FV, Ocvirk R, Najafee R et al. Improving the efficiency of the formalin test. Pain 1999; 83: 561–9.

49. Butkevich IP, Vershinina EA. Prenatal stress alters characteristics and intensity of formalin-induced pain responses in juvenile rats. Brain Res 2001; 915: 88–93.

50. Butkevich IP, Vershinina EA. Maternal stress differently alters nociceptive behaviors in the formalin test in adult female and male rats. Brain Res 2003; 961: 159–65.

51. Aloisi AM, Albonetti ME, Carli G. Sex differences in the behavioral response to persistent pain in rats. Neurosci Lett 1994; 179: 79–82.

52. Butkevich IP. Sex differences in effects of prenatal stress on specific biphasic behavioral response in the nociceptive formalin test in adult rats. Zhurn Evol Biochim Fiziol 2003; 39: 173–8 (in Russian).

53. Lauder JM, Towle AC, Patrick K et al. Decreased serotonin content of embryonic raphe neurons following maternal

administration of p-chlorophenylalanine: a quantitative immunocytochemical study. Dev Brain Res 1985; 20: 107–14.

54. Otellin VA, Khozhay LI. Role of serotonin in prenatal development and pathology of mammalian brain. In: Theoretical and Applied Aspects of Embryonic Histogenesis. St Petersburg: Pediatric Medical Academy, 2002: 25–32 (in Russian).

55. McLaughlin CR, Lichtman AH, Fanselow MS et al. Tonic nociception in neonatal rats. Pharmacol Biochem Behav 1990; 36: 859–62.

56. Guy ER, Abbott FV. The behavioral response to formalin in preweanling rats. Pain 1992; 51: 81–90.

57. Barr GA. Maturation of the biphasic behavioral and heart rate response in the formalin test. Pharmacol Biochem Behav 1998; 60: 329–35.

58. Fitzgerald M, Koltzenburg M. The functional development of descending inhibitory pathways in the dorsolateral funiculus of the newborn rat spinal cord. Dev Brain Res 1986; 24: 261–70.

59. Coderre TJ, Katz J, Vaccarino AL et al. Contribution of central neuroplasticity to pathological pain: review of clinical and experimental evidence. Pain 1993; 52: 259–85.

60. Dallel R, Raboisson P, Clavelou P et al. Evidence for a peripheral origin of the tonic nociceptive response to subcutaneous formalin. Pain 1995; 61: 11–16.

61. Puig S, Sorkin LS. Formalin-evoked activity in identified primary afferent fibres: systemic lidocaine suppresses phase 2 activity. Pain 1996; 64: 345–57.

62. Goroll D, Arias P, Wuttke W. Ontogenic changes in the hypothalamic levels of amino acid neurotransmitters in the female rat. Dev Brain Res 1994; 77: 183–8.

63. Knoll J, Miklya I. Enhanced catecholaminergic and serotonergic activity in rat brain from weaning to sexual maturity: rationale for prophylactic (-)deprenyl (selegiline) medication. Life Sci 1995; 56: 611–20.

64. Henry JL, Yashpal K, Pitcher GM et al. Physiological evidence that the 'interphase' in the formalin test is due to active inhibition. Pain 1999; 89: 57–63.

65. Pitcher GM, Henry JL. Second phase of formalin-induced excitation of spinal dorsal horn neurons in spinalized rats

is reversed by sciatic nerve block. Eur J Neurosci 2002; 15: 1509–15.

66. Wu WL, Ziskind-Conhaim L, Sweet MA. Early development of glycine- and GABA-mediated synapses in rat spinal cord. J Neurosci 1992; 12: 3935–45.

67. Desjardins C, Macmillan KL, Hafs HD. Reproductive organ DNA and RNA of male and female rats from birth to 100 days of age. Anat Rec 1968; 161: 17–22.

68. Fillingim RB, Ness TJ. Sex-related hormonal influences on pain and analgesic responses. Neurosci Biobehav Rev 2000; 24: 485–501.

69. Lauder JM. Ontogeny of the serotonergic system in the rat: serotonin as a developmental signal. Ann N Y Acad Sci 1990; 600: 297–313.

70. Whitaker PM, Whitaker-Azmitia M, Druse P et al. Serotonin as a developmental signal. Behav Brain Res 1996; 73: 19–29.

71. Otellin VA. Tissue mechanisms of prenatal development of human brain, Institute of Experimental Medicine on the Eve of New Millenium. In: Achievements in the Field of Experimental Biology and Medicine. St Petersburg: Nauka, 2000: 102–11 (in Russian).

72. Butkevich IP, Khozhai LI, Mikhailenko VA et al. Decreased serotonin level during pregnancy alters morphological and functional characteristics of tonic nociceptive system in juvenile offspring of the rat. Reprod Biol Endocrinol 2003; 1: 96 (http://www.RBEj.com/articles/browse.asp).

73. Lauder JM, Krebs H. Effects of p-chlorophenylalanine on time of neuronal origin during embryogenesis in the rat. Brain Res 1976; 107: 638–44.

74. Bell J, Zhang X, Whitaker-Azmitia PM. 5-HT$_3$ receptor-active drugs alter development of spinal serotonergic innervation: lack of effect of other serotonergic agents. Brain Res 1992; 571: 293–7.

75. Lauder JM, Liu J, Grayson DR. In uterus exposure to serotonergic drugs alters neonatal expression of 5-HT1A receptor transcripts: a quantitative RT-PCR study. Int J Dev Neurosci 2000; 18: 171–6.

Section V – Perinatal factors altering behavioral outcomes

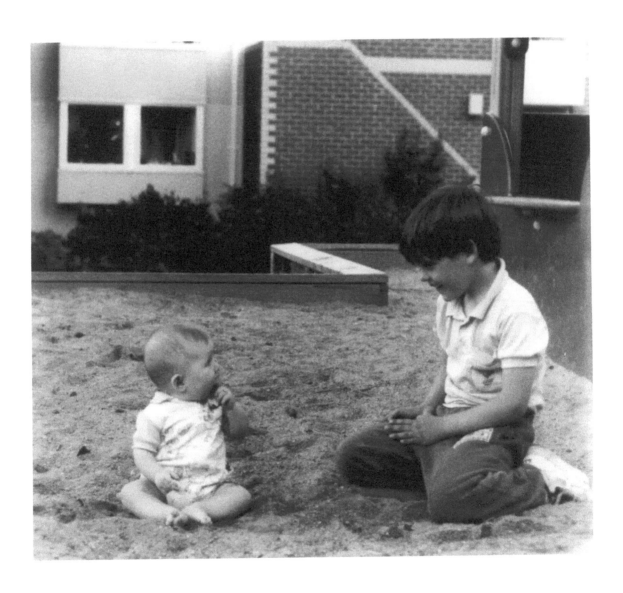

'The seed of a tree has the nature of a branch or twig or bud. It is a part of the tree, but if separated and set in the earth to be better nourished, the embryo or young tree contained in it takes root and grows into a new tree' Isaac Newton

17

Prenatal androgens and the ontogeny of behavior

Sheri A Berenbaum

INTRODUCTION

Studies in human and nonhuman species make clear that events occurring early in development can have lifelong effects. Many chapters in this book describe how early events affect health and disease throughout the lifespan. Several chapters show that these effects are not limited to physical characteristics, but extend to behavior. For example, physical and emotional stressors experienced by pregnant rodent, monkey, and human females are associated with behavioral problems in offspring;[1–3] maternal anxiety during pregnancy is associated with a variety of childhood problems in offspring.[4] The physical and behavioral effects of prenatal stress and anxiety appear to be mediated by hormone-induced actions on the developing hypothalamic-pituitary-adrenal (HPA) axis.[3,5]

Long-term physical and behavioral effects also occur after another type of prenatal event: exposure to sex hormones, particularly androgens. With respect to physical development, sexual differentiation of the mammalian reproductive system depends largely on the amount of androgens that are present early in development. In human beings, this period begins at about 7–8 weeks of gestation when the testes develop and begin to secrete testosterone.[6] The amount of testosterone (or other androgens) present at that time determines whether the undifferentiated external genitalia develop in a male-typical or a female-typical fashion. When levels of testosterone are high (as is typical for males), the genitalia become the penis, scrotum, and urogenital sinus; when testosterone levels are low (as is typical for females), the genitalia become the clitoris, labia majora, and separate vaginal and urethral canals. When levels of testosterone are moderate (in between those typical for males and those typical for females), the genitalia are ambiguous, e.g. an enlarged clitoris

with fused labia or a small penis. Prenatal exposure to sex hormones also affects the development of the internal reproductive structures and probably the hypothalamic-pituitary-gonadal axis, which influences later reproductive function.[6]

With respect to behavioral effects of prenatal androgen exposure, studies in a variety of nonhuman mammalian species very clearly demonstrate that behavioral variations across the lifespan are related to androgen exposure early in life, either from experimental manipulation or from naturally occurring variations such as gestating close to an animal of the opposite sex (for reviews, see refs 7–11). Rodents exposed during the neonatal period to androgen levels that are atypical for their sex also show behavior that is atypical for their sex, including alterations in juvenile rough play, adult aggressive and sexual behavior, and maze performance. Androgens also produce changes in parts of the brain, including the hypothalamus, which is involved in sexual behavior, and the hippocampus, involved in spatial learning.[7]

Primates also show long-lasting behavioral effects of exposure to early androgens: female monkeys treated early in development are masculinized with respect to sexual behavior, rough play, grooming,[12,13] and some learning abilities.[14,15] Studies in monkeys show that there may be several distinct sensitive periods – even within the prenatal period – for androgen effects on behavior, and that it is possible to masculinize the genitalia and behavior independently.[12] Further, the environmental context can modify how the behavioral effects of hormones are manifest.[13]

As described in this chapter, studies of the long-term behavioral effects of prenatal androgens in humans have generally confirmed the findings and principles derived from rodent and primate research. Much of this work has been done in clinical samples, i.e. where hormones were unusual because of disease or accident. Because such 'experiments of nature' have limitations related to alternative explanations and generalizability, it is important to note that recent work in typical populations has provided some convergence of the evidence regarding the behavioral importance of prenatal androgens.

METHODS FOR STUDYING PRENATAL ANDROGEN EFFECTS ON HUMAN BEHAVIORAL DEVELOPMENT

Clinical conditions

It is obviously not feasible or ethical to conduct experimental manipulations of prenatal androgens in human beings, but the field has benefited from natural experiments, i.e. studies of people with disorders of sexual differentiation whose prenatal androgen exposure is inconsistent with other aspects of biological sex such as sex chromosomes.[16] The studies vary in their methodological rigor, and it is important to temper generalizations in light of these limitations, particularly alternative explanations, sample bias (especially the possibility that those who participate in studies are not representative of the population of patients); objectivity, reliability, and validity of measures; comparison groups; and low statistical power for detecting differences between those with clinical conditions and controls (for further discussion of these issues, see refs 17–22).

Some clinical conditions have been studied more extensively than others, in part because of differences in prevalence and complications, and this chapter focuses on conditions where there is more substantive evidence regarding the behavioral effects of androgen. This includes congenital adrenal hyperplasia (CAH), complete androgen insensitivity syndrome (CAIS), and boys without a penis due to cloacal exstrophy (CE) or accidental ablation.

Congenital adrenal hyperplasia

CAH is the most extensively studied naturally occurring problem of sexual differentiation because it is common, occurring in 1 in 10 000 to 15 000 live births.[6,23] As a result of a single-gene defect in an enzyme that controls cortisol production, individuals with CAH produce high levels of adrenal androgens beginning very early in gestation. Postnatal treatment with corticosteroids (and mineralocorticoids for the 75% who are salt-losers) reduces hormone levels, generally to normal or subnormal levels.[24] Both sexes are affected by CAH, and both have been studied

behaviorally, but studies in nonhuman species indicate clearer findings for females than for males. Genetic females with CAH have external genitalia that are masculinized to varying degrees, but they have ovaries and a uterus and are fertile. They are usually diagnosed at birth and treated with cortisol to reduce androgen excess (otherwise, they will experience rapid growth and early puberty) and surgically to feminize their genitalia. If prenatal androgens affect human sex-typed behavior, then females with CAH should be behaviorally more masculine and less feminine than a comparison group of females without CAH. And they are in many, but not all ways, as described below and reviewed in detail elsewhere.[18,21,25]

Complete androgen insensitivity syndrome

CAIS is a rare genetic condition in which there is normal male-typical sexual differentiation – karyotype of 46, XY, *SRY* gene, testes, and normal male levels of testosterone – but androgen receptors are defective, so the body cannot respond to testosterone. Consequently, affected individuals have female-typical genitalia and are reared as girls, with most diagnosed in adolescence when menarche fails to occur. If human behavior is affected by early androgens, then individuals with CAIS should be female-typical because they do not have functioning receptors to respond to the high (normal male) levels present. It is important to note, however, that other influences on behavior are confounded with androgens in CAIS. Effects of genes on the Y chromosome could produce male-typical behavior, and social rearing as a female could produce female-typical behavior.

Boys without a penis

Much attention has been directed to rare clinical conditions in which boys are lacking a penis but all other aspects of sexual differentiation are male-typical, including exposure to high levels of androgens during early development. The first results from cloacal exstrophy, a very rare congenital defect (1 in 400 000 births[26]), in which the bladder and external genitalia are not properly formed. Although it occurs in both sexes, the effect is most pronounced in males, because an affected boy is born with a malformed or absent penis but with otherwise completely normal male-typical physical development. The second situation is ablatio penis, in which a boy is missing a penis because of an accident after birth, such as a mishandled circumcision.

Until recently, boys without a penis were reared as girls, because of two beliefs: (a) that development of satisfactory gender identity and overall psychological adjustment depend on having normal-looking genitalia (although some surgical correction is now possible, the penis will never look or function normally) and (b) that gender identity is determined predominantly by rearing.[16] The beliefs that have resulted in rearing these children as girls have been vigorously challenged in the past few years, primarily on the basis of scientific and popular reports about one child born a boy but raised as a girl and then self-reassigned to the male sex.[27,28] Although these reports have focused on the biological determination of gender identity, the systematic evidence described below reveals a complex picture. Because these children have been reared as girls, they provide the opportunity to examine the relative behavioral contributions of prenatal hormones (male-typical) vs sex of rearing (female-typical). If they behave and identify as girls, this suggests the importance of the social environment. If they are masculinized in their behavior, however, this provides evidence for the importance of prenatal androgens or genes on the Y-chromosome.

Studies in typical populations

Clinical populations have provided valuable information about the hormonal contributions to behavior, but they are not perfect experiments (because of methodological limitations and concerns about generalization) and they are also difficult to study (because of their relatively low frequency and sampling problems). Therefore, it is important to evaluate whether typical variations in prenatal androgen exposure have long-lasting consequences for behavior within the normal range.

Direct methods

An ideal study would involve direct measurements of fetal hormones, taken serially at many points in gestation, to ensure reliable measures of the hormones at several likely sensitive periods, and then a follow-up behavioral study in childhood and beyond. The ideal is obviously difficult to realize because of the risks associated with collecting specimens from living fetuses. But, some progress has been made with studies that obtain 'snapshots' of the fetal hormone environment, from samples of peripheral hormones (although none directly measure fetal hormone levels). These studies involved evaluations of childhood or adult behavior in relation to hormones obtained in early development from amniotic fluid, mother's blood during pregnancy or umbilical cord blood. Although these studies have limitations, primarily related to concerns about timing of collection and reliability of hormones, weaknesses

in behavioral assessments, and small samples with limited variability, they have provided useful information, as described below (for detailed review, see ref. 19).

Indirect methods

Given the difficulties of obtaining direct measures of sex hormones, indirect methods have been developed that are thought to reflect prenatal androgen exposure (detailed reviews of these methods and results can be found elsewhere).[19,29] The first method involves studies of opposite-sex human twins,[30,31] a logical extension of animal studies showing that behavior and physiology are influenced by naturally occurring variations in hormones that result from an animal's position in the uterus, particularly the sex of its littermates (intrauterine position, IUP).[9,11,32] Studies suggest that the physical and behavioral masculinization of female rodents that gestate between two males results directly from transfer of testosterone from the male fetus to the adjacent female fetus.[33]

There are a number of studies of sex-typed behavior in twins in relation to the sex of their co-twin, as described below. It is unclear, however, whether this is a good method for studying the behavioral effects of prenatal androgens in humans, because there is currently no evidence that human twins are exposed to hormones from their co-twins at all or at high enough levels or during sensitive periods. There is also reason to think that females are protected by a separate placenta from significant exposure to testosterone from their male womb mate. Females in other species are probably exposed to relatively higher levels than are human female twins, because the former have multiple littermates.

The second indirect method to assess behavioral effects of prenatal androgens involves examining associations between behavior and morphological measures thought to reflect prenatal androgen exposure by virtue of the fact that they show sex differences or associations with traits known to be influenced by androgen. These measures include otoacoustic emissions (sounds produced by the ear and reflecting auditory function), finger ratio (the relative lengths of the index and ring fingers), body asymmetry, and dermatoglyphics (fingerprints). Unfortunately, there is very little direct evidence relating these markers specifically to prenatal exposure to androgens, and associations between these markers and behavior do not yield clear results.

EVIDENCE FOR PRENATAL ANDROGEN EFFECTS ON HUMAN BEHAVIORAL DEVELOPMENT

Prenatal androgens are most likely to have effects on behaviors that differ between the two sexes, given their role in sexual differentiation of the body (and thus the brain). Studies in other species confirm this, showing that exposure to androgens during critical periods of brain development affects only those behaviors that show sex differences. Therefore, most human studies have focused on behavioral characteristics that differ between males and females. The nature of sex-related behaviors has been conceptualized in a number of ways, but most emphasize its multidimensionality. Table 17.1 lists the domains described in a widely used conceptualization of gender-typing.[34] Although all domains might theoretically be influenced by prenatal androgens, studies have generally focused only on some aspects of some domains.

Activities and interests

The earliest evidence regarding the behavioral effects of androgens came from girls with CAH, who were reported to be tomboys.[16] The interpretation was complicated, however, by the methods used (non-blind interviews, small samples, inadequate comparisons), factors associated with the disease and its treatment (especially other hormones) and, most seriously, the possibility that behavior resulted from parental treatment in response to the appearance of the girls' genitals.[35]

Subsequent studies have addressed many of these problems and extended assessments across age and across behavioral domains. There is now a considerable literature showing that exposure to androgens early in life (through CAH) has a large effect on activities that are differentially preferred by typical males and females. In childhood, girls with CAH play much more with boys' toys than do their unaffected sisters or other controls, as seen in direct observations of children's play, in girls' self-reports of their activities, and in parents' reports of the girls' activities.[36–41] For example, girls with CAH aged 3–12 played with boys' toys about 1.5–2 times as much as comparison girls. When choosing a toy to keep, about 50% of girls with CAH chose a transportation toy, whereas no control girl did.

Androgens continue to exert effects on sex-typed activities beyond childhood. Adolescent and adult females with CAH are interested in male-typical activities, as seen in self-reports and parents' reports of their daughters' activities (SA Berenbaum, unpublished data, 2003).[42,43] For example, teenage girls with CAH are more likely than their sisters to report interest in electronics and sports.

The male-typical interests of females with CAH extend to vocational interests. For example, teenage girls with CAH express interest in male-typical careers, such as engineer, construction worker, and airline pilot, whereas their unaffected sisters express interest in female-typical careers, such as X-ray technician, ice skater, and hair stylist.[41,42] Because interests show stability in typical males and females,[44] it is likely that adult females with CAH will choose male-typical occupations more often than their sisters, but this awaits empirical test.

Across age, these male-typical preferences are characteristic of (that is, they are found in almost all) girls with CAH, especially those with the greatest degree of prenatal androgen exposure, as reflected by clinical features[41,42,45,46] and genotype.[40] The increase in male-typical activity interests in females with CAH is paralleled by a decrease in female-typical interests, including play with girls' toys and interest in female-

---

Table 17.1 Primary dimensions of gender-related behavior[34]

Domain	Characteristics
Gender identity	Sense of self as male or female
Activities and interests	Toys, play activities, hobbies, occupations, household roles, tasks
Personality-social attributes	Personality traits (e.g. aggression), social behaviors (e.g. help-seeking)
Social relationships	Sex of peers, friends, lovers; preferred parent, models
Style and symbols	Gestures, speech patterns (e.g. tempo), play styles, fantasy
Values	Knowledge of and endorsement of greater value attached to one sex or gender role than the other

typical activities, hobbies, and careers.[36–38,41,42,45,46] Thus, the sex-atypical interests of females with CAH have been documented in several studies from different laboratories using multiple methods and sampling strategies.

The importance of prenatal androgen exposure for sex-typed interests is also suggested by data from other groups with sex-atypical hormone exposure, although these conditions have not been studied as extensively as CAH. Adult females with CAIS, who are insensitive to and unable to respond to androgens, have female-typical activity interests, as measured by reports of their current interests and by retrospective reports of their childhood interests.[47,48] Individuals with cloacal exstrophy who have high (male-typical) prenatal androgen exposure, but female rearing because of absent penis, are reported by themselves and their parents to have male-typical childhood activity interests.[26]

Although the data from clinical samples strongly implicate a role for prenatal androgens in the expression of sex-typed interests across development, they are not perfect experiments. Nevertheless, alternative explanations for the findings have generally not been supported. First, the behavioral changes observed in females with CAH might result from social responses to their masculinized genitalia,[35] but effects of parent socialization have not been demonstrated. For example, the amount of time that girls with CAH play with boys' toys is not increased when parents are present,[40] and parents wish that their daughters with CAH were *less* masculine than they are (whereas they wish that their daughters without CAH were more masculine than they are).[41] These results are consistent with those from androgenized female monkeys showing mothers' behaviors to be unrelated to their offsprings' masculine behavior.[12] Second, behavioral changes in CAH may reflect effects of increased androgen continuing into postnatal life. But behavior in females with CAH has been found to relate more to indicators of prenatal androgen excess, such as degree of enzyme deficiency reflected in genetic mutation[40] and severity of illness,[41,45,46] and not to indicators of postnatal androgen excess, such as advanced growth or hormones measured close in time to behavioral assessment.[45] Evidence from males with cloacal exstrophy also argues against the primacy of postnatal androgen. Although they are castrated in the perinatal period, they appear to have male-typical childhood activity interests.[26] Third, females with CAH have abnormalities beyond prenatal androgen, such as progesterone and corticosteroids, but these hormones have smaller and less consistent behavioral effects than androgen, and may actually prevent masculinization.[49]

Further, behavioral similarities between CAH and control males and between CAIS and control females make it unlikely that behavioral changes in CAH females reflect general disease characteristics or other hormonal abnormalities.[18]

There is also some question about the extent to which findings from CAH females can be generalized to the overall female population given that their androgen levels are considerably higher than those of any female without CAH. Thus, it is important to confirm findings in females with typical levels of prenatal androgen exposure. Such evidence comes from two studies which found higher testosterone in mother's blood during pregnancy to be associated with masculinized gender-role behavior in their daughters in later life. One study examined sex-typed activities in typical girls at age 3½ years in relation to testosterone in their mother's serum during pregnancy (blood samples were collected between weeks 5 and 36 of gestation). Girls who engaged in masculine activities had mothers with higher testosterone when the girls were *in utero* than did girls who engaged in feminine activities.[50] Another study examined a broad measure of gender-role behavior in adult females. Behavior was found to be associated with the women's own hormones in adulthood, hormones in mother's blood during pregnancy, and their interaction.[51–53] Consistent with suggestions that prenatal weeks 8–24 are the key sensitive period, behavior was related to hormones from maternal blood during the second trimester only. The only evidence inconsistent with androgen effects on sex-typical interests comes from females with a male co-twin who do not appear to differ from females with a female co-twin in childhood play[54–56] or adult interests,[57,58] although this may reflect problems with the twin method for assessing androgen effects.

Overall, then, the evidence from CAH, CAIS, cloacal exstrophy, and several typical samples shows clearly that exposure to elevated androgen during prenatal life is associated with increased interest in male-typical activities and reduced interest in female-typical activities in childhood, adolescence, and adulthood. Effects are large at moderate-to-high levels of androgen (as in females with CAH), but may be somewhat smaller when androgens are within the range of typical females.

Gender identity

There is considerable controversy over the extent to which prenatal androgen exerts long-lasting effects on gender identity (identification as male or female). For most people, gender identity is unquestioned and corresponds with both their biological sex and rearing sex. Gender identity is an issue in a relatively small number of people in the general population who are unhappy with their sex and, in some cases, seek sex-reassignment with or without surgery (transsexual individuals). Gender identity has also been an issue in individuals whose prenatal sex hormone exposure is not consistent with their genital appearance, e.g. boys without a penis due to cloacal exstrophy or accident, girls with CAH and very masculinized genitalia.

The evidence suggests that androgens may play a role in the establishment of gender identity, but that it is far from determinative. Females with CAH are most likely to have typical gender identity, although their degree of identification may be reduced compared with typical females.[39,59–61] Gender change in females with CAH is uncommon, but still more common than in the general population.[61,62] Importantly, variations in gender identity in females with CAH are *not* related to the degree of prenatal androgen excess or genital appearance.

Evidence from boys without a penis is not as systematic as in CAH, but also shows considerable variability in outcome that is not simply related to prenatal androgen exposure. As noted above, much has been written and inferred from a single individual born a boy but reared as a girl after a mishandled circumcision. Although early reports suggested that this child adapted well to the female assignment,[16] later reports revealed considerable unhappiness with the assignment, resulting in self-reassignment to the male sex.[27,28] This is widely interpreted to show the primacy of biology in determining gender identity, but close inspection of the evidence reveals important caveats. The child was reared as a boy early in life (the accident happened at age 7 months, reassignment was made in the second year, and initial feminizing genital surgery was not completed until 21 months), so there was a long and perhaps sensitive period when he was reared as a boy. Further, another individual with a similar history but with earlier female reassignment had a different gender identity, identifying as a female.[63]

Boys with cloacal exstrophy reared as girls are also heterogeneous with respect to gender identity,[64] but it is unclear what accounts for the variability because they have not been studied in sufficient detail. Much attention has been directed to a recent small study of 14 individuals,[26] of whom 6 or 8 (depending on the criteria) were stated to identify as male, with the results interpreted to demonstrate the biological determination of gender identity. The study is impressive in enlisting all potential participants (thus removing any concern about sample bias), but there is considerable ambiguity in interpretation of results because of unsystematic and subjective assessments, likely effects

of interviewer expectations, and some conflating of gender identity with male-typical activity interests.[65] Further, gender change may arise not just from biology, but in response to complex social conditions, e.g. a mismatch between behavior and parent expectations, peer stigmatization associated with atypical interests, internalized homophobia.[62,64] Case reports and other small-scale studies of individuals with cloacal exstrophy reveal a mixed picture with respect to gender identity, although most did not include good assessments of gender identity and likely did not have representative samples.[64,66]

Additional information about gender identity comes from other clinical conditions in which an individual with a male karyotype has been exposed to reduced levels of prenatal androgen, e.g. micropenis, partial androgen insensitivity syndrome. Some of these individuals were reared as male and some as female. Case reports and small-scale studies of these individuals show variation in gender identity that is not simply related to prenatal androgens or rearing sex.[64,67,68]

Overall, then, the evidence from males with male-typical androgens who were reared as females and individuals with intermediate levels of androgens reared as females or males show variability in gender identity that is not simply related to prenatal androgen. The evidence from females with CAH suggests that moderate levels of prenatal androgens are insufficient to masculinize gender identity. But it is unclear whether exposure to higher levels of androgens has a more pronounced effect, in light of the methodological limitations in studies of males with altered androgens or absent penis (primarily unrepresentative sampling and limited assessment of gender identity).

Sexual orientation

There has been considerable interest in prenatal 'programming' of sexual orientation by sex hormones. The best evidence about androgen effects on sexual orientation comes from studies of women with CAH. Social constraints limit the expression of homosexual behavior (in terms of opportunity and societal disapproval), so the best studies examine arousal and not just experiences. Two recent and methodologically careful studies show that, as a group, females with CAH are more likely to be sexually attracted to women than are their unaffected sisters.[60,61] Nevertheless, a majority of women with CAH report themselves to be exclusively heterosexual in both behavior and arousal, and it is unclear what differentiates them from the approximately one-third who are bisexual or homosexual. There is some reason to think, however, that androgen effects on sexual orientation might be larger than suggested from these studies, because of possible underreporting or sample bias (women with homosexual interests might be more reluctant to participate or to reveal their true interests than would women with a heterosexual orientation).

Evidence from other clinical conditions is consistent with data from females with CAH suggesting that prenatal exposure to elevated androgens increases sexual interest in women. The two individuals with ablatio penis described above had sexual interest in women (despite different gender identity outcomes).[28,63] Individuals with CAIS reared as females show sexual attraction to men. This preference could reflect either absence of exposure to androgen or female rearing.[47]

Indirect evidence for androgen effects on sexual orientation has been sought by examining orientation in relation to sexually dimorphic anatomical markers or functions. The premise of these studies is that homosexual individuals are sex-atypical: gay men are hypothesized to be 'hypomasculine,' that is, to have characteristics that are demasculinized and feminized compared with heterosexual men, whereas lesbians are hypothesized to be 'hypermasculine,' having masculinized and defeminized characteristics compared with heterosexual women. There is a sizable literature examining morphological markers in relation to sexual orientation, with some – but not nearly all – studies finding sex-atypical patterns in homosexual individuals (for review and discussion, see refs 19, 69). For example, lesbians, but not gay males, have been found to be intermediate to heterosexual males and females on an aspect of auditory function,[70] and on the relative length of the second and fourth fingers.[71] Homosexual men have been reported to have a pattern of fingerprint asymmetry more similar to heterosexual women than to heterosexual men,[72] but there are several failures to replicate this finding.[73] Homosexual individuals are also more likely than same-sex heterosexual comparisons to report sex-atypical interests measured concurrently in adulthood and retrospectively in childhood.[74–76]

Personality and social behaviors

Prenatal androgens also appear to be associated with personal and social attributes that show sex differences, including maternal behavior and aggression. Although androgens appear to affect these characteristics less than activities and interests, they have not been as well studied, so it is difficult to make definitive comparisons. As with other behaviors, much of the evidence for the effects of androgen comes from females with CAH. Compared to unaffected females,

females with CAH are less interested in babies and in having their own children.[38,77,78] It is possible that this reflects a psychological response to reduced fertility associated with the disease, but it seems unlikely because women with Turner syndrome (who are completely infertile) do not show reduced interest in babies,[16] nor do males with CAH.[78]

Females with CAH are also more likely than their unaffected sisters to report that they would use physical aggression in hypothetical conflict situations, especially when they are reporting as adults about their childhood behavior.[79] These results confirm an earlier study in females who were prenatally exposed to androgenizing progestins as a result of a preventive maternal treatment for miscarriage:[80] the daughters when aged 6–18 were more likely than their similar-age unexposed sisters to report that they would use aggression in conflict situations. It is important to note, however, the complexity of androgen effects on aggression in both human and nonhuman animals. For example, in both rodents and primates, aggression in adulthood is affected by treatment with androgens during prenatal, early postnatal, and adult life.[81–84] In humans, circulating testosterone is sometimes associated with aggression, with the effects most pronounced in adolescents and when aggression is measured as response to provocation, and aggression itself or a related trait, social dominance, may increase androgen levels.[84–88] Androgens may mediate aggression through direct brain effects and through facilitation of the learning of aggression.[83]

There are many other aspects of personality and social behavior that show sex differences, but few data to indicate whether they are related to prenatal androgens. There is some suggestion from twin studies that prenatal androgens influence sensation-seeking (a trait usually higher in males than females). Females with a male co-twin were reported to be masculinized as compared with females with a female co-twin on sensation-seeking[30] and rule-breaking,[57] although it is possible that the effects were due to sharing a postnatal social environment and other studies have failed to find differences on similar traits.[58,89] It will be interesting to look at these traits in females with CAH, as well as to determine whether the latter have lower scores on traits (besides maternal interest) on which females score higher than males, such as emotional expressivity, intimacy in friendships, and depression.[34]

A recent study focused on associations between social behavior (in young children) and prior testosterone levels in amniotic fluid.[90–92] The study was motivated by an interest in early precursors of developmental disorders that show sex differences (especially autism), which might be influenced by prenatal testosterone.[93,94] Sex differences were found with girls scoring higher than boys on vocabulary, eye contact, and mother-reported communication skills, social relationships, and breadth of interests. Several behaviors were associated with testosterone across sex, but this largely reflects the sex differences in testosterone and behavior. There were few within-sex associations between prenatal testosterone and behavior and they were in boys. Consistent with the idea that androgens masculinize/defeminize behavior, higher testosterone in boys was associated with restricted interests[90] and lower amounts of eye contact.[91] It will be important to replicate these results and seek confirmation in other samples, e.g. to assess these behaviors in girls with CAH. It is unclear why there were no significant associations between prenatal testosterone and behavior in girls, but likely explanations include small sample (and thus low statistical power) and limited variability in testosterone.

Cognitive abilities

Early androgen also appears to play a role in aspects of cognition. There are no sex differences in general intelligence, but there are differences in the *pattern* of intellectual abilities. Males, on average, outperform females on measures of spatial, mechanical, and mathematical abilities, whereas females, on average, outperform males on measures of verbal fluency, verbal memory, emotional perception, and perceptual speed.[95] Several lines of evidence from clinical and typical samples converge to suggest that the sex difference in at least one of these abilities – spatial – is influenced by prenatal androgen acting to organize the brain early in development.

Females with CAH have been reported to have greater spatial ability than their unaffected female relatives in childhood, adolescence, and adulthood.[96–98] The aspects of spatial ability that appear to be enhanced include spatial orientation and visualization, and targeting. Although this difference has not always been found,[97,99,100] it is important to note that the nonreplications are generally associated with small samples and insensitive measures (those that do not show sex differences). Given that the sex differences in spatial ability are smaller than the differences in other psychological traits such as activity interests, it may be difficult to discern differences in androgen-exposed groups, especially with the size of the samples typically studied.[25]

Consistent with data from females with CAH, males with low early androgen levels (due to idiopathic hypogonadotropic hypogonadism, IHH) have lower spatial ability than controls. This difference

likely reflects reduced androgen early in development, because spatial ability was correlated with testicular volume and did not improve with androgen replacement in males with IHH, and was not reduced in males with acquired (late-onset) hypogonadism.[101] Unfortunately, cognitive abilities have not been well studied in individuals with other clinical conditions, such as CAIS and cloacal exstrophy.

There is also some suggestion from nonclinical samples that typical variation in prenatal androgen is related to spatial ability, although the results are not straightforward. In one study, testosterone in amniotic fluid was related to spatial ability in girls at age 7. Girls with higher amniotic testosterone levels had faster (but not necessarily more accurate) performance on a mental rotation task than did girls with lower levels, but effects were found only in a subgroup of girls who used a rotation strategy, and, unexpectedly, girls were faster at rotation than boys.[102] A study of female dizygotic twins showed females with a male co-twin to have higher spatial ability than females with a female co-twin.[103] These studies, if replicated, suggest that enhanced spatial ability in females with CAH results directly from the effects of androgen on the developing brain, and not from social responses to the girls' virilized genitalia or other abnormalities of the disease.

There is not much known about the effect of prenatal androgen on other sex-typed cognitive abilities, including those on which males are superior (e.g. mechanical and mathematical abilities) and those on which females are superior (e.g. verbal fluency and memory). It will be interesting to study, for example, whether females with CAH have lower (more male-typical) verbal memory than unaffected females. It may be difficult to get good answers to these questions, however, because sex differences in these abilities are smaller than those in spatial ability, so that large samples will be necessary to detect any effects of early androgens.

Summary of the evidence

It is clear that androgen affects behavior in human beings, and that these effects are complex, confirming findings in other species. Much of what we know comes from females with CAH, although there is convergence of evidence from typical samples. Figure 17.1 summarizes the size of the effects in the context of the major domains of gender-typing, although it is important to remember that some domains have been studied more extensively than others. Androgen has large facilitative effects on interest in male-typical activities across the lifespan, from childhood through adolescence and into adulthood. It also has moderate

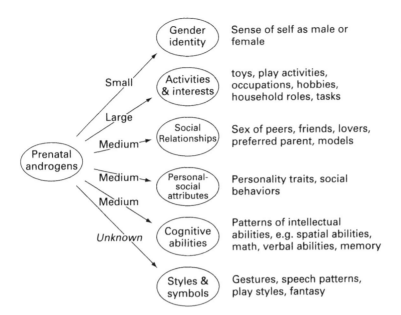

Figure 17.1 Summary of androgen effects on the major domains of sex-typed behavior.

facilitative effects on aspects of social relationships (sexual arousal to females), personal and social attributes (aggression and perhaps sensation-seeking), and cognitive abilities (spatial ability). Androgen also has a moderate inhibitory effect on behaviors in these domains, reducing interest in female-typical activities across the lifespan, and at least one personal-social attribute (interest in babies). There is less evidence regarding androgen effects on behaviors on which females score higher than males than on those with the opposite sex difference. Androgen appears to have a weak effect on gender identity, but this requires additional study.

Details of androgen effects on behavior

There is now little question that there are long-term behavioral effects of the fetal hormone environment, particularly with respect to androgens. But, there is still much that is unknown about these effects, with key questions concerning the precise details of hormone action (see elsewhere for additional discussion).[19,20,104]

First, the *specific sensitive periods* have yet to be delineated. Weeks 8–24 of gestation have been considered the important sensitive period for behavior, given the reported surge in testosterone in males that occurs during that time, but there may be multiple sensitive periods, and different brain regions (and thus different behaviors) may be affected by hormones at different times. Ample data from other species, including primates, confirm this point.[10] There are no relevant data in human beings, although there are speculations, e.g.

that the early postnatal period is important for masculinization of spatial ability.[96,97]

Second, there are many *specific details about hormone effects* yet to be described in human beings, although many have been clearly specified in other species.[7,10] It is unclear what form of androgen is involved in the modulation of human behaviors, how much androgen is needed to masculinize different behaviors, whether associations between androgen and behavior are always linear, and the extent to which androgen effects might be moderated by exposure to other hormones. For example, is a lower dose of androgen needed to masculinize interests than gender identity? For any behavior, is there a threshold of androgen exposure sufficient for masculinization?

Third, much of the focus has been on hormone levels and very little on *hormone responsiveness*. It is clear that mutations in the human androgen receptor gene have consequences for physical traits, producing variations in men ranging from complete insensitivity to androgens (and thus female differentiation, as discussed above) to infertility and minor undervirilization.[105,106] It seems likely that there will be parallel effects for behavioral traits and that the behavioral effects of a given level of androgens will depend on a person's androgen sensitivity. Such effects might be partly responsible for variations in androgen effects within and across studies.

MECHANISMS MEDIATING LONG-TERM BEHAVIORAL EFFECTS OF PRENATAL ANDROGENS

The most compelling question about the behavioral effects of androgen concerns the mechanisms whereby exposure to a single class of hormones during prenatal development can have such profound and long-lasting effects. Most attempts to address questions of mechanism focus on the brain. But, even when we know more about brain mediators of androgen effects on behavior, we will still need to understand how the 'prenatal program' is carried out and how it is modified as the individual navigates through his or her social and physical environment.

Neural mechanisms

How does androgen exposure change brain regions in specific ways to alter behavior later in life? In the past decade, there have been many studies showing sex differences in brain structure and function, including regions involved in behaviors that show sex differences, e.g. the hippocampus and spatial learning, the amygdala and emotion. But all the links between the brain and behavior have not yet been made: it is still unclear how brain differences translate into behavioral differences. Further, sex differences in the brain might arise from a number of sources, including prenatal exposure to androgens, but also in response to other factors, such as sex-differential experience and sex hormones circulating at puberty. It seems reasonable to examine brain structure and function in individuals with known prenatal androgen exposure, e.g. females with CAH. Initial brain imaging studies of such individuals have not shown them to differ from controls in ways that would be expected on the basis of sex differences seen in parallel studies.[107] It is likely that neuroimaging studies will be more informative when there are more data directly linking individual differences in the brain to individual differences in behavior and when they assess brain activation in response to tasks known to be related to androgen exposure, e.g. spatial ability or activity interests.

Mechanisms between the brain and behavior

What are the psychological mechanisms mediating associations between prenatal androgens and behavior? For example, how and why do high levels of early androgen result in high scores on tests of spatial ability, or interest in playing with toy trucks, or reduced attention to babies? Behavioral effects of androgens might be mediated in several ways. First, there might be effects through *physical morphology*, as has been shown in rodents.[8,9] In people, for example, this might include effects on peripheral musculature.

Second, effects might be mediated by *basic perceptual or sensory processes*. Consider two examples of behaviors that are influenced by androgens. Attraction to trucks and Lincoln Logs in children who have been exposed to high androgens might reflect androgen effects on perceptual or affective preferences, such as motion, color, shape, and texture.[108,109] Sex differences in higher cognitive function might result from hormones operating at specific cortical sites and at peripheral sites that contribute to the activation of the cortical sites.[110]

Third, effects might be mediated by differences in *basic cognitive processes* and the neural substrates that subserve them. Sex differences in spatial ability appear to depend, in part, on sex differences in the use of landmarks vs geometric cues. In one study, men and women were found to differ in brain activation during a navigation task; this may reflect men's use of geometric cues vs women's use of working memory to keep landmark cues active.[111] In rodents, these processes appear to be differentially sensitive to hormones.[112]

Developmental pathways

What are the developmental processes by which the effects of hormones are mediated or moderated by aspects of the environment, both social (e.g. parental child-rearing practices) and physical (e.g. prenatal exposure to alcohol)? Some clues are available from studies in monkeys showing that behavioral sex differences result from hormonally influenced predispositions to engage in certain behaviors, even though their ultimate expression is shaped by the social environment in which the animal develops.[13] For example, androgen-induced sex differences in rough-and-tumble play occur in all rearing environments, with the *size* of the difference affected by the situational context. Differences in aggressive and submissive behaviors in androgenized female monkeys were found only in certain rearing environments. Behaviors showing consistent sex differences across social context are most affected by prenatal androgens. Some evidence from human children is consistent with this evidence from monkeys: activities and interests show large sex differences across cultures and are strongly affected by prenatal androgens, whereas aggression levels vary as a function of context and are not as strongly influenced by hormones.

Joint effects of hormones and the social environment might occur in several ways. Individuals with differing levels of hormones may be exposed to different environments because they select different environments or because others provide them with different environments. Consider a speculative example of such a hormone–environment correlation in the development of maternal behavior,[78] as illustrated in Figure 17.2 for typical boys and girls and girls with CAH. A child with a predisposition to be interested in infants (because of prenatal exposure to low levels of androgen) chooses to be around babies and seeks exposure to babies, e.g. babysitting, and obtains rewards from such contact, thereby seeking out additional experience with babies, further developing the interest, and practicing mothering skills. Other factors may affect the trajectory, such as pubertal hormones (which would make females with CAH similar to their sisters) and actual parenting experience (which would increase the experiences of males).

Individuals with different levels of hormones may also respond differently to the same environment. Consider a speculative example of such a hormone–environment interaction in the development of spatial ability, as illustrated in Figure 17.3 for typical boys and girls and girls with CAH. The groups start out at somewhat different levels because of different prenatal exposure to androgens (and thus differences in brain structure related to spatial ability) and they are all exposed to the same environment, e.g. classroom instruction. But, even with the same environment, the differences become magnified with age because those with moderate to high androgen exposure benefit more from their environment than do those with low exposure. The group differences in spatial ability would become even larger if the relevant environments differed for the groups, e.g. playing with spatial toys.

CLINICAL IMPLICATIONS

It is clear that prenatal androgens affect the ontogeny of normal behavior, and it is likely that they also affect the ontogeny of abnormal behavior, but there is no evidence on this issue. Across the lifespan, there are behavioral and mental disorders that are more prevalent in one sex than the other. For example, in childhood and adolescence, there is preponderance of speech and language disorders, autism, ADHD, oppositional and conduct disorder in males, and a female preponderance of separation anxiety disorder. In adulthood, males predominate in substance abuse, females in dysthymic disorder, generalized anxiety disorder, and certain phobias (for specific data see ref. 113). It is reasonable to speculate that at least part of these differences are due to a differential prenatal exposure to androgens.[93,94,114] But this is not an easy issue to study, given the methodological constraints involved in studying behavioral effects of exposure to prenatal androgens, and thus the difficulty of obtaining the large samples that would be necessary to look at these less common events.

SUMMARY AND CONCLUSIONS

Prenatal exposure to androgens has long-lasting masculinizing and defeminizing effects on behavior across the lifespan. Effects are most pronounced at moderate-to-high levels of exposure and for some behavioral domains more than others. Thus, androgens have a large effect on sex-typed interests, a moderate effect on sexual orientation, aspects of personality, and spatial ability, and a weak effect on gender identity. We are on the verge of a more complete understanding of behavioral effects of hormones (in humans) and the mechanisms that mediate the behavioral effects of androgens, including neural substrates and the

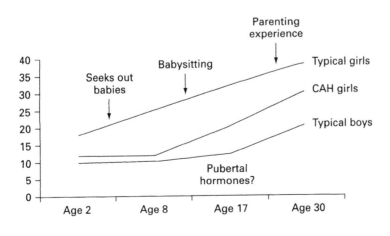

Figure 17.2 Hypothetical example of hormone–environment correlation: development of interest in babies.

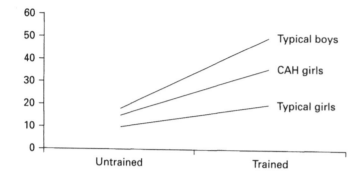

Figure 17.3 Hypothetical example of hormone–environment interaction: development of spatial ability.

developmental pathways. Future work will also indicate how prenatal androgens affect developmental disorders and mental illnesses that occur with different prevalence in males and females.

ACKNOWLEDGMENTS

Preparation of this chapter and my own research reported here were supported by a grant from the National Institutes of Health, grant HD19644. A number of people have contributed to my research and I would particularly like to thank Kristina Korman Bryk for providing outstanding research assistance, the pediatric endocrinologists who generously provided access to their patients and answered medical questions, the graduate and undergraduate students who have helped to collect and process data, and Drs Stephen Duck, Michael Bailey, and Susan Resnick for their collaborations. I am particularly grateful to the families who have participated in my studies.

REFERENCES

1. Gordon HW. Early environmental stress and biological vulnerability to drug abuse. Psychoneuroendocrinology 2002; 27: 115–26.
2. O'Connor TG, Heron J, Golding J, Glover V. Maternal antenatal anxiety and behavioural/emotional problems in children: a test of a programming hypothesis. J Child Psychol Psychiatry 2003; 44: 1025–36.
3. Schneider ML, Moore CF, Kraemer GW, Roberts AD, DeJesus OT. The impact of prenatal stress, fetal alcohol exposure, or both on development: perspectives from a primate model. Psychoneuroendocrinology 2002; 27: 285–98.
4. Van den Bergh BRH, Marcoen A. High antenatal maternal anxiety is related to ADHD symptoms, externalizing problems, and anxiety in 8- and 9-year-olds. Child Dev 2004; 75: 1085–97.
5. Weinstock M. Does prenatal stress impair coping and regulation of hypothalamic-pituitary-adrenal axis? Neurosci Biobehav Rev 1997; 21: 1–10.
6. Grumbach MM, Hughes IA, Conte FA. Disorders of sex differentiation. In: Williams Textbook of Endocrinology, 10th edn (Larsen PR, Kronenberg HM, Melmed S, Polonsky KS, eds). Philadelphia: WB Saunders, 2002.
7. Becker JB, Breedlove SM, Crews D, McCarthy MM, eds. Behavioral Endocrinology, 2nd edn. Cambridge, MA: MIT Press, 2002.
8. Breedlove SM. Sexual dimorphism in the vertebrate nervous system. J Neurosci 1992; 12: 4133–42.
9. Clark MM, Galef BG. Effects of intrauterine position on the behavior and genital morphology of litter-bearing rodents. Dev Neuropsychol 1998; 14: 197–211.
10. Goy RW, McEwen BS. Sexual Differentiation of the Brain. Cambridge: MIT Press, 1980.
11. Ryan BC, Vandenbergh JG. Intrauterine position effects. Neurosci Biobehav Rev 2002; 26: 665–78.
12. Goy RW, Bercovitch FB, McBrair MC. Behavioral masculinization is independent of genital masculinization in prenatally androgenized female rhesus macaques. Horm Behav 1988; 22: 552–71.
13. Wallen K. Nature needs nurture: the interaction of hormonal and social influences on the development of behavioral sex differences in rhesus monkeys. Horm Behav 1996; 30: 364–78.
14. Bachevalier J, Hagger C. Sex differences in the development of learning abilities in primates. Psychoneuroendocrinology 1991; 16: 177–88.
15. Clark AS, Goldman-Rakic PS. Gonadal hormones influence the emergence of cortical function in nonhuman primates. Behav Neurosci 1989; 103: 1287–95.
16. Money J, Ehrhardt AA. Man and Woman, Boy and Girl. Baltimore: Johns Hopkins University Press, 1972.
17. Berenbaum SA. Management of children with intersex conditions: psychological and methodological perspectives. Growth, Genetics & Hormones 2003; 19: 1–6.
18. Berenbaum SA. Androgen and behavior: implications for the treatment of children with disorders of sexual differentiation. In: Pediatric Endocrinology: Mechanisms, Manifestations, and Management (Pescovitz OH, Eugster EA, eds). Philadelphia: Lippincott Williams & Wilkins, 2004: 275–84.
19. Cohen-Bendahan CCC, van de Beek C, Berenbaum SA. Prenatal sex hormone effects on child and adult sex-typed behavior: methods and findings. Neurosci Biobehav Rev 2005; 29: 353–84.
20. Collaer ML, Hines M. Human behavioral sex differences: a role for gonadal hormones during early development? Psychol Bull 1995; 11: 55–107.

21. Meyer-Bahlburg HFL. Gender and sexuality in congenital adrenal hyperplasia. Endocrinol Metab Clin North Am 2001; 30: 155–71.

22. Hampson E. Sex differences in human brain and cognition: The influence of sex steroids in early and adult life. In: Behavioral Endocrinology, 2nd edn (Becker JB, Breedlove SM, Crews D, McCarthy MM, eds). Cambridge, MA: MIT Press; 2002: 579–628.

23. Therrell BL, Berenbaum SA, Manter-Kapanke V et al. Results of screening 1.9 million Texas newborns for 21-hydroxylase-deficient congenital adrenal hyperplasia. Pediatrics 1998; 101: 583–90.

24. Speiser PW, White PC. Congenital adrenal hyperplasia. N Engl J Med 2003; 349: 776–88.

25. Berenbaum SA. Cognitive function in congenital adrenal hyperplasia. Endocrinol Metab Clin North Am 2001; 30: 173–92.

26. Reiner WG, Gearhart JP. Discordant sexual identity in some genetic males with cloacal exstrophy assigned to female sex at birth. N Engl J Med 2004; 350: 333–41.

27. Colapinto J. As Nature Made Him: The Boy Who Was Raised as a Girl. New York: Harper Collins, 2000.

28. Diamond M, Sigmundson HK. Sex reassignment at birth: long-term review and clinical implications. Arch Pediatr Adolesc Med 1997; 151: 298–304.

29. Putz DA, Gaulin SJC, Sporter RJ, McBurney DH. Sex hormones and finger length. What does 2D: 4D indicate? Evol and Hum Behav 2004; 25: 182–99.

30. Resnick SM, Gottesman II, McGue M. Sensation-seeking in opposite-sex twins: an effect of prenatal hormones? Behav Genet 1993; 23: 323–9.

31. Miller EM. Prenatal sex hormone transfer: a reason to study opposite-sex twins. Pers and Indiv Differ 1994; 17: 511–29.

32. vom Saal FS. Sexual differentiation in litter-bearing mammals: influence of sex adjacent fetuses in utero. J Anim Sci 1989; 67: 1824–40.

33. Even MD, Dhar MG, vom Saal FS. Transport of steroids between fetuses via amniotic fluid in relation to the intrauterine position phenomenon in rats. J Reprod Fertil 1992; 96: 709–16.

34. Ruble DN, Martin CL. Gender development. In: Handbook of Child Psychology, Vol. 3. Social, Emotional, and Personality Development, 5th edn (Damon W, Eisenberg N, eds). New York: Wiley, 1998: 993–1016.

35. Quadagno DM, Briscoe R, Quadagno JS. Effects of perinatal gonadal hormones on selected nonsexual behavior patterns: a critical assessment of the non-human and human literature. Psychol Bull 1977; 84: 62–80.

36. Berenbaum SA, Hines M. Early androgens are related to childhood sex-typed toy preferences. Psychol Sci 1992; 3: 203–6.

37. Berenbaum SA, Snyder E. Early hormonal influences on childhood sex-typed activity and playmate preferences: implications for the development of sexual orientation. Dev Psychol 1995; 31: 31–42.

38. Ehrhardt AA, Baker SW. Fetal androgens, human central nervous system differentiation and behavior sex differences. In: Sex Differences in Behavior (Friedman RC, Richart RM, Vande Wiele RL, eds). New York: Wiley, 1974: 33–51.

39. Meyer-Bahlburg HFL, Dolezal C, Baker S et al. Prenatal androgenization affects gender-related behavior but not gender identity in 5–12-year-old girls with congenital adrenal hyperplasia. Arch Sex Behav 2004; 33: 94–104.

40. Nordenström A, Servin A, Bohlin G, Larsson A, Wedell A. Sex-typed toy play behavior correlates with the degree of prenatal androgen exposure assessed by CYP21 genotype in girls with congenital adrenal hyperplasia. J Clin Endocrinol Metab 2002; 87: 5119–24.

41. Servin A, Nordenström A, Larsson A, Bohlin G. Prenatal androgens and gender-typed behavior: a study of girls with mild and severe forms of congenital adrenal hyperplasia. Dev Psychol 2003; 39: 440–50.

42. Berenbaum SA. Effects of early androgens on sex-typed activities and interests in adolescents with congenital adrenal hyperplasia. Horm Behav 1999; 35: 102–10.

43. Dittmann RW, Kappes MH, Kappes ME et al. Congenital adrenal hyperplasia I: gender-related behaviors and attitudes in female patients and their sisters. Psychoneuroendocrinology 1990; 15: 401–20.

44. Swanson JL. Stability and change in vocational interests. In: Vocational Interests: Meaning, Measurement, and Counseling Use (Savickas ML, Spokane AR, eds). Palo Alto, CA: Davies-Black Publishers, 1999: 135–58.

45. Berenbaum SA, Duck SC, Bryk K. Behavioral effects of prenatal versus postnatal androgen excess in children with 21-hydroxylase-deficient congenital adrenal hyperplasia. J Clin Endocrinol Metab 2000; 85: 727–33.

46. Dittmann RW, Kappes MH, Kappes ME et al. Congenital adrenal hyperplasia: II. Gender-related behavior and attitudes in female salt-wasting and simple-virilizing patients. Psychoneuroendocrinology 1990; 15: 421–34.

47. Hines M, Ahmed F, Hughes IA. Psychological outcomes and gender-related development in complete androgen insensitivity syndrome. Arch Sex Behav 2003; 32: 93–101.

48. Wisniewski AB, Migeon CJ, Meyer-Bahlburg HFL et al. Complete androgen insensitivity syndrome: long-term medical, surgical, and psychosexual outcome. J Clin Endocrinol Metab 2000; 85: 2664–9.

49. Hull EM, Franz JR, Snyder AM, Nishita JK. Perinatal progesterone and learning, social and reproductive behavior in rats. Physiol Behav 1980; 24: 251–6.

50. Hines M, Golombok S, Rust J, Johnston KJ, Golding J. Testosterone during pregnancy and gender role behavior of preschool children: a longitudinal, population study. Child Dev 2002; 73: 1678–87.

51. Udry JR. The nature of gender. Demography 1994; 31: 561–73.

52. Udry JR, Morris NM, Kovenock J. Androgen effects on women's gendered behavior. J Biosoc Sci 1995; 27: 359–68.

53. Udry JR. Biological limits of gender construction. Am Sociol Rev 2000; 65: 443–57.

54. Elizabeth PH, Green R. Childhood sex-role behaviors: similarities and differences in twins. Acta Genet Med Gemellol (Roma) 1984; 33: 173–9.

55. Henderson BA, Berenbaum SA. Sex-typed play in opposite-sex twins. Devel Psychobiol 1997; 31: 115–23.

56. Rodgers CS, Fagot BI, Winebarger A. Gender-typed toy play in dizygotic twins: a test of hormone transfer theory. Sex Roles 1998; 39: 173–84.

57. Loehlin JC, Martin NG. Dimensions of psychological masculinity-femininity in adult twins from opposite-sex and same-sex pairs. Behav Genet 2000; 30: 19–28.

58. Rose RJ, Kaprio J, Winter T et al. Femininity and fertility in sisters with twin brothers: prenatal androgenization? Cross-sex socialization? Psychol Sci 2002; 13: 263–7.

59. Berenbaum SA, Bailey JM. Effects on gender identity of prenatal androgens and genital appearance: evidence from girls with congenital adrenal hyperplasia. J Clin Endocrinol Metab 2003; 88: 1102–6.

60. Hines M, Brook C, Conway GS. Androgen and psychosexual development: core gender identity, sexual orientation, and

recalled gender role behavior in women and men with congenital adrenal hyperplasia (CAH). J Sex Res 2004; 41: 75–81.

61. Zucker KJ, Bradley SJ, Oliver G et al. Psychosexual development of women with congenital adrenal hyperplasia. Horm Behav 1996; 30: 300–18.

62. Meyer-Bahlburg HFL, Gruen RS, New MI et al. Gender change from female to male in classical congenital adrenal hyperplasia. Horm Behav 1996; 30: 319–32.

63. Bradley SJ, Oliver GD, Chernick AB, Zucker KJ. Experiment of nurture: ablatio penis at 2 months, sex reassignment at 7 months, and a psychosexual follow-up in young adulthood. Pediatrics 1998; 102: e9.

64. Zucker KJ. Intersexuality and gender identity differentiation. Annu Rev Sex Res 1999; 10: 1–69.

65. Berenbaum SA, Sandberg DE. Sex determination, differentiation, and identity. N Engl J Med 2004; 350: 2204.

66. Schober JM, Carmichael PA, Hines M, Ransley PG. The ultimate challenge of cloacal exstrophy. J Urol 2002; 167: 300–4.

67. Migeon CJ, Wisniewski AB, Gearhart JP et al. Ambiguous genitalia with perineoscrotal hypospadias in 46,XY individuals: long-term medical, surgical, and psychosexual outcome. Pediatrics 2002; 110: e31.

68. Wisniewski AB, Migeon C, Gearhart JP et al. Congenital micropenis: long-term medical, surgical and psychosexual follow-up of individuals raised male or female. Horm Res 2001; 56: 3–11.

69. Mustanski BS, Chivers ML, Bailey JM. A critical review of recent biological research on human sexual orientation. Annu Rev Sex Res 2002; 13: 89–140.

70. McFadden D, Pasanen EG. Comparison of the auditory systems of heterosexuals and homosexuals: click-evoked otoacoustic emissions. Proc Natl Acad Sci 1998; 95: 2709–13.

71. Williams TJ, Pepitone ME, Christensen SE et al. Finger-length ratios and sexual orientation. Nature 2000; 404: 455–6.

72. Hall JAY, Kimura D. Dermatoglyphic asymmetry and sexual orientation in men. Behav Neurosci 1994; 108: 1203–6.

73. Mustanski BS, Bailey JM, Kaspar S. Dermatoglyphics, handedness, sex, and sexual orientation. Arch Sex Behav 2002; 31: 113–32.

74. Bailey JM, Zucker KJ. Childhood sex-typed behavior and sexual orientation: a conceptual and quantitative review. Dev Psychol 1995; 31: 43–55.

75. Bailey JM, Oberschneider MJ. Sexual orientation and professional dance. Arch Sex Behav 1997; 26: 433–44.

76. Lippa R. Gender-related traits of heterosexual and homosexual men and women. Arch Sex Behav 2002; 31: 83–98.

77. Helleday J, Edman G, Ritzen EM, Siwers B. Personality characteristics and platelet MAO activity in women with congenital adrenal hyperplasia (CAH). Psychoneuroendocrinology 1993; 18: 343–54.

78. Leveroni CL, Berenbaum SA. Early androgen effects on interest in infants: evidence from children with congenital adrenal hyperplasia. Dev Neuropsychol 1998; 14: 321–40.

79. Berenbaum SA, Resnick SM. Early androgen effects on aggression in children and adults with congenital adrenal hyperplasia. Psychoneuroendocrinology 1997; 22: 505–15.

80. Reinisch JM. Prenatal exposure to synthetic progestins increases potential for aggression in humans. Science 1981; 211: 1171–3.

81. Beatty WW. Gonadal hormones and sex differences in non-reproductive behaviors. In: Handbook of Behavioral Neurobiology, Vol. 11, Sexual differentiation (Gerall AA, Moltz H, Ward IL, eds). New York: Plenum, 1992: 85–128.

82. Eaton GG, Goy RW, Phoenix CH. Effects of testosterone treatment in adulthood on sexual behavior of female pseudohermaphrodite rhesus monkeys. Nat New Biol 1973; 242: 119–20.

83. Joslyn WD. Androgen-induced social dominance in infant female rhesus monkeys. J Child Psychol Psychiatry 1973; 14: 137–45.

84. Monaghan EP, Glickman SE. Hormones and aggressive behavior. In: Behavioral Endocrinology (Becker JB, Breedlove SM, Crews D, eds). Cambridge: MIT Press, 1992: 261–85.

85. Albert DJ, Walsh ML, Jonik RH. Aggression in humans: what is its biological foundation? Neurosci Biobehav Rev 1993; 17: 405–23.

86. Bernhardt PC, Dabbs JM, Fielden JA, Lutter CD. Testosterone changes during vicarious experiences of winning and losing among fans at sporting events. Physiol Behav 1998; 65: 59–62.

87. Booth A, Shelley G, Mazur A, Tharp G, Kittok R. Testosterone, and winning and losing in human competition. Horm Behav 1989; 23: 556–71.

88. Olweus D, Mattsson A, Schalling D, Low H. Testosterone, aggression, physical, and personality dimensions in normal adolescent males. Psychosom Med 1980; 42: 253–69.

89. Cohen-Bendahan CCC, Buitelaar JK, van Goozen SHM, Orlebeke JF, Cohen-Kettenis PT. Is there an effect of prenatal testosterone on aggression and other behavioral traits? A study comparing same-sex and opposite-sex twin girls. Horm Behav 2005; 47: 230–7.

90. Knickmeyer R, Baron-Cohen S, Raggatt P, Taylor K. Foetal testosterone, social relationships, and restricted interests in children. J Child Psychol Psychiatry 2005; 46: 198–210.

91. Lutchmaya S, Baron-Cohen S, Raggatt P. Foetal testosterone and eye contact in 12-month-old human infants. Infant Behav Dev 2002; 25: 327–35.

92. Lutchmaya S, Baron-Cohen S, Raggatt P. Foetal testosterone and vocabulary size in 18- and 24-month-old infants. Infant Behav Dev 2002; 24: 418–24.

93. Baron-Cohen S. The cognitive neuroscience of autism: Implications for the evolution of the male brain. In: The Cognitive Neurosciences, 2nd edn (Gazzaniga M, ed). Cambridge, MA: MIT Press, 2000.

94. Geschwind N, Galaburda AM. Cerebral Lateralization: Biological Mechanisms, Associations, and Pathology. Cambridge, MA: MIT Press, 1987.

95. Halpern DF. Sex Differences in Cognitive Abilities, 3rd edn. Mahwah, NJ: Erlbaum, 2000.

96. Hampson E, Rovet JF, Altmann D. Spatial reasoning in children with congenital adrenal hyperplasia due to 21-hydroxylase deficiency. Dev Neuropsychol 1998; 14: 299–320.

97. Hines M, Fane BA, Pasterski VL et al. Spatial abilities following prenatal androgen abnormality: targeting and mental rotations performance in individuals with congenital adrenal hyperplasia. Psychoneuroendocrinology 2003; 28: 1010–26.

98. Resnick SM, Berenbaum SA, Gottesman II, Bouchard TJ. Early hormonal influences on cognitive functioning in congenital adrenal hyperplasia. Dev Psychol 1986; 22: 191–8.

99. Helleday J, Bartfai A, Ritzen EM, Forsman M. General intelligence and cognitive profile in women with congenital adrenal hyperplasia. Psychoneuroendocrinology 1994; 19: 343–56.

100. McArdle P, Wilson BE. Hormonal influences on language development in physically advanced children. Brain Lang 1990; 38: 410–23.

101. Hier DB, Crowley WF. Spatial ability in androgen-deficient men. N Engl J Med 1982; 302: 1202–5.

102. Grimshaw GM, Sitarenios G, Finegan JA. Mental rotation at 7 years: relations with prenatal testosterone levels and spatial play experience. Brain Cogn 1995; 29: 85–100.

103. Cole-Harding S, Morstad AL, Wilson JR. Spatial ability in members of opposite-sex twin pairs (abstract). Behav Genet 1988; 18: 710.

104. Berenbaum SA. How hormones affect behavioral and neural development. Dev Neuropsychol 1998; 14: 175–96.

105. Casella R, Maduro MR, Lipshultz LI, Lamb DJ. Significance of the polyglutamine tract polymorphism in the androgen receptor. Urology 2001; 58: 651–6.

106. McPhaul MJ, Marcelli M, Zoppi S, Griffin JE, Wilson JD. Genetic basis of endocrine disease 4. The spectrum of mutations in the androgen receptor gene that causes androgen resistance. J Clin Endocrinol Metab 1993; 76: 17–23.

107. Merke DP, Fields JD, Keil MF et al. Children with classic congenital adrenal hyperplasia have decreased amygdala volume: Potential prenatal and postnatal hormonal effects. J Clin Endocrinol Metab 2003; 88: 1760–5.

108. Iijima M, Arisaka O, Minamoto F, Arai Y. Sex differences in children's free drawings: a study on girls with congenital adrenal hyperplasia. Horm Behav 2001; 40: 99–104.

109. Landy CL. Characteristics of boys' and girls' toys. Thesis, University Park, PA: The Pennsylvania State University, 2003.

110. McFadden D. Sex differences in the auditory system. Dev Neuropsychol 1998; 14: 261–98.

111. Grön G, Wunderlich AP, Spitzer M, Tomczak R, Riepe MW. Brain activation during human navigation: gender-different neural networks as substrate of performance. Nature Neurosci 2000; 3: 404–8.

112. Williams CL, Meck WH. The organizational effects of gonadal steroids on sexually dimorphic spatial ability. Psychoneuroendocrinology 1991; 16: 155–76.

113. Hartung CM, Widiger TA. Gender differences in the diagnosis of mental disorders: conclusions and controversies of the DSM-IV. Psychol Bull 1998; 123: 260–78.

114. Sikich L, Todd RD. Are the neurodevelopmental effects of gonadal hormones related to sex differences in psychiatric illnesses? Psychiatr Dev 1988; 6: 277–309.

18

The role of prenatal stress in the programming of behavior

Marta Weinstock

INTRODUCTION

The brain undergoes rapid growth during fetal and early postnatal life that is characterized by a high turnover of neuronal connections. This rapid growth rate makes the fetal brain especially vulnerable to stress hormones that can reach it in excess amounts from the maternal circulation as a result of infection, chronic illness, or psychological stress. These stress hormones may impede the formation of correct neural connections and reduce plasticity in the developing fetal brain. Maternal stress could also have adverse effects on fetal brain development by causing a reduction in placental blood flow and oxygen supply.[1] Thus, periods of transient hypoxia have been shown to have a detrimental influence on the brain and have been implicated in the etiology of schizophrenia.[2] Alterations in neural plasticity and neurotransmitter activity can induce subtle changes in cognitive function and behavior, the nature and intensity of which appears to depend on the genetic vulnerability of the individual, the severity of the stress, its duration and the time during pregnancy when experienced by the mother. This chapter will evaluate the evidence for prenatal stress as a predisposing factor for alterations in the programming of behavior and its contribution to mental disorders.

GESTATIONAL STRESS, EARLY DEVELOPMENT, CHILDHOOD, ADOLESCENT, AND ADULT BEHAVIORAL PATHOLOGY

The consequences of maternal stress that are most overt are those on gestation length and birth weight because they are not influenced by postnatal events. A number of studies have reported a higher incidence of preterm birth (before 37th week) and lower birth weight (less than 2.5 kg) in babies whose mothers had experienced periods of prolonged psychological stress during pregnancy.[3,4] However, in several of these, concomitant drug intake, smoking, poor nutrition or ill health could also have contributed to the findings. Low birth weight and preterm delivery have themselves been associated with developmental impairments and motor disabilities and were also suggested to be risk factors for schizophrenia.

Other research has assessed the early behavior and physical development of prenatally-stressed (PS) infants during the first years of life. These studies reported developmental delays, seen in a later onset of walking, speech, toilet training, and attainment of other milestones. There have also been reports of a greater incidence of emotional problems, such as persistent crying and clinging to the mother, low frustration threshold, and unsociable and inconsiderate behavior.[3] In a preliminary study, maternal stress during pregnancy also appeared to have an adverse effect on perinatal temperament of the infant and later scholastic achievements at the age of 6.[5] However, the interpretation of the findings may be confounded by the continuing presence of maternal anxiety and its influence on the degree of attention the mother gives to her infant, which can affect development and behavior.[6]

One project attempted to relate increased emotional behavior in the newborn infants to circulating maternal hormone levels in late gestation. It was found that the infants of mothers who had relatively high salivary cortisol displayed a greater incidence of crying, fussing, and negative facial expressions than those with low levels, but the differences between infants were no longer seen by the age of 4 months. A negative correlation was also found between maternal salivary cortisol and mental and motor development at 3 months, which suggested that perceived maternal stress could influence temperament in the infants.[7]

In older children, it has been reported that maternal emotional problems and perinatal complications may increase the incidence of attention deficits[8] and of Tourette's syndrome, a familial, neuropsychiatric disorder of childhood onset characterized by motor tics.[9] However, these too could have resulted from, or been compounded by genetic factors, maternal smoking, alcohol or drug intake.[8] When rhesus monkeys were subjected to stress of noise and cage transport early in gestation, a greater incidence of emotional and attention deficits was found in their offspring than in those in which the mothers were stressed at mid-gestation.[10] These experimental data suggest that prenatal stress may play a role in attention deficits.

Information about the involvement of maternal stress in the etiology of neurological and psychiatric disorders in adulthood has of necessity been obtained from retrospective studies. A higher incidence of schizophrenia was found in young adults born to mothers exposed during pregnancy to the stress of war and widowhood, the Dutch hunger winter, radiation, or overcrowding in inner cities.[3] In the offspring of mothers that experienced war stress during the first trimester, a significantly greater number of schizophrenic individuals of each sex were found than in the controls of the same age. In those experiencing the stress during the second trimester, a higher incidence of schizophrenic symptoms occurred only in men. This gender difference in susceptibility may be due to the slower rate of cortical development in males than in females, thereby making the male brain vulnerable to insult for a longer period.

An increase in the incidence of depression and drug abuse has also been described in subjects whose mothers reported intense psychological stress during pregnancy.[3] The difficulty in replicating the observations of abnormalities in behavior in most studies arises from their prospective design, which makes it impossible to control for the complex interactions between prenatal, genetic, and postnatal factors acting in consort or in different directions. The infants and children of stressed mothers may either have received appropriate maternal care that reduced the likelihood of developing psychopathology, or the effects may have been exacerbated by inadequate care and attention. Therefore, the only way it has been possible to isolate gestational stress from other postnatal factors as a cause of behavioral pathology is by well-controlled experimental studies in animals. The majority of this research has been carried out in rats, with a few in domestic animals

and nonhuman primates. In such studies, it is easier to control for genetic factors, timing of stress, parity and the maternal pre- and postnatal environment and specifically document an effect of prenatal stress on the development and behavior of the offspring.[3,11,12] Knowledge of the timing of the development of neuronal systems is also essential in order to provide a biochemical basis for a putative role of maternal stress hormones in the etiology of the behavioral pathology in the offspring.

HORMONAL RESPONSE TO STRESS

In response to perceived stress, corticotrophin releasing hormone (CRH) and arginine vasopressin (AVP) are released from the paraventricular nuclei (PVN) of the hypothalamus into the portal circulation from which they stimulate the release of adrenocorticotropic hormone (ACTH) and β-endorphin from the anterior pituitary. ACTH activates the adrenal gland to increase circulating cortisol (corticosterone, CORT in rodents) and catecholamines.[13] The response to stress is regulated through primary feedback loops within the hypothalamic-pituitary-adrenal (HPA) axis, but also through mineralocorticoid (MR) and glucocorticoid (GR) receptors. The former are found in high concentrations in the hippocampus and have a higher affinity for CORT within the range of normal circulating levels. GR are present in several brain regions including the hippocampus, hypothalamus, pituitary, cingulate cortex, and amygdala and are activated by higher levels of glucocorticoids in response to stress. Through these receptors in the hippocampus and at different levels of the HPA axis, glucocorticoids exert a negative feedback on this axis. In addition, CORT enhances the stress response to fear conditioning and fear-potentiated startle, at least in rodents, by activating GR in the amygdala.[14] Anxiogenic and fear-related behavior is also increased by CRH in its neurotransmitter role, through activation of appropriate noradrenergic and glutamatergic systems.[15]

Response to acute stress in pregnancy

In pregnant humans, the placenta provides an additional source of CRH and other neuropeptides which can influence the response of the HPA axis to stress. Plasma levels of CRH increase several-fold during gestation, but its biological activity is curtailed by a binding protein (CRH-BP) in plasma and amniotic fluid until just before gestation, when levels of CRH-BP fall, thereby releasing free CRH. CRH can be detected in the fetal hypothalamus from the 12th week of gestation but unlike that in the mother, the fetal blood level of CRH does not increase significantly during gestation. Although cortisol crosses the placenta from the maternal blood, about 80% is metabolized to cortisone *en route*, but a rise of 10–20% in maternal plasma cortisol could still cause significant increases in the fetal blood and influence brain development and plasticity. Placental CRH is secreted into the fetal circulation and may release hormones from the fetal adrenal, as the CRH type 1 receptor is present in human adrenal tissue from mid-gestation. In contrast to its inhibitory action in the brain, cortisol stimulates the release of CRH from the placenta, thereby establishing a positive placental-adrenal feedback loop, resulting in an amplification of the hormonal response to stress.[16]

From mid-gestation the human fetal pituitary is capable of responding to the stress of blood sampling through the abdominal wall independently of the mother. This response was shown by an increase in circulating levels of cortisol, ACTH, and β-endorphin in the fetal but not in the maternal blood and indicated that it probably did not result from the placental release of CRH.[17] The fetus is also able to respond to maternal psychological stress. This was shown by changes in fetal heart rate and heart rate variability[18] and by the induction of prolonged motor hyperactivity.[19]

Response to chronic stress in pregnancy

Chronic psychological stress in humans, as in experimental animals, results in a significant elevation in plasma levels of CRH, ACTH, and β-endorphin early in the third trimester of gestation. Preterm births or low birth weight infants were more likely to occur when plasma concentrations of CRH exceeded 90 pM at 26 weeks of gestation or were about double those in pregnancies that reached full term (35 pM). The finding of high circulating levels of these peptide hormones suggests that normal regulation of the HPA axis can be overcome by prolonged periods of uncontrollable or inescapable stress, resulting in excess maternal hormonal activity.[16]

Elevation of CRH in association with perceived maternal stress suppressed the normal habituation response to an acoustic stimulus, demonstrating its ability to affect the functioning of the nervous system.[20] CRH could have been interacting with specific CRH receptors which are present in the amygdala, hippocampus, and limbic cortical areas in the rat fetus,[21] but have not yet been identified in humans. Alternatively, failure of the fetus to habituate to an acoustic stimulus could have been due to increased cortisol released from the adrenal. A similar alteration in fetal response was found after the administration of the synthetic glucocorticoid, betamethasone to the mother.[22] Taken together, these data suggest that repeated exposure of the human fetus to excess hormones of the HPA axis as a result of maternal stress could permanently alter the programming arousal responses in the infant.

Although most of our information has been obtained from studies in experimental animals, it is important to be aware of species differences between rodents and primates in the regulation of the stress response. These must be taken into consideration when attempting to extrapolate from rat data to humans. Among these differences is the absence of a placental source of CRH in rodents and the fact that a considerable amount of neuroendocrine and neural development takes place in the rat during the postnatal period, in contrast to humans, other primates, and guinea pigs. This developmental difference probably makes the rat more sensitive to the influence of maternal care and postnatal environmental conditions.[23]

RESPONSE OF RAT FETUS TO MATERNAL STRESS

Acute stress

The fetal HPA axis in the rat is able to respond to changes in maternal stress hormones and to release ACTH and CORT from around day 15–16 of gestation that is 21–22 days in most strains. When the pregnant rat was stressed on day 10, ACTH increased in the maternal but not in the fetal blood, but CORT increased in both the maternal and fetal circulation. While β-endorphin can cross the placental barrier and influence the developing fetal brain, ACTH acts indirectly by releasing hormones from the maternal adrenal gland with the actions mediated by placental transfer of CORT. GR receptor mRNA can be detected in several areas in the fetal rat brain from day 13 of gestation, but MR mRNA appears only in the hippocampus on day 16. Thus, changes in maternal steroid levels occurring after day 13 could influence neuronal activity and the function of the HPA axis in the offspring by interacting with GR receptors. The number of these receptors increases considerably at the time of parturition.[16] Direct evidence that the rat fetal brain can respond to maternal stress was provided by the finding that the expression of CRH mRNA was increased in PVN on day 15 of gestation.[24] In another experiment, maternal stress on day 20 resulted in a reduction in the levels of

CRH, β-endorphin, noradrenaline (NA) and dopamine in the hypothalamus, and those of β-endorphin and ACTH in the pituitary.[25]

Chronic stress

A variety of stressful procedures have been used in pregnant rats to determine whether these can induce changes in hormonal regulation and behavior in the offspring. Saline injections, unpredictable noise, electric shocks to the tail or feet, or restraint with or without elevated temperature, were applied daily or three times weekly throughout gestation, or only from day 14 or 15 until gestation.[3,11] A few researchers subjected pregnant rats to two stressors simultaneously or varied the type of stress from day-to-day to prevent the rat from adapting to it.[26] Prenatal stress induced a reduction in birth weights and/or growth rate and slowed motor development like that seen in some but not all human studies.[16] Changes in the regulation of the HPA axis and behavior of the offspring were reported, even in the absence of an effect on growth.

Maternal restraint stress in rats during the last week of gestation induced a 2–4-fold increase in plasma CORT in the mothers and their fetuses (see Figure 18.1).[27] In other studies, it was shown that after four daily sessions of electric shocks applied to the tail of the pregnant rats, plasma CORT no longer returned to pre-stress levels within 1–2 hours, but remained 30% above normal in the maternal and fetal blood 2 days after the last stress was applied.[28] The prolonged elevation of CORT was probably due to a combination of a decrease in plasma CORT binding globulin (CBG) and down-regulation of brain GR, thereby decreasing the negative feedback of CORT on the HPA axis. These data point to the likelihood that the fetal brain is exposed to excessive levels of glucocorticoid for much longer periods if the mother is subjected to repeated stress rather than to a single episode. If such an elevation of cortisol also occurs in human pregnancies, it could explain why more significant correlations with infant morbidity and later psychopathology are seen after prolonged psychosocial stress rather than after a single stressful episode.[3,16]

EFFECT OF PRENATAL STRESS ON THE REGULATION OF THE HPA AXIS IN THE OFFSPRING

Many studies have been performed in prenatally stressed (PS) offspring of different ages to determine whether exposure of the fetal brain to high levels of CORT during a specific developmental period resulted in an impairment in HPA regulation. Some studies reported higher resting levels of CORT and ACTH in young (3–23-day-old) but not in older PS males.[16] The lack of a difference in resting CORT in the older animals may have depended on the time of day the measurements were made relative to the light cycle under which the rats were maintained. However, most authors failed to mention when their studies were performed. Circadian periodicity of the HPA axis only becomes established in the rat between 21 and 25 days of age and thereafter CORT levels are highest at the end of the light period. Since PS rats show an earlier peak in the circadian rhythm in the early afternoon,[29] basal CORT levels can be expected to be higher than

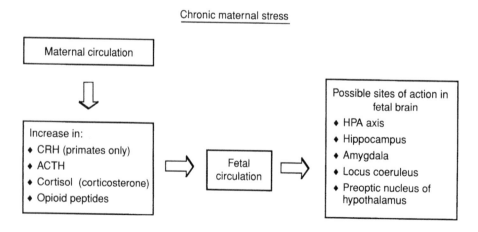

Figure 18.1 Relationship between circulating maternal stress hormones and their possible sites of action in the developing fetal brain.

in controls if measured at this time in rats older than 25 days of age.

In response to stress, HPA activation also only appeared to be greater in PS than in control males between the ages of 3 and 23 days. In older males, there was either no difference from controls in the peak CORT response to stress, or PS rats showed a slower rate of decline in CORT from these levels.[12,16] By contrast, PS females usually showed both higher resting and increased peak levels with a prolonged duration of the stress response at all ages. A delayed HPA recovery was associated with decreased hippocampal MR and GR, testifying to the impairment of feedback regulation.[12,30] This effect of prenatal stress was mimicked by daily maternal injection of dexamethasone (0.05 mg/kg) on days 15–19 of gestation,[31] indicating that it probably resulted from an action of excess CORT on the fetal brain.

While control rats will typically adapt to repeated exposure of the same stressor and no longer release high CORT on each occasion, PS rats were shown to adapt more slowly. Their plasma CORT still remained elevated after eight successive exposures to the same open field.[32] It is likely therefore that PS rats would also fail to adapt to other mildly stressful situations and the excess CORT might further impair regulation of the HPA axis. This suggestion is supported by our finding that 3 weeks after exposure to novelty or a saline injection, they displayed higher morning (trough) CORT than did controls treated similarly.[33] Elevated morning CORT was also found in control rats that had been repeatedly stressed in adulthood. However, while these rats compensated for the raised morning CORT by reducing levels in the afternoon and evening,[34] hormone levels of the steroid were also higher in the afternoon in PS rats.[29]

Two studies were designed in an attempt to provide direct evidence that excess CORT is the mediator of PS effects on the developing brain and HPA axis. In one experiment, carbenoxolone was injected daily to pregnant rats from the beginning of gestation to inhibit placental 11β-hydroxysteroid dehydrogenase (11β-HSD) and prevent inactivation of CORT, allowing higher concentrations to reach the fetus. Although this treatment resulted in an increase in basal morning plasma CORT in the neonates and at the age of 6 months, it did not alter the response of the HPA axis to 20-minute restraint stress, or produce a significant reduction in GR or MR in the hippocampus.[35] The lack of the expected effect of maternal carbenoxolone treatment like PS may have been because the control animals in this study also appeared different. Mothers were injected with saline, which itself has been shown to alter both the activity of the HPA axis and the

behavior of offspring.[36] In the second study, excess steroid release in stressed pregnant rats was prevented by adrenalectomy on day 13 of gestation, and normal levels of circulating CORT were replaced by implantation of a sustained release pellet. The adult offspring of these CORT-regulated females did not show the delay in the decline of CORT levels in response to stress or the decrease in brain MR and GR.[37] In addition, injection of CORT to the adrenalectomized, stressed mothers in amounts that simulated stress responses in intact rats, reproduced the dysregulation of the HPA axis in the pups. While these data provide additional support for the role of maternal CORT, they do not entirely preclude a contribution of other hormones. Since the effect of maternal adrenalectomy and replacement of CORT on the behavior of PS rats has not been tested, we do not know whether maternal CORT is also responsible for the behavioral alterations.

CHANGES IN THE ACTIVITY OF OTHER MATERNAL HORMONES AS A RESULT OF STRESS

Psychological and physical stressors release a spectrum of hormones and neurotransmitters in addition to CORT.[38] The pregnant rat also releases ACTH, oxytocin, opioid peptides, vasopressin, and catecholamines, depending on the nature and severity of the stress.[39] Several of these hormones could contribute to the changes in development and behavior of the offspring. Met-enkephalin can reach the fetus through the placental circulation and may inhibit DNA synthesis in the fetal brain.[40] Other opioid peptides can affect maturation in a cell type-dependent manner, depending on the receptor through which they act and how it is coupled to intracellular signaling.[41]

A role of increased opioid activity during gestational stress was demonstrated by the chronic administration of naltrexone, an opioid antagonist, to the stressed pregnant rat via a slow release minipump. This treatment prevented the stress-induced reduction in anogenital distance in 1-day-old PS males[42] and normalized their typically impaired sexual activity in adulthood, without affecting the behavior of controls. Prenatal stress has been shown to reduce aromatase activity in the hypothalamic preoptic area. This effect could explain both the impaired sexual activity in adulthood and the alteration in some sexual dimorphic behaviors like sweet preference. Maternal naltrexone injection in the pregnant rat during the period of stress restored aromatase activity in 10-day-old pups.[43] Opioid receptor blockade also improved growth rate and selectively reduced the hyperanxiety of PS rats without affecting the controls.[42] Although these data provide support for a possible role of excess opioid activity in PS rats, we do not know whether these effects are related to or independent of the effects on the fetal HPA axis.

MORPHOLOGICAL AND NEUROTRANSMITTER CHANGES IN PRENATALLY STRESSED RATS

The prefrontal cortex (PFC) is known to play an important role in the regulation of emotion and in the integration of affective states by modulating the activity of the neuroendocrine system.[44] A greater release of dopamine in the PFC may alter the behavioral and physiological response to stress. This association was confirmed by the finding that local injection of dopamine antagonists in the PFC reduced the HPA response to different stressors.[45] The rat brain shows substantial hemispheric specialization. The right PFC is normally dominant in the activation of stress-related systems, while the left may play a role in countering this activation through inter-hemispheric inhibition. The finding of a reduction in inter-hemispheric coupling in PS rats[46] and that of a higher dopamine release in the right PFC[47] could partly explain the greater HPA activation in response to stress.

Prenatal stress also induces changes in the structural and functional organization of the orbitofrontal and anterior cingulate cortices. Three-week-old PS male rats showed a significant decrease of 25–28% both in dendritic spine density and in spine length in these cortical areas.[48] In adult rats, a decrease was found in the frontal pole of the brain in genes and proteins involved in calcium/calmodulin signaling and with neurotransmitter vesicles or vesicle recycling, like synapsin 2 and vamp2/synaptobrevin II.[49] The PS rats in this study showed a delayed return to basal CORT levels after stress exposure, indicating that they had an impaired regulation of the HPA axis.

ALTERATIONS IN BEHAVIOR INDUCED BY PRENATAL STRESS

Increased anxiety and impaired coping in adversity

A chronic anxiety state in humans may be considered to be the result of inappropriate activation of defensive responses arising from an erroneous assessment of danger. This wary state has been modeled in experimental animals in tests involving fear-like reactions, which can be elicited in unfamiliar open spaces like the 'open field' or in the elevated plus maze (EPM), and is usually accompanied by an increase in CORT. The EPM has two open and two closed arms, presenting the rat with a conflict between the desire to explore a novel situation and its fear of height and open spaces. Anxiolytic agents like diazepam increase the time spent in the open arms of the maze, and conversely the exploratory behavior is decreased by anxiogenic agents. A number of studies have shown that adult male and female PS rats spend less time than controls in the open arms of the EPM, particularly if the experiment is carried out in dim light to encourage control rats to venture into the open arms.[3] Other measures of heightened anxiety in PS rats include a decrease in exploration, voiding of more fecal pellets in the open field, and an increased latency to enter a brightly lit arena from a small dark holding box (defensive withdrawal test).[50] The increased anxiety of PS rats was abolished by intracerebroventricular injection of CRH receptor antagonists, which had no effect on the behavior of control rats. These data suggested that the greater anxiogenic behavior of PS rats resulted from more CRH activity in specific brain regions, like the amygdala and/or cortex (see below). PS rats also showed a decrease in ^{3}H flunitrazepam binding in the hippocampus, consistent with fewer benzodiazepine receptors.[51] This finding may indicate that there are reduced GABA-mediated inhibitory connections between the hippocampus and other brain areas.

Similar signs of higher anxiety were also evident in PS monkeys and evinced as increased irritability, more clinging to companions, and less exploration in a novel situation after the mothers were subjected to unpredictable noise during gestation.[52] Like rats (see below) the young PS monkeys also showed poorer cognitive performance.[53]

The amygdala is bidirectionally related to the frontal cortex and hippocampus, and is involved in mood regulation, especially the mediation of fear and anxiety.[54] Functional neuroimaging has shown activation of the right amygdala during negative affective states, such as anxiety and depression in humans.[55]

Stimulation of CRH1 receptors in the basolateral nucleus of the amygdala by local injection of CRH increases fear-like responses and draws greater attention to events and cues that could threaten survival,[56] while discrete lesions of the amygdala blunt anxiety and unconditioned fear responses.[57] Since the neurons in the basolateral nucleus of the amygdala are generated during days 14 and 17 of gestation in the rat,[58] alterations in their development could be triggered by CRH liberated during this sensitive period. The importance of those developmental processes was demonstrated by the finding of an enlarged amygdala with a greater number of neurons and glia in the basolateral nucleus in adult PS rats.[59] The increased fear that these rats have of novel or intimidating situations could therefore result from more sensory information from the environment being processed via the enlarged basolateral nucleus.

Relationship between anxiogenic behavior and changes in brain neurotransmitter activity

The pathophysiology of mood disorders and neuropsychiatric diseases involves the disruption of the activity of a number of neurotransmitters. These neural changes could reflect in part the excessive release of CRH as a result of chronic stress, or increased sensitivity of the amygdala and other brain regions to CRH, as found in PS rats.[50,60] Chronic inescapable stress in adult rats increases the synthesis and release of NA in the prefrontal cortex through activation by CRH of NAergic cell bodies in the locus coeruleus.[61] Consistent with these findings are data from two studies on NA release in the brain of PS rats. NA turnover in PS males aged 40–45 days was increased in the whole brain. In a second study, NA turnover was increased in cortex and locus coeruleus, and this change was associated with behavioral suppression of PS rats in novel intimidating situations (see Table 18.1).[3,11]

Behavior consistent with depression

The core symptoms of clinical depression involve changes in mood, which cannot be readily assessed in animals. However, behavioral parameters clearly related to human depression such as loss of active coping, social withdrawal, and an inability to feel pleasure (anhedonia) can be measured in rats under appropriate conditions. Loss of coping in the face of adversity was demonstrated in adult PS rats that were food deprived for 23 hours. They showed a greater delay than controls in responding to the challenges of food

reward being offered under mildly aversive conditions.[32] Similarly, PS females separated from their 4-day-old offspring by a meter-long tunnel returned them to the nest at the same rate as controls. However, under a slightly aversive condition induced by cold air puffs, which had little effect on the behavior of controls, most of the PS rats failed to do so in the allotted time.[51] Loss of coping was also seen in the more rapid development by PS rats of behavioral despair induced by chronic variable stress and in a forced swim test, which is frequently used for predicting the clinical potential of antidepressant drugs (see Table 18.1).[3]

Anhedonia can be assessed by a loss of preference for sweet solutions. It is dependent on activation of endogenous opioid systems and can be abolished by administration of an opiate antagonist, naloxone. Prenatal stress reduced sweet preference in female rats, but increased it in males.[42] This selective effect in females concurs with the reduction in pro-opiomelanocortin mRNA in the hypothalamus that was seen only in female PS rats[30] and the fact that opioid-dependent behavior was also more evident in PS females than in males. The increase in sweet preference in PS males may be explained by a relative lack of testosterone[27] and of aromatase activity[43] at a critical time during development, making them appear to behave more like females (see Table 18.1).

Alterations in sleep patterns and circadian rhythm have been described in some forms of human depressive illness. Prenatal stress in rats caused a phase shift in the circadian rhythm of CORT[29] reminiscent of that in humans with unipolar depression. As in humans with depressive symptoms, PS rats show changes in paradoxical sleep that are directly related to alterations in their plasma CORT.[62]

DA regulates the emotional and behavioral sequelae of exposure to unavoidable aversive events, and excess amounts may be responsible for learned helplessness and the escape deficit seen in adult rats subjected to repeated inescapable stress. Both inescapable stress in adult rats and prenatal stress induced a higher release of DA in the PFC and also depressed the release of DA in the nucleus accumbens.[3] The latter was associated with an increased susceptibility to self-administer amphetamine,[63] which is in keeping with reports of an increased likelihood for drug abuse in the human offspring of mothers stressed during pregnancy.[64] A reduction in DA release in the accumbens could also explain the greater tendency for PS rats[42] and those stressed chronically in adulthood to develop anhedonia.

Table 18.1 Structural and functional alterations in brain of prenatally stressed offspring

Brain area	Structural changes	Alteration in neurotransmitters	Change in behavior
PFC	Decrease in number of dendritic spines and spine length	Increase in DA release in right PFC Increase in NA release in cortex	Activation of HPA axis Attention deficits Behavioral suppression in a novel situation
Orbitofrontal and anterior cingulate	Decrease in number of genes associated with neurotransmitter release and vesicle recycling	Decrease in DA release in nucleus accumbens	Anhedonia Increased propensity for amphetamine self-administration
Hippocampus	Decrease in synaptic density Neurogenesis (rats and monkeys) Decrease in BDNF Rim-1 and neuroregulators of exocytosis and neurotransmitter release	Decrease in BDZ binding	Impaired spatial memory Increased anxiety
Amygdala	Increase in volume of basolateral nucleus	. . .	Increase in fear-like behavior
Hypothalamic preoptic nucleus	Decrease in aromatose activity	. . .	Decrease in sexual activity in males
HPA axis	Decrease in GR and MR	Increase in release of CORT and ACTH in response to stress	Prolongation of HPA axis response to stress

BDNF, brain-derived neurotrophic factor; BDZ, benzodiazepine; CORT, corticosterone; DA, dopamine; GR, glucocorticoid receptor; HPA, hypothalamic-pituitary-adrenal; MR, mineralocorticoid receptor; NA, noradrenaline; PFC, prefrontal cortex.

Impairment of memory and cognitive function

Prenatal stress has been shown to enhance learning and memory in adult rats (3–5 months of age) in the radial arm maze,[65] or impair spatial learning in the Morris water maze in males.[66,67] These tests of spatial memory depend on intact dorsal hippocampal activity for normal execution. The design of the particular test of spatial memory used by the authors enabled them to detect a difference between control and PS rats, which indicated a less flexible strategy for solving the spatial orientation task.[66] The maternal restraint stress procedure, 30–45 minutes three times daily on days 15–19 of gestation used in the studies by Lemaire et al.,[67] increased maternal CORT 2–3-fold above that in control pregnant rats. On the other hand, Fujioka et al.[65] exposed the pregnant rats to restraint for only 30 minutes once daily on days 15–17. Although its effect was not measured on maternal plasma hormones, it was shown that the HPA response to stress in the PS offspring did not differ from that in controls. By contrast, the more prolonged maternal stress resulted in increased fetal adrenal weight and evidence of HPA dysregulation.[67] Thus, the detection of learning deficits in PS rats appears to be related to the intensity of the maternal stress and its duration, whether or not it altered HPA regulation. These data are in agreement with reports on the effects of stress on the performance of adult rats in hippocampal-dependent tasks, which may be either facilitated or impaired depending on the nature and intensity of the stress procedure.

We have recently assessed the effect of prenatal stress (three times daily restraint during the last week of gestation), on episodic memory in adult rats by an object recognition test which depends on intact cortical and hippocampal function. While we found no differences in object discrimination in naïve PS and control rats, a significant reduction in episodic memory was detectable only in PS rats several weeks after a stress exposure. This finding agrees with other observations that a difference in behavior between PS and control rats can be more readily detected after subsequent postnatal exposure to a stressful situation.[33,50]

EFFECT OF PRENATAL STRESS ON NEUROPLASTICITY

Neurogenesis occurs in the dentate gyrus of the hippocampus throughout the lifetime of animals and humans and may be impaired by a decrease in serotonin transmission and increase in glucocorticoid activity resulting from stress. Serotonin release in the hippocampus can be reduced by CRH activation of a gamma-aminobutyric acid (GABA) inhibitory input to the dorsal raphe region. This type of change is expected to occur in PS rats, as well as in those chronically stressed, in addition to other alterations of CRH interactions with neurotransmitters. Excess CORT acting on GR further decreases serotoninergic transmission by reducing the expression of 5HT1A receptors in the granule layer of the dentate gyrus in rats. The greater sensitivity of the dentate gyrus to CORT can be explained by the fact that it contains the highest densities in the brain of GR and MR for glucocorticoids.[68]

Long-term potentiation (LTP) is a mechanism by which the hippocampus is able to regulate the storage of information. It involves the activation of a subtype of NMDA receptors in the CA1 region of the hippocampus, which act as a critical switch for synaptic plasticity. Activation of these receptors promotes signalling to the nucleus in response to elevation of cytoplasmic cAMP or Ca^{2+} that culminates in the phosphorylation of cyclic AMP response-element binding protein (CREB). CREB controls many genes including that of brain-derived neurotrophic factor (BDNF), which are directly involved in the regulation of protein machinery at postsynaptic nerve terminals.[69] Chronic, unavoidable stress in normal rats depresses LTP and produces deficits in spatial learning and memory. The deficits are associated with a reduction in the expression of BDNF in the hippocampus and in the rate of proliferation of granule precursor cells in the dentate gyrus (see Table 18.1). We have found that prenatal stress significantly reduced LTP (10–60 minutes post-high frequency stimulation

(HFS)) induced by HFS in hippocampal slices of 3-week-old male rats.[70] Analysis of hippocampal RNA from littermates of these rats using the Affymetrix DNA array showed a reduction in mRNA of BDNF and Rim-1 and their proteins, which are involved in neurogenesis.[71] There was also a reduction in several proteins, like syntaxin, synaptobrevin, complexin, munc 18 and 13, that are important regulators of exocytosis in glutamatergic neurons.[71] As in the cortical areas, prenatal stress also decreased dendritic spines in the hippocampus and suppressed neurogenesis and cell proliferation in the dentate gyrus in young rats that continued throughout the lifespan.[67] Using a similar technique to quantify neurogenesis, Coe and his colleagues[72] found a significant (10–12%) reduction in hippocampal volume and cell proliferation in PS rhesus monkeys. These changes in hippocampal structure and function could have resulted from excess glucocorticoid activity starting during embryonic life and continuing postnatally. While certain forms of learning and memory are dependent on intact functioning of the dorsal hippocampus, anxiety-related behaviors may be mediated by neurons arising in the ventral hippocampus. The reduction in synaptic density, neurogenesis, and in specific genes related to exocytosis and plasticity in the whole hippocampus could explain both the memory impairment and greater anxiety in PS offspring. A decrease in neurogenesis has also been shown to occur in conjunction with lower levels of CREB and BDNF in the brains of human subjects with depressive dis-order[73] and in chronically stressed adult rats.[74] Both neurogenesis and levels of CREB and BDNF can be restored to normal by antidepressant treatment which alleviates the depressive symptomatology.[74,75] Chronic treatment of young PS rats has also been shown to prevent the appearance of anxiety and depressive-like behavior. The behavioral effect of antidepressant treatment was associated with normalization of the regulation of the HPA axis, an observation that supports the potential of these drugs to restore GR and neurogenesis.[76]

CONCLUSIONS

The ability of an individual to adapt to stressful situations is determined by genetic, environmental, and developmental factors. Embryonic life is a period of high vulnerability to stress-related hormones that may affect development, personality and behavior, and physiological functions. By altering the strength of synaptic connections and neurogenesis in cortical and limbic areas, and the action of neurotransmitters like NA, DA, serotonin, and glutamate, stress hormones can make the organism hyperresponsive to environmental cues and impending danger. An impairment of the regulation of the HPA axis that occurs in PS offspring and results in greater postnatal exposure to its own stress hormones, could lead to a maladaptive response to the environment, anxiety, and depression.

CLINICAL IMPLICATIONS

Many of the experiments described in this chapter provide evidence that maternal stress at critical periods of development may alter the programming of the fetal brain, thereby increasing susceptibility to psychopathology. The role of stress hormones like glucocorticoids in neuronal programming is becoming increasingly clear, although many questions still remain to be answered. By increasing the awareness of obstetricians, social workers, and the general public of the potential consequences of gestational stress, there will be more effort to develop responsive programs. For example, interventions could be instituted to increase support by social workers or family members for pregnant women with depression or chronic anxiety. In preliminary studies such support has been reported to reduce preterm CRH levels and the incidence of preterm birth.[77] The emotional development of the infant is greatly influenced by the strength of the relationship with its mother during early infancy.[6] Therefore, interventions designed to improve parenting skills that begin during pregnancy and continue throughout childhood could reduce maladaptive behavioral outcomes. If educational and psychosocial treatments are insufficient to ameliorate anxiety and depressive symptoms, more research will be needed to explore the efficacy of appropriate antidepressant medications.

REFERENCES

1. Myers RE. Maternal psychological stress and fetal asphyxia: a study in the monkey. Am J Obst Gyn 1975; 122: 47–59.
2. McDonald C, Murray RM. Early and late environmental risk factors for schizophrenia. Brain Res Rev 2000; 31: 130–7.
3. Weinstock M. Alterations induced by gestational stress in brain morphology and of the offspring. Prog Neurobiol 2001; 65: 427–51.
4. Rondo PH, Ferreira RF, Nogueira F et al. Maternal psychological stress and distress as predictors of low birth weight, prematurity and intrauterine growth retardation. Eur J Clin Nutr 2003; 57: 266–72.
5. Niederhofer H, Reiter A. Prenatal maternal stress, prenatal fetal movements and perinatal temperament factors influence behavior and school marks at the age of 6 years. Fetal Diagn Ther 2004; 19: 160–2.
6. Leckman JF, Feldman R, Swain JE et al. Primary parental preoccupation: circuits, genes, and the crucial role of the environment. J Neural Transm 2004; 111: 753–71.
7. Buitelaar JK, Huizink AC, Mulder EJ et al. Prenatal stress and cognitive development and temperament in infants. Neurobiol Aging 2003; 24 suppl 1: S53–60.
8. Milberger S, Biederman J, Faraone SV et al. Pregnancy, delivery and infancy complications and attention deficit hyperactivity disorder: issues of gene-environment interaction. Biol Psychiatry 1997; 41: 65–75.
9. Leckman JF, Dolnansky ES, Hardin MT et al. Perinatal factors in the expression of Tourettes's syndrome: an exploratory study. J Am Acad Child Adolesc Psychiatry 1990; 29: 220–6.
10. Schneider ML, Roughton EC, Koehler AJ et al. Growth and development following prenatal stress exposure in primates: an examination of ontogenetic vulnerability. Child Dev 1999; 70: 263–74.
11. Weinstock M. Does prenatal stress impair coping and regulation of the hypothalamic-pituitary-adrenal axis? Neurosci Biobehav Rev 1997; 21: 1–10.
12. Maccari S, Darnaudery M, Morley-Fletcher S et al. Prenatal stress and long-term consequences: implications of glucocorticoid hormones. Neurosci Biobehav Rev 2003; 27: 119–27.
13. Chrousos G, Gold PW. The concepts of stress and stress system disorders. JAMA 1992; 267: 1244–52.
14. LeDoux JE. Emotion: clues from the brain. Annu Rev Psychol 1995; 46: 209–35.
15. Makino S, Hashimoto K, Gold PW. Multiple feedback mechanisms activating corticotropin-releasing hormone system in the brain during stress. Pharmacol Biochem Behav 2002; 73: 147–58.
16. Weinstock M. The potential influence of maternal stress hormones on development and mental health of the offspring. Brain Behav Immun 2005; 19: 296–308.
17. Gitau R, Fisk NM, Teixeira JMA et al. Fetal hypothalamic-pituitary-adrenal stress responses to invasive procedures are independent of maternal responses. J Clin Endocrinol Metab 2001; 86: 104–9.
18. Monk C, Fifer WP, Myers MM et al. Maternal stress responses and anxiety during pregnancy: effects on fetal heart rate. Dev Psychobiol 2000; 36: 67–77.
19. Ianniruberto A, Tajani E. Ultrasonographic study of fetal movements. Semin Perinatol 1981; 5: 175–81.
20. Sandman CA, Kastin AJ. The influence of fragments of the LPH chains on learning, memory and attention in animals and man. Pharmacol Ther 1981; 13: 39–60.
21. Avishai-Eliner S, Brunson KL, Sandman CA et al. Stressed-out, or in (utero)? Trends Neurosci 2002; 25: 518–24.
22. Rotmensch S, Celentano C, Liberati M et al. The effect of antenatal steroid administration on the fetal response to vibroacoustic stimulation. Acta Obstet Gynecol Scand 1999; 78: 847–51.
23. Matthews SG. Early programming of the hypothalamo-pituitary-adrenal axis. Trends Endocrinol Metabol 2002; 13: 373–80.
24. Fujioka T, Sakata Y, Yamaguchi K et al. The effects of prenatal stress on the development of hypothalamic paraventricular neurons in fetal rats. Neuroscience 1999; 92: 1079–88.
25. Ohkawa T, Takeshita S, Murase T et al. The effect of an acute stress in late pregnancy on hypothalamic catecholamines of the rat fetus. Nippon Sanka Fujinka Gakkai Zasshi 1991; 43: 783–7.

26. Secoli SR, Teixeira NA. Chronic prenatal stress affects development and behavioral depression in rats. Stress 1998; 2: 273–80.

27. Ward IL, Weisz J. Differential effects of maternal stress on circulating levels of corticosterone, progesterone and testosterone in male and female rat fetuses and their mothers. Endocrinology 1984; 114: 1635–44.

28. Takahashi LK, Turner JG, Kalin NH. Prolonged stress-induced elevation in plasma corticosterone during pregnancy in the rat: implications for prenatal stress studies. Psychoneuroendocrinology 1998; 23: 571–81.

29. Koehl M, Darnaudéry M, Dulluc J et al. Prenatal stress alters circadian activity of the hypothalamo-pituitary-adrenal axis and hippocampal corticosteroid receptors in adult rats of both gender. J Neurobiol 1999; 40: 302–15.

30. Weinstock M, Matlina E, Maor GI. et al. Prenatal stress selectively alters the reactivity of the hypothalamic-pituitary-adrenal system in the female rat. Brain Res 1992; 595: 195–200.

31. Muneoka K, Mikuni M, Ogawa T et al. Prenatal dexamethasone exposure alters brain monoamine metabolism and adrenocortical response in rat offspring. Am J Physiol 1997; 273: R1669–75.

32. Fride E, Dan Y, Feldon J et al. Effects of prenatal stress on vulnerability to stress in prepubertal and adult rats. Physiol Behav 1986; 37: 681–7.

33. Weinstock M. Long-term effects of gestational stress on and pituitary-adrenal function. In: New Frontiers in Stress Research, Modulation of Brain Function (Levy A, Grauer E, Ben Nathan D et al., eds). Chur, Switzerland: Harwood Academic, 1998: 155–61.

34. Akana SF, Dallman MF. Feedback and facilitation in the adrenocortical system: unmasking facilitation by partial inhibition of the glucocorticoid response to prior stress. Endocrinology 1992; 131: 57–68.

35. Welberg LA, Seckl JR, Holmes MC. Inhibition of 11beta-hydroxysteroid dehydrogenase, the foeto-placental barrier to maternal glucocorticoids, permanently programs amygdala GR mRNA expression and anxiety-like in the offspring. Eur J Neurosci 2000; 12: 1047–54.

36. Peters DAV. Prenatal stress: effects on brain biogenic amines and plasma corticosterone levels. Pharmacol Biochem Behav 1982; 17: 721–6.

37. Barbazanges A, Piazza PV, Le Moal M et al. Maternal glucocorticoid secretion mediates long-term effects of prenatal stress. J Neurosci 1996; 16: 3963–9.

38. Pacak K, Palkovits M, Yadid G et al. Heterogeneous neurochemical responses to different stressors: a test of Selye's doctrine of nonspecificity. Am J Physiol 1998; 275: R1247–55.

39. Neumann ID, Johnstone HA, Hatzinger M et al. Attenuated neuroendocrine responses to emotional and physical stressors in pregnant rats involve adenohypophysial changes. J Physiol 1998; 508: 289–300.

40. Zagon IS, Wylie JD, Hurst WJ et al. Transplacental transfer of the opioid growth factor, [Met(5)]-enkephalin, in rats. Brain Res Bull 2001; 55: 341–6.

41. Hauser KF, Mangoura D. Diversity of the endogenous opioid system in development. Novel signal transduction translates multiple extracellular signals into neural cell growth and differentiation. Perspect Dev Neurobiol 1998; 5: 437–49.

42. Keshet GI, Weinstock M. Maternal naltrexone prevents morphological and behavioral alterations induced in rats by prenatal stress. Pharmacol Biochem Behav 1995; 50: 413–19.

43. Reznikov AG, Nosenko ND, Tarasenko LV. Participation of endogenous opioids in pathogenesis of early neuroendocrine manifestations of prenatal stress syndrome. Bull Exp Biol Med 2003; 135: 421–3.

44. Sullivan RM. Hemispheric asymmetry in stress processing in rat prefrontal cortex and the role of mesocortical dopamine. Stress 2004; 7: 131–43.

45. Spencer SJ, Ebner K, Day TA. Differential involvement of rat medial prefrontal cortex dopamine receptors in modulation of hypothalamic-pituitary-adrenal axis responses to different stressors. Eur J Neurosci 2004; 20: 1008–16.

46. Fride E, Weinstock M. Increased interhemispheric coupling of the dopamine systems induced by prenatal stress. Brain Res Bull 1987; 18: 457–61.

47. Fride E, Weinstock M. Prenatal stress increases anxiety-related behavior and alters cerebral lateralization of dopaminergic activity. Life Sci 1988; 42: 1059–65.

48. Murmu SM, Bock J, Weinstock M, Salomon S, Braun K. Development of dendritic spines in the rodent anterior cingulate cortex is modulated by prenatal stress. Neural Plasticity 2004; 12: 42–3.

49. Kinnunen AK, Koenig JI, Bilbe G et al. Repeated variable prenatal stress alters pre- and postsynaptic gene expression in the rat frontal pole. J Neurochem 2003; 86: 736–48.

50. Ward HE, Johnson EA, Salm AK et al. Effects of prenatal stress on defensive withdrawal behavior and corticotropin releasing factor systems in rat brain. Physiol Behav 2000; 70: 359–66.

51. Fride E, Dan Y, Gavish M et al. Prenatal stress impairs maternal behavior in a conflict situation and reduces hippocampal benzodiazepine receptors. Life Sci 1985; 36: 2103–9.

52. Schneider ML, Moore CF, Kraemer GW et al. The impact of prenatal stress, fetal alcohol exposure, or both on development: perspectives from a primate model. Psychoneuroendocrinology 2002; 27: 285–98.

53. Schneider ML. Delayed object permanence development in prenatally stressed Rhesus monkey infants (Macaca mulatta). Occup Ther J Res 1992; 12: 96–110.

54. Davis M. The role of the amygdala in fear and anxiety. Annu Rev Neurosci 1992; 15: 353–75.

55. Abercrombie HC, Schaefer SM, Larson C et al. Metabolic rate in the right amygdala predicts negative affect in depressed patients. Neuroreport 1998; 9: 3301–7.

56. Merali Z, Khan S, Michaud DS et al. Does amygdaloid corticotropin-releasing hormone (CRH) mediate anxiety-like behaviors? Dissociation of anxiogenic effects and CRH release. Eur J Neurosci 2004; 20: 229–39.

57. Kalin NH, Shelton SE, Davidson RJ et al. The primate amygdala mediates acute fear but not the behavioral and physiological components of anxious temperament. J Neurosci 2001; 21: 2067–74.

58. Bayer SA, Altman J, Russo RJ et al. Timetables of neurogenesis in the human brain based on experimentally determined patterns in the rat. Neurotoxicology 1993; 14: 83–144.

59. Salm AK, Pavelko M, Krouse EM et al. Lateral amygdaloid nucleus expansion in adult rats is associated with exposure to prenatal stress. Dev Brain Res 2004; 148: 159–67.

60. Day JC, Koehl M, Deroche V et al. Prenatal stress enhances stress- and corticotropin-releasing factor-induced stimulation of hippocampal acetylcholine release in adult rats. J Neurosci 1998; 18: 1886–92.

61. Van Bockstaele EJ, Colago EE, Valentino RJ. Corticotropin-releasing factor-containing axon terminals synapse onto catecholamine dendrites and may presynaptically modulate other afferents in the rostral pole of the nucleus locus coeruleus in the rat brain. J Comp Neurol 1996; 364: 523–34.

62. Dugovic C, Maccari S, Weibel L et al. High corticosterone levels in prenatally stressed rats predict persistent paradoxical sleep alterations. J Neurosci 1999; 19: 8656–64.

63. Henry C, Guegant G, Cador M et al. Prenatal stress in rats facilitates amphetamine-induced sensitization and induces long-lasting changes in dopamine receptors in the nucleus accumbens. Brain Res 1995; 685: 179–86.

64. Huttunen MO, Niskanen P. Prenatal loss of father and psychiatric disorders. Arch Gen Psychiatry 1978; 35: 429–31.

65. Fujioka T, Fujioka A, Tan N et al. Mild prenatal stress enhances learning performance in the non-adopted rat offspring. Neuroscience 2001; 103: 301–7.

66. Aleksandrov AA, Polyakova ON, Batuev AS. The effects of prenatal stress on learning in rats in a Morris maze. Neurosci Behav Physiol 2001; 31: 71–4.

67. Lemaire V, Koehl M, Le Moal M. Prenatal stress produces learning deficits associated with an inhibition of neurogenesis in the hippocampus. Proc Natl Acad Sci USA 2000; 97: 11032–37.

68. Weinstock M. Convergence of antidementia and antidepressant pharmacology. In: Cognition and Mood Interactions, (Sun M-K, ed.) New York: Nova Science Publisher, 2005: 185–224.

69. Popoli M, Gennarelli M, Racagni G. Modulation of synaptic plasticity by stress and antidepressants. Bipolar Disord 2002; 4: 166–82.

70. Bogoch Y, Nachum-Biala Y, Salomon S et al. Prenatal stress in rats attenuates hippocampal long-term potentiation (LTP) and induces deficits in synaptic plasticity and spatial memory. Neural Plasticity 2004; 12: 9.

71. Ziv N, Garner CG. Cellular and molecular mechanisms of presynaptic assembly. Nature Rev Neurosci 2004; 5: 385–99.

72. Coe CL, Kramer M, Czéh B et al. Prenatal stress diminishes neurogenesis in the dentate gyrus of juvenile Rhesus monkeys. Biol Psychiatry 2003; 54: 1025–34.

73. Duman RS. Pathophysiology of depression: the concept of synaptic plasticity. Eur Psychiatry 2002; 17 (Suppl 3): 306–10.

74. Drigues N, Poltyrev T, Bejar C et al. cDNA gene expression profile of rat hippocampus after chronic treatment with antidepressant drugs. J Neural Transm 2003; 110: 1413–36.

75. Dowlatshani D, MacQueen GM, Wang JF et al. Increased temporal cortex CREB concentrations and antidepressant treatment in major depression. Lancet 1998; 352: 1754–5.

76. Poltyrev T, Gorodetsky E, Bejar C et al. Effect of chronic treatment with ladostigil (TV-3326), on anxiogenic and depressive-like behavior and on activity of the hypothalamic pituitary adrenal axis in male and female prenatally stressed rats. Psychopharmacology 2005; 181: 118–25.

77. Feldman PJ, Dunkel-Schetter C, Sandman CA et al. Maternal social support predicts birth weight and fetal growth in human pregnancy. Psychosom Med 2000; 62: 715–25.

19

Antenatal programming of child behavior and neurodevelopment: links with maternal stress and anxiety

Vivette Glover and Thomas G O'Connor

INTRODUCTION

Symptoms of anxiety and depression are frequent during pregnancy. Indeed, they are more common in late pregnancy than in the postpartum period.[1] It is now apparent that these conditions are important to recognize and treat, both for the woman herself, and for the sake of her child.

It is a commonly held belief in many societies that the mood of a mother during pregnancy can affect the development of the child she is bearing. Hippocrates was already aware in 400 BC of the importance of emotional attitudes for the outcome of pregnancy. In China, more than a thousand years ago, recognition of the importance of prenatal attitudes led to the institution of the first antenatal clinic.[2] In the middle of the twentieth century, Sontag (1941) proposed a biological explanation that could account for this presumed strong connection.[3] However, it is only relatively recently that this idea has been investigated rigorously in basic and applied research.

The evidence from animal studies that maternal stress in pregnancy has a long-term effect on the behavior of offspring is now very strong, both for rodents[4] and nonhuman primates.[5] The rodent experiments started in the late 1950s, with experiments that showed that the offspring of mothers made more anxious in pregnancy behaved in a more anxious manner themselves.[6,7] Several conclusions can be drawn from this animal research.[4,5,8] The first is that the effects of prenatal stress extend to a wide range of outcomes, including behavioral inattention and anxiety, activity of the hypothalamic-pituitary-adrenal (HPA) axis, cognitive and neuronal development, cardiovascular and immune functioning, sex-typical behaviour, and sleep regulation, among others. Second, in the absence of any intervention, the effects can persist into adulthood and may even provide a model of environmentally induced intergenerational transmission. Third, the effects of prenatal stress may be moderated and even reversed by positive postnatal rearing, suggesting that although there may be persisting effects of prenatal stress, it is not inevitable (although the developmental window in which the effects may be reversed is not yet clear). Finally, there is evidence that the HPA axis is an important mediating mechanism. For example, in rodents adrenalectomy blocks the effect of prenatal stress, and in primates injections of adrenocorticotrophin hormone (ACTH) in the absence of prenatal stress produces similar effects.[9] Among the many outcomes shown in the offspring is an elevated cortisol or corticosterone responses to stress,[10,11] which may be 'set' by exposure to maternal stress during pregnancy.[8] In summary, these findings strongly support a causal connection between prenatal stress and the later physiology and health of offspring.

The animal studies provide a powerful rationale for research into the consequences of prenatal stress or anxiety in humans. If parallel effects occur, then there are profound implications for understanding behavioral development, for our concepts of risk and resilience, and the importance of when to schedule prevention and intervention. There would also be substantial clinical implications. The HPA axis is the major stress response system in the body and a dysregulation of HPA activity is associated with a range of disorders, including those of mood.[12,13]

In this review, we examine the major studies that have recently examined the links between maternal anxiety/stress or depression in pregnancy and outcomes for the child. We also consider possible mechanisms underlying the findings in humans, including the likelihood of fetal programming. We conclude by discussing the clinical implications of the findings and their public health significance.

STUDIES SHOWING A LINK BETWEEN ANTENATAL STRESS AND ANXIETY AND THE BEHAVIORAL AND COGNITIVE DEVELOPMENT OF THE CHILD

Early studies

A pioneering study linking antenatal stress with effects on the child was published by DH Stott in 1973.[14] Information was collected from 200 women in Scotland in 1965–6, at the end of their pregnancy. Stott reported that the design was not to test any specific hypothesis, but an inductive one to examine associations. The questions asked of the mother concerned her physical and mental health, the course of the pregnancy, and her social circumstances. The health, development, and behavior of the child were followed for the next 4 years. His major conclusion was that stresses during pregnancy involving severe and continuing personal tensions, in particular marital discord, were closely associated with child morbidity in the form of ill health, neurological dysfunction, developmental delays and behavior disturbance.

In a study carried out in Washington DC, with predominantly primaparous, African American women, it was found that several psychosocial variables, including stress, anxiety, and partner interaction, were associated with reduced behavioral scores on the Brazelton Neonatal Behavior Assessment Scale (NBAS) when the newborns were 2 days of age.[15] An Israeli study examined the outcome for two cohorts of boys, one group consisting of those born in the year of the Six-Day War and a second group born 2 years later. The children from the 'war exposed pregnancies' had significant developmental delays and evinced regressive behavior,[16] although antenatal and postnatal stress effects were not distinguished in the analyses. A retrospective study by McIntosh et al.[17] showed that if the mother experienced moderate emotional stress, or smoked cigarettes during pregnancy, her child was more likely to be diagnosed with an attention deficit disorder. These studies laid the important groundwork and shaped the nature of the inquiries in better controlled studies described below.

Major studies linking antenatal stress/anxiety with child behavioral and cognitive outcomes

Major recent studies examining the relationship between maternal mood in pregnancy and the child's neonatal, cognitive, and behavioral outcomes are listed in Tables 19.1, 19.2, and 19.3, respectively.[18–31] Even though these studies used a wide range of different methods, both for measuring antenatal stress or anxiety, and for assessing the child, they all found links in a way that revealed an effect on the development of the brain. The evidence for such a connection is compelling. The findings, as well as some of the strengths and weaknesses of the studies, are discussed below.

Size and setting of the samples

These studies are mainly European with two in North America;[20,24] none are from developing countries. The sample size varies considerably from 58[24] to 7448 in the Avon Longitudinal Study of Parents and Children (ALSPAC),[26] one of the few longitudinal and prospective community studies to examine this issue. The size of the study sample has predictable effects on the methods that can be used for assessment and analysis. Whereas the larger studies have had to rely on maternal report for both ratings of maternal stress/anxiety and for assessing the child, the smaller studies typically have the advantage of direct observation of the children and, in some cases, measures from several raters.[24,30] Methodological differences in sampling and measurement are noteworthy, but what is perhaps more important is how robust the findings are across the different settings and research strategies.

Defining the risk

Virtually all studies focus on anxiety or stress using self-rating questionnaires. There is variation in the type of questionnaire administered, however, as some studies assessed daily hassles,[22] whereas others focused on life events[18,24,29] or perceived stress.[22,31] It seems from these studies that developmental effects can be observed with relatively low levels of anxiety and frequent stresses, at least for the kinds of cognitive, behavioural/emotional, and neurodevelopmental outcomes shown in Tables 19.1–19.3. In the case of child physical development, however, Hansen et al.[32] found that only the most severe life stresses, such as death of an older child, were associated with more teratogenic types of effects on the developing fetus, cranial-neural-crest malformations, and even this observation needs to be replicated.

Table 19.1 Studies linking antenatal stress/anxiety with neonatal outcome

Population	Stress/anxiety	Outcome	Comments	Reference
Danish cohort $n = 3021$ 120 selected for this study	70 with moderate/severe life events and inadequate social support compared with 50 controls	Neonates Smaller head circumference, lower birth weight, worse Prechtl neurological score	Observer rating of babies No gestational times given No breakdown of nature of life events	18
Dutch sample $n = 105$	Spielberger Anxiety Scales compared those with state and/or trait anxiety > 1 SD above mean Given at 32 weeks gestation	Anxious subgroup lower Brazelton orientation scores at 3 weeks	Small numbers Objective measure of child development Multivariate analyses	19
American sample $n = 166$	Antenatal anxiety, depression and anger	Antenatal anxiety linked with worse performance on the Brazelton Neonatal Behavior Assessment Scale (motor maturity, autonomic stability and withdrawal)	Possible antenatal confounders such as smoking or alcohol consumption not examined	20

A separate set of studies used anxiety questionnaires rather than measures of stress or life events, and reported similar findings.[26,30] These results raise the question of whether prenatal stress or anxiety is the key risk factor for offspring. Stress and anxiety are different concepts, but the questionnaires used to assess them often blur the distinctions. Broadly defined, as in the case of 'generalized anxiety disorder', anxiety reflects anticipatory worry about the future. However, general anxiety questionnaires such as the Spielberger State Anxiety questionnaire,[33] used in several of these studies,[19,30] asks respondents to rate items such as 'I feel calm'; 'I feel secure'; 'I am relaxed'; 'I feel pleasant', on a scale from 'not at all' to 'very much'. These questions would also seem to be appropriate in a questionnaire that measured how stressed someone was feeling. They are also quite different from the items included on inventories that focus on the assessment of stressful life events.

Other types of anxiety and stress have been discussed by some authors. For example, it has been suggested that pregnancy-specific worries (e.g. worries that the baby is normal) may be particularly impor-

tant,[22,34] although it is not yet clear that pregnancy-specific anxiety/stress differs from more 'routine' anxiety/stress or that it has different effects on the physiology of the mother or the baby.

Many subtypes of anxiety disorder are recognized, including generalized anxiety, panic, specific phobia, post-traumatic stress, acute stress, and obsessive-compulsive disorders. These disorders may involve quite different physiological processes.[35] None of the published studies have used clinical interviews and, consequently, none can demonstrate if there are differences among these disorders with respect to the effect on the fetus and child. As a result, it is unclear whether most of the findings relate to an anxiety disorder or, for example, to more general concept of 'worry', or to the distress associated with lack of support by the partner. It is interesting that the actual life events found in one study to be most linked with low scores on the Bayley Mental Developmental Index (MDI), were 'separation/divorce' and 'cruelty by the partner' (Bergman, O'Connor and Glover, unpublished data). This finding is similar to the conclusion by Stott[14] that continuing personal tensions (in particular, marital discord)

Table 19.2 Studies linking antenatal stress/anxiety with child cognitive outcome

Population	Stress/anxiety	Outcome	Comments	Reference
Dutch sample $n = 105$	Spielberger Anxiety Scales compared those with state and/or trait anxiety > 1 SD above mean Given at 32 weeks gestation	Lower Bayley MDI score at 2 years	Small numbers Objective measure of child development Maternal depression measured at 1 and 2 years postpartum Multivariate analyses	19
Dutch sample $n = 170$	Daily hassles scale Pregnancy Related Anxiety and Perceived Stress scale Given at early, mid and late pregnancy Logistic regression	Daily hassles in early pregnancy (15–17 weeks) linked with lower Bayley's MDI score at 8 months High fear of giving birth at 27–28 weeks linked with low PDI at 8 months	Rather complicated measures of antenatal stress/anxiety Co-varied maternal postnatal stress/depression	21, 22, 23
Canadian sample $n = 58$	Varying exposure to a life event – ice storm	Bayley's MDI and language abilities 17% of variance accounted for by prenatal stress	. . .	24
Austrian sample $n = 227$	Antenatal stress questionnaire, e.g. 'do you have financial problems?'	Maternal antenatal stress linked child's school marks at 6 years	Correlational analysis No allowance for possible other antenatal or postnatal maternal factors	25
English sample $n = 61$	Compare antenatal and postnatal life events	Significant (c10 points) reduction in MDI scores with 3 or more antenatal life events, not postnatal	Observer-rated Postnatal effects co-varied No information on gestational age of sensitivity	Bergman, O'Connor and Glover, unpublished data

were a particular risk factor for later 'neurological dysfunction, developmental delays and behaviour disturbance in the child'.

The high co-occurrence of symptoms of anxiety and depression raise questions about the specific predictions from maternal anxiety. In terms of understanding the effects on the child, the key issue is not whether anxiety and depression are both manifest in the mother, but whether the effects of each on the developing baby can be distinguished. There is some evidence that the effect on the child derives more from prenatal anxiety rather than depression. O'Connor et al.[26] found that although antenatal depression was associated with child behavioral problems in a similar way to prenatal anxiety, the effect was smaller; furthermore, when prenatal anxiety was covaried, the association was not significant. In contrast, the prediction from prenatal anxiety to child behavioural problems was substantial and not reduced when prenatal depression was co-varied. The authors also

Table 19.3 Studies linking antenatal stress/anxiety with child behavioral problems

Population	Stress/anxiety	Outcome	Comments	Reference
Community English cohort n = 7448	Maternal anxiety (Crown Crisp questionnaire) Given at 18 and 32 weeks Top 15% compared with rest	More behavioral problems at ages 4 and 7 years, especially ADHD, but also anxiety and depression Effect stronger at 32 weeks than 18 weeks	Large numbers Multiple co-variates Co-varied out postnatal anxiety Maternal report	26, 27, 28
Danish sample n = 4031	Number of life events	More symptoms of ADHD at 9–11 years linked with life events in second trimester	Large numbers Only antenatal period co-variates Maternal report	29
Belgian sample n = 71	Spielberger State anxiety Measured at 12–22 weeks and 32–40 weeks	More ADHD and externalizing problems in children 8/9 years Largest effect at 12–22 weeks gestation	Small numbers Child observer rated Co-varied postnatal anxiety	30
Swedish sample n = 286	Perceived stress scale	More ADHD in 7-year-olds Largest effects at 10 weeks gestation	Child assessed by both mother and teacher No postnatal stress/anxiety assessments	31

found that the link between antenatal anxiety and child behavioral problems was separate and additive to the effects of postnatal depression.[27]

In summary, there is growing evidence that the risk most closely linked with adverse child outcomes is maternal anxiety/stress. There is also evidence that the effects on the child are not restricted to extreme anxiety or stress in the mother, but can occur across quite a wide range.[26] On the other hand, there is some uncertainty about what type(s) of anxiety/stress may be most predictive of later developmental and health problems. The consistent findings across studies, despite different measures of anxiety and stress, may indicate that the risk derives from a broad range of negative emotions that occur in stressed and anxious individuals. It remains to be seen how refinement in the measurement of prenatal anxiety/stress improves the prediction of child outcomes, and how the inclusion of biological measures of stress may help us to understand the nature of the risk for children.

The effect on the child

These studies have examined children at a wide range of ages from the newborn to 11 years.[18,20,29] Examining the newborn may eliminate the additional effect of parenting, although not necessarily genetic contributions, or other possible confounders such as alcohol or drug consumption during pregnancy. Two studies found impairment in the newborn using the Brazelton NBAS[19,20] and one study used the Prechtl neurological assessment.[18] Field et al.[20] reported that the newborns of mothers with high anxiety had greater relative right frontal brain activation (as measured by EEG) and lower vagal tone. The babies also spent more time in deep sleep and less time in quiet and active alert states, and showed more state changes and less optimal performance on the NBAS (motor maturity, autonomic stability, and withdrawal). Lou et al.[18] proposed that there may be a 'fetal stress syndrome' analogous to the 'fetal alcohol syndrome', on the basis of their study which showed that antenatal life events resulted in a smaller head circumference, lower birth weight and lower neurological scores on the Prechtl scale.

The studies listed in Table 19.2 all show an effect of prenatal stress or anxiety on the cognitive development of the child, as assessed by scores on the Bayley MDI, or by school grades. The MDI is a widely used standardized tool for the assessment of cognitive development in infants and young children. Scores on this test have been shown to modestly predict later ability. Findings on the MDI are interesting, therefore, but need to be complemented with measures of cognitive functioning from middle childhood, at a point at which individual differences in cognitive abilities are more differentiated and stable. It is possible that at this young age an impaired score relates to other developmental problems, such as a failure in attention.

The four prospective studies in Table 19.3 have all found a link between antenatal stress/anxiety and behavioral/emotional problems in the child. The most consistent adverse outcome is in symptoms of attention deficit hyperactivity disorder (ADHD), and this association has been found in children from 4 to 11 years old. However other effects have also been observed, such as an increase in anxiety[26,30] and in externalizing problems.[30] It is of interest that in the non-human primate studies of prenatal stress, a consistent effect has been an impairment of attention.[5]

What has not yet been investigated, given the constraints of a limited follow-up period, is whether antenatal anxiety/stress predicts depression, a psychiatric outcome that is relatively rare in children prior to puberty. This will be a particularly important goal for further research because depression is the psychiatric disorder most closely linked with the neuroendocrine system implicated in mediating prenatal stress, namely, disturbance in the HPA axis.[36] Another specific area for further follow-up is cognitive functioning, especially in domains known to be affected by high cortisol, such as working memory.[37] Finding evidence that antenatal stress can impair later working memory in children and adults would provide an important extension of the more limited research so far on cognitive functioning.

Gestational age of stress/anxiety effect

There is little agreement about the gestational age most sensitive to antenatal maternal stress or anxiety with respect to the childhood outcomes discussed here. This situation is different when it comes to the effects of stress on physical development. Hansen et al.[32] found, in a very large cohort, that an extreme life event such as the unexpected death of an older child,

increased the frequency of cranial-neural crest malformations eight-fold. Other severe life events also caused an increased incidence of malformations. These effects were limited to the first trimester, which makes sense as this is the stage of fetal development when organogenesis is occurring.

Of the four studies that investigated symptoms of ADHD as the outcome, one found some evidence for greater sensitivity in the first trimester,[31] two in mid-gestation,[29,30] and one at 32 weeks.[26] There are several possible reasons for these discrepancies. One is that anxiety/stress is, in most cases, hard to time precisely. For example, even major life events outside the control of the individual – such as earthquakes or ice storms – might be expected to have lingering effects beyond the immediate event. Given that the timing of onset and offset of anxiety/stress are not precise, we might expect to find inconsistencies between studies. In addition, each study used different gestational windows and there may be more overlap than is apparent. In the study of O'Connor et al.,[26] anxiety was measured only at 18 and 32 weeks gestation, and the associations were stronger with the latter time point. It remains possible that the effects were actually maximal at mid-gestation, for example, about 24 weeks, and this would concur with other studies. There may also be similar effects on other nonspecific outcomes, such as attention, by multiple mechanisms operating at different gestational ages. Another possibility is that the studies did not have enough power to effectively examine sensitive periods. More research is clearly needed to clarify these issues.

Sex differences

Most studies have not reported results for boys and girls separately. This is potentially a serious limitation because animal studies often find different risks for males and females. The studies of O'Connor et al.[26] and Van Den Bergh and Marcoen[30] did examine both sexes, and found a greater effect of antenatal anxiety on ADHD symptoms in boys than in girls. However, in a follow-up study of O'Connor et al.[28] when the children were 7 years old, the increased risk due to antenatal anxiety was similar for both, suggestive of an interactive effect of gender and maturation.

Magnitude of effect

The size of the effects found in many of these studies is considerable. O'Connor et al. reported that women in the top 15% for symptoms of anxiety at 32 weeks gestation had double the risk of having children with behavioral problems at 4 and 7 years of age even after allowing for multiple co-variates.[26,28] It raised the risk for a child with symptoms of ADHD from 5% to 10%. Van den Bergh and Marcoen[30] found that maternal anxiety during pregnancy accounted for 22% of the variance in symptoms of ADHD in 8–9-year-old children. Exposure to stressful events doubled the risk for ADHD problems in the study by Obel et al.[29] Huizink and colleagues found a smaller effect.[22] Laplante et al.[24] showed that the level of prenatal stress exposure accounted for 11.4% and 12.1% of the variance in the toddlers' Bayley MDI and productive language abilities, respectively, and accounted for 17.3% of the variance of their receptive language abilities. In all, 3–8% of the variance in behavioral regulation and mental and motor development at 3 and 8 months were explained by anxiety/stress in pregnancy.[22] Bergman, O'Connor and Glover (unpublished data) discerned an even larger effect of antenatal life events at 18 months of age, accounting for 22% of the variance in the Bayley's MDI scores.

Most of these are substantial effects, but there remains considerable variation across children. It is quite possible that there is a gene–environment interaction so that the effects of antenatal stress/anxiety become apparent only in those children who also have a genetic susceptibility. This concept of vulnerability has been shown convincingly with the interaction between a polymorphism in the serotonin (5HT) transporter gene and the child's exposure to adverse life events, in creating the risk for the development of depression.[38] It is likely that there are also protective influences. For example, a warm mothering style may help to prevent behavior problems, such as ADHD, in low birth weight children.[39]

Other developmental effects

One of the more interesting conclusions from the animal data is that there appear to be wide-ranging effects of prenatal stress. For example, it has been shown that prenatal stress is linked with altered laterality of the brain in the offspring.[4,40] Glover et al.[41] used the ALSPAC cohort to test the hypothesis that antenatal maternal anxiety might be associated with altered lateralization in humans, as demonstrated by mixed handedness. Child handedness was assessed at 42 months of age using an established maternal report scale. Multivariable analyses indicated that maternal anxiety at 18 weeks of pregnancy predicted an increased likelihood of mixed handedness in the child (OR = 1.23, 95% CI 1.02–1.48, $p < 0.05$), independent of parental handedness, obstetric and other antenatal risks, and postnatal anxiety. For this outcome measure, there was no link with anxiety at 32 weeks or postnatal anxiety.

Obel et al.[42] have also shown that antenatal life events are associated with a higher prevalence of mixed handedness in the child. They used a sample of 824 individuals followed from pregnancy until the children were assessed at 42 months of age. Findings from both studies were similar in several key respects. Both demonstrated links between antenatal anxiety and mixed handedness rather than left handedness, and observed that this effect was stronger with antenatal anxiety/stress than with antenatal depression. However, the effect of anxiety/stress in the study by Obel et al. was stronger in later pregnancy (defined as 30 gestation weeks) rather than during early pregnancy (defined as 12 gestation weeks). More work is clearly needed to delineate the possibility of variation in vulnerability at different stages of fetal development.

Atypical laterality has been found in children with autism, learning disabilities, and other psychiatric conditions, including problems with attention, as well as in adult schizophrenia.[41] There is anecdotal evidence for a link between antenatal maternal stress and both autism and dyslexia, in addition to the evidence discussed already for ADHD. It is an interesting possibility that many of these symptoms or disorders, which are associated with mixed handedness, share some neurodevelopmental components in common, which may be exacerbated by antenatal maternal stress or anxiety.

EVIDENCE FOR PROGRAMMING

The studies highlighted in Tables 19.1–19.3 have all reported associations between antenatal stress or anxiety and impaired outcomes in children. However, even this consistency across studies and the persistence into late childhood does not prove that fetal programming is occurring. There could still be some genetic mediation; a mother prone to anxiety may pass on genes to her children, making them more likely to develop behavioral problems. If a mother is stressed or anxious during pregnancy, she may also continue to be stressed or anxious during the postpartum period, and this could impair her parenting, and thus have later impact on the child's behavior. Furthermore, anxiety/stress in the pre- and postnatal period could also affect her perceptions of her child and so influence her answers to the researchers' questions about her child's development. This methodological consideration does not apply to those studies in which the child was examined by an impartial observer, such as with the NBAS.[34,43] However, there still could be effects of other persistent maternal behaviors and environmental conditions, such as smoking. Most studies, although not all, co-varied out maternal smoking and drinking, which may be associated with stress and also may have a direct effect on the development of the fetus. None of the studies listed in Tables 19.1–19.3 examined any genetic factors directly. The studies on handedness did not have this limitation in that they were able to co-vary out parental handedness, and the findings were most unlikely to be due to postnatal parenting effects[41,42] although forced switching of handedness was once more common.

Fetal programming would presumably result in a permanent alteration of the developmental pattern. The comparatively short follow-up in the human studies leaves open the question of whether there are lasting changes that persist into adulthood. It would also be that the case for fetal programming is stronger if the associations can be specifically linked with antenatal stress/anxiety and can be shown to be not due to postnatal effects. Several studies co-varied out maternal postnatal anxiety or depression, and still found an association.[19,26,30] Bergman, O'Connor and Glover (unpublished data) determined the frequency of both antenatal and postnatal life events, and found that the reduction in Bayley's MDI score was associated only with the antenatal life events. It would appear to provide further evidence for antenatal programming.

POSSIBLE MECHANISMS

We do not know how maternal stress affects fetal development in humans, although various mecha-

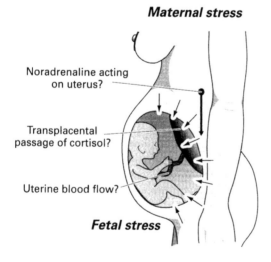

Maternal stress

Noradrenaline acting on uterus?

Transplacental passage of cortisol?

Uterine blood flow?

Fetal stress

Figure 19.1 Mechanisms by which maternal stress may affect the fetus.

nisms have been suggested (see Figure 19.1). Sontag wrote in 1941 that 'deeply disturbed maternal emotion produces a marked increase in activity of the fetus, probably as a result of increased adrenalin level in the maternal, and therefore the fetal, blood'.[3] The link between disturbed antenatal maternal mood and fetal motoric activity has been confirmed in several subsequent studies,[44,45] but it is most unlikely to be due to the direct transfer of adrenaline or noradrenaline from mother to fetus. However, Sontag's general conclusion remains credible. The effect of maternal hormones on the uterus, and the *in utero* exposure of the fetus to abnormally high levels of maternal hormones, especially cortisol, are plausible mechanisms by which maternal stress may affect the fetus.

The two main stress systems of the body are the HPA axis, which results in the secretion of cortisol, and the sympathetic-adrenomedullary system, which results in the release of noradrenaline and adrenaline. Stress and anxiety are associated with elevated activity in both systems, although the relationships are complex, and depend on the nature and chronicity of the stressful events and experiences. In general, the sympathetic system responds quickly, in seconds, whereas the HPA axis takes 10–20 minutes for significant elevations in cortisol to occur. Noradrenaline may have indirect effects via changes in maternal muscular or vascular tone. Elevated noradrenaline levels in the maternal circulation can stimulate uterine contractions in later pregnancy, whereas high adrenaline levels can be inhibitory.[46] Neuroendocrine-induced changes in blood flow to the uterus and placenta can cause hypoxia in the fetus, which may in turn be a vector of fetal programming.[47]

Transfer of hormones across the placenta

The correlation between maternal and fetal hormonal activity has been examined in several studies that simultaneously determined the levels of five hormones (see Table 19.4).[48–52] Small quantities of extra blood were obtained when fetal blood sampling was being carried out for clinical purposes, and maternal samples were taken at the same time. Most of these fetuses were subsequently found to be normal and the values could thus be included in the analyses. The correlation between maternal and fetal cortisol levels was found to be very strong (0.58, $p < 0.001$).[48] In contrast, the correlation between maternal and fetal noradrenaline levels was negligible.[52] Adrenaline was not measured, but one would expect a low association like noradrenaline. Testosterone levels were moderately correlated, corticotrophin releasing hormone (CRH) less so, and no significant correlation was

Table 19.4 Correlations between maternal and fetal plasma hormone levels

Hormone	Correlation	Maternal-fetal ratio	Reference
Cortisol	0.58 $p > 0.01$	11.8	48 49
Testosterone	0.42 $p > 0.01$	1.25	50
CRH	0.36 $p = 0.03$	1.7	51
β-Endorphin	−0.2 NS	0.61	49
Noradrenaline	0.08 NS	10.5	52

found for β-endorphin. There were large differences found in the maternal-fetal ratio for these hormones. Cortisol and noradrenaline were about 10-fold higher in the mother, whereas β-endorphin was somewhat higher in the fetus.

Steroid hormones such as cortisol and testosterone are lipophilic and can cross cell membranes easily. Testosterone and cortisol were highly correlated in the two compartments. This is not true of peptide hormones such as β-endorphin or CRH, or for the catecholamines such as noradrenaline and adrenaline. CRH was correlated in maternal and fetal blood, but it should be noted that the placenta is the primary source of CRH during pregnancy.[51]

Part of the function of the placenta is to be an effective barrier between the mother and fetus, to protect the latter from potentially toxic compounds. It is rich in protective enzymes such as monoamine oxidase A, that metabolizes adrenaline and noradrenaline, peptidases that metabolize β-endorphin, and 11β-hydroxysteroid dehydrogenase type 2, that converts cortisol to the less active cortisone.[53] As maternal cortisol levels are substantially higher than fetal levels, this difference is compatible with substantial (80–90%) metabolism of maternal cortisol during passage across the placenta.

It is unlikely that the transfer of maternal cortisol underlies the immediate links between changes in maternal mood, e.g. in anxiety while doing a cognitive test, and fetal behavior[45,54] because of the slow response time of the HPA axis. The effect of noradrenaline on the uterine muscle may play a role here. Nevertheless, we need to know more about what happens when cortisol levels are raised in the human fetus.

Does this affect the development of the nervous and other systems as in the animal models, and if so, at which gestational ages?

The maternal HPA axis during pregnancy

There have been very few studies examining the functioning of the maternal HPA axis during pregnancy in relation to emotional state. Obel et al.[55] observed that evening but not morning saliva cortisol was raised in women with high perceived life stress at 30 weeks, but not at 16 weeks of gestation. Huizink et al.[22] found that early morning values of cortisol in late pregnancy were negatively related to both mental and motor development in infants at 3 months and motor development at 8 months.

Maternal cortisol rises markedly as pregnancy progresses.[56] We do not know the extent to which this affects the pattern of antenatal responses, although we do know that the mother's HPA axis becomes less responsive to acute stressors at the end of pregnancy.[57] Also, one study has found that women rated their subjective response to an earthquake as less severe if it occurred later in their pregnancy.[58] However, much remains to be learned. No study has yet linked maternal HPA activity during pregnancy with the functioning of the HPA axis in the child. Some studies that found an association between antenatal anxiety and impaired child development[19,26] have found the effect late in pregnancy, at 32 weeks, which is at a stage when the maternal HPA axis is desensitized.[57] We need to know more about the HPA correlates of high anxiety, stress, and the response to life events in the pregnant woman at different periods of gestation.

Fetal exposure to testosterone

The level of fetal exposure to testosterone *in utero* may also be important for programming later behavior. Animal models have shown that fetal testosterone acts in a dose-dependent manner to program the male fetal brain for its masculine role.[59] In humans, girls with congenital adrenal hyperplasia (CAH), which results in a deficiency of cortisol but an excess of testosterone, show some masculinization, including a greater tendency to 'rough and tumble' play and selection of masculine toys.[60] They also evince alterations in laterality.[61] It has been suggested that certain neurodevelopmental disorders that are more common in males, such as dyslexia and autism, may result in part from excessive exposure to testosterone *in utero*.[62] Language development at 18 months and 2 years has been found to correlate with the amniotic fluid testosterone levels, which suggests a possible role in autistic spectrum disorders where impairments in language are prominent.[63]

Recently, it has also been shown that, unlike the norm in the adult, there is a positive correlation between plasma cortisol and testosterone levels in the fetus.[50] Fetal testosterone levels are higher in males than females, but there is no difference in cortisol between the two sexes. However, it may be that in the fetus some of the factors that raise fetal cortisol may also cause an increase in testosterone. This explanation is compatible with the hypothesis that maternal antenatal stress may have some masculinizing effects.

Other systems

Many other fetal systems are likely to be affected by antenatal stress. Prenatal stress in rats has been found to increase the responsiveness of the cardiovascular system to a novel stressor, suggesting fetal programming of the sympathetic system.[64] Animal studies have shown alterations in several brain neurotransmitters, including the dopaminergic pathways, by prenatal stress. The alterations found in brain dopamine asymmetry in rodents after prenatal stress are similar to those found in boys with ADHD, as determined by positron emission tomography (PET).[40]

Uterine blood flow

Another mechanism by which maternal anxiety or stress may affect the development of the fetus is via blood flow in the uterine arteries. It has been found that women in a higher anxiety group (Spielberger's State Anxiety scores of 40 or more) had significantly different uterine flow velocity waveform patterns than those in the lower anxiety groups, suggesting less blood flow to the placenta and fetus.[65] This finding was recently confirmed in a larger cohort where an association between maternal anxiety and uterine blood flow was present at 30, but not at 20 weeks gestation (Jackson, Fisk, and Glover, unpublished observations).

A study by Sjostrom and colleagues,[66] aimed at determining whether fetal circulation was affected by maternal anxiety in the third trimester, found that women with high trait anxiety scores had altered blood flow in the umbilical artery and their fetuses exhibited differences in their middle cerebral artery, suggesting a change in blood distribution in favor of brain circulation in the fetus. These results indicate that maternal anxiety, even within a normal population, can influence fetal cerebral blood flow.

We do not know whether these associations between maternal anxiety and blood flow are sustained, or whether they are of sufficient magnitude to be of clinical significance. Further work is needed to determine if stress or anxiety in early pregnancy can affect later blood flow patterns, or whether the associations are seen only with current emotional state.

CLINICAL IMPLICATIONS

Concerns about mental health in the perinatal period have tended to focus on postnatal depression. This emphasis reflects the high prevalence of depression in the postnatal period (about 10%)[67] and concerns about the particular vulnerabilities and stresses that confront depressed mothers and their newborns.[68] Because of these efforts, postnatal depression is now recognized by psychiatrists, psychologists, nurses, pediatricians, social workers, and obstetricians to be an important clinical issue. On the other hand, other perinatal mental health problems, such as antenatal anxiety, have received comparatively little attention.

Anxiety/stress in pregnancy should receive more attention.[18] We now know that symptoms of anxiety are common and, like depression, even more frequent in pregnancy than in the postnatal period.[1] Antenatal anxiety predicts not only postnatal anxiety, but also postnatal depression, independently of maternal depression during pregnancy. As reviewed in this chapter, there is now substantial research showing connections between antenatal anxiety/stress and potentially important indicators of healthy fetal and child development.

The studies discussed above suggest that effective interventions to reduce maternal stress and/or anxiety during pregnancy may help to reduce the occurrence of cognitive/behavioral problems in children. A major problem with treating stress, anxiety or depression in pregnant women is the understandable reluctance of clinicians to prescribe, and women to accept, standard pharmacologic treatments. Although the safety of the selective serotonin uptake inhibitors (SSRIs) has been investigated in a number of studies, the follow-up period is very limited and there is some evidence of abnormalities, albeit mild.[69] It is thus premature to advocate wide-scale use of such drugs to treat anxiety and depression during pregnancy. Psychological therapies would appear to be better suited to this situation. However, evidence to document the benefits of psychosocial intervention of 'counseling' or 'support' in high-risk groups is still sparse.

In the United Kingdom, there have been no randomized controlled trials examining the efficacy of any established psychological therapies designed to reduce anxiety and depression during pregnancy. Only one small randomized, controlled trial of 16 sessions of interpersonal psychotherapy for antenatal depression has been conducted in the US.[70] Moreover, the Cochrane Pregnancy and Childbirth Group trials register database on assessments of programs offering additional social support for pregnant women believed to be at risk for having preterm or low birthweight babies, failed to find any benefit on these outcomes.[71] This result may well have been because these interventions were not sufficient to prevent the previously discussed effects on the hormonal status of these women.

In a small unpublished study (Teixeira, Adams, and Glover), we assessed whether a short period of directed or passive relaxation would reduce maternal self-rated anxiety, heart rate, plasma catecholamines, cortisol and uterine artery blood flow in pregnant women. Both methods reduced maternal state anxiety and heart rate, the directed therapy more so. Passive relaxation while sitting on a chair had a greater effect in reducing cortisol and noradrenaline. Nevertheless, there was a striking lack of correlation between the psychological effects and all the biological indices measured. In order to reduce the physiological effects of anxiety, different methods may be needed from those that are effective at ameliorating subjective anxiety.

The most promising studies in this area have been conducted by Olds and co-workers.[72,73] The participants were an especially deprived group. Nurses completed an average of 6.5 home visits during pregnancy and 21 visits from birth to the children's second birthdays, and the outcomes were compared with standard care. The nurse visitations produced significant effects on a wide range of maternal and child outcomes.

Nurse-visited mothers and children interacted with one another more responsively, and 6-month-old infants were less likely to exhibit emotional distress in response to fear stimuli. At 21 months, nurse-visited children born to women with low psychological resources were less likely to exhibit language delays and at 24 months, they exhibited superior mental development on the MDI. From the data reported so far, it is not clear that a reduction of maternal stress during pregnancy accounted for the positive gains in the intervention group, but that is a plausible hypothesis that requires further investigation. Additional studies to evaluate the efficacy of similar types of interventions starting during pregnancy should be part of the agenda for new public health research.

CONCLUSION

- There is now strong evidence for a link between maternal stress and anxiety during pregnancy and later cognitive and behavioral problems in the child.
- There is some evidence from studies assessing antenatal life events, and from analysis that co-varied out postnatal depression, stress and/or anxiety, that these relationships are due at least in part to fetal programming.
- The biological basis of the effects of antenatal maternal stress on fetal development is little understood; noradrenaline, the HPA axis and testosterone may be involved.
- Effective interventions to reduce maternal stress and/or anxiety during pregnancy may help to lower the occurrence of cognitive/behavioral problems in children. Evaluation of the efficacy of such interventions should be a new focus for public health research.

REFERENCES

1. Heron J, O'Connor TG, Evans J, Golding J, Glover V. The course of anxiety and depression through pregnancy and the postpartum in a community sample. J Affect Disord 2004; 80: 65–73.
2. Ferreira AJ. Emotional factors in prenatal environment. Journal of Nerv Ment Dis 1965; 141: 108–18.
3. Sontag LW. The significance of fetal environmental differences. Am J Obst Gynecol 1941; 42: 996–1003.
4. Weinstock M. Alterations induced by gestational stress in brain morphology and behaviour of the offspring. Prog Neurobiol 2001; 65: 427–51.
5. Schneider ML, Moore CF, Kraemer GW, Roberts AD, DeJesus OT. The impact of prenatal stress, fetal alcohol exposure, or both on development: perspectives from a primate model. Psychoneuroendocrinology 2002; 27: 285–98.

6. Thompson WR. Influence of perinatal maternal anxiety on emotionality in young rats. Science 1957; 125: 698–99.
7. Ader R, Belfer M. Prenatal maternal anxiety and offspring emotionality in the rat. Physiological Reports 1962; 10: 711–18.
8. Maccari S, Darnaudery M, Morley-Fletcher S et al. Prenatal stress and long-term consequences: implications of gluco-corticoid hormones. Neurosci Biobehav Rev 2003; 27: 119–27.
9. Roughton EC, Schneider ML, Bromley LJ, Coe CL. Maternal endocrine activation during pregnancy alters neurobehavioral state in primate infants. Am J Occup Ther 1998; 52: 90–8.
10. Henry C, Kabbaj M, Simon H, Le Moal M, Maccari S. Prenatal stress increases the hypothalamo-pituitary-adrenal axis response in young and adult rats. J Neuroendocrinol 1994; 6: 341–5.
11. Clarke AS, Wittwer DJ, Abbott DH, Schneider ML. Long-term effects of prenatal stress on HPA axis activity in juvenile rhesus monkeys. Dev Psychobiol 1994; 27: 257–69.
12. Checkley S. The neuroendocrinology of depression and chronic stress. Br Med Bull 1996; 52: 597–617.
13. Gold PW, Chrousos GP. Organization of the stress system and its dysregulation in melancholic and atypical depression: high vs low CRH/NE states. Mol Psychiatry 2002; 7: 254–75.
14. Stott DH. Follow-up study from birth of the effects of prenatal stresses. Dev Med Child Neurol 1973; 15: 770–87.
15. Oyemade U, Cole O, Johnson A et al. Prenatal predictors of performance on the Brazelton Neonatal Behavioral Assessment Scale. J Nutr 1994; 124 (6 Suppl): 1000S–1005S.
16. Meijer A. Child psychiatric sequelae of maternal war stress. Acta Psychiatr Scand 1985; 72: 505–11.
17. McIntosh DE, Mulkins RS, Dean RS. Utilization of maternal perinatal risk indicators in the differential diagnosis of ADHD and UADD children. Int J Neurosci 1995; 81: 35–46.
18. Lou HC, Hansen D, Nordenfoft M et al. Prenatal stressors of human life affect fetal brain development. Dev Med Child Neurol 1994; 36: 826–32.
19. Brouwers E, van Baar A, Pop V. Maternal anxiety during pregnancy and subsequent infant development. Infant Behav Dev 2001; 24: 95–106.
20. Field T, Diego M, Hernandez-Reif M et al. Pregnancy anxiety and comorbid depression and anger: effects on the fetus and neonate. Depress Anxiety 2003; 17: 140–51.
21. Buitelaar JK, Huizink AC, Mulder EJ, de Medina PG, Visser GH. Prenatal stress and cognitive development and temperament in infants. Neurobiol Aging 2003; 24 (Suppl 1): S53–S60; discussion S67–S68.
22. Huizink AC, Robles de Medina PG, Mulder EJ, Visser GH, Buitelaar JK. Stress during pregnancy is associated with developmental outcome in infancy. J Child Psychol Psychiatry 2003; 44: 810–18.
23. Huizink AC, de Medina PG, Mulder EJ, Visser GH, Buitelaar JK. Psychological measures of prenatal stress as predictors of infant temperament. J Am Acad Child Adolesc Psychiatry 2002; 41: 1078–85.
24. Laplante DP, Barr RG, Brunet A et al. Stress during pregnancy affects general intellectual and language functioning in human toddlers. Pediatr Res 2004; 56: 400–10.
25. Niederhofer H, Reiter A. Prenatal maternal stress, prenatal fetal movements and perinatal temperament factors influence behavior and school marks at the age of 6 years. Fetal Diagn Ther 2004; 19: 160–2.
26. O'Connor TG, Heron J, Golding J, Beveridge M, Glover V. Maternal antenatal anxiety and children's behavioural/emotional problems at 4 years. Report from the Avon Longitudinal Study of Parents and Children. Br J Psychiatry 2002; 180: 502–8.
27. O'Connor TG, Heron J, Glover V. Antenatal anxiety predicts child behavioral/emotional problems independently of postnatal depression. J Am Acad Child Adolesc Psychiatry 2002; 41: 1470–7.
28. O'Connor TG, Heron J, Golding J, Glover V. Maternal antenatal anxiety and behavioural/emotional problems in children: a test of a programming hypothesis. J Child Psychol Psychiatry 2003; 44: 1025–36.
29. Obel C, Henriksen TB, Dalsgaard S et al. [Does gestational anxiety result in children's attention disorders?] Ugeskr Laeger 2003; 165: 479.
30. Van Den Bergh BR, Marcoen A. High antenatal maternal anxiety is related to ADHD symptoms, externalizing problems, and anxiety in 8- and 9-year-olds. Child Dev 2004; 75: 1085–97.
31. Rodriguez A, Bohlin G. Are maternal smoking and stress during pregnancy related to ADHD symptoms in children? J Child Psychiat 2005; 46: 246–54.
32. Hansen D, Lou HC, Olsen J. Serious life events and congenital malformations: a national study with complete follow-up. Lancet 2000; 356: 875–80.
33. Spielberger CD, Gorusch RL, Lushene RE. STAI Manual for the State-trait Anxiety Inventory. Pao Alto, CA: Consulting Psychologists Press, 1970.
34. Mancuso RA, Schetter CD, Rini CM, Roesch SC, Hobel CJ. Maternal prenatal anxiety and corticotropin-releasing hormone associated with timing of delivery. Psychosom Med 2004; 66: 762–9.
35. Tsigos C, Chrousos GP. Hypothalamic-pituitary-adrenal axis, neuroendocrine factors and stress. J Psychosom Res 2002; 53: 865–71.
36. Ryan ND. Psychoneuroendocrinology of children and adolescents. Psychiatr Clin North Am 1998; 21: 435–41.
37. Newcomer JW, Selke G, Melson AK et al. Decreased memory performance in healthy humans induced by stress-level cortisol treatment. Arch Gen Psychiatry 1999; 56: 527–33.
38. Caspi A, Sugden K, Moffitt TE et al. Influence of life stress on depression: moderation by a polymorphism in the 5-HTT gene. Science 2003; 301: 386–9.
39. Tully LA, Arseneault L, Caspi A, Moffitt TE, Morgan J. Does maternal warmth moderate the effects of birth weight on twins' attention-deficit/hyperactivity disorder (ADHD) symptoms and low IQ? J Consult Clin Psychol 2004; 72: 218–26.
40. Kofman O. The role of prenatal stress in the etiology of developmental behavioural disorders. Neurosci Biobehav Rev 2002; 26: 457–70.
41. Glover V, O'Connor TG, Heron J, Golding J. Antenatal maternal anxiety is linked with atypical handedness in the child. Early Hum Dev 2004; 79: 107–18.
42. Obel C, Hedegaard M, Henriksen TB, Secher NJ, Olsen J. Psychological factors in pregnancy and mixed-handedness in the offspring. Dev Med Child Neurol 2003; 45: 557–61.
43. Field T, Diego M, Hernandez-Reif M et al. Prenatal anger effects on the fetus and neonate. J Obstet Gynaecol 2002; 22: 260–6.
44. Van den Bergh BRH. Maternal emotions during pregnancy and fetal and neonatal behaviour. In: Fetal Behaviour (Nijhuis, JN, ed.). London: OUP, 1992: 157–78.
45. DiPietro JA, Hilton SC, Hawkins M, Costigan KA, Pressman EK. Maternal stress and affect influence fetal neurobehavioral development. Dev Psychol 2002; 38: 659–68.

46. Pennefather JN, Paull JD, Story ME, Ziccone SP. Supersensitivity to the stimulant action of noradrenaline on human myometrium near term. Reprod Fertil Dev 1993; 5: 39–48.

47. Herlenius E, Lagercrantz H. Development of neurotransmitter systems during critical periods. Exp Neurol 2004; 190 (Suppl 1): 8–21.

48. Gitau R, Cameron A, Fisk NM, Glover V. Fetal exposure to maternal cortisol. Lancet 1998; 352: 707–8.

49. Gitau R, Fisk NM, Teixeira JM, Cameron A, Glover V. Fetal hypothalamic-pituitary-adrenal stress responses to invasive procedures are independent of maternal responses. J Clin Endocrinol Metab 2001; 86: 104–9.

50. Gitau R, Adams D, Fisk NM, Glover V. Fetal plasma testosterone correlates positively with cortisol. Arch Dis Child 2005; 90: F166–9.

51. Gitau R, Fisk NM, Glover V. Human fetal and maternal corticotrophin releasing hormone responses to acute stress. Arch Dis Child Fetal Neonatal Ed 2004; 89: F29–32.

52. Giannakoulopoulos X, Teixeira J, Fisk N, Glover V. Human fetal and maternal noradrenaline responses to invasive procedures. Pediatr Res 1999; 45(4 Pt 1): 494–9.

53. Seckl JR. Glucocorticoid programming of the fetus; adult phenotypes and molecular mechanisms. Mol Cell Endocrinol 2001; 185: 61–71.

54. Monk C, Myers MM, Sloan RP, Ellman LM, Fifer WP. Effects of women's stress-elicited physiological activity and chronic anxiety on fetal heart rate. J Dev Behav Pediatr 2003; 24: 32–8.

55. Obel C, Hedegaard M, Henriksen TB et al. Stress and salivary cortisol during pregnancy. Psychoneuroendocrinology 2005; 30: 647–56.

56. Mastorakos G, Ilias I. Maternal and fetal hypothalamic-pituitary-adrenal axes during pregnancy and postpartum. Ann N Y Acad Sci 2003; 997: 136–49.

57. Kammerer M, Adams D, Castelberg Bv B, Glover V. Pregnant women become insensitive to cold stress. BMC Pregnancy Childbirth 2002; 2: 8.

58. Glynn LM, Wadhwa PD, Dunkel-Schetter C, Chicz-Demet A, Sandman CA. When stress happens matters: effects of earthquake timing on stress responsivity in pregnancy. Am J Obstet Gynecol 2001; 184: 637–42.

59. Goy RW, McEwen BS. Sexual differentiation of the brain. Cambridge Mas: MIT Press, 1980.

60. Berenbaum SA, Hines M. Early androgens are related to childhood sex-typed toy preferences. Psychol Sci 1992; 3: 203–6.

61. Nass R, Baker S, Speiser P et al. Hormones and handedness: left-hand bias in female congenital adrenal hyperplasia patients. Neurology 1987; 37: 711–15.

62. Baron-Cohen S. The extreme male brain theory of autism. Trends Cogn Sci 2002; 6: 248–54.

63. Lutchmaya S, Baron-Cohen S, Raggatt P. Foetal testosterone and vocabulary size in 18 and 24 month old infants. Infant Behav Dev 2002; 25: 327–35.

64. Igosheva N, Klimova O, Anishchenko T, Glover V. Prenatal stress alters cardiovascular responses in adult rats. J Physiol 2004; 557 (Pt 1): 273–85.

65. Teixeira JM, Fisk NM, Glover V. Association between maternal anxiety in pregnancy and increased uterine artery resistance index: cohort based study. BMJ 1999; 318: 153–7.

66. Sjostrom K, Valentin L, Thelin T, Marsal K. Maternal anxiety in late pregnancy and fetal hemodynamics. Eur J Obstet Gynecol Reprod Biol 1997; 74: 149–55.

67. Cox JL, Connor Y, Kendell RE. Prospective study of the psychiatric disorders of childbirth. Br J Psychiatry 1982; 140: 111–17.

68. Murray L, Fiori-Cowley A, Hooper R, Cooper P. The impact of postnatal depression and associated adversity on early mother-infant interactions and later infant outcome. Child Dev 1996; 67: 2512–26.

69. Laine K, Heikkinen T, Ekblad U, Kero P. Effects of exposure to selective serotonin reuptake inhibitors during pregnancy on serotonergic symptoms in newborns and cord blood monoamine and prolactin concentrations. Arch Gen Psychiatry 2003; 60: 720–6.

70. Spinelli MG, Endicott J. Controlled clinical trial of interpersonal psychotherapy versus parenting education program for depressed pregnant women. Am J Psychiatry 2003; 160: 555–62.

71. Hodnett ED, Fredericks S. Support during pregnancy for women at increased risk of low birthweight babies. Cochrane Database Syst Rev 2003: CD000198.

72. Olds DL. Prenatal and infancy home visiting by nurses: from randomized trials to community replication. Prev Sci 2002; 3: 153–72.

73. Olds DL, Robinson J, O'Brien R et al. Home visiting by paraprofessionals and by nurses: a randomized, controlled trial. Pediatrics 2002; 110: 486–96.

20

Cytokines, social development, and psychopathology: an empirical and theoretical integration

Douglas A Granger and Nancy A Dreschel

INTRODUCTION

The past three decades have witnessed exponential growth in our knowledge of the interactions among the central and peripheral nervous systems and the immune system.[1-3] The signals and routes via which psychological and physical stressors lead to endocrine and immune responses have been studied extensively.[4-7] This chapter focuses on the implications of another leading edge of psychoneuroimmunologic research;[8-10] specifically, new findings that sparked a scientific revolution regarding the direction of effects: immune on brain and behavior.[11,12] Our objective is to reveal the implications of this new knowledge on theories about the origins of individual differences in social behavior and psychopathology. As a starting point, a historical overview of our understanding regarding the neuroendocrine-immune network is provided. We introduce the immune system as our 'sixth sense'. Then, the influence of the regulatory cellular molecules of the neuroendocrine-immune network (e.g. cytokines) on the brain and ultimately behavior are described. Next, we review studies indicating that immune-stimulated changes in the nervous and endocrine systems during early development cause permanent alterations in social behavior that persist into adulthood. We conclude that there may be a large class of ubiquitous and omnipresent stimuli (i.e. viruses, bacteria, and toxins) that may have been overlooked in the search for environmental factors that shape microevolution and the development of psychopathology.[13,14] We present a theoretical model of how psychoneuroimmunologic processes affect developmental plasticity, and make recommendations for research to integrate such ideas into developmental science.

THE NEUROENDOCRINE-IMMUNE NETWORK

The history of ideas linking behavior or psychological states and immune function is punctuated by three major eras.[2,15] The first spans the turn of the last century through the early 1950s. During this period, immunologists made discoveries that defined our understanding of cell function, antibody production and activity, and the basic features of the immune system. The scientists of this time considered the brain an immunologically privileged site because the central nervous system (CNS) lacks lymphatic ducts to drain tissues and capture potential antigens, and the blood-brain barrier (BBB) is impermeable to many soluble substances (i.e. cytokines) and restricts the migration of lymphoid cells into the CNS.[16] The dominant assumption was that the immune system operated in isolation from the CNS, and the possibility that it might be influenced by psychological states or behavior, or that immune activity may affect the brain or behavior attracted, little empirical attention (except see Kopeloff et al.[17]).

A number of observations in the 1960–70s ushered in the second era. Solomon et al. reported that symptoms of autoimmune arthritis varied as a function of social-psychological features of the family environment.[18,19] In the late 1970s anatomical pathways were discovered that physiochemically linked the central nervous and lymphoid systems (see Figure 20.1). Specific nerve tracts were identified that terminated in lymphoid tissues and organs.[20] Receptors were also found on lymphoid cells for a variety of the products (e.g., epinephrine, norepinephrine) secreted by these nerve terminals,[20] and released by the hypothalamic-pituitary-adrenal (HPA)

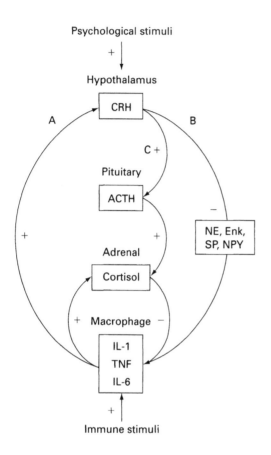

Psychological stimuli

Figure 20.1 Schematic representation of the neuroendocrine-immune pathways and signaling molecules. Pathway A indicates immune-to-brain communication via the activity of cytokines (IL-1, interleukin-1; TNF, tumor necrosis factor; IL-6, interleukin-6). Pathway B indicates the communication route between the autonomic nervous system (ANS) and the immune system (NE, norepinephrine; ENK, enkephalin; SP, substance P; NPY, neuropeptide Y). Pathway C indicates the communication link between the hypothalamic-pituitary-adrenal axis and the immune system (CRF, corticotropin releasing hormone; ACTH, adrenocorticotropic hormone; CORT, cortisol or corticosterone). + and (−) identify pathways with primarily excitatory or inhibitory effects.

axis (i.e. adrenocorticotropic hormone, glucocorticoids) and autonomic nervous systems (i.e. substance P, neuropeptide Y, norepinephrine).[21] The primary focus of psychoneuroimmunology (PNI) research at this time was on links between stress and negative health outcomes mediated via the effect of psychological states on immune function.[1,3,22]

In parallel, basic research on the immune system progressed at a very rapid pace. Experiments in the 1960s and 1970s[23,24] revealed that lymphoid cells secreted soluble chemical messengers to initiate, maintain, and regulate immune responses. Later it was discovered that these 'lymphokines'[25] also had effects on nonlymphoid cells (cells in the CNS and endocrine system) at considerable distances away from the cells that secreted them.[26,27] In recognition of this 'functional diversity' the molecules were relabeled 'cytokines' in the early 1980s. Most importantly, for present purposes, these discoveries completed a communication loop: the immune system could both receive and send signals to the CNS (see Figure 20.1).

The contemporary emphasis of much PNI research is now intensively focused on topics in molecular biology and neuroscience.[2] Studies have unequivocally revealed that cells of the lymphoid, CNS, and endocrine systems can use the same effector molecules to send and receive signals.[3,8,11,28] The brain, endocrine system, and immune system constitute an interactive information network with each capable of affecting and being affected by the activity of the others.[2,29,30] A schematic of these interactive systems with representative signaling molecules and communication routes is depicted in Figure 20.1.

IMMUNE SYSTEM AS OUR 'SIXTH SENSE'

Decoding the biochemical syntax of the neuroendocrine-immune axis has enabled theorists to attribute new sensory and regulatory features to the immune system's functions. Blalock[11] advocated the view that the immune system recognizes unique environmental stimuli (i.e. microbes, toxins) that are undetectable by our visual, auditory, olfactory, and gustatory senses. One cannot see, hear, smell, taste, or feel an individual microbe, but when immune recognition occurs, the encounter is converted into a cascade of biochemical messages. These signals are responsible for inducing changes in the host's metabolic, thermogenic, and behavioral states. Increased sleepiness and the reduced activity, arousal and motivation seen with systemic infection may be an adaptive physiological response to conserve energy. Fever stimulated by the release of proinflammatory cytokines and acute phase proteins produces an unfavorable environment for the growth of many microbial pathogens.[31] In addition, the afflicted individual's expression of sickness behaviors (see below) may include social withdrawal, conveying benefits to the immediate social group by limiting their exposure to the pathogen. Advances in our understanding of the sensory functions of the immune system raise the possibility that immune-to-brain communications represent a largely unexplored pathway through which biochemical signals triggered by environmental factors continually reshape the structure and function of biological systems underlying atypical behavior. With few exceptions[32–35] these novel ideas attracted only minimal attention from developmentally oriented researchers.

A PRIMER ON CYTOKINES

Here we describe the general properties of some of the critical effector molecules that mediate the aforementioned sensory functions and review how they communicate with and affect the brain, endocrine system, and behavior.

Basic properties and functions

Cytokines are small protein molecules that act as both intra- and intercellular messengers. They range in molecular weight from 8 to 30 kDa and induce their effects by binding to high affinity receptors on cell membranes. Monocytes and macrophages are especially efficient producers of cytokines. Some cytokines are stored preformed in the intracellular granules for instantaneous release, but most cytokine secretion involves *de novo* protein synthesis; a process that takes hours.

Cytokines are pleiotropic, meaning they have multiple target cells and multiple actions, and their effects are often redundant, sometimes synergistic, and less frequently antagonistic. Cytokines are grouped by their

structure and whether they have anti-inflammatory, proinflammatory, or growth-promoting functions. Within the immune system, interleukins (e.g. IL-1, IL-2, IL-4, IL-6, IL-10, IL-13) act as messengers between white blood cells, colony-stimulating factors (e.g. IL-3, G-CSF, m-CSF, GM-CSF) promote cell proliferation; tumor necrosis factors (TNF-α, TNF-β) initiate inflammation and cause necrosis and cachexia; and interferons (e.g. IFN-α, IFN-γ) act to interfere with viral replication.

Regulation and inhibition

Cytokines even in very low pg/ml levels can induce substantial biological activity, and not surprisingly several processes exist to prevent these potent substances from doing damage to the host. They include receptor antagonists (e.g. IL-1ra), molecules homologous to the ligand and able to bind cytokine receptors without leading to signal transduction; shed receptors (e.g. s-TNF-R type I and II), that bind cytokines in the intercellular fluid space and stop them from reaching cells or tissues;[36,37] and other molecules that act through independent receptors to exert opposite effects on the cell.[38] Some cytokines also inhibit each other (e.g. IL-10 inhibits synthesis of TNF, IL-1, IL-6, and others).

Inadequate production of cytokines will result in an insufficient cellular response and potentially negative consequences related to enhanced pathogenesis of the microbe, bacteria, or virus (see Figure 20.2). Without medical intervention, individuals who consistently under-produce cytokines would not be likely to survive. It is probable that this phenotype would be rapidly removed from the gene pool as these individuals would succumb to illness in nature. On the other hand, excessive cytokine secretion has been linked to abnormal 'sickness behaviors' (see below), autoimmune disorders (i.e. arthritis), neurological disease (e.g. multiple sclerosis), toxic shock, and even death (i.e. sepsis) (see Figure 20.2). It is plausible that the forces of natural selection would also remove individuals who over-produce cytokines from the gene pool. That is, when challenged by immune stimuli, these individuals would experience severe fatigue, fever, loss of appetite, inactivity, social withdrawal, weight loss, and cognitive slowing, which significantly increase risk of pathology and/or predation. Thus, under natural circumstances, selective pressure from microorganisms as well as predators serves to regulate the gene pool such that reproductively fit individuals would also optimally regulate their cytokine activity (see Figure 20.2).

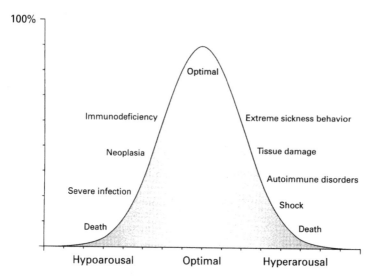

Figure 20.2 Individual differences in the activity of the cytokine network are related to variation in physical and mental health. Regulation of cytokine activity within an optimal range is essential to avoid the negative biobehavioral consequences linked with either hypoarousal or hyperarousal of the immune system.

Cytokines and the CNS

The most well-characterized pathway through which peripheral stimuli induce immune signals that change the CNS begins with the macrophage. When activated, macrophages secrete a cascade of chemical messengers (see Figure 20.1). Importantly, it is the cytokine products released, not the microbial stimulus (e.g. bacterial or viral pathogenesis), that mediate the resulting changes in the brain.[39–41] Molecular, cellular, and in vivo evidence suggests that macrophage-derived IL-1 has the most pervasive and hormone-like effects of the cytokines[25] with widespread consequences for the brain.[42] Peripheral administration of nanogram amounts of IL-1β stimulates corticotropin-releasing factor (CRF) release from hypothalamic neurons,[43,44] resulting in increased circulating levels of adrenocorticotrophic hormone (ACTH) and corticosterone.[45] Many others, including Berkenbosch et al.[46,47] and Dunn[48–50] also reported that peripheral administration of IL-1β potentiates the response of the HPA axis to environmental challenge.

Cytokines have a variety of effects on neurotransmission.[51,52] IL-1β acts to stimulate cerebral norepinephrine (NE) metabolism, probably reflecting increased synaptic release. IL-1, IL-6, and TNF also stimulate indolamine metabolism of tryptophan and decrease the concentration of serotonin (5HT). Through their action on indolamines, cytokines affect the synthesis of quinolinic (QUIN) and kynurenic acid (see Figure 20.3). QUIN is an agonist of the N-methyl-D-aspartate (NMDA) receptor and other excitatory amino acid receptors. These receptors mediate excitatory amino acid neurotransmission within the hippocampus, basal ganglia, and cerebral cortex and have been implicated in nerve cell death and dysfunction.[53,54] On the other hand, kynurenic acid is an antagonist of NMDA receptors and could modulate the neurotoxic effects of QUIN as well as disrupt excitatory amino acid transmission. A schematic of one type of cerebral effects induced by cytokines is depicted in Figure 20.3.

Many of the changes in the CNS occur because of simultaneous activation of IL-1β production in various regions of the brain.[55] That is, within hours after peripheral immune activation, expression of IL-1β transcripts is induced in the hippocampus, hypothalamus, and pituitary.[56,57] IL-1 receptors are widely distributed throughout the brain and endocrine tissues,[58] with high densities observed in the hippocampal area and the choroid plexus.[59] Thus, it is not surprising that the behavioral and physiological effects can be mimicked by administration of IL-1β directly into the brain,[42] and that they can be attenuated by intracerebroventricular (i.c.v.) injection of the receptor antagonist to IL-1 (IL-1ra).[60]

The first studies on the cytokine–brain interactions emphasized the more permissive parts of the BBB (the circumventricular organs) that allow proinflammatory cytokines to pass and act on brain. However, in the mid-1990s, it was discovered that the subdiaphragmatic section of the vagus nerve attenuates the brain effects of systemic cytokines, suggesting that neural transmission and inducible cytokines in the brain played a major role. This observation shifted research attention away from the circumventricular organs to

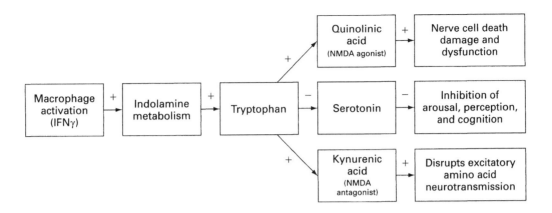

Figure 20.3 Immune activation has many effects on cerebral neurotransmission. Infections result in macrophage release of cytokines that activate indoleamine-2,3-dioxygenase (IDO). Increases in IDO activity accelerate the degradation of L-tryptophan to neuroreactive kynurenines, including the excitotoxin quinolinic acid (QUIN), and the antagonist of excitatory amino acid receptors, kynurenic acid (KYNA). QUIN and KYNA act on N-methyl-D-aspartate (NMDA) receptors. Degradation of L-tryptophan via this kynurenic pathway results in reduced serotonin levels. This immune-to-brain pathway can result in neural damage and dysfunction, neurologic deficits and neurodegeneration, and can inhibit arousal, perception, and cognition.

possible neural pathways. Since then, considerable research has confirmed that a faster route of communication from the immune system to the brain is via the vagus nerves. This neural afferent pathway complements a humoral pathway that involves cytokines produced locally at the circumventricular organs and in the brain parenchyma.[61,62]

In summary, biological pathways via which cytokines affect the CNS have been well characterized. The effects of cytokines in the brain involve changes in neurotransmission in regions (such as the hippocampus, hypothalamus), with well-established links to learning and memory, emotion regulation, and the stress response. We speculate that elimination of predators and widespread medical interventions to eradicate infectious diseases (i.e. antibiotics, immunizations) may have created an opportunity for a wide range of individual differences in the activity of the cytokine network in the modern human population. The next sections detail our understanding of the links between immune activation and behavior, and cytokines and psychopathology.

CYTOKINE EFFECTS AT THE BEHAVIORAL SURFACE

Numerous studies in animals have shown that IL-1β administration elicits anorexia,[63] increases sleep time,[64] decreases social and nonsocial exploration,[65]

decreases sexual activity,[66] increases defensive withdrawal, and affects other behaviors characteristic of sickness symptoms.[12,39] Some suggest that sickness behavior also disrupts motivation and arousal in ways that reorganize the organism's priorities to better cope with infectious pathogens.[12,67,68]

Mild-to-moderate adverse behavioral effects of peripherally released cytokines such as IL-1β can be recognized in any person with an active influenza infection. Tyrell and colleagues documented adverse effects of experimentally induced respiratory virus infection and cytokine administration on human psychomotor performance, mood, and memory.[69–71] Evidence of moderate-to-severe psychological effects of cytokines was also revealed in clinical trials of interleukins and interferons as therapeutic biological response modifiers. Many oncology patients treated with cytokines complained of headache, fever, anorexia, fatigue, and social withdrawal.[72,73] Repeated prolonged exposure of cancer patients to cytokines resulted in increased irritability, short temper, agitation, aggressiveness, extreme emotional lability, depression, fearfulness, and severe cognitive changes, including disorientation, paranoia, and suicidal ideation.[74] Results from that study also indicated that while these adverse effects generally resolved with termination of the protocol, some participants remained emotionally impacted for weeks.[75–79]

The experimental animal and clinical human studies provide strong support for the conclusion that endogenous cytokine production and administration of exogenous cytokines are causally linked to the expression of atypical emotional, behavioral, and cognitive function. The severity of the symptoms extends into the clinical range. Generally, the effects of cytokines on behavior are consistent with our knowledge about the physiological changes induced in the CNS and neuroendocrine axes.

There have been few comprehensive evaluations between psychiatric disorders and cytokine regulation. Some studies report that adult patients with severe depression, anxiety, and symptoms of stress-related psychiatric disorders have immune abnormalities.[80,81,82] The findings are not always consistent, but the pattern largely supports the hypothesis of an association between internalizing behavior problems and activation of the cytokine network.[83,84]

Depression

The hypothesis that cytokines play a role in the pathophysiology of major depression is based on assumptions that depression is: 1) closely associated with stress and can be an exaggerated response to stress, 2) often accompanied by atypical HPA axis activity, and 3) the cardinal manifestations include changes in sleep, appetite, sex drive, social withdrawal, and cognitive slowing.[85] Cytokines are associated with or influence many of these symptoms.[86,87] Maes et al. reported significant elevations of IL-1β and IL-6 in the plasma of depressed patients.[88,89] In recent studies, Owen et al. reported elevated levels of IL-1β in major depression and postviral depression.[90] Similarly, Musselman et al.[91] found that cancer patients with depression had markedly higher plasma concentrations of IL-6 than healthy subjects and cancer patients without depression. Berk et al.[92] had also shown that C-reactive protein and IL-6 levels were significantly raised with major depression.

On the other hand, Haack and colleagues[93] cautioned that the association between depressive symptoms and cytokines may in part be due to a number of other confounding influences. In the largest study to date (361 psychiatric patients, 64 healthy controls), they found little, if any, evidence for immunopathology in major depression, when age, body mass, gender, smoking habits, ongoing or recent infectious diseases, and medications are carefully taken into account.

Very few studies have explored relationships between psychiatric symptoms or problem behavior and cytokine levels in younger subjects. Birmaher et al.[94] studied 20 adolescents with major depressive disorder, 17 nondepressed subjects with conduct disorder, and 17 healthy controls. Blood samples were obtained to determine the numbers of total white blood cells and lymphocyte subsets and to conduct assays of natural killer (NK) cell activity and lymphocyte proliferation. Overall, there were no significant group differences, but this project did not measure cytokines. A preliminary study by our laboratories revealed that serum levels of cytokines were significantly correlated with behavior problems in clinic-referred youth, but not in nonreferred, age-matched comparisons. In this study (M age = 11.3 years, range 8–17) we observed that individual differences of IL-1 levels were positively correlated, r (17) = 0.59 and 0.55, $p < 0.05$, with self-reported anxiety/depression on the Youth Self-Report version of the Child Behavior Checklist and Children's Depression Inventory in a clinic-referred group ($n = 20$) but not in a control group of nondisturbed children ($n = 19$).[95] Similar findings were recently reported by Brambilla et al.[96] in children and adolescents with major depressive disorder.

Anxiety disorders

Depression is often accompanied by anxiety and other anxiety-related disorders, but in comparison to depression, the data linking cytokines and anxiety disorders are scant. There is a growing body of evidence suggesting a role for autoimmune-like processes in some specific cases of *obsessive compulsive disorder* (OCD).[97–99] Maes et al. noted a positive association between IL-6 and the severity of compulsive symptoms.[100] Mittleman et al.[101] reported atypical cytokine levels in the cerebrospinal fluid in patients with childhood-onset OCD. These studies do not consistently support a link between immune abnormalities and *panic disorders* (PD). Brambilla et al. reported that plasma IL-1β was significantly higher in patients with PD than controls.[102,103] In contrast, Rapaport and Stein[104] and Weizman et al. failed to find that immune measures differentiated patients with PD from normal controls.[105] Spivak et al.[106] found circulating levels of IL-1β were significantly higher in patients with combat-related *post-traumatic stress disorder* (PTSD), with IL-1β levels correlating with duration of PTSD, and severity of anxiety and depression. No studies to our knowledge have explored the links between anxiety and cytokine activity in children.

In summary, cytokines can cause a rapid reorganization in several behavioral domains. The intensity of these effects ranges from mild to extreme, and the duration of the effects can outlast the events that initially precipitated their release. The biobehavioral effects of cytokines underscore the possibility that their dysregulation might alter the organization of human physiology and behavior in ways that affect individual development and the evolutions of populations and species. In particular, the literature highlights the possibility that variation in the expression of cognitive, emotional, and behavioral symptoms associated with depression and/or socially inhibited behaviors may be partially explained by cytokines and differential sensitivities to the naturally occurring and ubiquitous immune stimuli.[12,82,107] However, the findings suggest that while cytokines are sufficient to cause psychiatric symptoms, it is also common that psychiatric symptoms occur in the absence of cytokine aberrations.

METHODS TO STUDY BEHAVIORAL EFFECTS OF CYTOKINES

Several methodological challenges confront researchers studying cytokine–behavior relationships. Under normal circumstances, in the healthy individual, the levels of many cytokines (particularly those responsible for the initiation and regulation of inflammation) are below the sensitivity of most assays, and thus nondetectable. This creates considerable obstacles to quantitatively correlating individual differences, as the range of values is restricted to present or absent. In addition, the variation in detectable cytokines is often not normally distributed. Thus, to explore the full range of individual differences in cytokine biology, investigators must evaluate cytokine responses in reaction to an immune challenge. This is most often accomplished in vitro with lymphoid cells that have been isolated from the body and cultured. The validity of such data for generalizing about functioning in vivo has been questioned.[108]

Another challenge is the difficulty of separating the effects of the infectious agent itself from the effects of the immune response to that agent. As reviewed above, our assumption is that some individuals generate more cytokines in response to immune challenges and/or that some have nervous and/or endocrine systems that are more sensitive to the effects of cytokines. An experimental paradigm commonly employed as a stimulus to induce cytokines is a nonreplicating component of bacterial cell walls, lipopolysaccharide (LPS), as a proxy for a viral or bacterial infection.[109] LPS (also referred to as endotoxin) is the immunologically active component of gram-negative bacteria cell walls and bacteria of this type are found in and commonly infect most mammalian species (Escherichia coli, Salmonella). The behavioral, neurochemical, and neuroendocrine response to administered LPS mimics the reaction to IL-1β very closely.[110] Use of LPS enables

standardized exposure to the immune stimulus, a control that is not easy to implement in human studies under natural circumstances. In one of the few studies conducted with humans, Reichenberg et al. employed a double-blind cross-over design with 20 healthy male volunteers.[111] Participants completed psychological questionnaires and neuropsychological tests 1, 3, and 9 hours after intravenous injection of endotoxin (0.8 ng/kg, Salmonella). After endotoxin administration, subjects showed a transient increase in anxiety and depressed mood, with decreased verbal and nonverbal memory, and these changes were associated with increased levels of IL-1β, TNF-α, and IL-6.

Substances like endotoxin have been used as adjuvants in vaccine preparations to boost the immunogenicity of vaccine and evoke a large response (e.g. whole-cell DTP vaccine). Investigators studying the effects of stress on immunity have frequently taken advantage of immunizations of many types as natural experiments.[112,113] The reaction to immunizations can also be used to explore individual differences in cytokine–behavior relationships.[114] Several studies conducted for other reasons also reported mild-to-moderate, short-term behavioral effects of immunizations in children.[115] The 'side effects' included fever, irritability, lack of appetite, and increased sleepiness, which correspond to nonspecific symptoms of sickness induced by cytokines. Research on the efficacy of most childhood vaccines was conducted largely before cytokines were known as regulators of the neuro-endocrine-immune network. Yet, even 15 years ago, a government-sponsored scientific panel in the United States called for more research on the biobehavioral predictors of individual differences in the severity of adverse responses to vaccines, as well as further investigations of the biological mechanisms responsible for vaccine-induced behavioral effects.[116]

CYTOKINES AND DEVELOPMENTAL PLASTICITY

Is it possible that activation of the cytokine network can also cause longer-term changes in biological systems that underlie more persistent alterations in behavioral, emotional, or cognitive capacities? Can cytokines even influence enduring aspects of our temperament or personality? At first glance, this possibility seems to contradict our everyday experience. That is, when adults have viral or bacterial infections, it is clear that the majority exhibit 'sickness behaviors', albeit to different degrees. But even those of us who become the most agitated, withdrawn, sleepy, and irritable when 'sick', seemingly return to our 'regular' selves soon after the infection subsides. Could there be developmental periods when humans are more susceptible to longer-term or permanent effects? To answer this question studies are needed that employ longitudinal designs and assess maturation of cytokine activity and the processes that influence their regulation, in parallel with evaluation of atypical behavior. To our knowledge, no such studies have been conducted with humans, but the evidence from animal studies is compelling.

Studies with rodents show conclusively that exposure to endotoxin or high levels of cytokines during early development permanently changes and can have organizational influences on the brain and behavior. O'Grady and colleagues reported that immune activation during pre- and neonatal periods affects the size of the adrenal glands, ovaries, and testes, and the differences persist into adulthood.[117–119] Shanks et al. showed that immune activation during the neonatal period critical to HPA axis development had profound effects on ACTH and corticosterone responsiveness to later environmental challenge during adulthood.[35] Specifically, administration of endotoxin (0.05 mg/kg) on days 3 and 5 of life resulted in decreased negative feedback of corticosterone of ACTH synthesis, thereby potentiating HPA responsiveness to restraint stress. These studies suggest that exposure to bacteria or large immune activations early in life can permanently alter neuroendocrine systems, i.e. HPA and hypothalamic-pituitary-gonadal (HPG) axes, in ways that continue to influence how environmental events interact with developmental processes.

This sensitivity of the immature host was also supported by Crnic and colleagues when they showed virally induced behavioral changes that persisted into adulthood.[34,120] Neonatal mice administered Herpes simplex virus (HSV-1) or interferon became spontaneously hyperactive for life.[121] This radical reorganization of behavior appeared to be mediated by the effects of cytokines on the migration of granule cells from the cerebellum. Crnic's findings are groundbreaking in that they provide evidence for the neuroanatomical basis of the permanent behavioral changes. Crnic postulated that other types of atypical behavior may be caused by common immunological stimuli that have 'uncommon effects' on the biological substrate of behavior.[34]

'UNCOMMON EFFECTS' OF IMMUNE STIMULI: INDIVIDUAL, DEVELOPMENTAL, AND SOCIAL INFLUENCES

We believe that studies on the uncommon effects of common immune stimuli may extend our understanding of individual development and microevolution.[13] In our laboratory we employed a well-established animal model of genotype–environment interactions as a means to investigate atypical social development, analogous to internalizing and externalizing behavior problems. The model uses two lines of mice that were selectively bred for differences in social interactions over more than 30 generations, as well as a control line of unselected mice. The advantages of the model included: 1) a known sensitive period for when early experiences most influenced later social behavior,[122] 2) documented line differences in the rate of development of aggressive behavior,[123] and 3) line differences in immune responsiveness that had been studied in detail at the cellular level.[124,125]

Individual differences

In the first study we explored genetic-developmental differences in the biobehavioral effects of induced illness.[126] Adult males from high and low aggressive behavior lines were injected with endotoxin (LPS: 0.25 mg/kg, 1.25 mg/kg or 2.5 mg/kg) or saline. Body temperature, weight, and locomotor activity were monitored before, and 8 and 24 hours after injection. At 24 hours, social behaviors were assessed in a 10-minute dyadic test, and then tissue (spleens and hypothalami) were collected. High-aggressive line males had a lower threshold to endotoxin-induced effects on body temperature, weight loss, spleen weight, hypothalamic norepinephrine, and corticosterone than did males from the low-aggressive line. In the high-aggressive line only, social reactivity increased (startle response to mild social investigation), and attack frequency and latency to attack decreased for endotoxin-treated as compared with saline-treated mice. Table 20.1 presents bivariate correlations among the physiological and behavioural effects of endotoxin for each selected line.

These genotype effects on the response to endotoxin treatment indicate the extent to which immune stimuli function differentially as 'biobehavioral' stressors.

In a companion set of studies, we explored the time course of the endotoxin effects in these selected lines (Granger, Hood, and Banta, unpublished observations). Adult male mice from the high- and low-aggressive lines were administered endotoxin (1.25 mg/kg) and their social behavior was assessed and

Table 20.1 Bivariate correlations among the biobehavioral effects of endotoxin in adult male mice selectively bred for differences in social behavior

Parameter	CORT	Spleen weight	Attack frequency	Behavioral immobility	Social exploration	Social reactivity
High-aggressive line						
8 h post-injection						
Activity	−0.68****	−0.50**	0.23	−0.22	0.05	−0.36
Weight	0.59***	0.49**	−0.50**	0.69****	−0.57***	0.68***
Temperature	−0.62***	−0.58***	0.51**	−0.62	0.39	−0.63***
24 h post-injection						
Activity	−0.64***	−0.47**	0.23	−0.19	0.03	−0.28
Weight	−0.70****	−0.56**	0.36	−0.47**	0.25	−0.47**
Temperature	−0.55***	0.25	0.30	−0.79****	0.51**	−0.47**
Corticosterone	. . .	0.28	−0.08	0.41*	−0.37	0.43**
Low-aggressive line						
8 h post-injection						
Activity	0.04	0.10	. . .	−0.32	0.00	0.56***
Weight	0.16	0.05	. . .	0.21	−0.35	−0.39
Temperature	−0.08	0.02	. . .	−0.34	0.38	0.16
24 h post-injection						
Activity	−0.11	−0.23	. . .	−0.44**	0.15	0.63***
Weight	−0.19	0.00	. . .	−0.29	0.42*	0.27
Temperature	0.16	0.19	. . .	−0.25	0.03	0.37
Corticosterone	. . .	0.53**	. . .	0.05	−0.45**	0.48**

Data were averaged across endotoxin dose. Activity, weight, and temperature scores represent percent change from baseline (pre-injection) levels at 8 and 24 h post-injection. Serum corticosterone (CORT) levels and social behaviors were assessed 24 h post-injection. *$p < 0.06$, **$p < 0.05$, ***$p < 0.01$, ****$p < 0.001$ (all dfs = 19, two-tailed tests). Reprinted from Granger et al.[126]

serum obtained at 12 time points (0.5–6, 18, and 24 hours) post-injection. In contrast to low-aggressive line mice, high-aggressive line mice showed an endotoxin-induced reduction in attack frequency and latency, more pronounced increases in behavioral immobility, socially reactive behavior, and more IL-1β in circulation. Endotoxin-related differences in levels of IL-1β, corticosterone and behavior change were positively associated in the high-aggressive line only (Figure 20.4).

Taken together with the findings on similar lines of mice (e.g. Pettito et al.[124]), these data suggest that behavioral differences across lines are due to variation in cytokine production. However, it cannot be ruled out that there may be line differences in the CNS or HPA axis sensitivity to the afferent signals of cytokines, or other acute phase proteins that respond to endotoxin. In the next experiment we further evaluated these possibilities. High- and low-aggressive line

mice were administered a standard dose of IL-1β (0.25–1.0 μg/ml) or saline. Consistent with Pettito's findings, high-aggressive line mice showed a larger increase in circulating levels of IL-6 that was associated with higher corticosterone, temperature loss, and more behavioral immobility in the observed social interactions (Figure 20.5, Table 20.2).

The underlying mechanisms responsible for the apparent linkage between these behavioral 'traits', and immune responsiveness are still unclear. Pettito and colleagues[127] raised two possibilities: that the association between selective line and immune responses (in their case NK cell activity) may be due to a linkage between subsets of genes involved in determining these complex behavioral and immune traits or that these results were caused by a fortuitous association that emerged during selective breeding. There is some independent evidence supporting the proposition that the aggression-immunity link is not restricted to

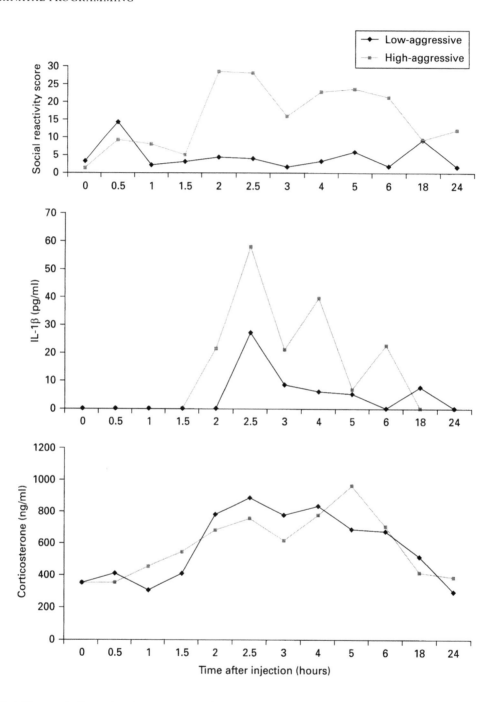

Figure 20.4 Temporal effects of endotoxin (1.25 mg/kg) on IL-1β and socially reactive (startle) behaviors are correlated, but distinctly differ in mice selectively bred for high versus low levels of aggressive behavior (Granger et al., unpublished observations).

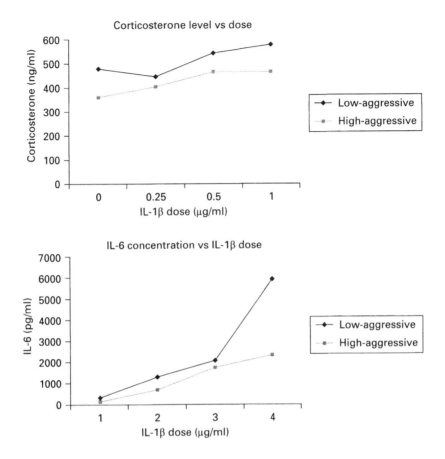

Figure 20.5 Administration of IL-1β (μg/ml) induces IL-6 and corticosterone differently in adult male mice selectively bred for high versus low levels of aggressive behavior (Granger et al., unpublished observations).

rodents. Experimental studies in a nonhuman primate species (*Macaca fascicularis*) revealed that changes in immune responses to viral infection caused by the stress of repeated reorganization of social groups were associated with individual differences in aggressive behavior.[128] High-aggressive monkeys also had higher lymphocyte counts than did low-aggressive monkeys.[129] These types of associations may also be seen in humans. Among men aged 30–48 years ($n = 4415$) there was a positive (albeit curvilinear) relationship found between individual differences in aggressive behavior and the numbers of B and T lymphocytes.[130]

Developmental effects

Other developmental consequences of immune activation in early life were also investigated in the lines of high- and low-aggressive mice.[131] Following Shanks et al.,[35] neonatal male mice were administered saline or 0.05 mg/kg endotoxin. There was a transient endotoxin-induced reduction in the growth rate of the neonates from the high-aggressive line only. At adulthood, social behavior was observed in a dyadic test and their hypothalami and sera were collected 20 minutes later. The frequency of socially reactive behaviors to other mice (i.e. kick, startle) was increased in the endotoxin-treated groups from both lines. For the high-aggressive line only, endotoxin treatment

Table 20.2 IL-1β-induced circulating levels of interleukin-6 (IL-6) are correlated with measures of HPA axis activation and social behavior

Parameter	Low-aggressive line			High-aggressive line		
	IL-1β	IL-6	Cort	IL-1β	IL-6	Cort
Temperature loss						
30 min post-injection	−0.20	−0.27	−0.21	−0.30	−0.20	−0.20
60 min post-injection	−0.13	−0.20	−0.27	−0.50*	−0.44*	−0.56*
120 min post-injection	−0.44*	−0.43+	−0.38	−0.52*	−0.45*	−0.37
Social reactivity	0.17	0.41+	−0.09	−0.24	−0.11	0.09
Behavioral immobility	0.51*	0.39	0.30	0.45*	0.68***	0.52*
Social exploration	−0.15	−0.30	0.08	−0.23	−0.43+	−0.22
IL-6	0.81***	. . .	. . .	0.91***	. . .	. . .
Corticosterone	0.33	0.56**	. . .	0.59**	0.64**	. . .

$+ p < 0.07$, $*p < 0.05$, $**p < 0.01$, $*** p < 0.001$. 'IL-1β' indicates dose condition (vehicle, 0.25 µg/ml, 0.50 µg/ml, 1.0 µg/ml). Corticosterone measured in ng/ml and IL-6 in pg/ml. Social behavior data are frequency scores during a 10-minute dyadic test.

increased behavioral immobility, decreased attack frequency, and decreased levels of hypothalamic CRF. The changes in socially reactive behavior were associated with individual differences in CRF levels in the high-aggressive but not low-aggressive line mice. These findings suggest that variation in the expression of social inhibited behaviors in later life may be partially explained by a differential sensitivity to immune stimuli in early life.

Early social environment

In mammalian species, early development is embedded in the context of maternal care,[132] and this social relationship may contribute to the lasting effects of immune challenges on offspring.[132–134] Two lines of evidence suggest that line-specific maternal responsiveness to endotoxin-treated pups may account for effects later in life. Shanks and colleagues reported anecdotal evidence that changes in mother–pup interactions occur following endotoxin administration to neonatal rats.[35] In addition, Gariepy et al.[135] showed that dams from the high-aggressive line are naturally more active (more licking, handling of pups, more social contacts) in maternal caregiving than are dams from the low-aggressive line.

The possible role of maternal behavior in mediating the effects of immune challenge was tested in this genetic-developmental model[136] (see Table 20.3).[137] Neonatal mice from the selectively bred lines received saline or 0.05 mg/kg LPS and were reared either by a

dam from the same genetic line or by a foster dam from an unselected line of mice. As before, adult social behaviors were assessed in a dyadic test. Mice from the high-aggressive line again showed more developmental sensitivity to immune challenge than did mice from the low-aggressive line. Line differences persisted regardless of the early maternal environment. As adults, endotoxin-treated mice from the high-aggressive line had lower levels of aggressive behavior, a longer latency to attack, and higher rates of socially reactive and inhibited behaviors as compared with saline controls (see Table 20.4).

Implications for an integrated theory of social development

The literature suggests two complementary models regarding selective breeding for social behavior and the developmental consequences of early immune challenge. One model posits that the relationship stems from an intrinsic difference in sensitivity to immune stimuli, which is associated with social behavioral predispositions (i.e. selective breeding for differences in social behavior). The second model assumes that the milieu of early social development may contribute to the effects of immune challenge on offspring. Based on the findings reported by Granger et al,[136] and presented in Table 20.4, we believe that when intrinsic genetic differences in immune responsiveness are pronounced, maternal responsiveness contributes to behavioral outcomes later in life. Alternatively,

Table 20.3 Predictions on developmental integration of early immune exposure: effects on adult social behaviors

Family of origin	Maternal caregiving	Intrinsic sensitivity to immune challenge	Adult social behavioral outcome
High-aggressive Low inhibition	Low caregiving	More sensitive	Lower externalizing Higher internalizing
Low-aggressive High inhibition	High caregiving	Less sensitive	Higher internalizing

Externalizing behaviors in the model include attack frequency and latency. Internalizing behaviors include social inhibition and social reactivity. Reprinted from Hood et al.[137]

Table 20.4 Differential effects of endotoxin exposure by selectively bred line: mean (and standard deviations) for social behaviors

	Low-aggressive line		High-aggressive line	
	Saline ($n = 18$)	Endotoxin ($n = 21$)	Saline ($n = 22$)	Endotoxin ($n = 19$)
Attack frequency	0.00 (00.00)	0.00 (00.00)	48.86 (17.87)	32.68** (22.32)
Attack latency	. . .	. . .	28.41 (28.09)	137.37** (197.46)
Behavioral immobility	21.17 (12.97)	25.81 (16.70)	0.68 (1.78)	4.95** (6.68)
Social reactivity	0.72 (0.89)	2.71* (3.20)	1.54 (2.72)	6.26* (8.32)
Social exploration	71.00 (18.69)	67.05 (18.74)	16.68 (14.11)	26.74 (24.45)

*$p < 0.05$, **$p < 0.01$; t tests (two-tailed) comparing neonatal edotoxin vs saline exposure conditions within selected line. The unit of measurement for attack latency is the number of 5-s observation periods to first attack. All other behaviors are scored as the number of 5-s periods in which the specific behavior was observed. Reprinted from Granger et al.[136]

when intrinsic differences in immunologic reactivity are not as extreme (or within the 'normal range', as depicted in Figure 20.2) the ontogenic process should be more open to the influence of social environmental forces.

A recent study examined the latter possibility. Neonatal mice bred without selection for behavior or differences in immune reactivity were fostered to dams from two lines of mice that show distinct differences in maternal caregiving behavior.[136] Naturalistic obser-

vations of maternal behavior were conducted on postnatal days 2, 4, 5, 6, and 8. On postnatal day 5, the pups were administered saline or 0.05 mg/kg endotoxin. Within minutes of return to the nest, endotoxin-treated pups emitted fewer ultrasonic vocalizations than did the saline-treated controls. At the peak intensity of the endotoxin response (3 hours post-injection), dams engaged in more licking and decreased time off-nest than did those with saline-treated pups. In addition, when intrinsic individual differences in immune reactivity are within the 'normative range', maternal responsiveness to stressed neonates can ameliorate the developmental effects of early illness on social behavior.[137] Taken together, the findings demonstrate two ways that intrinsic differences in immunologic reactivity can interact with the social environment to determine adult outcomes.

CONCLUDING COMMENTS AND FUTURE RESEARCH DIRECTIONS

Contemporary theorists place behavioral adaptation in a pivotal position with respect to the bidirectional nature of environmental and biological influences on individual development. Cognitive and behavioral responsiveness to environmental events is thought to mediate or moderate the impact of environmental events on rapid (physiological) and slower (genetic) acting biological processes.[13] Ultimately, the effects become manifest in behavioral organization or individual variation in responsiveness, or both. These

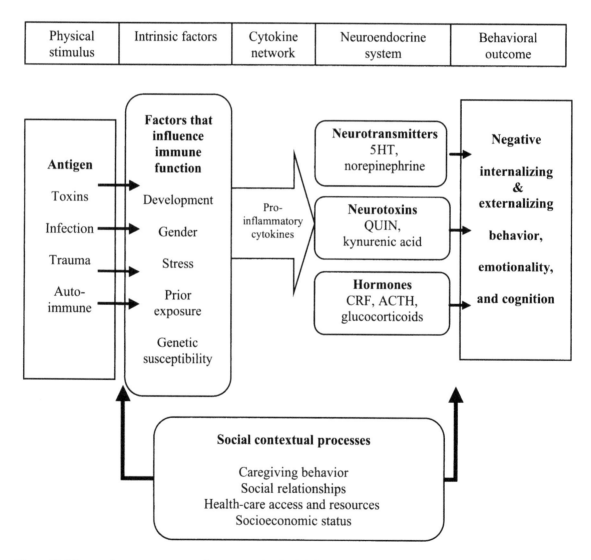

Figure 20.6 Interacting processes contributing to individual differences in the developmental effects of cytokine network activation.

processes enable individuals to continuously adapt to the ever-changing topography of environmental demands and the social landscapes, as well as appropriately match developmental processes to the optimal adult outcomes.

It seems reasonable that cytokines may contribute via their potential to impact on adaptive behavioral and cognitive processes. As reviewed above, there is unequivocal evidence that cytokines alter many behavioral domains and can induce some maladaptive states. Cytokine-induced changes may activate stress systems and augment responsiveness. Still another possibility is that cytokines restrict individual plasticity including social contexts that nurture behavioral and emotional development. For instance, cytokine-induced social and defensive withdrawal or cognitive slowing would limit experiences in ways that hamper learning and benefiting from social interactions.

In the field of child development, the most important etiologic factors determining risk of atypical developmental outcomes have been difficult to resolve. We have proposed a novel perspective that a common set of biobehavioral processes may be involved in biological and behavioral plasticity. This 'common initial pathway' may modify developmental processes impacting a range of adult outcomes.

A theoretical model summarizing the numerous direct and indirect pathways between dysregulation of the cytokine network and developmental psychopathology is presented in Figure 20.6. At least five levels of analysis are relevant to understanding individual differences in the 'uncommon effects' of immune stimuli: 1) features of the physical environment or socioeconomic factors that increase risk or exposure to immune stimuli (e.g. population density, hygiene, water and food quality, heath-care access or quality); 2) psychological factors that influence antigen exposure, susceptibility, and severity of consequences; 3) physiological predispositions or states that affect the synthesis of immune-derived substances or the sensitivity of target tissues; 4) the capacity of the social environment to facilitate recovery once a susceptible individual is exposed; or 5) the competence of individuals in gregarious species to elicit assistance and support from social companions.[136] This biosocial model leads to testable hypotheses at several levels of analysis.

To adequately investigate this model, studies are needed that employ prospective longitudinal designs and focus on the links between the cytokines and the development of onset, maintenance or discontinuation of typical and atypical behavior. Research focused on the uncommon effects of childhood immunizations, early infections or inflammatory diseases in childhood, and in special populations at high risk of pathogen exposure early in life will be especially informative.

ACKNOWLEDGMENTS

The projects were supported in part by the Pennsylvania State University Behavioral Endocrinology Laboratory, the Center for Developmental Science at UNC Chapel Hill, the National Institute of Mental Health (MH 57035–02), and the UCLA Task Force on Psychoneuroimmunology.

REFERENCES

1. Ader R. Psychoneuroimmunology. San Diego: Academic Press, 1981.
2. Ader R. On the development of psychoneuroimmunology. Eur J Pharmacol 2000; 405: 167–76.
3. Ader R, Felten DL, Cohen DJ. Psychoneuroimmunology. San Diego: Academic Press, 1991.
4. Cohen S, Herbert TB. Health psychology: psychological factors and physical disease from the perspective of human psychoneuroimmunology. Annu Rev Psychol 1996; 47: 113–42.
5. Herbert TB, Cohen S. Stress and immunity in humans: a meta-analytic review. Psychosom Med 1993; 55: 364–79.
6. Kemeny ME, Laudenslager ML. Introduction beyond stress: the role of individual difference factors in psychoneuroimmunology. Brain Behav Immun 1999; 13: 73–5.
7. Kiecolt-Glaser JK, Glaser R. Psychoneuroimmunology and health consequences: data and shared mechanisms. Psychosom Med 1995; 57: 269–74.
8. Maier SF, Watkins LR. Bidirectional communication between the brain and the immune system: implications for behavior. Anim Behav 1998; 57: 741–51.
9. Maier SF, Watkins LR. Cytokines for psychologists: implications of bidirectional immune-to-brain communication for understanding behavior, mood, and cognition. Psychol Rev 1998; 105: 83–107.
10. Maier SF, Watkins LR, Fleshner M. Psychoneuroimmunology. The interface between behavior, brain, and immunity. Am Psychol 1994; 49: 1004–17.
11. Blalock JE. The immune system: our sixth sense. The Immunologist 1994; 2: 8–15.
12. Dantzer R. Cytokine-induced sickness behavior: where do we stand? Brain Behav Immun 2001; 15: 7–24.
13. Gottlieb G. Individual Development and Evolution: The Genesis of Novel Behavior. New York: Oxford University Press, 1992.
14. Sameroff AJ. Developmental systems: context and evolution. In: Handbook of Child Psychology, Vol. 1. History, Theory, and Methods, Vol. 1 (Mussen PM, ed.). New York: Wiley, 1983.
15. Ader R, Cohen N, Felten D. Psychoneuroimmunology: interactions between the nervous system and the immune system. Lancet 1995; 345: 99–103.
16. Benveniste EN. Inflammatory cytokines within the central nervous system: sources, function and mechanism of action. Cell Physiol 1992; 32: 1–16.

17. Kopeloff N, Kopeloff LM, Raney ME. The nervous system and antibody production. Psychiatry Quarterly 1993; 7: 84.

18. Solomon GF. Emotions, stress, the central nervous system, and immunity. Ann N Y Acad Sci 1969; 164: 335–43.

19. Solomon GF, Amkraut AA, Kasper P. Immunity, emotions and stress. With special reference to the mechanisms of stress effects on the immune system. Ann Clin Res 1974; 6: 313–22.

20. Felten SY, Felten DL, Bellinger DL, Olschowka JA. Noradrenergic and peptidergic innervation of lymphoid organs. Chem Immunol 1992; 52: 25–48.

21. Carr DJ, Radulescu RT, DeCosta BR, Rice KC, Blalock JE. Opioid modulation of immunoglobulin production by lymphocytes isolated from Peyer's patches and spleen. Ann N Y Acad Sci 1992; 650: 125–7.

22. Kiecolt-Glaser JK, Glaser R. Psychoneuroimmunology: past, present, and future. Health Psychol 1989; 8: 677–82.

23. Granger GA, Williams TW. Lymphocyte cytotoxicity in vitro: activation and release of a cytotoxic factor. Nature 1968; 218: 1253–4.

24. Hessinger DA, Daynes RA, Granger GA. Binding of human lymphotoxin to target-cell membranes and its relation to cell-mediated cytodestruction. Proc Natl Acad Sci USA 1973; 70: 3082–6.

25. Smith E. Hormonal effects of cytokines. In: Neuroimmunoendocrinology (Blalock JE, ed.). New York: Krager, 1992: 154–69.

26. Besedovsky H, del Rey A, Sorkin E et al. The immune response evokes changes in brain noradrenergic neurons. Science 1983; 221: 564–6.

27. Besedovsky HO, del Rey A. Mechanism of virus-induced stimulation of the hypothalamus-pituitary-adrenal axis. J Steroid Biochem 1989; 34: 235–9.

28. Blalock JE. The syntax of immune-neuroendocrine communication. Immunol Today 1997; 15: 504–11.

29. Black PH. Psychoneuroimmunology: brain and immunity. Scientific American Science and Medicine 1995; 1: 16–25.

30. Cotman CW, Brinton RE, Glaburda A, McEwen BS, Schneider DM. The Neuro-immune-endocrine connection. New York: Raven Press, 1987.

31. Kluger MJ. Fever: Its Biology, Evolution, and Function. Princeton, NJ: Princeton University Press, 1979.

32. Adamson-Macedo EN. Neonatal psychoneuroimmunology: emergence, scope and perspectives. Neuroendocrinol Lett 2000; 21: 175–86.

33. Coe CL. Developmental psychoneuroimmunology revisited. Brain Behav Immun 1996; 10: 185–7.

34. Crnic LS. Behavioral consequences of viral infection. In: Psychoneuroimmunology, 2nd edn. (Ader R, Felten DL, Cohen N, eds). New York: Academic Press, 1991: 749–70.

35. Shanks N, Larocque S, Meaney MJ. Neonatal endotoxin exposure alters the development of the hypothalamic-pituitary-adrenal axis: early illness and later responsivity to stress. J Neurosci 1995; 15 (1 Pt 1): 376–84.

36. Gatanaga T, Hwang CD, Kohr W et al. Purification and characterization of an inhibitor (soluble tumor necrosis factor receptor) for tumor necrosis factor and lymphotoxin obtained from the serum ultrafiltrates of human cancer patients. Proc Natl Acad Sci USA 1990; 87: 8781–4.

37. Gatanaga T, Lentz R, Masunaka I et al. Identification of TNF-LT blocking factor(s) in the serum and ultrafiltrates of human cancer patients. Lymphokine Res 1990; 9: 225–9.

38. Thomson A, Lotze MT. The Cytokine Handbook, 4th edn. San Diego, CA: Academic Press, 2003.

39. Dantzer R, Bluth R-M, Goodall G. Behavioral effects of cytokines: an insight into mechanisms of sickness behavior. Methods Neurosci 1983; 16: 130–50.

40. Dinarello CA. Interleukin 1 as mediator of the acute-phase response. Surv Immunol Res 1984; 3: 29–33.

41. Dinarello CA. Interleukin-1. Rev Infect Dis 1984; 6: 51–95.

42. Weiss JM, Quan N, Sundar SK. Widespread activation and consequences of interleukin-1 in the brain. Ann N Y Acad Sci 1994; 741: 338–57.

43. Sapolsky R, Rivier C, Yamamoto G, Plotsky P, Vale W. Interleukin-1 stimulates the secretion of hypothalamic corticotropin-releasing factor. Science 1987; 238: 522–4.

44. Woolski BMRNJ, Smith E, Meyer WJ, Fuller GM, Blalock JE. Corticotrophin-releasing activity of monokines. Science 1985; 230: 1035–7.

45. Dunn AJ. Interleukin-1 as a stimulator of hormone secretion. Prog Neuroimmunol 1990; 3: 26–34.

46. Berkenbosch F, de Goeij DE, Rey AD, Besedovsky HO. Neuroendocrine, sympathetic and metabolic responses induced by interleukin-1. Neuroendocrinology 1989; 50: 570–6.

47. Berkenbosch F, de Rijk R, Del Rey A, Besedovsky, H. Neuroendocrinology of interleukin-1. Adv Exp Med Biol 1990; 274: 303–14.

48. Chuluyan HE, Saphier D, Rohn WM, Dunn AJ. Noradrenergic innervation of the hypothalamus participates in adrenocortical responses to interleukin-1. Neuroendocrinology 1992; 56: 106–11.

49. Dunn AJ. Endotoxin-induced activation of cerebral catecholamine and serotonin metabolism: comparison with interleukin-1. J Pharmacol Exp Ther 1992; 261: 964–9.

50. Dunn AJ. The role of interleukin-1 and tumor necrosis factor alpha in the neurochemical and neuroendocrine responses to endotoxin. Brain Res Bull 1992; 29: 807–12.

51. Dunn AJ, Wang J. Cytokine effects on CNS biogenic amines. Neuroimmunomodulation 1995; 2: 319–28.

52. Dunn AJ, Wang J, Ando T. Effects of cytokines on cerebral neurotransmission. Comparison with the effects of stress. Adv Exp Med Biol 1999; 461: 117–27.

53. Heyes MP, Quearry BJ, Markey SP. Systemic endotoxin increases L-tryptophan, 5-hydroxyindoleacetic acid, 3-hydroxykynurenine and quinolinic acid content of mouse cerebral cortex. Brain Res 1989; 491: 173–9.

54. Heyes MP, Saito K, Crowley JS et al. Quinolinic acid and kynurenine pathway metabolism in inflammatory and non-inflammatory neurological disease. Brain 1992; 115 (Pt 5): 1249–73.

55. Quan N, Sundar SK, Weiss JM. Induction of interleukin-1 in various brain regions after peripheral and central injections of lipopolysaccharide. J Neuroimmunol 1994; 49: 125–34.

56. Ban EM, Haour FG, Lenstra R. Brain interleukin-1 gene expression induced by peripheral lipopolysaccharide administration. Cytokine 1992; 4: 48–54.

57. Laye S, Parnet P, Goujon E, Dantzer R. Peripheral administration of lipopolysaccharide induces the expression of cytokine transcripts in the brain and pituitary of mice. Brain Res Mol Brain Res 1994; 27: 157–62.

58. Cunningham ET, De Souza EB. Interleukin-1 receptors in the brain and endocrine tissues. Immunol Today 1993; 14: 171–6.

59. Takao T, Tracy DE, Mitchell WM, De Souza EB. Interleukin-1 receptors in the mouse brain – characterization and neuronal localization. Endocrinology 1990; 127: 3070–8.

60. Bluthe RM, Dantzer R, Kelley KW. Effects of interleukin-1 receptor antagonist on the behavioral effects of lipopolysaccharide in rat. Brain Res 1992; 573: 318–20.

61. Dantzer R, Bluthe RM, Gheusi G et al. Molecular basis of sickness behavior. Ann N Y Acad Sci 1998; 856: 132–8.

62. Dantzer R, Konsman JP, Bluthe RM, Kelley KW. Neural and humoral pathways of communication from the immune system to the brain: parallel or convergent? Auton Neurosci 2000; 85: 60–5.

63. Hart BL. Biological basis of the behavior of sick animals. Neurosci Biobehav Rev 1988; 12: 123–37.

64. Opp MR, Orbal F, Kreuger JM. Interleukin-1 alters rat sleep: temporal and dose-related effects. Am J Physiol 1991; 260: 52–8.

65. Sparado F, Dunn AJ. Intracerebrovascular administration of interleukin-1 to mice alters investigation of stimulus in a novel environment. Brain Behav Immun 1990; 4: 308–22.

66. Avitsur R, Yirmiya R. The immunobiology of sexual behavior: gender differences in the suppression of sexual activity during illness. Pharmacol Biochem Behav 1999; 64: 787–96.

67. Aubert A. Sickness and behaviour in animals: a motivational perspective. Neurosci Biobehav Rev 1999; 23: 1029–36.

68. Gahtan E, Overmier JB. Performance more than working memory disrupted by acute systemic inflammation in rats in appetitive tasks. Physiol Behav 2001; 73: 201–10.

69. Smith AP, Tyrell DA, Al-Nakib W et al. Effects of experimentally induced respiratory virus infection and illness on psychomotor performance. Neuropsychobiology 1987; 18: 144–8.

70. Smith A, Tyrell D, Coyle K, Higgins P. Effects of interferon alpha on performance in man: a preliminary report. Psychopharmacology 1988; 96: 414–16.

71. Smith RW, Tyrell D, Coyle K, Willman JS. Selective effects of minor illnesses on human performance. Br J Psychol 1987; 78: 183–8.

72. Gutterman JU, Fine S, Quesada J et al. Recombinant leukocyte A interferon: pharmacokinetics, single dose tolerance, and biological effects in cancer patients. Ann Intern Med 1982; 96: 549–56.

73. Mannering GJ, Deloria LB. The pharmacology and toxicity of the interferons: an overview. Ann Rev Pharmacol Toxicol 1986; 26: 455–515.

74. Renault PF, Hoofnagle JH, Parky Y et al. Psychiatric complications of long-term interferon-alpha therapy. Arch Intern Med 1987; 147: 1577–80.

75. Capuron L, Bluthe RM, Dantzer R. Cytokines in clinical psychiatry. Am J Psychiatry 2001; 158: 1163–4.

76. Capuron L, Ravaud A, Dantzer R. Early depressive symptoms in cancer patients receiving interleukin 2 and/or interferon alfa-2b therapy. J Clin Oncol 2000; 18: 2143–51.

77. Capuron L, Ravaud A, Dantzer R. Timing and specificity of the cognitive changes induced by interleukin-2 and interferon-alpha treatments in cancer patients. Psychosom Med 2001; 63: 376–86.

78. Capuron L, Ravaud A, Gualde N et al. Association between immune activation and early depressive symptoms in cancer patients treated with interleukin-2-based therapy. Psychoneuroendocrinology 2001; 26: 797–808.

79. Scheibel RS, Valentine AD, O'Brien S, Meyers CA. Cognitive dysfunction and depression during treatment with interferon-alpha and chemotherapy. J Neuropsychiatry Clin Neurosci 2004; 16: 185–91.

80. Kelly RH, Ganguli R, Rabin BS. Antibody to discrete areas of the brain in normal individuals and patients with schizophrenia. Biol Psychiatry 1987; 22: 1488–91.

81. Kronfol Z. Immune dysregulation in major depression: a critical review of existing evidence. Int J Neuropsychopharacol 2002; 5: 333–43.

82. Kronfol Z, Remick DG. Cytokines and the brain: implications for clinical psychiatry. Am J Psychiatry 2000; 157: 683–94.

83. Connor TJ, Leonard BE. Depression, stress and immunological activation: the role of cytokines in depressive disorders. Life Sci 1998 62: 583–606.

84. Dantzer R, Wollman E, Vitkovic L, Yirmiya R. Cytokines and depression: fortuitous or causative association? Mol Psychiatry 1999; 4: 328–32.

85. Kronfol Z. Depression and immunity: the role of cytokines. In: Cytokines: Stress and Immunity (Plotnikoff NP, Faith RE, Murgo AJ, Good RA, eds). New York: CRC Press, 1999: 51–60.

86. Anderson JA, Lentsch AB, Hadjiminas DJ, et al. The role of cytokines, adhesion molecules, and chemokines in interleukin-2-induced lymphocytic infiltration in C57BL/6 mice. J Clin Invest 1996; 97: 1952–9.

87. Herbert, TB, Cohen S. Depression and immunity: a meta-analytic review. Psychol Bull 1993; 113: 472–86.

88. Maes M, Bosmans E, Meltzer HY, Scharpe S, Suy E. Interleukin-1 beta: a putative mediator of HPA axis hyperactvity in major depression? Am J Psychiatry 1993; 150: 1189–93.

89. Maes M, Meltzer HY, Bosmans E. et al. Increased plasma concentrations of interleukin-6, soluble interleukin-6, soluble interleukin-2 and transferrin receptor in major depression. J Affect Disord 1995; 34: 301–9.

90. Owen BM, Eccleston D, Ferrier IN, Young AH. Raised levels of plasma interleukin-1beta in major and postviral depression. Acta Psychiatr Scand 2001; 103: 226–8.

91. Musselman DL, Miller AH, Porter MR et al. Higher than normal plasma interleukin-6 concentrations in cancer patients with depression: preliminary findings. Am J Psychiatry 2001; 158: 1252–7.

92. Berk M, Wadee AA, Kuschke RH, O'Neill-Kerr A. Acute phase proteins in major depression. J Psychosom Res 1997; 43: 529–34.

93. Haack M, Hinze-Selch D, Fenzel T et al. Plasma levels of cytokines and soluble cytokine receptors in psychiatric patients upon hospital admission: effects of confounding factors and diagnosis. J Psychiatr Res 1999; 33: 407–18.

94. Birmaher B, Rabin BS, Garcia MR et al. Cellular immunity in depressed, conduct disorder, and normal adolescents: role of adverse life events. J Am Acad Child Adolesc Psychiatry 1994; 33: 671–8.

95. Granger DA, Ikeda S, Block MB. Developmental, psychoneuroimmunology: integrating effects of environmental, biological, and behavioral processes on child development. Presented at the Annual Meeting of the Society for Research in Child Development, Washington, DC, 1997.

96. Brambilla F, Monteleone P, Maj M. Interleukin-1beta and tumor necrosis factor-alpha in children with major depressive disorder or dysthymia. J Affect Disord 2004; 78: 273–7.

97. Garvey M, Giedd J, Swedo SE. PANDAS: the search for environmental triggers of pediatric neuropsychiatric disorders. Lessons from rheumatic fever. J Child Neurol 1998; 13: 413–23.

98. Leonard HL, Swedo SE, Garvey M et al. Postinfectious and other forms of obsessive-compulsive disorder. Child Adolesc Psychiatr Clin North Am 1999; 8: 497–511.

99. Swedo SE, Leonard HL, Garvey M et al. Pediatric autoimmune neuropsychiatric disorders associated with streptococcal infections: clinical description of the first 50 cases. Am J Psychiatry 1998; 155: 264–71.

100. Maes M, Meltzer HY, Bosmans E. Psychoimmune investigation in obsessive-complusive disorder: assays of plasma transferrin, IL-2 and IL-6 receptor, and IL-1β and IL-6 concentrations. Neuropsychobiology 1994; 30: 57.

101. Mittleman BB, Castellanos FS, Jacobsen LK et al. Cerebrospinal fluid cytokines in pediatric neuropsychiatric disease. J Immunol 1997; 159: 2994–9.

102. Brambilla F, Bellodi L, Perna G, et al. Psychoimmunoendocrine aspects of panic disorder. Neuropsychobiology 1992; 26: 12–22.

103. Brambilla F, Bellodi L, Perna G et al. Plasma interleukin-1 beta concentrations in panic disorder. Psychiatry Res 1994; 54: 135–42.

104. Rapaport MH, Stein MB. Serum cytokine and soluble interleukin-2 receptors in patients with panic disorder. Anxiety 1994; 1: 22–5.

105. Weizman R, Laor N, Wiener Z, Wolmer L, Bessler H. Cytokine production in panic disorder patients. Clin Neuropharmacol 1999; 22: 107–9.

106. Spivak B, Shohat B, Mester R et al. Elevated levels of serum interleukin-1 beta in combat-related posttraumatic stress disorder. Biol Psychiatry 1997; 42: 345–8.

107. Watson JB, Mednick SA, Huttunen M, Wang X. Prenatal teratogens and the development of adult mental illness. Dev Psychopathol 1999; 11: 457–66.

108. Kiecolt-Glaser JK, Glaser R. Methodological issues in behavioral immunology research with humans. Brain Behav Immun 1988; 2: 67–78.

109. Tilders FJH, DeRuk RH, VanDam A-M et al. Activation of the hypothalamus-pituitary-adrenal axis by bacterial endotoxins: routes and intermediate signals. Psychoneuroendocrinology 1994; 19: 209–32.

110. Dunn AJ. Psychoneuroimmunology, stress and infection. In: Psychoneuroimmunology, Stress and Infection (Friedman H, Klein TW, Friedman A eds). New York: CRC Press, 1996: 25–46.

111. Reichenberg A, Yirmiya R, Schuld A et al. Cytokine-associated emotional and cognitive disturbances in humans. Arch Gen Psychiatry 2001; 58; 445–52.

112. Bonneau RH, Sheridan JF, Feng N, Glaser R. Stress-induced modulation of the primary cellular immune response to herpes simplex virus infection is mediated by both adrenal-dependent and independent mechanisms. J Neuroimmunol 1993; 42: 167–76.

113. Kiecolt-Glaser JK, Glaser R, Gravenstein S, Malarkey WB, Sheridan J. Chronic stress alters the immune response to influenza virus vaccine in older adults. Proc Natl Acad Sci USA 1996; 93: 3043–7.

114. Morag M, Yirmiya R, Lerer B, Morag A. Influence of socioeconomic status on behavioral, emotional and cognitive effects of rubella vaccination: a prospective, double blind study. Psychoneuroendocrinology 1998; 23: 337–51.

115. Cody CL, Baraff LJ, Cherry JD, Marcy SM, Manclark CR. Nature and rates of adverse reactions associated with DTP and DT immunizations in infants and children. Pediatrics 1981; 68: 650–9.

116. Howson CP, Howe CJ, Fineberg HV. Adverse effects of pertussis and rubella vaccines: A report of the committee to review the adverse consequences of pertussis and rubella vaccines. Unpublished manuscript. Washington, DC: National Academy Press, 1991.

117. O'Grady MP, Hall NRS. Postnatal exposure to Newcastles disease virus alters endocrine development. Teratology 1990; 41: 623–4.

118. O'Grady MP, Hall NRS. Long-term effects of neuroendocrine-immune interactions during early development. In: Psychoneuroimmunology (Ader R, Felten DL, Cohen N, eds). 2nd edn. New York: Academic Press, 1991: 561–72.

119. O'Grady MP, Hall NRS, Goldstein AL. Developmental consequences of prenatal exposure to thymosin: long term changes in immune and endocrine parameters. Soc Neurosci 1987; 13: 1380.

120. Segall MA, Crnic LS. An animal model for the behavioral effects of interferon. Behav Neurosci 1990; 104: 612–8.

121. Crnic LS, Pizer LI. Behavioral effects of neonatal herpes simplex type 1 infection of mice. Neurotoxicol Teratol 1988; 10: 381–6.

122. Cairns BD, Hood K, Midlam J. On fighting mice: Is there a sensitive period for isolation effects? Anim Behav 1985; 33: 166–80.

123. Cairns RB, Gariepy JL, Hood KE. Development, microevolution, and social behavior. Psychol Rev 1990; 97: 49–65.

124. Pettito JM, Lysle DT, Gariepy J, Lewis M. The expression of genetic differences in social behavior in ICR mice correlates with differences in cellular immune responsiveness. Clin Neuropharmacol 1992; 15: 658–9.

125. Pettito JM, Lysle DT, Gariepy J, Lewis M. Association of genetic differences in social behavior and cellular immune responsiveness. Brain Behav Immun 1994; 8: 111–2.

126. Granger DA, Hood K, Ikeda S et al. Effects of peripheral immune activation on social behavior and adrenocortical activity in aggressive mice. Aggressive Behavior 1997; 23: 93–105.

127. Pettito JM, Gariepy J, Gendreau PL et al. Differences in NK cell function in mice bred for high and low aggression: genetic linkage between complex behavior and immunological traits? Brain Behav Immun 1999; 13: 175–86.

128. Cohen S, Line S, Manuck SB et al. Chronic stress, social status, and susceptibility to upper respiratory infections in nonhuman primates. Psychosom Med 1997; 59: 213–21.

129. Line S, Kaplan JR, Heise E et al. Effects of social reorganization on cellular immunity in male cynomolgus monkeys. Am J Primatol 1996; 39: 235–49.

130. Granger DA, Booth A, Johnson D. Human aggression and enumerative measures of immunity. Psychosom Med 2000; 62: 583–90.

131. Granger DA, Hood KE, Ikeda SC, Reed CL, Block ML. Neonatal endotoxin exposure alters the development of social behavior and the hypothalamic-pituitary-adrenal axis in selectively bred mice. Brain Behav Immun 1996; 10: 249–59.

132. Hofer MA. Early relationships as regulators of infant physiology and behavior. Acta Paediatr Suppl 1994; 397: 9–18.

133. Liu D, Dioria J, Tannenbaum B et al. Maternal care, hippocampal, glucocorticoid receptors, and hypothalamic-pituitary-adrenal responses to stress. Science 1997; 277: 1659–62.

134. Meaney MJ, Aitken DH, Bhatnagar S, Van Berkel C, Sapolsky RM. Postnatal handling attenuates neuroendocrine, anatomical, and cognitive impairments related to the aged hippocampus. Science 1988; 238: 766–8.

135. Gariepy J-L, Nehrenberg D, Mills-Koonce R. Maternal care and separation stress in high- and low-aggressive mice. Presented at the Annual Meeting of the International Society for Developmental Psychobiology, New Orleans, LA, 2000.

136. Granger DA, Hood KE, Dreschel NA, Sergeant E, Likos A. Developmental effects of early immune stress on aggressive, socially reactive, and inhibited behaviors. Dev Psychopathol 2001; 13: 599–610.

137. Hood K, Dreschel N, Granger DA. Maternal behavior changes after immune challenge of neonates with developmental effects on adult social behavior. Dev Psychobiol 2003; 42: 17–34.

Section VI – Future directions: pre- and postnatal modulation of the genetic program

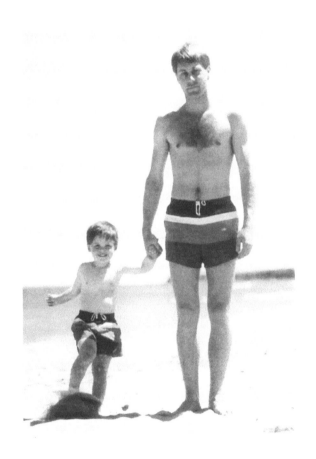

'When one tugs at a single thing in nature, he finds it attached to the rest of the world' John Muir

21

Genomic imprinting and epigenetic programming of fetal development

Marie Dziadek

INTRODUCTION

The growth and development of a human fetus *in utero*, and the acquisition of physiological and behavioral functions after birth and into adult life, depend on the processing of information that is encoded in the genetic material in the nucleus of every cell. Each individual has a precise DNA sequence that is determined at fertilization and then replicated through successive cell divisions. This DNA sequence is unique to that individual if they do not have a monozygotic twin. We know from many examples that single base mutations and chromosomal aberrations (e.g. trisomies, unbalanced translocations, deletions) that are either inherited or acquired in cells during the life of the individual can have a range of effects, from very subtle to quite profound, on the functioning of cells and tissues at different stages of human development. A major effort in human genetics has been to associate early and late onset disease with genetic defects, and this has been extremely successful in identifying the genetic basis of a large number of human diseases.

However, we now know that there is another layer of heritable information for gene regulation, which is epigenetic rather than genetic in basis. Epigenetics is defined as the covalent modifications of DNA and associated proteins (histones) that regulate gene activity without altering the DNA sequence itself. Many genes are silenced by epigenetic modifications that include DNA methylation, histone modification, and association of noncoding RNA. Together, these control mechanisms are involved in both initiating and sustaining epigenetic silencing of specific genes. Epigenetic modifications are inherited through cell division, but unlike DNA mutations, are not irreversible alterations, and can be added or removed by developmental signals as well as environmental factors throughout life. Epigenetic mechanisms of gene regulation result in different subsets of genes being expressed in the different types of cells of the developing embryo, such as in blood cells, neurons, and hepatocytes. Such modifications provide a complex regulatory framework by which environmental signals can generate heritable, but yet reversible, changes in the activity of genes. Epigenetics thus sits at the molecular nexus of gene–environment interactions, and has excited scientists because it can explain phenotypic differences between monozygotic twins,[1] age-related diseases such as cancer,[2–4] and parent-of-origin genetic influences through genomic imprinting.[5,6] It is also very likely to explain some fundamental aspects of perinatal programming. Epigenetic processes provide a mechanism for preserving information on environmental exposure, and may one day be used as diagnostic markers of that exposure. This field of research is still in its infancy, but will make as much impact over the next decades as genetics has on our understanding of phenotypic variation in humans and on direct causes or predispositions to human disease.

This chapter will outline what is currently understood regarding the molecular basis of epigenetic gene regulation and factors that influence it, focusing particularly on epigenetic programming in fetal development. While much of the molecular information comes from mouse studies, the high degree of conservation between mice and humans in the identity of genes that are regulated by epigenetic modifications and the precise biochemical nature of these modifications mean that similar, if not identical, mechanisms will undoubtedly apply to human development. Finally, the still scant, but nevertheless intriguing data will be presented to suggest that epigenetic programming could underlie the perinatal origins of some adult disease.

THE MOLECULAR NATURE OF EPIGENETIC MODIFICATIONS

DNA methylation

The methylation of cytosine (C) residues is the major epigenetic modification of DNA in eukaryotes, involving the addition of a methyl (CH_3) group to the 5-carbon position in the pyrimidine ring (Figure 21.1A).[7] This covalent chemical modification occurs predominantly at CpG dinucleotides, where a methylated cytosine has a guanine (G) as its 3′ neighbor (Figure 21.1B). The CpG dinucleotide pairs with a CpG in the complementary strand of the double-stranded DNA molecule (C pairs with G, A pairs with T), and the C in this CpG dinucleotide is also methylated, such that both DNA strands are methylated at the symmetric CpG site (Figure 21.1B). It has been estimated that 70% of CpG dinucleotides within the mammalian genome are methylated, and these account for the

4–8% of cytosines in the entire genome being methylated.[7] However, stretches of CpG-rich sequences of at least 500 base pairs (called CpG islands) are found in the regulatory promoters of functional genes, and these are mostly unmethylated.[7] Changes in the level of DNA methylation at specific sites are associated with the level of gene expression, with high levels of methylation (hypermethylation) usually associated with gene silencing and low levels of methylation (hypomethylation) being associated with active gene expression. The density of methylation within a given region contributes to the degree of promoter repression, such that the methylation of several CpG dinucleotides is required rather than a single CpG site.[8] DNA methylation is involved in allele-specific gene expression (genomic imprinting), X chromosome inactivation, and transcriptional silencing of transposable viral elements.[6,9] The latter function is thought to be an initial defense mechanism to inactivate viruses and prevent movement of transposable elements

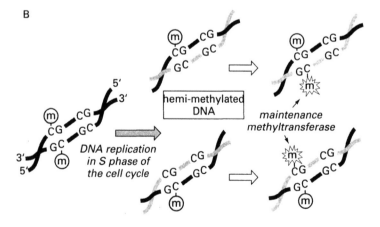

Figure 21.1 DNA methylation is the modification of cytosine residues by enzymatic addition of a methyl group. (A) The chemical structure of cytosine and methyl-cytosine nucleotides. Cytosine is methylated by enzymatic (methyltransferase) addition of a methyl (-CH3) group at the 5-carbon position of the pyrimidine ring. This methyl group can be actively removed by a process of demethylation. (B) The pattern of CpG dinucleotide (5′–3′) methylation (C-m) is maintained after DNA replication. The newly synthesized DNA strand (light gray) is not methylated, so the paired parental (black) and new strands are hemi-methylated. The maintenance methyltransferase has a specificity for hemi-methylated CpG pairs and methylates CpGs (star) that are paired with a methylated CpG on the parental strand. Nonmethylated CpGs on the parental strands are not recognized by the enzyme, and the CpG pair on the new strand remains unmethylated. Thus the pattern of methylated and nonmethylated CpG dinucleotides is replicated at each cell division.

throughout the genome.[9] The mechanisms underlying this modulation of transcription are outlined in a later section.

DNA methylation occurs by an enzymatic addition of a methyl group to cytosine residues by DNA methyltransferases (DNMTs). DNMTs are classified into two types: de novo methyltransferases which use nonmethylated DNA as a substrate; and maintenance methyltransferases which replicate previously methylated sites and use hemi-methylated DNA as a substrate.[10] The de novo methyltransferases, such as DNMT3A and DNMT3B, are important in establishing new patterns of DNA methylation, having a major role in embryonic development in determining which genes will be silenced. How de novo DNMTs recognize sites for methylation is not known, but which sites do become methylated does not appear to be random. Studies of methylation patterns in cancer have demonstrated that some genes/regions are frequently methylated while others remain unmethylated.[2] Evidence suggests that repetitive DNA sequences are targeted for methylation, and structural features of chromatin at these sites may provide some level of recognition by DNMTs. DNMTs are likely to work in cooperation with other factors in establishing methylation patterns, including histones and noncoding RNAs.[10]

Once a particular CpG site has been methylated de novo, after DNA replication it is used as the hemi-methylated substrate for maintenance methyltransferases such as DNMT1, which is the major maintenance methyltransferase in mammals (Figure 21.1B). DNMT1 ensures that the methylation patterns are accurately perpetuated through consecutive cell divisions, and thus has a key role in maintaining the 'memory' of an epigenetic modification from the time of its establishment.[7] There is evidence that levels of DNMT1 diminish with aging, and account in part for the lower levels of genomic methylation seen in older individuals.[11] However, it is also clear that this is offset by increased activity of DNMT3A and DNMT3B,[12] which cause increased gene-specific methylation, and can cause inactivation of tumor suppressor genes.[3] There is substantial evidence now for an epigenetic basis of cancer, through age or environmental-related changes in DNA methylation.[2–4] This heritable change in the 'epigenetic programme' thus establishes a new pattern of gene expression which can directly cause a change in cell function or behavior and lead to disease. There is increasing interest in investigating whether there is an epigenetic basis to neurological disease, including mental disorders.[13]

It is obvious that levels of DNMTs need to be sustained in order to maintain an epigenetic program within any given tissue. Total elimination of any of these enzymes (e.g. by gene knockout technology in mice) causes embryo lethality, indicating an absolute requirement for DNA methylation events in embryonic development.[14] Reduced levels of enzyme activity will progressively reduce the degree of methylation by a passive process. However, cytosine methylation can also be reversed by an active process of demethylation (Figure 21.1A), which is the mechanism for erasure of epigenetic modifications in primordial germ cells and the early embryo. As will be discussed later, this erasure is crucial for the removal of DNA methylation at the start of embryonic development, so that tissue-specific patterns of methylation can be established to direct the developmental programme in each embryo. However, while it is clear that a process of 'active' demethylation does take place, it is interesting that no specific DNA demethylases have yet been isolated.

Regulation of DNA methylation

The process of DNA methylation requires sufficient methyl groups to be available for addition to cytosine residues by methyltransferases. These methyl groups are donated by the ubiquitous methyl donor S-adenosyl-methionine (SAM), and the availability of SAM is a key limiting factor in the regulation of methylation in a variety of biochemical reactions (Figure 21.2).[15] SAM is derived from methionine, which is obtained either directly from the diet, or by metabolic conversion of homocysteine to methionine by methionine synthase (Figure 21.2). Additional essential sources of methyl donors in the diet are folate and choline, which through separate pathways contribute methyl groups for methionine production from homocysteine.[15] Methylenetetrahydrofolate (methyl-THF) produced via one-carbon metabolism, and betaine produced from choline provide these sources of methyl groups for methylation of homocysteine (Figure 21.2).[16] Methionine is then converted to SAM by the enzyme methionine adenosyl transferase. Dietary methyl donors thus contribute significantly to the process of DNA methylation by providing the substrates for de novo synthesis of methyl groups through one-carbon metabolism (folate) and by transmethylation pathways whereby methyl groups are exchanged between molecules (betaine) to ultimately generate SAM as the principal methyl donor for DNA methylation. A large number of genetic and nutritional studies have demonstrated that the metabolic pathways involved in methionine and SAM production are essential to maintain DNA methylation. Animal studies have tested the effects of deficiencies in individual methyl donors or a combination of all three, and have demonstrated reduced levels of global DNA methylation and

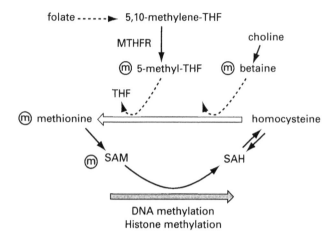

Figure 21.2 Pathways that provide methyl donors for DNA and histone methylation. S-Adenosyl methionine (SAM) is the key methyl donor for many methylation reactions in the cell. Its methyl group is donated by methionine, derived by addition of a methyl group to homocysteine. Choline is a major dietary methyl donor that provides a methyl group via betaine. Dietary folate contributes methyl groups via one-carbon metabolism, requiring methylenetetrahydrofolate reductase (MTHFR) to produce 5-methyl-tetrahydrofolate (5-methyl-THF), which contributes a methyl group to homocysteine and forms THF. Methionine is also provided directly from the diet.

hypomethylation of specific genes in as little as 1–2 weeks of severe deficiency.[17] Deficiencies in choline and methionine, and/or folate, result in reduction of hepatic SAM concentrations and significantly increased levels of plasma homocysteine, indicative of major disruptions to the metabolic pathways that produce SAM.[15] The interrelationship between folate, choline, and methionine metabolism means that a deficiency in a single dietary component may have no overall effect on DNA methylation, and that levels of homocysteine and SAM are more reliable indicators of methyl group insufficiency than the levels of each independent methyl donor. Of significance in terms of disease development associated with methyl deficiency is that DNA hypomethylation can be reversed rapidly when animals are given a methyl-supplemented diet.[17]

The necessity of the dietary supply of methyl group donors provides a clear link between nutrient supply and epigenetic modification. The implications of this association for perinatal programming will be discussed towards the end of this chapter. But the added complexity of genetic variation in such gene–environment interactions also needs to be highlighted in this context. An excellent example of this variability is the role of polymorphisms in genes involved in methyl metabolism. The MTHFR gene is one such example. It codes for methylene tetrahydrofolate reductase, a key enzyme in folate metabolism, where it irreversibly converts 5,10-methylenetetrahydrofolate to methyl-THF (Figure 21.2).[16] A variant of this gene has been identified which produces a less stable (thermolabile) protein that has reduced enzyme activity. The thermolabile variant is due to a missense mutation at base pair 677 (C677T) where the

cytosine-to-thymine base change results in an alanine-to-valine substitution in the MTHFR amino acid sequence that causes a structural change in the enzyme.[16] The prevalence of this variant in the population is quite high, with 20% of individuals being homozygous for the thermolabile TT variant. Homozygous individuals were found to have elevated levels of plasma homocysteine, indicative of altered one-carbon metabolism and reduced conversion of homocysteine to methionine (see Figure 21.2). However, this elevated homocysteine is most significant in individuals with lower blood folate levels.[18] Studies have shown a clear correlation between the TT variant and reduced DNA methylation only in individuals with low blood folate levels. This nutritional–genetic interaction appears to influence the susceptibility of individuals to development of colon cancer and cardiovascular disease.[19,20] Identification of additional genetic variants and their combined effects on epigenetic modification and disease under different dietary influences is a key area of research into the genetic/environmental interface in perinatal programming.

Transcriptional silencing through DNA methylation

The major importance of DNA methylation is its role in the transcriptional silencing of genes, providing a mechanism by which a given gene can be silenced in one cell type and expressed in a different cell type.[7,10] The effect of DNA methylation on gene transcription is mediated in a number of different ways. Firstly, the protruding methyl groups can affect DNA–protein interactions. Protein factors have been characterized that recognize and bind to specific DNA sequences containing either methylated or unmethylated CpGs. For example, the methylation-sensitive CTCF regulator protein will only bind to specific DNA sequences if they are not methylated.[21] Specific transcriptional regulators are influenced by methylated CpGs within the gene promoter region, and this has a direct effect on transcription (Figure 21.3B). Thus, some transcription factors, such as CREB, E2F, and c-myc, are methyl-sensitive and will not bind to methylated CpGs, while many others are methyl-insensitive and will bind and activate transcription irrespective of the methylation status.[7] Binding of methyl-binding proteins to methylated DNA in a sequence-independent manner can also interfere with association of the transcriptional complex to the promoter and directly inhibit transcription (Figure 21.3C). Four such methyl-binding proteins have been identified: MeCP2, MBD1, MBD2, and MBD3.[10] Changes in DNA methylation are commonly linked to changes in chromatin structure that are influenced by proteins associated with DNA. A highly condensed chromatin structure, called heterochromatin, is not accessible for binding of RNA polymerase and transcriptional regulators, leading to transcriptional silencing (Figure 21.3D). Histones are the most abundant proteins found to complex with DNA to form chromatin and these proteins play a major role in

organizing the packing structure of DNA. The way in which a length of DNA is packaged influences the transcriptional activity of the genes that are included in that region. Five different histone proteins have been identified – H1, H2A, H2B, H3, and H4. Octameric histone complexes comprising two molecules of each of H2A, H2B, H3, and H4 constitute the central core of the nucleosomes that are the building blocks of the chromatin structure, while H1 binds to the outside of the nucleosome (Figure 21.4).[22] The amino-terminal tails of the histone proteins contain several positively charged lysine residues which bind to phosphate groups in DNA. Histones can be chemically modified (reversibly) after the protein has been synthesized, by post-translational acetylation, methylation, and phosphorylation at specific amino acid residues within the amino-terminal tail of the protein that influences binding to DNA.[23] Acetylation of lysines removes the positive charge and reduces their interaction with DNA. A highly condensed chromatin structure that is not accessible for binding of transcriptional regulators is characterized by both a high density of DNA methylation and the association of histones that are deacetylated.[23] Acetylated core histones are generally associated with transcriptionally active gene loci found in regions of chromatin which have an extended conformation. Methylated histones, on the other hand, are associated with either transcriptionally

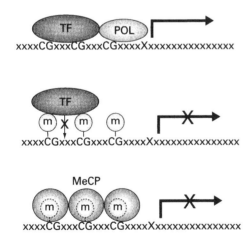

Figure 21.3 Influence of CpG methylation on gene transcription. (A) Transcription factors (TF) bind directly to recognition sequences in the regulatory region of genes and facilitate the formation of transcriptional complexes between RNA polymerase (POL) and other factors that activate transcription (arrow). (B) Methylated CpGs at these recognition sites can directly interfere with the binding of methyl-sensitive TFs and prevent transcription (crossed arrow). (C) Methyl-binding proteins (MeCP) bind to any CpG sites and block the binding of transcriptional regulators, thus preventing transcription. (D) Methyl-binding proteins can attract histone deacetylases which modify histones and induce condensation of DNA that becomes inaccessible to transcription.

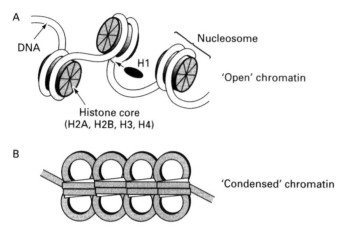

Figure 21.4 The conformation of chromatin is dependent on histones. (A) Acetylated histones H2A, H2B, H3, and H4 form an octameric histone complex around which the DNA is wound twice to form a nucleosome. Nucleosomes are linked by a stretch of linker DNA, and this beaded structure represents an 'open' chromatin structure that is accessible to transcriptional regulators. (B) Deacetylated histones together with attachment of histone H1 to the outer surface of the nucleosome mediate close interactions between neighboring nucleosomes and cause 'condensation' of the chromatin into a tightly packed structure that is inaccessible to transcriptional regulators.

active or inactive chromatin, depending to some degree on which particular lysines are methylated (lysine 4 or lysine 9 in H3).[23–25] Because of the role of modified histones in determining the conformation and transcriptional activity of chromatin, histone modifications are considered to be significant epigenetic modifiers in addition to DNA methylation. The variation in acetylation and methylation of histones, in addition to other modification such as phosphorylation, provides a large number of possible functional isoforms that constitute what has been called a 'histone code'.[25] It is becoming increasingly clear that there are mechanistic links between DNA methylation, histone modification, and chromatin structure. DNA methylation can recruit histone deacetylases, and DNA methyltransferases can be attracted to chromatin regions by complexes of histone deacetylases, histone methyltransferases, and methyl-binding proteins, to initiate new patterns of epigenetic modification.[21–26] This interplay between the regulators of DNA and histone modification provides for a highly variable and reversible framework of epigenetic modification, which is utilized to regulate gene expression during development, and in response to environmental stimuli.

Additional regulators of gene expression that are now also classified as 'epigenetic regulators' are noncoding RNA molecules which are not translated into proteins.[27] Some noncoding RNAs have sequences that are anti-sense to an RNA that does code for a protein, and by binding specifically to this RNA they can interfere directly with its translation into protein.[27] Other noncoding RNAs are able to bind to and 'coat' regions of DNA by mechanisms that are not yet understood, and function to repress gene expression. An example of such a noncoding RNA is the Xist gene product, which is transcribed from the X chromosome which will be inactivated, and binds along the length of the same chromosome to result in X chromosome inactivation.[28] Yet other noncoding RNAs have roles in RNA processing, and in regulation of protein translation.[27,28] Noncoding RNAs are now known to be abundant transcripts, and much of what has for a long time been considered as 'junk' DNA in the genome through which protein-coding genes are dispersed, is now known to be transcribed into noncoding RNAs.[29] While it is not yet clear exactly how all of these RNAs function, and what their significance will turn out to be, it has been proposed that their increased abundance during evolution contributes to the developmental programming of complex organisms.[29]

We thus have an epigenetic 'toolbox', containing the necessary components and the tools that work on DNA methylation, those that work on histone modification, and those that interlink both of these processes and influence chromatin structure. The ultimate outcome of such epigenetic modifications is the control of the pattern of gene expression in different cells, which is crucial for cell differentiation in different tissues and for normal embryonic growth and development. It is now well established that specific patterns of epigenetic modification are established and maintained during gametogenesis, preimplantation embryo development, and fetal and placental growth and development. This is most evident from genomic imprinting, a very specific form of epigenetic regulation that influences allele-specific gene silencing in a parent-of-origin manner. But while the tools that are used to modify DNA and histones are now quite well understood at the molecular level, it is not at all well understood how specific sites in the genome are selected for epigenetic modification in the first instance. The application of sensitive new techniques to study sequence-specific methylation in the analysis of genomic imprinting in humans and in animal models has shed some light on when and how various components of the epigenetic 'toolbox' are used to generate the 'epigenetic program' of an individual at birth.

GENOMIC IMPRINTING

Genomic imprinting refers to the parent-specific epigenetic regulation of genes that determines which parental allele, maternal or paternal, will be silenced and which will be expressed.[30] Not many genes in the genome appear to be regulated by genomic imprinting, with only about 80 genes so far identified that are expressed in a strict parental allele-specific pattern.[30,31] Silencing of one parental copy of the gene means that imprinted genes are monoallelically expressed, compared with the supposed biallelic expression of all other genes in the genome, so that genomic imprinting is in fact a mechanism of gene dosage regulation. This monoallelic expression is crucial for the normal developmental program, since abnormal development and embryo lethality are seen in cases of parthenogenesis and androgenesis when the entire diploid genome is derived from one parent (uniparental).[32] Parthenogenetic embryos (diploid maternal genome) develop very poorly, with limited trophoblast growth, and are the cause of human ovarian teratomas.[32] Androgenetic embryos (diploid paternal genome), on the other hand, have excessive trophoblast proliferation and differentiation, and are the origin of hydatidiform moles (trophoblastic disease) in humans.[32] Growth, developmental, and behavioral disorders are seen when both copies of individual chromosomes or parts of chromosomes that harbor imprinted genes are derived from only one parent caused by either the deletion of one parental copy or uniparental disomy (UPD) resulting from mis-segregation of chromosomes during meiosis or post-fertilization mitosis. For example, Beckwith-Wiedemann syndrome (BWS) is caused by paternal UPD or maternal deletion at chromosome 11p15.5.[5,32] BWS is characterized by fetal and placental overgrowth, multi-organ overgrowth including macroglossia, examphalos, and a predisposition to childhood tumors such as Wilm's tumor.[5,32] Two other syndromes are linked on chromosome 15q11–13 and exhibit neurological defects as well as growth disorders. Angelman syndrome (AS) is caused by paternal UPD or maternal deletion at 15q11–13, while Prader-Willi syndrome (PWS) is caused by maternal UPD or paternal deletion at 15q11–13.[5,32] Despite being associated with the same chromosome region these syndromes are very different phenotypically. Children with PWS were growth-retarded *in utero* and retain a short stature. They have hypotonia and feeding problems, but later become obese due to hyperphagia, and also have mild mental retardation with some behavioral problems.[5,32] Children with AS, on the other hand, have more severe mental retardation, have abnormal laughter but do not speak, are hyperactive, exhibit ataxia, and frequently have seizures. The different phenotypic effects seen in uniparental conceptuses or embryos having UPD of imprinted chromosomes such as 11p15.5 and 15q11–13 are due to the lack of expression of genes that are normally expressed on the parental chromosome which is missing. There are a number of different genetic and epigenetic mechanisms that cause aberrant patterns of imprinting, that result in similar phenotypic consequences for the individual.[32] In addition, loss of imprinting (LOI) can occur in somatic cells, and can contribute to cancer growth when it results in aberrant biallelic expression of genes that regulate cell proliferation.[33]

Which genes are imprinted?

The majority of imprinted genes are grouped in clusters on only a few chromosomes (e.g. chromosomes 11p15.5, 15q11–13) (Table 21.1),[31] rather than scattered throughout the genome. Some chromosomes appear to have no imprinted genes, raising the question of why specific chromosome regions or specific genes are targeted for imprinting. It seems to be significant that a large number of imprinted genes are involved in some way in the regulation of fetal and postnatal growth, development and survival (Table 21.1), because abnormalities in placental and fetal growth and postnatal development are seen when individual imprinted genes are mutated and not expressed.[5] It has thus been proposed that the key evolutionary role of imprinting is in parental coordination of the balance between growth of the fetus and growth of the placenta.[34] The major fetal growth factor, insulin-like growth factor II (IGF-II), was the first specific gene shown to be imprinted in both mice and humans.[35,36] A cell surface binding receptor for IGF-II, IGF-IIR, is also imprinted, as well as genes that are involved in cell signaling and cell cycle regulation (Table 21.1). Still other imprinted genes are expressed in the central nervous system and, in many cases, their precise cellular functions have not yet been established.[34] Quite a number of imprinted genes are expressed as noncoding RNAs, that are presumed to have some regulatory roles in the cell (Table 21.1). However, there are also an extremely large number of

Table 21.1 List of some known human imprinted genes, their chromosomal localization, and function of the gene product:[31] expression of the maternal (M) or paternal (P) allele is indicated

Gene	Chromosome localization	Expressed allele (M/P)	Protein/RNA function
ZAC	6q24	P	Regulator of apoptosis (cell death) and cell cycle arrest
HYMA1	6q24	P	Noncoding RNA
IGF-IIR	6q25	M*	Cell surface receptor for IGF-II
GRB10	7p11–12	P or M	Growth factor receptor binding and signaling
MEST/PEG1	7q32	P	Similar to hydroxylase enzyme
MESTIT1	7q32	P	Anti-sense RNA
H19	11p15.5	M	Noncoding RNA
IGF-II	11p15.5	P (or both)	Fetal growth factor
INS	11p15.5	P (or both)	Insulin: glucose regulation and growth factor
KCNQ1	11p15.5	M	Voltage-sensitive potassium ion channel
KCNQ1OT1/LIT1	11p15.5	P	Anti-sense RNA
CDKN1C	11p15.5	M	Cell cycle regulator – cyclin-dependent kinase inhibitor
TSSC5/SLC22A	11p15.5	M	Organic cation transporter
TSSC3/IPL	11p15.5	M	Potential tumor suppressor, apoptosis promoter
ZNF215	11p15.5	M	Predicted transcriptional regulator
GTL2	14q32	M	Noncoding RNA
DLK1	14q32	P	Transmembrane protein
ZNF127	15q11–13	P	Predicted transcriptional regulator
NDN	15q11–13	P	Neuronal cell differentiation
MAGEL2	15q11–13	P	Unknown
SNRPN	15q11–13	P	mRNA processing
PWCR1	15q11–13	P	Small nucleolar RNA
PAR5	15q11–13	P	Noncoding RNA
PAR1	15q11–13	P	Noncoding RNA
IPW	15q11–13	P	Noncoding RNA
UBE3A	15q11–13	M	Ubiquitin protein ligase
ATP10C	15q11–13	M	ATPase
GABRB3/A5/G3	15q11–13	P	GABA receptor
PEG3	19q13.4	P	Predicted transcriptional regulator
NNAT	20q11.2	P	Unknown
GNAS1locus:	20q13.11		
Gs-alpha	20q13.11	M (or both)	Small GTPase
XL-alpha s	20q13.11	P	G protein alpha-subunit
NESP55	20q13.11	M	Neuroendocrine secretory protein
Exon 1A	20q13.11	P	Noncoding RNA
GNAS-AS	20q13.11	P	Anti-sense RNA

*Polymorphic imprinting in humans.

genes known to regulate cell growth and development that are not imprinted. Therefore, it may not be the functional properties of the encoded proteins that determine which genes are subject to imprinting, but rather the specific structural features of the genome regions in which imprinted genes reside may be critical. It is interesting that imprinting has been largely conserved between mice and humans, between syngeneic chromosome domains, even though there has been rearrangement of these regions between different chromosomes and an increase in the total number of chromosomes in humans.[31,32] What is noteworthy, however, is that genomic imprinting occurs exclusively in placental mammals, and is not evident in egg-laying mammals or other vertebrates.[37] Whatever the real evolutionary significance of genomic imprinting, imprinted genes are clearly markers of an intrinsic regulatory framework of epigenetic modification. Because imprinted genes are so uniformly programmed, a close analysis of how and when imprinted genes become epigenetically modified reveals when and how these epigenetic processes are laid down during the life cycle.

Imprinting mechanisms

In some ways genomic imprinting can be most likened to X-chromosome inactivation, an epigenetic mechanism in mammals that inactivates one of the two X chromosomes in female embryos (XX). DNA methyl-

ation, histone modification, noncoding RNAs, and changes in chromatin structure are key characteristics of X-chromosome inactivation and of genomic imprinting.[28] However, unlike X-chromosome inactivation, which is random in all tissues apart from the placenta and fetal membranes, genomic imprinting is not random. For a particular imprinted gene, it is always the allele inherited from the one particular parent that is silenced while the other one is expressed (Figure 21.5). For example, the KCNQ1 gene inherited on the maternal chromosome 11 is active, and the paternal copy is inactive, while for the SNRPN gene on chromosome 15, the paternally inherited copy is active and the maternal copy is silenced (Table 21.1). This parental allele-specific gene expression pattern is essentially identical in all individuals regardless of gender and regardless of which grandparent contributed the chromosome (Figure 21.5). In order to maintain such a strict pattern of parent-specific gene expression through consecutive generations, mechanisms must exist to re-program the epigenetic modifications for each new individual. Thus at some stage in

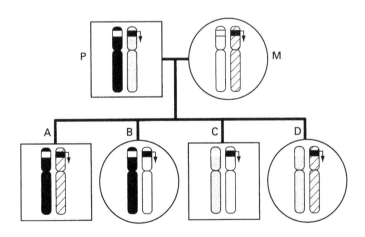

Figure 21.5 Inheritance pattern of genomic imprints. Diagrammatic representation of the inheritance of a maternally expressed gene on chromosome 11. The expressed gene is shown as a black box (with arrow) and the silenced genes as an unfilled box on the chromosomes. Both parents (P and M) have inherited chromosomes from their parents, shown in different colors. Four offspring are shown, two males (A and C) and two females (B and D). Chromosomes 11 from the two parents are distributed randomly between the four offspring, but each shows an identical pattern of expression of the imprinted gene: the maternally inherited gene copy is always expressed and the paternally inherited copy always silenced. This means that the inactive copy of chromosome 11 present in the mother (white) is activated in offspring B and C, and the active copy of chromosome 11 present in the father (gray) is inactivated in offspring C and D. The activity of each imprinted gene depends entirely on the parent contributing the chromosome.

the reproductive life cycle existing epigenetic modifications need to be removed and new patterns established.[30,38,39] As will be discussed below, it turns out that DNA methylation, the epigenetic modification that underlies imprinting, is erased in germ cells and then reset in male and female gametes to ensure transmission of the correct parental-specific epigenetic pattern to the next generation.

Imprinted genes in adult cells can, in many cases, be recognized by differentially methylated regions (DMRs) of DNA sequence on the two parental chromosomes, and these can be used to distinguish the alleles.[38,39] Some of these DMRs are modified during gametogenesis, and these are referred to as *primary imprints* that 'mark' the particular gene for permanent methylation during rounds of cell division after fertilization. Other DMRs are established during embryonic development, and this is referred to as *secondary imprinting*.[38,39] Primary imprints can act as imprinting centres (ICs) that are necessary for establishment of secondary methylation imprints within nearby regions of the chromosome that result in parental allele-specific expression in different cells of the embryo. However, this monoallelic expression can also be regulated by inhibitory noncoding RNAs that are produced near the IC and bind to neighboring genes. Primary and secondary imprinting will be discussed further in the following sections.

As discussed above, all normal individuals are non-mosaic for expression of autosomal genes that are imprinted, the only exception being that some genes are imprinted in a tissue-specific manner, such that both parental alleles are expressed in some tissues. A good example of this is the IGF-II gene, which is expressed from the paternal allele in all fetal tissues except the choroid plexus and leptomeninges around the brain, where both maternal and paternal copies are expressed.[35,36] In humans, but not mice, IGF-II expression becomes biallelic in the liver during infancy due to regulation by a promoter that is not imprinted, and this pattern is then maintained.[40] Other examples also exist (Table 21.1), and indicate that there are additional complexities to be considered with respect to the establishment, reading, and maintenance of genomic imprints that will not be discussed here. As a general rule though, in every cell that expresses the imprinted gene, it is always the same parental allele that is silenced. Thus, the two alleles on the two homologous chromosomes exist in the same cell nucleus and are subject to the same cellular environment, but behave very differently with respect to transcriptional activity. The detailed comparison of the biochemical modification of the expressed and silent alleles allows direct correlations to be made between specific epigenetic modifications and transcriptional regulation (as seen in Figure 21.3). Detailed analyses of the epigenetic modifications involved in establishment and maintenance of primary imprints, establishment and maintenance of secondary imprints, and erasure of imprints, have revealed the stages when these occur during the life cycle of an individual, and have highlighted the dynamic nature of epigenetic modification during gametogenesis and early fetal development.[38] These gene-specific data are corroborated by studies of genome-wide methylation levels that suggest that more widespread epigenetic modifications occur during development.[41]

ERASURE AND ESTABLISHMENT OF IMPRINTS DURING GAMETOGENESIS

Gametes are the only cells that can normally pass genetic information into the next generation, and the gametic stage of sexual reproduction is the only stage of the reproductive cycle when the genetic contribution from each parent is packaged in separate cells and is under the influence of different cellular factors. It is these separate environments that produce different patterns of epigenetic modification on the genomes of eggs and sperm, and account for the 'parent-of-origin' effects that underlie genomic imprinting. This process involves the erasure of existing DNA methylation at very early stages of gametogenesis, and establishment of new patterns of DNA methylation during both oogenesis and spermatogenesis.

Erasure of imprints

Detailed studies of germ cell development in the mouse embryo have shown that demethylation of the germ cell genome occurs during early fetal development, when primordial germ cells have just taken residence in the developing gonads after migration from the yolk sac.[41] Prior to being in the gonadal environment the primordial germ cells are highly methylated. This stage is when the embryos are phenotypically of indeterminate sex, prior to the onset of gonadal sexual differentiation, which is equivalent to 4–5 weeks of human fetal development. The rapid demethylation appears to be unique to primordial germ cells in the developing embryo, and is a developmental process that precedes sex-specific gametogenesis. Genome-wide demethylation includes total removal of methylation from imprinted genes and the inactive X chromosome, and results in biallelic expression of some imprinted genes in primordial germ cells.[30] While the precise mechanism by which this active demethylation occurs has not yet been identified, this process represents what has been considered to be total erasure of all epigenetic modifications, including parental-specific imprints. However, this view needs to be qualified, because there is now some evidence emerging of 'transgenerational epigenetic inheritance', which indicates that some epigenetic modifications are transmitted through the germ line in mice.[42] Some repetitive DNA sequences and retrotransposons appear to be resistant to demethylation in primordial germ cells, indicating there may be specific DNA sequences that escape the demethylation process.[43] Nonerasure of epigenetic modifications may prove to be the mechanism underlying observations of intergenerational programming of birth weight and adult disease.[44]

Establishment of sex-specific primary imprints

New imprints are subsequently established during gametogenesis in both sexes, but occur in a different time-frame and affect different chromosomal regions in the two sexes.[14,45] This distinction must presumably reflect and be part of the vastly different cellular and molecular programs of both germ cell and gonadal tissue development in male and female fetuses initiated by sex-determining genes on the Y chromosome. The mature gametes that are formed many years later after the onset of puberty are highly methylated in both sexes.[14,38] The timing and sequence-specificity of *de novo* DNA methylation events that occur in each sex have been followed by looking at acquisition of primary methylation imprints during oogenesis and spermatogenesis in mice. Two major differences between the sexes are evident from these analyses. Firstly, most of the germ-line methylation imprinting occurs during development of the egg, with only a few imprints so far shown to occur in sperm.[38] Secondly, in females *de novo* methylation imprints are established postnatally during the period of oocyte growth initiated at puberty, while in males *de novo* methylation is already apparent in premeiotic spermatogonia in the fetus before birth (Figure 21.6).[45]

Oocyte-specific DNA methylation has been demonstrated in sequences within or close to the mouse SNRPN, IGF-IIR, MEST, and PEG3 genes, while sperm-specific DNA methylation occurs close to the H19 promoter, and in a region between the GTL2 and DLK1 genes.[14,45] These DMRs represent the primary imprints, and most of these appear to represent ICs. Studies of human gametes have shown a specific region of the SNRPN gene to be methylated in maturing oocytes while the same region is completely unmethylated in sperm.[46] Oocyte-specific methylation has also been demonstrated for the KCNQ1OT1, MEST, and PEG3 genes in humans.[47] As in the mouse, the human H19 gene is methylated in spermatogonia and later stage germ cells but not in oocytes.[48,49] Quite detailed studies of postnatal oocyte growth demonstrate that primary imprints for all the genes are not all established at the same time, but in a specific sequence, with all being complete by the mature metaphase II oocyte stage.[48] More immature oocytes that have not yet established the full complement of primary imprints are developmentally compromised, as assessed by the inability of the oocyte nucleus to support embryo development after nuclear transfer to a mature egg.[50] These findings have raised concerns about the adequacy of *in vitro* oocyte maturation for human *in vitro* fertilization.[45] In the male, methylation of imprinted genes is initiated in spermatogonia that resume mitosis before birth and is completed by the end of meiosis when germ cells are at the round spermatid stage of development (Figure 21.6).[48,49]

The establishment of primary imprints in the two germ lines in a very specific manner indicates that *de novo* DNA methylation occurs in both types of gametes, but the target sequences differ. How the ICs are recognized and targeted for methylation is not yet understood, but the presence of tandem repeat sequence in close association with primary DMRs suggests that such repeat sequences may be recognition domains for methyltransferases and associated proteins.[30] It has also been suggested that binding of proteins to individual ICs might protect these sites for methylation in one germ line, but not in the other if the binding proteins are not expressed. For example, CTCF may bind to the H19 unmethylated IC region in the female germ line, thus preventing maternal methylation.[51] Additional factors such as sex-specific differences in chromatin organization or differences in enzyme specificities or activities may also contribute to the sex-specific methylation patterns. It has been speculated that specific proteins or noncoding RNAs are expressed from genes and DNA sequences close to the ICs in each germ line, and that these may recruit the necessary factors for DNA methylation,[30] but no evidence for such mechanisms is currently available. A specific methyltransferase-like protein, DNMT3L, has been shown to be required for establishment of primary imprints in mouse oocytes, but this protein does not possess any enzyme activity and therefore cannot be the oocyte-specific methylating agent by itself.[52] DNMT3L appears to cooperate with DNMT3A to target maternal ICs.[53] DNMT3A and DNMT3L are both also expressed in the male germ line, so these enzymes alone cannot account for sex-specific

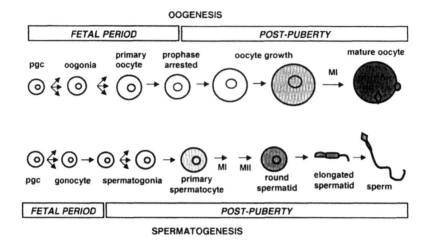

Figure 21.6 Comparison of the acquisition of methylated primary imprints during oogenesis and spermatogenesis. Primordial germ cells (pgcs) in both sexes are demethylated during early fetal development and all imprints are erased. The progressive acquisition of imprints during germ cell development in each sex is shown as increasing coloration. Methylated primary imprints are first detected during postnatal oocyte growth when oogenesis resumes after puberty, and primary maternal imprints are progressively established as the oocyte matures. Initial methylation of paternal imprints is already evident in male gonocytes at late stages of fetal development and become progressively established during postnatal spermatogenesis. Methylation of imprints is complete by the round spermatid stage of spermatogenesis.

methylation patterns.[54] DNMT3L deficiency in male mice causes failure of methylation on dispersed repeat sequences in spermatogonia, but not tandem repeat sequences, and the H19 gene IC becomes only partially methylated.[54] Some light may soon be shed on what the regulators of primary imprinting are in oocytes, from characterization of a genetically based imprinting defect recently identified in a family.[47] This maternal-effect mutation results in repeated cases of complete hydatidiform mole in affected females, caused by a global failure of primary maternal imprint establishment in oocytes. Fertilization of these oocytes results in embryos that lack maternal imprints and have an imprint pattern that is equivalent to a paternal-only androgenetic conceptus characteristic of hydatidiform moles. No mutations were found in known DNMTs in the affected women.[55] Identification of the specific gene product affected in this family will provide some important insights into the regulation of imprint establishment in the female germ line.

EPIGENETIC MODIFICATION IN THE EMBRYO

A series of major changes in DNA methylation takes place immediately after fertilization, which includes a phase of rapid demethylation of nonimprinted regions, *de novo* global DNA methylation, establishment of secondary methylation imprints, and establishment of a number of epigenetic processes that result in parental allele-specific expression.

Post-fertilization demethylation

Once the highly methylated haploid genomes in the sperm and the egg come together after fertilization a rapid wave of demethylation occurs that is followed by *de novo* methylation in a tissue-specific manner (Figure 21.7).[38,41] The demethylation process has two important features. First, the parental chromosomes undergo quite different processes of demethylation. The sperm-derived chromosomes are preferentially demethylated within a few hours after fertilization, before any DNA replication or transcription from the embryonic genome has taken place.[38] Maternally derived chromosomes are relatively resistant to this

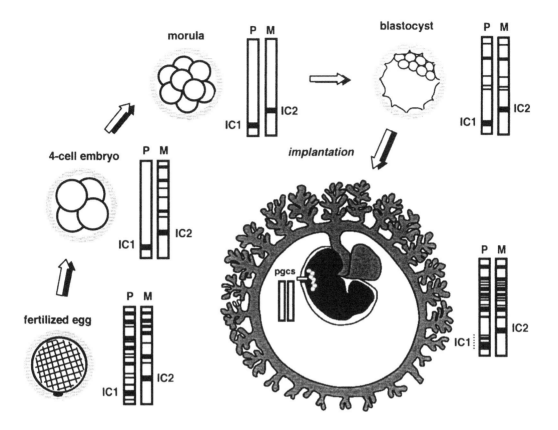

Figure 21.7 Changes in DNA methylation during embryonic development. The levels of global DNA methylation in embryos at different stages of development are represented by the degree of blue shading. The degree of methylation of paternal (P) and maternal (M) chromosomes is shown by the number of black lines along each chromosome. The genome of the fertilized egg is highly methylated (crosshatched), with both parental chromosomes showing high, but different patterns, of DNA methylation. Rapid demethylation occurs after fertilization, with preferential demethylation of the paternal chromosome (shown at the 4-cell stage). The imprinting centers (IC1 and IC2) on both parental chromosomes are protected from demethylation. By the 8–16-cell stage morula, the genome is demethylated except for the ICs. *De novo* methylation is initiated by the blastocyst stage, and increases after implantation. The placental DNA is generally less methylated than the fetal DNA. During placental and fetal development there is spreading of the initial primary imprint from the IC (shown by dotted line), which establishes secondary differentially methylated regions on the chromosomes. Primordial germ cells (pgcs) become entirely demethylated during early fetal development, including loss of IC methylation.

active demethylation, and become demethylated more slowly over the preimplantation period by passive demethylation due to absence of nuclear DNMT1 during the cleavage stages and hence no replication of the methylated CpG sites during cell division.[38] Second, the primary imprints established in each gamete before fertilization are protected from either of these demethylation processes, and retain their methylation pattern.[41] Both of these features are illustrated in Figure 21.7, and represent what must be quite

different chromatin conformations of the two sets of parental chromosomes, as well as some unique characteristics of ICs.[41] By the 8–16-cell stage of cleavage of the preimplantation embryo, little DNA methylation remains apart from that associated with the ICs (Figure 21.7).[41] What the mechanism is that protects all ICs from demethylation is not known, but it might involve methyl-binding proteins that recruit histone deacetylases.[6] There is evidence of differences in acetylation and methylation of histones that are associated with the methylated and unmethylated IC regions, and this may result in quite specific alterations in chromatin structure at these sites that protect from demethylation.[30,56] As is the case in primordial germ cells, certain types of repetitive sequences and retrotransposons are also protected from demethylation.[57] A unique methyltransferase, Dnmt1o, that is present in the nucleus only at the 8-cell stage may be responsible for maintaining the methylation of ICs in the absence of DNMT1.[58] Protection of IC methylation is crucial for preserving the gametic 'epigenetic memory' that ultimately confers monoallelic gene expression at later stages of embryogenesis.

De novo methylation

De novo methylation starts in the preimplantation mouse embryo after the fifth cleavage division and coincides with development of the blastocyst (Figure 21.7). The two cell lineages that differentiate in the blastocyst appear to be differently methylated at a global level, with the trophoblast cells that form the outer cell layer being methylated to a lower degree than the inner cell mass.[41,59] The inner cell mass is the stem cell population for all cell lineages that make up the fetus, including primordial germ cells. These different embryonic cell types become differentially methylated as part of the developmental program that regulates differential gene expression and cell diversification after implantation of the blastocyst into the uterine wall. All fetal and placental tissues become progressively methylated during development *in utero*, with placental tissue showing consistently lower levels of global methylation when compared with various fetal tissues (Figure 21.7).[60]

A specific type of *de novo* methylation is the 'secondary imprinting' of sequences adjacent to the DMR that specifies the IC, such that either additional sites in the same gene are methylated, or sites on neighboring genes within the imprinted chromosomal domain become methylated. This 'spreading' of DNA methylation can be over long distances, being several megabases along chromosome 15q11–13 from the maternally methylated SNRPN-IC.[38] The spread of methylation along the chromosome contributes to transcriptional silencing of a number of genes on the maternal chromosome that were not differentially methylated in the oocyte (Figure 21.8B).[61] However, epigenetic 'spreading' from the IC is not always due to spreading of DNA methylation. In some cases, absence of methylation at the IC site on one allele results in the expression of noncoding RNAs at that site that represses nearby genes on the same chromosome (Figure 21.8C). For example, a noncoding RNA

that overlaps part of the IGF-IIR gene (Air) is produced from the paternal allele that has a non-methylated IC, which represses the transcription of the IGF-IIR and adjacent genes (Slc22a2 and Slc22a3) on the paternal chromosome.[30,62] A similar mechanism has been reported for the KCNQ1, and in this case a noncoding RNA (KCNQ1OT1/LIT1) is produced from the paternal allele that contains the nonmethylated IC.[30] This quite localized process appears to be very similar to the more extensive inactivation of the X chromosome. Imprinted X-chromosome inactivation occurs in the mouse placenta, by a process whereby the entire paternal X chromosome is 'coated' by the Xist noncoding RNA expressed from the paternal IC.[6] A general role for noncoding RNA produced at ICs may be in the recruitment of proteins and enzyme complexes that modify chromatin and silence gene transcription.

There are, thus, at least two different ways in which an allele-specific primary methyl imprint can work to silence genes within an imprinted chromosome domain. First, the methylated IC associated with a given gene influences the methylation status of adjacent genes and results in gene silencing of methylated genes (Figure 21.8B). In this case, maternal methylation of an IC results in silencing of the maternal alleles. Second, the methylated IC has no direct role in gene silencing, but the other nonmethylated allele generates noncoding RNAs that silence genes on the nonmethylated chromosome. In this case, maternal methylation of an IC is associated with transcriptional activity of the genes on the maternal chromosome, while the genes on the nonmethylated chromosome are inactivated by RNA-mediated transcriptional repression (Figure 21.8C). This second type of epigenetic gene silencing helps reconcile the fact that while the majority of primary imprints are of maternal origin, about half of the transcriptionally inactive alleles of imprinted genes are of paternal origin (Table 21.1).

Parental allele-specific gene expression

The end result of genomic imprinting in the male and female germ lines is parental allele-specific gene expression. The differential methylation of ICs is the first step in this entire process, which is necessary for establishing a more complex pattern of methylation, histone modification, and expression of noncoding RNAs during embryonic development. It is these later modifications that repress gene transcription from one of the parental alleles. While analysis of genomic imprinting has revealed the key mechanisms underlying epigenetic regulation during gametogenesis and

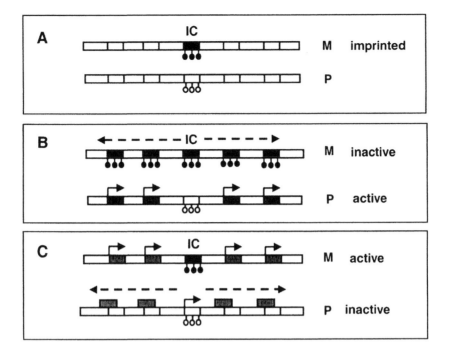

Figure 21.8 Two types of secondary imprinting. (A) Primary imprinting during gametogenesis establishes differential methylation at imprinting centers (IC), with most primary methylation imprints (black box and circles) acquired on the maternal chromosomes during oogenesis. (B) Secondary imprinting can be the 'spreading' (hashed line) of DNA methylation from the IC along the chromosome in both directions. This methylation silences genes along this region (inactive). The IC on the paternal chromosome is unmethylated, and so secondary methylation does not take place. The genes along the paternal chromosome are transcriptionally active (arrows). (C) A different mechanism of secondary imprinting can occur, whereby the noncoding RNAs are expressed from the unmethylated IC on the paternal chromosome (arrow). These RNAs bind to adjacent regions of the chromosome and silence expression of genes (inactive). No noncoding RNA is expressed from the methylated IC on the maternal chromosome, and adjacent genes are transcriptionally active (arrows).

embryogenesis, the expression of a large number of nonimprinted genes is also influenced by similar epigenetic modifications. The 'epigenetic toolbox' is thus used in complex ways throughout embryogenesis to manipulate the expression of the genome to create a fully developed human fetus. It means that imprinted genes will be expressed only from one parental copy in all cells (monoallelic silencing), while other nonimprinted genes will be silenced from both copies in specific cell types (biallelic silencing). How this epigenetic program of development is orchestrated will continue to challenge researchers in this field for many years to come. Both genetic and environmental factors, such as diet, can influence the contents and usage of the 'epigenetic toolbox' during early development, and will determine the epigenetic program acquired during fetal life. This program establishes the repertoire of genes that are expressed from the genome and

their levels of expression in different tissues. These tissue-specific patterns of gene expression regulate the growth and development of the fetus and placenta *in utero*, and ultimately the physiology and phenotype of the adult. Thus, the epigenetic modifications acquired during fetal development can generate phenotypic variation between individuals, and will reflect to some degree the nutritional environment *in utero*. Since epigenetic modifications are heritable through cell division, they will also determine adult health and predisposition to disease.

EPIGENETIC BASIS OF DISEASE

The availability and activity of components in the 'epigenetic toolbox' that affect both the metabolic process of DNA methylation and methylation-mediated gene regulation are predicted to have effects on the establishment, maintenance, and reading of epigenetic modifications. There are several examples of how genetic and environmental factors limit the availability and/or activity of critical epigenetic components and influence growth, development, and disease.

Genetic effects

In humans a number of genetic disorders of metabolism (hyperhomocysteinemia, homocysteinuria, and hypermethioninemia) arise from genetic variants and mutations. These mutations often affect enzymes involved in folate and homocysteine metabolism (e.g. MTHFR and cystathionine β-synthase) and are linked to decreased levels of global DNA methylation.[63,64] Conditions such as hyperhomocysteinemia are associated with increased risk of cardiovascular disease and neurological dysfunction in older individuals, and in pregnant females the risk of neural tube defects is increased.[63,64] These genetic metabolic disorders influence the availability of methyl groups for methyltransferases, and can be overridden by dietary supplementation, for example, with folate.[65] DNA methyltransferase activity can also be directly affected by mutations in the DNMT genes. A mutation in the DNMT3B gene in humans is the cause of ICF syndrome (immunodeficiency, centromeric region instability, facial anomalies).[14,66] ICF is a rare recessive disease, and affected individuals generally die in childhood from immune dysfunction caused by effects of DNA hypomethylation on the development of B lymphocytes.[66] A different genetic disorder, Rett syndrome, is caused by a mutation in the X-linked gene coding for the methyl-binding protein MeCP2.[67] Rett syndrome is a developmental disorder that causes mental retardation in girls. It is interesting that affected infants are quite normal until 6–18 months of life, when severe dementia and autistic behavior reveal the genetic disorder.[67] This postnatal onset appears to predominantly affect the central nervous system (CNS) despite the ubiquitous expression of MeCP2 in all tissues, indicating that gene silencing mechanisms mediated by MeCP2 binding are quite tissue-specific.[67] Different epigenetic mechanisms in different tissues will thus determine which ones are affected and which are not affected by specific mutations.

These few examples of genetic mutations, which give rise to epigenetic disorders illustrate that even though the mutated enzymes or methyl-binding proteins are widely expressed in different cells of the body, quite specific phenotypic effects are associated with the different mutations. While there is a great deal of heterogeneity in the disease phenotypes, the development of the immune system is principally affected in individuals with ICF, and the CNS is principally affected in girls with Rett syndrome. On this basis one can predict that environmental factors that influence these same epigenetic pathways might also give rise to tissue-specific phenotypic effects.

Nutritional deficiency

Growth and development of the fetus are dependent on an adequate nutritional supply through the placenta, and nutritional deficiency is considered to be the major cause of fetal growth restriction in the absence of known genetic or chromosomal defects. It is now starting to be recognized that nutrient supply is likely to have a fundamental impact on the epigenetic programming of the fetus, which will determine the phenotype after birth. While there is still very little direct evidence for this prediction, this situation is likely to change as more research is undertaken.

The most convincing evidence that nutrients influence epigenetic modification comes from culture of preimplantation embryos. It has been clearly demonstrated using animal embryos that different types of culture medium have significant effects on patterns of DNA methylation and the expression of imprinted genes.[68,69] Embryo culture is also associated with growth and developmental abnormalities *in utero* and after birth.[69] These observations have become of particular interest since the reported increased incidence of imprinting disorders in children born after *in vitro* fertilization (IVF) or related artificial reproductive technologies.[14] In a recent case-control study, the risk of BWS in IVF pregnancies has been calculated to be nine times that in the general population, and is predominantly due to a maternal methylation abnormality.[70] The influence of the culture environment on epigenetic modification seen *in vitro* suggests that a suboptimal nutrient environment in the oviduct may have a similar effect as suboptimal *in vitro* culture. However, studies to test this proposal are difficult to undertake. Analyses of the effects of nutritional status on the early human embryo have demonstrated the important role of methyl donors on birth weight and on the incidence of neural tube defects (NTDs).[71,72] A number of studies have now shown that mothers who have the highest dietary intake of folate, choline, and betaine, particularly around the time of conception, have significantly reduced risk of having babies with NTDs.[72] In countries where folate fortification of food has been introduced as a public health policy, a 78% reduction in NTDs has been achieved.[73] While there is yet no direct demonstration of changes in DNA methylation associated with human NTDs, analyses of mouse models of NTDs suggest that altered methylation is likely to be a contributing factor in these congenital defects.[74] These studies suggest that the brain might be particularly sensitive to the effects of methyl deficiency, and a range of neurodevelopmental disorders may arise from the effects of methyl deficiency on DNA methylation.[74] However, since methyl donors are required for a range of cellular processes other than DNA and histone methylation, it is not possible to make a direct link between dietary factors and epigenetic abnormalities.

Animal studies will be important in testing the prediction that specific alterations in epigenetic programming *in utero* determine adult health and disease. The first direct evidence of changes in epigenetic modification in an animal model of fetal programming has just been reported.[75] Reduced levels of DNA methylation and increased levels of histone acetylation were found in the livers of rats in a model of uteroplacental insufficiency.[75] This study is the start of what will undoubtedly be a major area of investigation into the mechanisms that underlie the perinatal origins of adult disease. Further research is needed to establish a direct link between dietary factors, epigenetic modifications, and adult onset disease. Advances in molecular technologies now allow specific epigenetic patterns to be ascertained, and will enable the development of methods to identify epigenetic 'fingerprints' that reflect any environmental impacts *in utero*. Direct evidence of an association between patterns of epigenetic modification and adult disease will inform public health recommendations for adequate nutrition during pregnancy.

CONCLUSIONS

- Expression or silencing of genes is regulated by epigenetic modifications that are heritable through cell division, and include an interaction between processes such as DNA methylation, histone modification, changes in chromatin conformation, and activity of noncoding RNAs.
- Epigenetic processes are influenced by the availability of methyl donors, being essentially methionine, folate, and choline, which come from the diet.
- During gametogenesis and early embryogenesis the genome undergoes dynamic changes in demethylation, *de novo* methylation, and maintenance of methylation, and these stages are particularly sensitive to lack of availability or activity of factors that regulate establishment and recognition of epigenetic modifications.

- The pattern of epigenetic modification reflects the history of environmental exposure, and molecular tools are now becoming available to 'fingerprint' these epigenetic patterns.
- Evidence of an association between patterns of epigenetic modification and adult disease will have enormous potential for directing public health recommendations for dietary interventions during pregnancy.

ACKNOWLEDGMENTS

I am very grateful to Peter Smith, Susan Ravelich, and Galina Konycheva for helpful comments on the manuscript. Imprinting studies in the author's laboratory are supported by the Marsden Fund, Royal Society of New Zealand.

REFERENCES

1. Singh SM, Murphy B, O'Reilly R. Epigenetic contributors to the discordance of monozygotic twins. Clin Genet 2002; 62: 97–103.
2. Liu L, Wylie RC, Andrews LG, Tollefsbol TO. Aging, cancer and nutrition: the DNA methylation connection. Mech Ageing Dev 2003; 124: 989–98.
3. Costello JF, Plass C. Methylation matters. J Med Genet 2001; 38: 285–303.
4. Bjornsson HT, Fallin MD, Feinberg AP. An integrated epigenetic and genetic approach to common human disease. Trends Genet 2004; 20: 350–8.
5. Walter J, Paulsen M. Imprinting and disease. Semin Cell Dev Biol 2003; 14: 101–10.
6. Jaenisch R, Bird A. Epigenetic regulation of gene expression: how the genome integrates intrinsic and environmental signals. Nat Genet 2003; 33: 245–54.
7. Singal R, Ginder GD. DNA methylation. Blood 1999; 93: 4059–70.
8. Boyes J, Bird A. Repression of genes by DNA methylation depends on CpG density and promoter strength: evidence for involvement of a methyl-CpG binding protein. EMBO J 1992; 11: 327–33.
9. Yoder JA, Walsh CP, Bestor TH. Cytosine methylation and the ecology of intragenomic parasites. Trends Genet 1997; 13: 335–40.
10. Newell-Price J, Clark AJ, King P. DNA methylation and silencing of gene expression. Trends Endocrinol Metab 2000; 11: 142–8.
11. Issa JP. Aging, DNA methylation and cancer. Crit Rev Oncol Hematol 1999; 32: 31–43.
12. Lopatina N, Haskell JF, Andrews LG et al. Differential maintenance and de novo methylating activity by three DNA methyltransferases in aging and immortalized fibroblasts. J Cell Biochem 2002; 84: 324–34.
13. Abdolmaleky HM, Smith CL, Faraone SV et al. Methylomics in psychiatry: modulation of gene-environment interactions may be through DNA methylation. Am J Med Genet 2004; 127B: 51–9.
14. Kelly TL, Trasler JM. Reproductive epigenetics. Clin Genet 2004; 65: 247–60.

15. Niculescu MD, Zeisel SH. Diet, methyl donors and DNA methylation: interactions between dietary folate, methionine and choline. J Nutr 2002; 132: 2333S–2335S.

16. Friso S, Choi SW. Gene-nutrient interactions and DNA methylation. J Nutr 2002; 132: 2382S–2387S.

17. Wainfan E, Dizik M, Stender M, Christman JK. Rapid appearance of hypomethylated DNA in livers of rats fed cancer-promoting, methyl-deficient diets. Cancer Res 1989; 49: 4094–7.

18. Friso S, Choi SW, Girelli D et al. A common mutation in the 5,10-methylenetetrahydrofolate reductase gene affects genomic DNA methylation through an interaction with folate status. Proc Natl Acad Sci USA 2002; 99: 5606–11.

19. Bailey LB. Folate, methyl-related nutrients, alcohol, and the MTHFR 677C→T polymorphism affect cancer risk: intake recommendations. J Nutr 2003; 133: 3748S–3753S.

20. Klerk M, Verhoef P, Clarke R et al. MTHFR Studies Collaboration Group. MTHFR 677C→T polymorphism and risk of coronary heart disease: a meta-analysis. JAMA 2002; 288: 2023–31.

21. Ohlsson R, Renkawitz R, Lobanenkov V. CTCF is a uniquely versatile transcription regulator linked to epigenetics and disease. Trends Genet 2001; 17: 520–7.

22. Felsenfeld G, Groudine M. Controlling the double helix. Nature 2003; 421: 448–53.

23. Peterson CL, Laniel MA. Histones and histone modifications. Curr Biol 2004; 14: R546–51.

24. Lachner M, O'Sullivan RJ, Jenuwein T. An epigenetic road map for histone lysine methylation. J Cell Sci 2003; 116: 2117–24.

25. Strahl BD, Allis CD. The language of covalent histone modifications. Nature 2000; 403: 41–5.

26. Weissmann F, Lyko F. Cooperative interactions between epigenetic modifications and their function in the regulation of chromosome architecture. Bioessays 2003; 25: 792–7.

27. Morey C, Avner P. Employment opportunities for non-coding RNAs. FEBS Lett 2004; 567: 27–34.

28. Goldmit M, Bergman Y. Monoallelic gene expression: a repertoire of recurrent themes. Immunol Rev 2004; 200: 197–214.

29. Mattick JS. RNA regulation: a new genetics? Nat Rev Genet 2004; 5: 316–23.

30. Delaval K, Feil R. Epigenetic regulation of mammalian genomic imprinting. Curr Opin Genet Dev 2004; 14: 188–95.

31. http://www.otago.ac.nz/IGC

32. Hitchins MP, Moore GE. Genomic imprinting in fetal growth and development. Expert Rev Mol Med 2002; http://www.expertreviews.org/0200457Xh.htm.

33. Feinberg AP, Cui H, Ohlsson R. DNA methylation and genomic imprinting: insights from cancer into epigenetic mechanisms. Semin Cancer Biol 2002; 12: 389–98.

34. Tycko B, Morison IM. Physiological functions of imprinted genes. J Cell Physiol 2002; 192: 245–58.

35. DeChiara TM, Robertson EJ, Efstratiadis A. Parental imprinting of the mouse insulin-like growth factor II gene. Cell 1991; 64: 849–59.

36. Ohlsson R, Nystrom A, Pfeifer-Ohlsson S et al. IGF2 is parentally imprinted during human embryogenesis and in the Beckwith-Wiedemann syndrome. Nat Genet 1993; 4: 94–7.

37. Murphy SK, Jirtle RL. Imprinting evolution and the price of silence. Bioessays 2003; 25: 577–88.

38. Reik W, Walter J. Genomic imprinting: parental influence on the genome. Nat Rev Genet 2001; 2: 21–32.

39. Rand E, Cedar H. Regulation of imprinting: a multi-tiered process. J Cell Biochem 2003; 88: 400–7.

40. Vu TH, Hoffman AR. Promoter-specific imprinting of the human insulin-like growth factor-II gene. Nature 1994; 371: 714–7.

41. Santos F, Dean W. Epigenetic reprogramming during early development in mammals. Reproduction 2004; 127: 643–51.

42. Rakyan VK, Preis J, Morgan HD, Whitelaw E. The marks, mechanisms and memory of epigenetic states in mammals. Biochem J 2001; 356: 1–10.

43. Lane N, Dean W, Erhardt S et al. Resistance of IAPs to methylation reprogramming may provide a mechanism for epigenetic inheritance in the mouse. Genesis 2003; 35: 88–93.

44. Drake AJ, Walker BR. The intergenerational effects of fetal programming: non-genomic mechanisms for the inheritance of low birth weight and cardiovascular risk. J Endocrinol 2004; 180: 1–16.

45. Lucifero D, Mann MR, Bartolomei MS, Trasler JM. Gene-specific timing and epigenetic memory in oocyte imprinting. Hum Mol Genet 2004; 13: 839–49.

46. Geuns E, De Rycke M, Van Steirteghem A, Liebaers I. Methylation imprints of the imprint control region of the SNRPN-gene in human gametes and preimplantation embryos. Hum Mol Genet 2003; 12: 2873–9.

47. Judson H, Hayward BE, Sheridan E, Bonthron DT. A global disorder of imprinting in the human female germ line. Nature 2002; 416: 539–42.

48. Hamatani T, Sasaki H, Ishihara K et al. Epigenetic mark sequence of the H19 gene in human sperm. Biochim Biophys Acta 2001; 1518: 137–44.

49. Kerjean A, Dupont JM, Vasseur C et al. Establishment of the paternal methylation imprint of the human H19 and MEST/PEG1 genes during spermatogenesis. Hum Mol Genet 2000; 9: 2183–7.

50. Obata Y, Kono T. Maternal primary imprinting is established at a specific time for each gene throughout oocyte growth. J Biol Chem 2002; 277: 5285–9.

51. Fedoriw AM, Stein P, Svoboda P, Schultz RM, Bartolomei MS. Transgenic RNAi reveals essential function for CTCF in H19 gene imprinting. Science 2004; 303: 238–40.

52. Hata K, Okano M, Lei H, Li E. Dnmt3L cooperates with the Dnmt3 family of de novo DNA methyltransferases to establish maternal imprints in mice. Development 2002; 129: 1983–93.

53. Chedin F, Lieber MR, Hsieh CL. The DNA methyltransferase-like protein DNMT3L stimulates de novo methylation by Dnmt3a. Proc Natl Acad Sci USA 2002; 99: 16916–21.

54. Bourc'his D, Bestor TH. Meiotic catastrophe and retrotransposon reactivation in male germ cells lacking Dnmt3L. Nature 2004; 431: 96–9.

55. Hayward BE, De Vos M, Judson H et al. Lack of involvement of known DNA methyltransferases in familial hydatidiform mole implies the involvement of other factors in establishment of imprinting in the human female germline. BMC Genet 2003; 4: 2.

56. Fournier C, Goto Y, Ballestar E et al. Allele-specific histone lysine methylation marks regulatory regions at imprinted mouse genes. EMBO J 2002; 21: 6560–70.

57. Kim SH, Kang YK, Koo DB et al. Differential DNA methylation reprogramming of various repetitive sequences in mouse preimplantation embryos. Biochem Biophys Res Commun 2004; 324: 58–63.

58. Howell CY, Bestor TH, Ding F et al. Genomic imprinting disrupted by a maternal effect mutation in the Dnmt1 gene. Cell 2001; 104: 829–38.

59. Santos F, Hendrich B, Reik W, Dean W. Dynamic reprogramming of DNA methylation in the early mouse embryo. Dev Biol 2002; 241: 172–82.

60. Fuke C, Shimabukuro M, Petronis A et al. Age related changes in 5-methylcytosine content in human peripheral leukocytes and placentas: an HPLC-based study. Ann Hum Genet 2004; 68: 196–204.

61. Buiting K, Saitoh S, Gross S et al. Inherited microdeletions in the Angelman and Prader-Willi syndromes define an imprinting centre on human chromosome 15. Nat Genet 1995; 9: 395–400.

62. Sleutels F, Zwart R, Barlow DP. The non-coding Air RNA is required for silencing autosomal imprinted genes. Nature 2002; 415: 810–13.

63. Selhub J. Homocysteine metabolism. Annu Rev Nutr 1999; 19: 217–46.

64. Singh SM, Murphy B, O'Reilly RL. Involvement of gene-diet/drug interaction in DNA methylation and its contribution to complex diseases: from cancer to schizophrenia. Clin Genet 2003; 64: 451–60.

65. Ingrosso D, Cimmino A, Perna AF et al. Folate treatment and unbalanced methylation and changes of allelic expression induced by hyperhomocysteinaemia in patients with uraemia. Lancet 2003; 361: 1693–9.

66. Ehrlich M. The ICF syndrome, a DNA methyltransferase 3B deficiency and immunodeficiency disease. Clin Immunol 2003; 109: 17–28.

67. Neul JL, Zoghbi HY. Rett syndrome: a prototypical neuro-developmental disorder. Neuroscientist 2004; 10: 118–28.

68. Mann MR, Lee SS, Doherty AS et al. Selective loss of imprinting in the placenta following preimplantation development in culture. Development 2004; 131: 3727–35.

69. Fernandez-Gonzalez R, Moreira P, Bilbao A et al. Long-term effect of in vitro culture of mouse embryos with serum on mRNA expression of imprinting genes, development, and behavior. Proc Natl Acad Sci USA 2004; 101: 5880–5.

70. Halliday J, Oke K, Breheny S, Algar E, J Amor D. Beckwith-Wiedemann syndrome and IVF: a case-control study. Am J Hum Genet 2004; 75: 526–8.

71. Wu G, Bazer FW, Cudd TA, Meininger CJ, Spencer TE. Maternal nutrition and fetal development. J Nutr 2004; 134: 2169–72.

72. Shaw GM, Carmichael SL, Yang W, Selvin S, Schaffer DM. Periconceptional dietary intake of choline and betaine and neural tube defects in offspring. Am J Epidemiol 2004; 160: 102–9.

73. Liu S, West R, Randell E, Longerich L et al. A comprehensive evaluation of food fortification with folic acid for the primary prevention of neural tube defects. BMC Pregnancy Childbirth 2004; 4: 20.

74. Juriloff DM, Harris MJ. Mouse models for neural tube closure defects. Hum Mol Genet 2000; 9: 993–1000.

75. MacLennan NK, James SJ, Melnyk S et al. Uteroplacental insufficiency alters DNA methylation, one-carbon metabolism, and histone acetylation in IUGR rats. Physiol Genomics 2004; 18: 43–50.

22

Maternal programming of glucocorticoid receptor expression and HPA responses to stress through DNA methylation in the rat

Michael J Meaney, Ian CG Weaver, Tao Wu, Ian Hellstrom, Josie Diorio, Patrick McGown, and Moshe Szyf

THE DEVELOPMENT OF INDIVIDUAL DIFFERENCES IN STRESS RESPONSES

In the late 1950s and early 1960s the pages of *Science* and *Nature* were frequently dedicated to articles reporting the effects of postnatal handling (aka, infantile stimulation) on the development of responses to adverse stimuli, or stressors.[1–3] The handling paradigm involves a brief (i.e. ~15 minutes) separation of the pups from the dam. This period falls well within the range of normal mother–pup separations that occur between nursing bouts and does not constitute any major deprivation of parental care. In infant rats and mice, handling during infancy decreases the magnitude of both behavioral and hypothalamic-pituitary-adrenal (HPA) responses to stress in adulthood. These findings demonstrated that the early environment influences the development of even rudimentary defensive responses to threat and provided a model for the study of environmental programming. Such effects are defined by enduring alterations in physiology and behavior that are caused by exposure to stimuli during a specific period in early development.

Levine and others suggested that the effects of handling are actually mediated by changes in maternal care. Indeed, handling increases the licking/grooming of pups by the mother.[4,5] Subsequent studies supported this maternal-mediation hypothesis. One approach has been to examine the consequences of naturally occurring variations in maternal licking/grooming. In this context, the term 'naturally occurring' simply refers to variation in maternal behavior in the absence of any experimental manipulation. These studies indicate that the adult offspring of high

licking/grooming (LG) mothers resembled postnatally handled animals on measures of behavioral and endocrine responses to stress, while those of low LG mothers were comparable to nonhandled animals. Cross-fostering studies, where pups born to high LG mothers were fostered at birth to low LG mothers (and vice versa), suggest a direct relationship between maternal care and the postnatal development of individual differences in behavioral and HPA responses to stress.[6,7] Finally, these studies suggest that variations within a normal range of parental care can dramatically alter development. The potency of such effects is likely due to the fact that natural selection has shaped offspring to respond to subtle variations in parental behaviors as a forecast of the environmental conditions they will ultimately face following independence from the parent.[8]

MATERNAL CARE IN THE RAT: BEHAVIORAL AND HPA RESPONSES TO STRESS

Central corticotropin-releasing factor (CRF) systems furnish the critical signal for the activation of behavioral, emotional, autonomic, and endocrine responses to stressors. There are two major CRF pathways regulating the expression of these stress responses. First, a CRF pathway from the parvocellular regions of the paraventricular nucleus of the hypothalamus (PVNh) to the hypophyseal-portal system of the anterior pituitary, which serves as the principal mechanism for the transduction of a neural signal into a pituitary-adrenal response.[9–12] In responses to stressors, CRF, as well as co-secretagogues such as arginine and vasopressin, are released from PVNh neurons into the portal blood supply of the anterior pituitary where they stimulate the synthesis and release of adrenocorticotropin hormone (ACTH). Pituitary ACTH, in turn, causes the release of glucocorticoids from the adrenal gland. CRF synthesis and release is subsequently inhibited through a glucocorticoid negative-feedback system mediated by both mineralocorticoid and glucocorticoid receptors in a number of brain regions including and perhaps especially in the hippocampus.[13]

CRF neurons in the central nucleus of the amygdala project directly to the locus coeruleus and increase the firing rate of locus coeruleus neurons, resulting in increased noradrenaline release in the vast terminal fields of this ascending noradrenergic system. Thus, intracerebroventricular (i.c.v.) infusion of CRF increases extracellular noradrenaline levels.[14–17] The amygdaloid (BNST) CRF projection to the locus coeruleus[17–21] is also critical for the expression of behavioral responses to stress.[22–29] Hence, the CRF neurons in the PVNh and the central nucleus of the amygdala serve as important mediators of both behavioral and endocrine responses to stress.

We examined the relation between maternal care and the development of behavioral and endocrine responses to stress using a rather simple model of naturally occurring variations in maternal behavior over the first 8 days after birth.[30] Individual differences in maternal behavior were characterized through direct observation of mother–pup interactions in normally reared animals. These observations revealed considerable variation in two forms of maternal behavior – licking/grooming of pups and arched-back nursing (ABN). Licking/grooming includes both body and anogenital licking. ABN, also referred to as 'crouching', is characterized by a dam nursing her pups with her back conspicuously arched and legs splayed outward.[31] While common, it is not the only posture from which dams nurse. A blanket posture represents a more relaxed version of the arched-back position where the mother is almost lying on the suckling pups. This provides substantially less opportunity for movement by the pups, such as nipple switching. Dams also nurse from their sides and often will move from one posture to another over the course of a nursing bout. Interestingly, the frequency of licking/grooming and ABN is correlated across animals and thus we are able to define mothers according to both behaviors; high or low LG-ABN mothers. For the sake of most of the studies described here, high and low LG-ABN mothers are females whose scores on both measures were $\pm$ 1

SD above (high) or below (low) the mean for their cohort. Importantly, high and low LG-ABN mothers do not differ in the amount of contact time with pups; differences in the frequency of licking/grooming or ABN do not occur simply as a function of time in contact with pups. High and low LG-ABN mothers raise a comparable number of pups to weaning and there are no differences in the weaning weights of the pups, suggesting an adequate level of maternal care across the groups. These findings also suggest that we are examining the consequences of variations in maternal care that occur within a normal range. Indeed, the frequency of both pup licking/grooming and ABN are normally distributed across large populations of lactating female rats.[30]

The critical question concerns the potential consequences of these differences in maternal behavior for the development of behavioral and neuroendocrine responses to stress. As adults, the offspring of high LG-ABN mothers show reduced plasma ACTH and corticosterone responses to acute stress by comparison to the adult offspring of low LG-ABN mothers.[5,32] Circulating glucocorticoids act at glucocorticoid and mineralocorticoid receptor sites in corticolimbic structures, such as the hippocampus, to regulate HPA activity. Such feedback effects commonly target CRF synthesis and release at the level of the PVNh. The high LG-ABN offspring showed significantly increased hippocampal glucocorticoid receptor mRNA expression, enhanced glucocorticoid negative feedback sensitivity and decreased hypothalamic CRH mRNA levels. Moreover, Liu et al.[5] found that the magnitude of the corticosterone response to acute stress was significantly correlated with the frequency of both maternal licking/grooming ($r = -0.61$) and ABN ($r = -0.64$) during the first week of life, as was the level of hippocampal glucocorticoid receptor mRNA and hypothalamic CRH mRNA expression (all r values > 0.70).

The offspring of the high LG-ABN mothers exhibit decreased CRF receptor levels in the locus coeruleus and increased GABA$_A$/BZ receptor levels in the basolateral and central nucleus of the amygdala, as well as in the locus coeruleus[7,33] and decreased CRF mRNA expression in the CnAmy (Francis, Diorio, and Meaney, unpublished observations). BZ agonists suppress CRF expression in the amygdala.[34] Predictably, stress-induced increases in PVNh levels of noradrenaline that are normally stimulated by CRF were significantly higher in the offspring of the low LG-ABN offspring.[35] Noradrenaline serves as a major stimulus in the PVNh for the synthesis and release of CRF, and the activation of HPA responses to stress.

Maternal care during the first week of life is associated with stable individual differences in $GABA_A$ receptor subunit expression in brain regions that regulate stress reactivity. The adult offspring of high LG-ABN mothers show significantly higher levels of $GABA_A$/BZ receptor binding in the basolateral and central nuclei of the amygdala as well as the locus coeruleus. These findings provide a mechanism for increased GABAergic inhibition of amygdala–locus coeruleus activity. Importantly, maternal care also affects the behavioral sensitivity to acute BZ administration.[36] A series of *in situ* hybridization studies[7] illustrate the molecular mechanism for these differences in receptor binding and suggest that variations in maternal care might actually permanently alter the subunit composition of the $GABA_A$ receptor complex in the offspring. The offspring of the high LG-ABN mothers show increased levels of the mRNAs for the $\gamma 1$ and $\gamma 2$ subunits, which contribute to the formation of a functional BZ binding site. Such differences are not unique to the γ subunits. Levels of mRNA for the $\alpha 1$ subunit of the $GABA_A$/BZ receptor complex are significantly higher in the amygdala and locus coeruleus of high compared with low LG-ABN offspring. The $\alpha 1$ subunit appears to confer higher affinity for GABA, providing the most efficient form of the $GABA_A$ receptor complex, through increased receptor affinity for GABA. The adult offspring of the low LG-ABN mothers actually show increased expression of the mRNAs for the $\alpha 3$ and $\alpha 4$ subunits in the amygdala and the locus coeruleus. Interestingly, $GABA_A$/CBZ receptor composed of the $\alpha 3$ and $\alpha 4$ subunits show a reduced affinity for GABA, in comparison with the $\alpha 1$ subunit. Moreover, the $\alpha 4$ subunit does not contribute to the formation of a BZ receptor site. These differences in subunit expression are tissue-specific; no such differences are apparent in the hippocampus, hypothalamus or cortex. Thus, differences in $GABA_A$/BZ receptor binding are not simply due to a deficit in subunit expression in the offspring of the low LG-ABN mothers, but of an apparently 'active' attempt to maintain a specific $GABA_A$/BZ receptor profile in selected brain regions.

Taken together with the findings from earlier handling studies, the results of these studies suggest that the behavior of the mother towards her offspring can 'program' behavioral and neuroendocrine responses to stress in adulthood. These effects are associated with sustained changes in the expression of genes in brain regions that mediate responses to stress, and form the basis for stable individual differences in stress reactivity. These findings provide a potential mechanism for the influence of parental care on vulnerability/resistance to stress-induced illness over the lifespan.

CROSS-FOSTERING STUDIES: EVIDENCE FOR DIRECT MATERNAL EFFECTS

Individual differences in behavioral and neuroendocrine responses to stress in the rat are associated with naturally occurring variations in maternal care. Such effects might serve as a possible mechanism by which selected traits might be transmitted from one generation to another. Indeed, low LG-ABN mothers are more fearful in response to stress than are high LG-ABN dams.[37] Individual differences in stress reactivity are apparently transmitted across generations: fearful mothers beget more stress reactive offspring. The obvious question is whether the transmission of these traits occurs only as a function of genomic-based inheritance. If this is the case, then the differences in maternal behavior may simply be an epiphenomenon, and not causally related to the development of individual differences in stress responses. The issue is not one of inheritance, but the mode of inheritance.

The results of recent studies provide evidence for a nongenomic transmission of individual differences in stress reactivity and maternal behavior.[38] One study involved a reciprocal cross-fostering of the offspring of low and high LG-ABN mothers. The primary concern here was that the wholesale fostering of litters between mothers is known to affect maternal behavior.[39] To avert this problem and maintain the original character of the host litter, no more than 2 of 12 pups were fostered into or from any one litter.[40] The critical groups of interest are the biological offspring of low LG-ABN mothers fostered onto high LG-ABN dams, and vice versa. The limited cross-fostering design did not result in any effect on group differences in maternal behavior. Hence, the frequency of pup licking/grooming and ABN across all groups of high LG-ABN mothers was significantly higher than that for any of the low LG-ABN dams regardless of litter composition.

The results of the behavioral studies are consistent with the idea that variations in maternal care are causally related to individual differences in the behavior of the offspring. The biological offspring of low LG-ABN dams reared by high LG-ABN mothers were significantly less fearful under conditions of novelty than were the offspring reared by low LG-ABN mothers, including the biological offspring of high LG-ABN mothers.[38] Subsequent studies reveal similar findings for hippocampal glucocorticoid receptor expression and for the differences in both the $\alpha 1$ and γ2 GABA$_A$ receptor subunit expression in the amygdala. These findings suggest that individual differences in patterns of gene expression and behavior can be directly linked to maternal care over the first week of life.

MOLECULAR BASIS FOR THE EFFECT OF MATERNAL CARE ON HPA RESPONSES TO STRESS

Both postnatal handling, which increases maternal licking/grooming, and increased levels of licking/grooming, increase serotonin (5HT) turnover in the hippocampus in day 6 rat pups.[41,42] Interestingly, postnatal handling results in specific increases in 5HT in the hippocampus and prefrontal cortex, where glucocorticoid receptor expression is increased.[42] Serotonin levels in the hypothalamus, septum, and amygdala are unaffected and glucocorticoid receptor levels in these regions are not altered by handling.

In vitro, the treatment of primary hippocampal cell cultures with 5HT increases glucocorticoid receptor expression and this effect is mediated by 5HT7 receptor activation.[41,43–45] The 5HT7 receptor is positively coupled to cAMP and glucocorticoid receptor expression in cultured hippocampal neurons is significantly increased after treatment with 8-bromo cAMP or with various doses of the specific 5-HT7 receptor agonist, 5-carboxamidotryptamine (5-CT) for 4 days. The effect of 5-CT is blocked by methiothepin and 5-CT produces a significant increase in cAMP levels, which is also blocked by methiothepin. These results further implicate the 5HT7 receptor. Agonists of the 5HT1A receptor have no effect on glucocorticoid receptor expression.[44] The increase in glucocorticoid receptor expression is also mimicked with 5-methoxytryptamine (5-MeOT); an effect blocked with methiothepin as well as H8, an inhibitor of PKA (cyclic nucleotide-dependent protein kinase). Over the course of these studies we found that other serotonergic agonists (quipazine, TFMPP, DOI) partially mimicked the 5HT effect on GR levels; however, this was the first evidence that a more selective serotonergic agonist, 5-CT, could fully mimic the 5HT effect. Across all studies, the magnitude of the serotonergic effect on cAMP concentrations is highly correlated ($r = 0.97$) with that on glucocorticoid receptor expression.[46] This observation is consistent with the idea that the effect of 5HT on glucocorticoid receptor expression in hippocampal neurons is mediated by a 5HT7 receptor via activation of cAMP.

Importantly, the increase in glucocorticoid receptor binding capacity following 5HT treatment persists following 5HT removal from the medium; for as long as the cultures can be maintained, there is a sustained increase in glucocorticoid receptor levels as long as 50 days beyond the removal of 5HT from the medium. Thus, 5HT can act directly on hippocampal neurons to increase glucocorticoid receptor expression and the effect of 5HT on glucocorticoid receptor density observed in hippocampal culture cells mimics the long-term, 'programming' effects of early environmental events.

Activation of cAMP pathways regulates gene transcription through effects on a number of transcription factors, including of course, the cAMP-response element binding protein (CREB) via an enhanced phosphorylation of CREB. pCREB regulates gene transcription through pathways that involve the transcriptional cofactor, CREB-binding protein (CBP). Primary hippocampal cell cultures treated with 8-bromo cAMP, 5-CT or 5-HT show a significant increase in CBP expression.

In vivo, both handling and increased maternal licking/grooming result in an increased level of hippocampal cAMP concentrations and the activation of PKA over the first week of postnatal life.[44] Activation of PKA results in the tissue-specific induction of a number of transcription factors. The day 6 offspring of high LG mothers or pups of the same age exposed to handling show increased hippocampal expression of NGFI-A (also known as zif-268, krox-24, egr-1, zenk, etc).[47] *In vitro*, 5HT increases NGFI-A expression in cultured hippocampal neurons and the effect of 5HT on glucocorticoid receptor expression in hippocampal cultures is completely blocked by concurrent treatment with an oligonucleotide anti-sense directed at the NGFI-A mRNA.[48]

These studies suggest that maternal licking/grooming results in an increased expression of NGFI-A, which in turn might then regulate glucocorticoid receptor expression. Other rodent models examining environmental regulation of hippocampal glucocorticoid receptor expression also suggest a correspondence between NGFI-A levels and glucocorticoid receptor expression.[49] In each case, increased levels of NGFI-A are associated with enhanced glucocorticoid receptor expression. However, the critical site for glucocorticoid receptor regulation remained to be defined.

We assumed that a potential target for regulation is the promoter region of the glucocorticoid receptor gene. We identified and characterized several new glucocorticoid receptor mRNAs cloned from rat hippocampus.[50] All encode a common protein, but differ in their 5′-leader sequences, presumably as a consequence of alternative splicing of, potentially, several different sequences from the 5' non-coding exon 1 region of the glucocorticoid receptor gene. Of the 10 alternate exon 1 sequences identified, four correspond to alternative exon 1 sequences previously identified in mouse, exons 1_1, 1_5, 1_9 and 1_{10}.[51,52] There is a consensus 5' splice site immediately downstream of each of these exon 1 sequences. Thus, each alternative exon 1 is spliced onto the first coding exon to create diverse glucocorticoid receptor mRNAs. Most alternative exons are located in a 3-kb CpG island upstream of exon 2 that exhibits substantial promoter activity in transfected cells. Ribonuclease protection assays demonstrate significant levels of six alternative exon 1 sequences *in vivo* in the rat, with differential expression in the liver, hippocampus, and thymus, presumably reflecting tissue-specific differences in promoter activity. Hippocampal RNA contains significant levels of the exon 1_7-containing glucocorticoid receptor mRNA variants expressed at undetectable levels in liver and thymus.

In transient transfection experiments, a construct encoding the whole CpG island of the glucocorticoid receptor gene, including eight of the alternate exon 1 sequences, fused to a luciferase reporter gene within exon 2, exhibited substantial promoter activity in all cell lines tested.[50] This activity results from transcripts originating at any point within the CpG island and, we presume, represents the sum of the activity of individual promoters on the genomic DNA fragment. Promoter activity is also associated with particular regions of the CpG island, where the fusion to luciferase was made within specific exon 1 sequences. In these cases, luciferase activity reflects transcription through the specific exon 1 sequences. Relative activity of these constructs in different cell types is similar with one notable exception, the exon 1_7 promoter sequence. The exon 1_7, fused to luciferase, has the highest activity of any single promoter construct in B103 and C6 cells, both of which are central nervous system (CNS)-derived. The activity of this construct is lower in hepatic cells. *In vivo*, glucocorticoid receptor mRNA transcripts containing exon 1_7 are present at significant levels in hippocampus, but absent from liver, suggesting that factors present in cells of CNS origin are responsible for transcription initiation at the promoter upstream of exon 1_7 in rat hippocampus.

Interestingly, exon 1_7 activity is altered by postnatal handling, which increases glucocorticoid receptor expression in the hippocampus. Handling selectively elevated glucocorticoid receptor mRNA containing exon 1_7; there is, for example, no effect on exon 1_{10}.[50] Predictably, maternal care also affected the expression of glucocorticoid receptor splice variants: variants containing the exon 1_7 sequence were significantly increased in the adult offspring of high LG-ABN mothers.

The CpG island of the glucocorticoid receptor gene contains GC boxes (GCGGGGGCG), which form the core consensus site for NGFI-A; indeed, there is a sequence exactly matching the consensus binding site for the family of zinc finger proteins that includes NGFI-A within exon 1_7.[53] Thus, increases in NGFI-A induced by maternal licking/grooming could increase transcription from a promoter adjacent to exon 1_7, leading to increased glucocorticoid receptor mRNA. Indeed, handling increases the binding of both NGFI-A to a promoter sequence for the human glucocorticoid receptor containing consensus sequences for both transcription factors.[54] Since neonatal handling increases maternal licking/grooming, these findings suggest that variations in maternal behavior might regulate glucocorticoid receptor expression in neonatal offspring through a 5HT-induced increase in NGFI-A expression, and the subsequent binding of NGFI-A to the exon 1_7 promoter. Recent findings support this idea, including studies using chromatin immunoprecipitation (ChIP) assay in which the *in vivo* formation of protein–DNA complexes is examined using cross-linking with paraformaldehyde perfusion and subsequently precipitated from soluble hippocampal samples using specific antibodies. Protein binding, defined by the specificity of the antibody, to specific DNA sequences is then quantified following PCR amplification with targeted primers and Southern blotting. ChIP analysis of hippocampal samples from postnatal day 6 pups reveals dramatically increased NGFI-A binding to the exon 1_7 promoter in the offspring of high compared with low LG-ABN mothers. These findings confirm that maternal care regulates the binding of NGFI-A to the exon 1_7 promoter sequence in pups.

More recent studies confirm the transactivational effect of NGFI-A at the exon 1_7 sequence. We used a co-transfection model with human embryonic kidney (HEK) cells (intentionally aiming as far from the neural target as possible) with an NGFI-A expression vector and an exon 1_7-luciferase construct. Co-transfection of the NGFI-A vector and the exon 1_7-luciferase construct resulted in a robust increase in luciferase activity, reflecting NGFI-A-induced-activation of transcription through the exon 1_7 promoter. As noted, an NGFI-A anti-sense completely blocks the effects of 5HT on glucocorticoid receptor expression in hippocampal cell cultures.[48]

These findings suggest that NGFI-A might increase glucocorticoid receptor expression in hippocampal neurons, and provide a mechanism for the effect of maternal care over the first week of life. However, while there are striking differences in NGFI-A expression in the offspring of high and low LG mothers at day 6 of postnatal life, hippocampal NGFI-A expression in adulthood is unaffected by maternal care: there is no difference in hippocampal NGFI-A expression in the adult offspring of high and low LG-ABN dams. We are thus left with the defining question of early experience studies: how are the effects of early life events sustained into adulthood?

THE EPIGENOME AND EPIGENETIC PROGRAMMING OF STRESS RESPONSES

The familiar linear models of DNA and protein–DNA interactions typically ignore the fact that most of the DNA is tightly packaged into nucleosomes that involve a close relationship between DNA wrapped around a core of histone proteins. The conformation or structure of the histone–DNA configuration regulates gene expression.[55] The relation between DNA and histone is maintained, in part, by electrostatic bonds occurring between the positively charged histones and the negatively charged DNA. This chromatin structure commonly reduces the probability of transcription factor binding to DNA and underscores the importance of enzymes that modify histone–DNA interactions. One class of such proteins, histone acetyltransferase (HAT),[56] catalyzes the acetylation of selected amino acids of histone tails that protrude from the nucleosome, most commonly the lysines or arginines of histone 3 (H3) or H4. Histone acetylation modifies the histone–DNA relation. For example, acetylation of the lysine (K) residue on H3 serves to neutralize the positively charged histone, opening the histone–DNA relationship, and facilitating transcription factor binding to DNA. Thus, H3-K9 acetylation serves as a marker of active gene transcription. Many known transcriptional cofactors, such as CBP, are HATs. Histone acetylation is dynamic and is regulated by histone deacetylases (HDACs) that block histone acetylation and suppress gene expression. Thus, chromatin structure is dynamic and subject to modification through intracellular signals that trigger either HATs or HDACs downstream.[57–59] Indeed, in addition to CBP, several known transcriptional cofactors act as histone acetylases. The study of histone acetylation provides a remarkable advance in our understanding of the dynamic and complex regulation of gene expression. Likewise, histone modifications involving methylation, phosphorylation, ribosylation, and ubiquitination can all modify chromatin structure and thus gene expression.[55]

THE CHEMISTRY OF DNA METHYLATION

In addition to chromatin, which is associated with DNA, the DNA molecule itself is chemically modified by methyl residues at the 5′ position of the cytosine rings in the sequence CG in vertebrates.[60,61] What distinguishes DNA methylation in vertebrate genomes is the fact that not all CGs are methylated in any given cell type.[65] Different CGs are methylated in different cell types, generating cell-specific patterns of methylation. Thus, the DNA methylation pattern confers cellular identity upon a genome. It was originally believed that the DNA methylation pattern is established during development and is then maintained faithfully through life by the maintenance of DNA methyltransferase.[62,63] The DNA methylation reaction was believed to be irreversible and that the only way methyl residues were lost was through replication in the absence of DNA methyltransferase, a process of passive demethylation.[60,61] This mechanism is not applicable to postmitotic tissue such as neurons in the brain. However, our recent data and findings reviewed here support an alternative model, which suggests that the DNA methylation pattern is dynamic and is an equilibrium of methylation and demethylation reactions.[64] We propose that DNA methylation is a reversible signal like any other biological signal and could therefore potentially change in response to environmental and physiological signals.[65] The notion that DNA methylation is reversible in postmitotic cells has immense implications for our understanding of the potential role of DNA methylation in marking gene expression in the brain.

The hallmark of DNA methylation is the correlation between chromatin and the DNA methylation pattern. Active chromatin is usually associated with unmethylated DNA, while inactive chromatin is associated with methylated DNA.[58,66,67] This relation between DNA methylation and chromatin structure has important implications for our understanding of the function of DNA methylation, as well as for the processes responsible for generating, maintaining, and altering DNA methylation patterns under physiological and pathological conditions. It was originally believed that DNA methylation precedes and is dominant over chromatin structure changes.[68] Methylation was thought to be generated independently of chromatin structure. Indeed, methylated DNA attracts methylated DNA binding proteins, which recruit repressor complexes containing histone deacetylases, which results in inactive chromatin.[69,70] The model positioning DNA methylation as driving chromatin inactivation is widespread and profoundly influences our understanding of how altered DNA methylation is involved in cancer. Nevertheless, there are currently data suggesting that the state of chromatin structure can also determine patterns of DNA methylation in both directions, triggering either *de novo* DNA methylation or demethylation.[71–73] These data revise the classic model of a DNA methylation pattern that is predetermined during development and is then maintained through life in favor of a more dynamic view of the DNA methylation pattern as an interface between the dynamic environment and the static genome. Thus, although DNA methylation is an extremely stable signal, it can be altered later in life when there is a sufficiently potent and consistent signal to activate the chromatin. Transient changes in chromatin structure are not accompanied by changes in DNA methylation. The DNA methylation pattern is proposed to guard the epigenome from random noise and protect it from drifting.[64,74] This relation between chromatin state and DNA methylation forms a molecular link through which environmental signals might alter DNA methylation in specific genes in post mitotic neurons. Behavioral signals trigger cellular signaling pathways whose downstream consequence is activation of *trans*-acting factors. These trans-acting factors recruit HAT to the target gene resulting in increased histone acetylation, chromatin opening and increased accessibility to DNA demethylases. Since methylation of cytosine is an extremely stable chemical bond on DNA, this modification will remain stable for years. For methylation signals to serve as stable marks, they should not be responsive to chromatin noise or short-term signals. The mechanism proposed here also allows for a reversal of the methylation mark by a similar intense change in chromatin structure later in life.[64,74] This model has important implications for our understanding of how environmental signals can stably alter glucocorticoid gene expression and how these stable marks in the genome are potentially reversible later in life by specific interventions in spite of their remarkable stability.

DNA methylation marks genes for silencing by a number of mechanisms. The first mechanism is indirect and links DNA methylation to inactive chromatin structure. A region of methylated DNA juxtaposed to regulatory regions of genes attracts different members of a family of methylated DNA binding proteins. The better-studied member of this class is MeCP2, which recruits HDACs[69,70] and histone methyltransferases[75] to methylated genes.[58,76] This results in a modification of chromatin around the gene precipitating an inactive chromatin structure. A different mechanism, which is relevant to our discussion here, involves direct inter-ference of a specific methylated CG residing within a cis recognition sequence for a transcription factor with the interaction of a transcription factor, such as the inhibition of binding of cMyc to its recognition element when it is methylated.[77] The methylated cytosine essentially serves as a mutation of the recognition element. A third mechanism involves a combination of binding of a methylated DNA binding protein and inhibition of activity of a transcription factor.[78] While the first mechanism is dependent on the general density of methyl cytosines within the region associated with a gene rather than methylation of a specific CG, the second mechanism requires a discrete methylation event and is relevant to the mechanism proposed here.

The important consideration is the stability of cytosine methylation, which is preserved by covalent carbon-carbon bonds and could serve, therefore, as a long-term memory of early life behavioral signaling, leading to chromatin activation of the glucocorticoid receptor promoter in offspring of high LG-ABN mothers and a lack of chromatin activation in low LG-ABN mothers. DNA methylation changes might provide *one* mechanism for environmental programming effects occurring in early development. Glucocorticoid receptor gene expression is increased throughout the hippocampus in the adult offspring of high compared with low LG-ABN mothers.[5] The exon 1_7 glucocorticoid receptor promoter sequence appears to be significantly more active in the adult offspring of high compared with low LG-ABN mothers and was therefore the focus of initial studies of possible maternal effects on DNA methylation. We examined the level of methylation across the entire exon 1_7 glucocorticoid receptor promoter sequence in the hippocampus using the sodium bisulfite mapping technique in the adult offspring of high and low LG-ABN mothers.[32] Sodium bisulfite (NaBis) treatment of DNA samples converts nonmethylated cytosines to uracils, which are then detected as thymidine on subsequent sequencing gels.[79] Methylated cytosines are unaffected by NaBis and the differences in methylation status are thus apparent and easily quantifiable on sequencing gels. We found significantly greater methylation of the exon 1_7 glucocorticoid receptor promoter sequence in the offspring of the low LG-ABN mothers. These findings are consistent with the hypothesis that maternal effects alter DNA methylation patterns in the offspring.

To determine whether DNA methylation of specific target sites on the glucocorticoid receptor promoter changes in response to maternal care, we mapped the differences in methylation using the NaBis mapping technique, focusing on a region around the NGFI-A consensus sequence within the exon 1_7 promoter. The results reveal significant differences in the methylation of specific regions of the exon 1_7 glucocorticoid receptor promoter sequence. Notably, the cytosine within the 5′ CpG dinucleotide of the NGFI-A consensus sequence is always methylated in the offspring of low LG-ABN mothers, and rarely methylated in the offspring of high LG-ABN dams. This is consistent with site-specific DNA methylation silencing of the GR promoter.

To directly examine a causal relation between maternal behavior and DNA methylation changes within the exon 1_7 glucocorticoid receptor promoter, we performed an adoption study[32] in which the biological offspring of high or low LG-ABN mothers were cross-fostered to either high or low dams within 12 hours of birth (as described above).[7,38] This experiment examined a purely genetic or a prenatal basis for the variation in DNA methylation in the offspring of high LG-ABN versus low LG-ABN mothers. Cross-fostering the biological offspring of high or low LG-ABN mothers produced a pattern of exon 1_7 glucocorticoid receptor promoter methylation associated with the rearing mother. The cross-fostering procedure reverses the difference in methylation at specific cytosines. The cytosine within the 5′ CpG dinucleotide of the NGFI-A consensus sequence is hypomethylated following cross-fostering of offspring of low LG-ABN to high LG-ABN dams, with no effect at the cytosine within the 3′ CpG dinucleotide. Thus, the pattern of methylation of the cytosine within the 5′ CpG dinucleotide of the NGFI-A consensus sequence within the exon 1_7 glucocorticoid receptor promoter of the biological offspring of low LG-ABN mothers cross-fostered to high LG-ABN dams is indistinguishable from that of the biological offspring of high LG-ABN mothers. The reverse is true for the offspring of high LG-ABN mothers fostered to low LG-ABN dams. Interestingly, cross-fostering does not have the same effect on the CpG methylation status on each individual dinucleotide in the exon 1_7 sequence. For example, the CpG dinucleotide of the AP-1 consensus sequence within the exon 1_7 glucocorticoid receptor promoter of the biological offspring of high LG-ABN mothers cross-fostered to low LG-ABN dams remains hypomethylated. In contrast, the CpG dinucleotide of the AP-1 consensus sequence within the exon 1_7 glucocorticoid receptor promoter of the biological offspring of low LG-ABN mothers cross-fostered to high LG-ABN dams remains hypermethylated. The molecular basis for such selectivity is unknown. These findings suggest that variations in maternal care alter the methylation status within specific sites of the exon 1_7 promoter of

the glucocorticoid receptor gene and represent the first demonstration of a DNA methylation pattern established through a behavioral mode of programming. Parental imprinting,[80] a well-established paradigm of inheritance of an epigenomic mark, requires germ-line transmission.[59,63]

SITE-SPECIFIC METHYLATION OF THE NGFI-A SITE BLOCKS NGFI-A BINDING

DNA methylation affects gene expression either by attracting methylated DNA binding proteins to a densely methylated region of a gene or by site-specific interference with the binding of a transcription factor to its recognition element.[58,76] Our data showing site-specific demethylation of the cytosine within the 5′ CpG dinucleotide of the NGFI-A response element are consistent with the hypothesis that methylation at this site interferes with the binding of NGFI-A protein to its binding site. To address this question, we determined the *in vitro* binding of increasing concentrations of purified recombinant NGFI-A protein[81] to its response element under different states of methylation using the electrophilic mobility shift assay (EMSA) technique with four ^{32}P-labeled synthetic oligonucleotide sequences bearing the NGFI-A binding site that was: a) nonmethylated, b) methylated in the 3′ CpG site, c) methylated in the 5′ CpG site, d) methylated in both sites, or e) mutated at the two CpGs with an adenosine replacing the cytosines. NGFI-A formed a protein–DNA complex with the nonmethylated oligonucleotide, while the protein was unable to form a complex with either a fully methylated sequence or a sequence methylated at the 5′ CpG site. NGFI-A binding to its reponse element was reduced only slightly with the sequence methylated at the 3′ CpG site. The effect of selective cytosine methylation on NGFI-A binding was further confirmed by competition experiments. NGFI-A recombinant protein was incubated with a labeled, nonmethylated oligonucleotide in the presence of increasing concentrations of nonlabeled oligonucleotides containing the NGFI-A consensus sequence that were either 3′ CpG methylated, 5′ CpG methylated, methylated at both sites, or mutated at the two CpGs with an adenosine replacing the cytosines. The nonmethylated oligonucleotide completely eliminates the formation of labeled oligonucleotide protein–DNA complex, while the mutated oligonucleotide is unable to compete away the labeled oligonucleotide protein–DNA complex. Neither the oligonucleotide methylated in both the 3′ and 5′ CpGs nor the 5′ CpG methylated oligonucleotide were able to compete. Importantly, the

3' CpG methylated oligonucleotide – which mimics the sequence observed in the offspring of high LG-ABN mothers – exhibited substantial competition, suggesting that binding activity is retained despite the methylation at this site. The results indicate that while methylation of the cytosine within the 5' CpG dinucleotide reduces NGFI-A protein binding to the same extent as methylation in both CpG sites, methylation of the cytosine within the 3' CpG dinucleotide only partially reduces NGFI-A protein binding. These data support the hypothesis that methylation of the cytosine within the 5' CpG dinucleotide in the NGFI-A response element of the exon 1_7 glucocorticoid receptor promoter region in the offspring of low LG-ABN mothers inhibits NGFI-A protein binding.

This finding is important for our understanding of the processes by which maternal care programs hippocampal glucocorticoid receptor expression and thus HPA responses to stress. While there are substantial differences in NGFI-A expression between the offspring of high and low LG-ABN mothers in early postnatal life, no such differences are apparent in adulthood. Our hypothesis is that the cytosine methylation in the binding site for NGFI-A interferes with NGFI-A binding to the GR exon 1_7 promoter. We predicted, therefore, that the lower cytosine methylation in the adult offspring of high compared to low LG-ABN mothers would result in greater NGFI-A binding to the exon 1_7 promoter. This prediction was confirmed using a ChIP assay examining *in vivo* formation of protein–DNA complexes in hippocampal tissue from adult animals.[32] Animals were perfused with paraformaldehyde to fix protein–DNA complexes at the time of sacrifice. NGFI-A-bound DNA complexes were then immunoprecipitated using a selective antibody. The protein–DNA complexes were uncrosslinked, and the precipitated genomic DNA was subjected to PCR amplification with primers specific for the exon 1_7 glucocorticoid receptor promoter sequence. The results indicated a three-fold greater binding of NGFI-A protein to the hippocampal exon 1_7 glucocorticoid receptor promoter in the adult offspring of high compared with low LG-ABN mothers. Using the same tissue samples and an antibody against the acetylated form of H3, we also found dramatically increased acetylated H3 association with the exon 1_7 glucocorticoid receptor promoter in the offspring of the high LG-ABN mothers. As described above, histone acetylation is associated with active states of gene expression. These findings are therefore consistent with the idea of increased NGFI-A binding to the exon 1_7 promoter, and increased transcriptional activation.

We confirmed that DNA methylation inhibits the ability of NGFI-A to activate the exon 1_7 promoter in isolation from other potential differences between adult offspring of high and low LG-ABN dams using a transient co-transfection assay in human HEK 293 cells. These cells are not of hippocampal origin and thus allow us to measure the transcriptional consequences of interaction of NGFIA with either a methylated or non-methylated version of the GR exon 1_7 promoter *per se*. While transfection of HEK cells containing an exon 1_7-luciferase reporter construct with an NGFI-A expression vector significantly increases luciferase activity, this effect is dramatically reduced if the CpG dinucleotides within the exon 1_7 sequence are methylated. Moreover, the effect of NGFI-A on transcription through an exon 1_7-luciferase reporter construct was almost completely abolished with a point mutation at the 5' cytosine (a cytosine to adenosine mutation). Taken together, these findings suggest that an 'epimutation' at a single cytosine within the NGFI-A consensus sequence alters the binding of NGFI-A and might therefore explain the sustained effect of maternal care on hippocampal glucocorticoid receptor expression and HPA responses to stress.

HOW DOES MATERNAL CARE ALTER CYTOSINE METHYLATION?

Maternal behavior could either inhibit *de novo* methylation or stimulate demethylation. To address this question, we performed a developmental study of the methylation pattern of GR exon 1_7 promoter from embryonic day 20 to day 90. High and low LG-ABN mothers differ in the frequency of pup licking/grooming and ABN only during the first week of life. Importantly, this period corresponds to the appearance of the difference in DNA methylation in the offspring in studies using NaBis mapping to precisely map the methylation status of the cytosines within the exon 1_7 glucocorticoid receptor promoter over multiple developmental time points. This analysis demonstrates that just before birth, on embryonic day 20, the entire exon 1_7 region is unmethylated in both groups. Strikingly, 1 day following birth (postnatal day 1) the exon 1_7 glucocorticoid receptor promoter is *de novo* methylated in both groups. The 5' and 3' CpG sites of the exon 1_7 glucocorticoid receptor NGFI-A response element in the offspring of both high and low LG-ABN mothers, which exhibit differential methylation later in life, are *de novo* methylated to the same extent. These data show that both the basal state of methylation and the first wave of *de novo* methylation after birth occur similarly in both groups. Whereas it is generally accepted that DNA methylation patterns are formed prenatally and that *de novo* methylation occurs early in development, there is at least one documented example of postnatal *de novo* methylation of the HoxA5 and HoxB5 genes.[82] Since similar analyses have not been documented for other genes, it is unknown yet whether changes in methylation are common around birth or whether they are unique to this glucocorticoid receptor promoter. One aspect of these findings that is important is that of the complete absence of cytosine methylation on embryonic day 20. Since the majority of the pyramidal cells of Ammon's horn are created between embryonic day 16 and 20, it seems unlikely that methylation patterns, at least on the exon 1_7 promoter of the glucocorticoid receptor, are generated at the time of DNA replication and cell division, as would normally be the case with imprinted genes.

The differences in the status of methylation of the exon 1_7 glucocorticoid receptor between the two groups emerges between postnatal day 1 and 6, which is precisely the period when differences in the maternal behavior of high and low LG-ABN dams are apparent. There are no differences in maternal licking/grooming between high and low LG-ABN mothers beyond day 8.[30,33] By postnatal day 6, the 5′ CpG dinucleotide of the NGFI-A response element is demethylated in the high, but not in the low LG-ABN group. These findings are consistent with data from the cross-fostering experiment, which illustrates that the differences between the two groups developed following birth in response to maternal behavior. The group difference in CpG dinucleotide methylation then remains consistent through to adulthood. Our findings suggest that the group difference in DNA methylation occurs as a function of maternal behavior over the first week of life. The results of earlier studies indicated that the first week of postnatal life is indeed a 'critical period' for the effects of early experience on hippocampal glucocorticoid receptor expression.[83]

REVERSAL OF THE MATERNAL EFFECT ON GR EXPRESSION AND HPA RESPONSES TO STRESS.

These findings suggest that maternal behavior produces an active demethylation process at selected and presumably targeted sites. The resulting demethylation of the 5′ CpG dinucleotide within the NGFI-A response element of the exon 1_7 promoter enhances NGFI-A binding, increasing GR gene transcription and HPA responses to stress.

These findings beg the question of how maternal high LG-ABN might activate a demethylation of the GR exon 1_7 promoter. As discussed above, a testable

working hypothesis is that high LG-ABN leads to activation of NGFI-A as a downstream effector of activation of 5HT signaling through increased CAMP and PKA. Increased NGFI-A increases the frequency of occupancy of the GR exon 1_7 promoter. NGFI-A interaction with the GR exon 1_7 promoter leads to increased acetylation and increased accessibility of the GR exon 1_7 promoter to demethylase resulting in DNA demethylation. This hypothesis predicts that pharmacological activation of chromatin using HDAC inhibitors should result in activation of GR exon 1_7 promoter demethylation. However, the question is whether this reversibility will be limited to early life exclusively or whether it is possible to reverse these alterations later in life as well if the appropriate signals to activate the chromatin structure are applied or by a pharmacological activation of chromatin structure.

Our hypothesis is that the DNA methylation is a steady state of DNA methylation and demethylation in which direction is determined by the state of chromatin structure.[64,74] This hypothesis predicts that both DNMTs and demethylases are present in adult neurons and that if the chromatin state is altered by either persistent physiological or pharmacological signals one should be able to change the state of methylation of a gene in postmitotic tissue such as adult hippocampal neurons. We previously established that pharmacological activation of chromatin structure by HDAC inhibitors could trigger replication-independent active demethylation of DNA.[71–73] We tested our hypothesis that the demethylation of the GR exon 1_7 promoter is driven by histone acetylation and could be activated in adult neurons. This understanding leads to an obvious prediction: HDAC inhibition should reverse the effects of cytosine methylation on NGFI-A binding to the exon 1_7 promoter, GR expression and HPA responses to stress. We tested this idea with central infusion of adult offspring of high or low LG/ABN mothers with the HDAC inhibitor, trichostatin A (TSA), for 4 consecutive days. As expected, ChIP assays revealed that TSA infusion significantly increased the level of acetylated H3 at the exon 1_7 site (i.e. HDAC inhibition resulted in increased histone acetylation) in the offspring of low LG/ABN mothers to levels comparable to those observed in the offspring of high LG-ABN mothers. The increased histone acetylation is associated with enhanced NGFI-A binding to the exon 1_7 promoter sequence and completely eliminates the effect of maternal care. As expected, enhanced NGFI-A binding to the exon 1_7 promoter increased hippocampal glucocorticoid receptor expression. Hippocampal glucocorticoid receptor expression in the TSA-treated adult offspring of low LG/ABN mothers is indistinguishable from that of the high LG-ABN groups. Most important, TSA infusion also eliminates the effect of maternal care on HPA responses to stress. During and following exposure to acute stress, plasma corticosterone levels in TSA-treated offspring of low LG-ABN mothers are indistinguishable from those of TSA- or vehicle-treated high LG-ABN mothers. There was no effect of TSA on any measure in the offspring of high LG/ABN animals. This is understandable, since under normal circumstances, there is considerable H3 acetylation and NGFI-A binding at the exon 1_7 sequence in these animals.

These findings have important implications for our understanding of the mechanisms linking early maternal behavior and stable changes in behavior later in adulthood, as well as for our understanding of the mechanisms responsible for maintaining the DNA methylation pattern in adult postmitotic tissues. First, our data support the idea that demethylation is driven by activation of chromatin and that HDAC inhibitors produce demethylation even in nondividing cells (i.e. in a replication-independent manner). Second, our data are consistent with the hypothesis that the demethylation of GR exon 1_7 in offspring of high LG-ABN rats early after birth is driven by increased histone acetylation as discussed above. Third, these data provide the first evidence that molecular mechanisms that underlie the effects of early life experience on neural function are potentially reversible in adulthood. This consideration has obvious social and therapeutic implications. Fourth, these data provide the first *in vivo* evidence for our hypothesis that the DNA methylation pattern is dynamic even in postmitotic tissues and that its steady state is maintained by the state of chromatin acetylation.[64] Finally, our data provide a general mechanism for how external signals could change the DNA methylation pattern and thus the chemistry of the genome itself even during adulthood.

MOLECULAR MECHANISMS LINKING MATERNAL BEHAVIOR AND ACTIVE DEMETHYLATION

The data discussed above support the hypothesis that histone acetylation could produce active demethylation of the GR exon 1_7 promoter, yet several questions remain unanswered. How, for example, is histone acetylation targeted to the exon 1_7 promoter as a consequence of maternal behavior? We propose that maternal behavior stimulates 5HT, which stimulates NGFI-A, and that NGFI-A then targets HATS and eventually demethylases to the GR exon 1_7 promoter.

To dissect the different molecular components of this hypothesis we took advantage of both hippocampal primary neuronal cell cultures and non-neuronal cell lines. The two systems have different strengths and could be used to test different components of the model. First, we tested the hypothesis that 5HT acts through cAMP to produce hypomethylation. Hippocampal cell cultures treated with either 5HT or 8-bromo-cAMP, a stable cAMP analog, show increased glucocorticoid receptor expression following 4 days of treatment. Treatment of hippocampal cells in culture with 5HT also results in the hypomethylation of the 5′ CpG dinucleotide of the NGFI-A consensus sequence within the exon 1_7 promoter of the glucocorticoid receptor gene, with no effect at the 3′ site. Treatment with 8-bromo-cAMP produces an even more pronounced effect on cytosine methylation at the 5′ CpG site. In both studies, cultures maintained under control conditions show complete methylation of both the 5′ and 3′ CpG sites of the NGFI-A consensus sequence. Bromo-deoxyuridine (BrdU) labeling, which marks newly generated cells, reveals little or no cell replication in the cultures at the time of 5HT treatment. These findings reinforce the idea that the alterations in cytosine methylation occur independently of cell replication and in response to intracellular signals associated with variations in maternal care. These cells establish that 5HT signaling induced by maternal care triggers replication-independent changes in methylation of GR exon 1_7 promoter through an increase in cAMP. Since increased cAMP activates NGFI-A, it seems that ectopic expression of NGFI-A can target the demethylation process to the GR exon 1_7 promoter. However, this would not explain the selective effect at the 5′ cytosine.

To test the hypothesis that NGFI-A targets demethylation to GR exon 1_7 promoter, we resorted to non-neuronal cell line HEK 293. Here we can isolate the direct effect of NGFI-A from other neuron-specific events that might confound the interpretation of data from the hippocampal cultures. By comparing the fate of a transiently transfected methylated GR exon 1_7 promoter-luciferase vector in the presence and absence of NGFI-A, we could better determine the specific effects of NGFI-A on demethylation. Since the nonintegrated plasmid does not bear an origin of replication and does not replicate in HEK 293 cells, the assay measures the effects of NGFI-A on active replication-independent demethylation. Whereas *in vitro* methylated GR exon 1_7 promoter-luciferase vector remains methylated in HEK 293 cells, co-expression of NGFI-A results in active demethylation of a significant fraction of the transfected plasmids. To demonstrate that this DNA demethylation requires direct contact between NGFI-A and its recognition element, we performed site-directed mutagenesis of the two CGs included in the NGFI-A recognition element. Our preliminary results suggest that these manipulations abolished the ability of NGFI-A to activate and demethylate the GR exon 1, promoter (Weaver et al., unpublished data, 2005). These experiments provide a molecular mechanism on how demethylation is triggered to specific sequences. The outstanding question is to determine how NGFI-A triggers demethylation upon binding to specific sequences. One possibility is that NGFI-A directly recruits a demethylase to the gene or that, as proposed before, it recruits a HAT which increases acetylation, thus increasing the accessibility to demethylase as proposed before.[71–73]

The results of the studies with hippocampal cell cultures, the HEK 293 cells, and the developmental time course study, suggest a process of active demethylation. In the developmental studies, the 5′ CpG site is initially methylated to the same extent in the offspring of high and low LG-ABN mothers. Over the course of the first week following birth, the methylation mark is functionally removed from the 5′ site in the offspring of high LG-ABN mothers. Prevailing models of DNA methylation propose that the methylation pattern of newly synthesized DNA is exclusively determined by the methylation pattern of the parental strand, and thus is thought to be preserved in somatic cells. This model cannot explain the data described here, nor recent data demonstrating demethylation in response to changes in chromatin structure, such as those induced by TSA.[72] Szyf and colleagues[65,84,85] proposed that DNA methylation is enzymatically reversible and that DNA methylation is dynamic in fully differentiated cells. This idea remains controversial. Active demethylation was nevertheless clearly demonstrated early in embryogenesis and the parental genome undergoes replication-independent, active demethylation hours after fertilization, well before the initiation of replication. Demethylation at very early stages in development has been relatively accepted, but the possibility of postnatal demethylation, and especially in fully differentiated somatic cells, has been hotly disputed. However, active replication demethylation was demonstrated in Epstein–Barr virus (EBV)-infected B cells and more recently it was repeatedly demonstrated in HEK 293 cells. The HEK 293 transient transfection provided direct evidence that active replication-independent demethylation takes place in somatic cells and that it is dependent on chromatin state. Fully *in vitro* methylated plasmid is transiently transfected into the cells. The plasmid, which does not bear an origin of replication, does not replicate in these cells and that has been validated using a *DpnI* restriction

analysis.[72] Upon treatment of the cells with TSA, the plasmid undergoes complete demethylation that could only be accomplished by a processive demethylase. A recent paper on altered expression of interleukin (IL)-2 expression by T lymphocytes following activation clearly implicates an active process of demethylation in a normal nontransformed somatic cell. Bruniquel and Schwartz[86] found that a region in a promoter of the IL-2 gene demethylates following activation in the absence of DNA replication and results in a profound increase in the production of IL-2. Our results[32] are the first demonstration of active demethylation in postmitotic neurons *in vivo*.

Earlier studies from Szyf's laboratory extracted active DNA demethylase activity from a human lung cancer cell line[65] and identified a protein with demethylase activity,[85] which was cloned concurrently by Bird's group and named MBD2.[87] Interestingly, the protein, MBD2, was found by Bird's group and others to also associate with a chromatin remodeling complex containing HDAC, which is involved in silencing of gene expression through the recruitment of a repressor complex. The assignment of a demethylase (dMTase) function to a protein that was independently discovered as a recruiter of repressor complexes triggered the expected controversy in the field and reports that MBD2 failed to produce demethylase activity. However, the observation that MBD2/dMTase expression produces the demethylation of some but not all promoters in a dose- and time-dependent manner has been confirmed.[88,89] Clearly, the contextual factors that determine MBD2 demethylase activity remain to be fully explained. Interestingly, MBD2 increased gene expression in those instances where promoter demethylation occurred, suggesting that not all promoters respond in the same orderly manner. Indeed, the same is true for DNA methylation, which impedes the DNA binding of most, but not all transcription factors; SP1 binds to methylated DNA. Anti-sense knock-down of MBD2 resulted in inhibition of active demethylation induced by valproate and caused hypermethylation and silencing of the prometastatic gene uPA in metastatic breast cancer cells. Another group reported that ectopic expression of MBD2/dMTase in a hepatocyte cell line caused demethylation and activation of the hexokinase type 2 gene.[90] Additional support for the demethylase activity of MBD2/dMTase emerges from the finding that expression of MBD2/dMTase is correlated with demethylation within the promoters of *C-ERBB-2* and *SURVIVIN* genes in ovarian cancers[91,92] and hypomethylated *CMYC* in gastric cancer.[93] In addition, the *Drosophila* homolog of MBD2, dMBD2/3, formed foci that associated with DNA at the cellular blastoderm stage, concurrent with the activation of the embryonic genome, and also associated with the active Y chromosome.[94]

To test the hypothesis that MBD2 is associated with maternally induced demethylation, we performed an *in situ* hybridization assay with probes for the mRNAs for a number of methylated binding proteins at day 6 postpartum. Our analysis revealed that MBD2/dMTase expression is elevated in the hippocampus at this point in time in offspring of high versus low LG-ABN mothers. A ChIP analysis with an antiMBD2/dMTase antibody demonstrates significantly increased binding of MBD2/dMTase to the exon 1$_7$ GR promoter in day 6 offspring of high versus low LG-ABN mothers. We also found increased NGFI-A binding to the same sequence in day 6 offspring of high LG-ABN offspring. We then performed a bisulfite mapping of the state of methylation of the exon 1$_7$ GR promoter bound to MBD2 and precipitated in the ChIP assay with anti-MBD2 antibody. If MBD2 is the demethylase involved in this process, or if it is part of the demethylase complex, then MBD2-bound exon 1$_7$ sequences at day 6 should be found in the process of demethylation. Indeed, most of the MBD2-bound DNA was unmethylated or partially unmethylated.

In summary, our findings suggest that shortly after birth, there is a wave of *de novo* methylation that results in the methylation of both CpG sites within the NGFI-A consensus sequence. Such events would impede the binding of NGFI-A to the exon 1$_7$ promoter. However, in the offspring of the high LG-ABN mothers, NGFI-A expression is increased to the point where binding occurs despite the 'low affinity' status of the binding site. The binding of NGFI-A is associated with histone acetylation and the subsequent availability of the site to demethylase. In support of this idea, the treatment of the adult offspring of the low LG-ABN mothers with TSA increases H3 acetylation and NGFI-A binding (see above) and results in the demethylation of the 5′ CpG site of the NGFI-A consensus sequence.[32] While this model remains speculative (and controversial) at this time, these findings do suggest that modifications to the DNA methylation status in fully differentiated cells are clearly possible and pharmacologically reversible, an idea that holds considerable potential therapeutic implications.

EXPERIENCE-DEPENDENT CHROMATIN PLASTICITY?

The defining question of early experience studies concerns the mechanism by which environmental effects occurring in early development are 'biologically embedded' and thus sustained into adulthood (i.e. so-called 'environmental programming' effects). The offspring of high LG-ABN mothers exhibit increased hippocampal glucocorticoid receptor expression from the exon 1$_7$ promoter and dampened HPA responses to stress that persist into adulthood. We propose that the differential epigenomic status of the exon 1$_7$ glucocorticoid receptor promoter in the offspring of high LG-ABN mothers serves as a mechanism for this maternal effect. It is important to note that these findings are restricted to the study of a single promoter of but one gene in one region of the brain. The degree to which such results might generalize to other instances of environmental programming remains to be determined. Moreover, further studies are required to determine how maternal behavior alters the epigenomic status of the exon 1$_7$ glucocorticoid receptor promoter. The developmental time course study is critical. As noted, the 5′ CpG dinucleotide of the NGFI-A consensus sequence of the exon 1$_7$ promoter is methylated to the same, elevated level in the newborn offspring of high and low LG-ABN mothers. It is only over the first week of life that the difference emerges, with the decline in the methylation of the 5′ CpG site in the offspring of high, but not low LG-ABN mothers. Note, no such demethylation occurs at the neighboring 3′ CpG site. The impressive selectivity suggests a demethylation process that is targeted in some manner. It is critical to define the processes by which such apparently active demethylation might occur. Regardless of these yet unanswered questions, these findings provide the first evidence that maternal behavior stably alters the epigenome of the offspring, providing a mechanism for the long-term effects of early experience on gene expression in the adult. These studies offer an opportunity to clearly define the nature of gene–environment interactions during development and how such effects result in the sustained 'environmental programming' of gene expression and function over the lifespan. Finally, it is important to note that maternal effects on the expression of defensive responses, such as increased HPA activity, are a common theme in biology,[95] such that the magnitude of the maternal influence on the development of HPA and behavioral responses to stress in the rat should not be surprising. Maternal effects on defensive responses to threat are apparent in plants, insects, and reptiles. Such effects commonly follow from the exposure of the mother to the same or similar forms of threat and may represent examples where the environmental experience of the mother is translated through an epigenetic mechanism of inheritance into phenotypic variation in the offspring. Indeed, maternal effects could result in the transmission of adaptive responses across generations.[96] Epigenomic modifications of targeted regulatory sequences, in response to even reasonably subtle variations in environmental conditions, might serve as a major source of epigenetic variation in gene expression and function and ultimately as a process mediating such maternal effects. We propose that epigenomic changes serve as an intermediate process that imprints dynamic environmental experiences on the fixed genome resulting in stable alterations in phenotype. Such variations may then serve as a source of individual differences in vulnerability/resistance to chronic illness over the lifespan depending upon the conditions of the prevailing environment. It's a question of fit.

REFERENCES

1. Levine S. Infantile experience and resistance to physiological stress. Science 1957; 126:405–6.
2. Levine S. Plasma-free corticosteroid response to electric shock in rats stimulated in infancy. Science 1962; 135: 795–96.
3. Denenberg VH. Critical periods, stimulus input, and emotional reactivity: a theory of infantile stimulation. Psychol Rev 1964; 71:335–51.
4. Lee MHS, Williams DI. Long term changes in nest condition and pup grouping following handling of rat litters. Dev Psychobiol 1975; 8: 91–5.
5. Liu D, Tannenbaum B, Caldji C et al. Maternal care, hippocampal glucocorticoid receptor gene expression and hypothalamic-pituitary-adrenal responses to stress. Science 1997; 77: 1659–62.
6. Francis DD, Meaney MJ. Maternal care and the development of stress responses. Curr Opin Neurobiol 1999; 9: 128–34.
7. Caldji C, Diorio J, Meaney MJ. Variations in maternal care alter GABAA receptor subunit expression in brain regions associated with fear. Neuropsychopharmacology 2003; 28: 150–9.
8. Hinde RA. Some implications of evolutionary theory and comparative data for the study of human prosocial and aggressive behaviour. In: Development of Anti-social and Prosocial Behaviour. (Olweus D, Block J, Radke-Yarrow M, eds). Orlando: Academic Press, 1986: 13–32.
9. Rivier C, Plotsky PM. Mediation by corticotropin-releasing factor of adenohypophysial hormone secretion. Annu Rev Physiol 1986; 48: 475–89.
10. Plotsky PM. Pathways to the secretion of adrenocorticotropin: a view from the portal. J Neuroendocrinology 1991; 3: 1–9.
11. Antoni FA. Vasopressinergic control of pituitary adrenocorticotropin secretion comes of age. Front Neuroendocrinol 1993; 14: 76–122.
12. Whitnall MH. Regulation of the hypothalamic corticotropin-releasing hormone neurosecretory system. Prog Neurobiol 1993; 40: 573–629.
13. De Kloet ER, Vregdenhil E, Oitzl MS, Joels M. Brain corticosteroid receptor balance in health and disease. Endocrinol Rev 1998; 19: 269–301.
14. Lavicky J, Dunn AJ. Corticotropin-releasing factor stimu-

15. Emoto H, Yokoo H, Yoshida M, Tanaka M. Corticotropin-releasing factor enhances noradrenaline release in the rat hypothalamus assessed by intracerebral microdialysis. Brain Res 1993; 601: 286–8.
16. Page ME, Valentino RJ. Locus coeruleus activation by physiological challenges. Brain Res Bull 1994; 35: 557–60.
17. Valentino RJ, Curtis AL, Page ME, Pavcovich LA, Florin-Lechner SM. Activation of the locus coeruleus brain noradrenergic system during stress: circuitry, consequences, and regulation. Adv Pharmacol 1998; 42: 781–4.
18. Moga MM, Gray TS. Evidence for corticotropin-releasing factor, neurotensin, and somatostatin in the neural pathway from the central nucleus of the amygdala to the parabrachial nucleus. J Comp Neurol 1989; 241: 275–84.
19. Koegler-Muly SM, Owens MJ, Ervin GN, Kilts CD, Nemeroff CB. Potential corticotropin-releasing factor pathways in the rat brain as determined by bilateral electrolytic lesions of the central amygdaloid nucleus and paraventricular nucleus of the hypothalamus. J Neuroendocrinol 1993; 5: 95–8.
20. Van Bockstaele EJ, Colago EE, Valentino RJ. Corticotropin-releasing factor-containing axon terminals synapse onto catecholamine dendrites and may presynaptically modulate other afferents in the rostral pole of the nucleus locus coeruleus in the rat brain. J Comp Neurol. 1996; 364: 523–34.
21. Gray TS, Bingaman EW. The amygdala: corticotropin-releasing factor, steroids, and stress. Crit Rev Neurobiol 1996; 10: 155–68.
22. Butler PD, Weiss JM, Stout JC, Nemeroff CB. Corticotropin-releasing factor produces fear-enhancing and behavioural activating effects following infusion into the locus coeruleus. J Neurosci 1990; 10: 176–83.
23. Liang KC, Melia KR, Miserendino MJ et al. Corticotropin releasing factor: long-lasting facilitation of the acoustic startle reflex. J Neurosci 1992; 12: 2303–12.
24. Swiergiel AH, Takahashi LK, Kahn NH. Attenuation of stress induced by antagonism of corticotropin-releasing factor receptors in the central amygdala in the rat. Brain Res 1993; 623: 229–34.
25. Koob GF, Heinrichs SC, Menzaghi F, Pich EM, Britton KT, Corticotropin-releasing factor, stress and behavior. Semin Neurosci 1994; 6: 221–9.
26. Schulkin J, McEwen BS, Gold PW. Allostasis, the amygdala and anticipatory angst. Neurosci Biobehav Rev 1994; 18: 385–96.
27. Stenzel-Poore MP, Heinrichs SC, Rivest S, Knob GF, Vale WW. Overproduction of corticotropin-releasing factor in transgenic mice: a genetic model of anxiogenic behavior. J Neurosci 1994; 14: 2579–84.
28. Bakshi VP, Shelton SE, Kalin NH. Neurobiological correlates of defensive behaviors. Prog Brain Res 2000; 122: 105–15.
29. Davis M, Whalen PJ, The amygdala: vigilance and emotion. Mol Psychiatry 2001; 6: 13–34.
30. Champagne FA, Francis DD, Mar A, Meaney MJ. Naturally-occurring variations in maternal care in the rat as a mediating influence for the effects of environment on the development of individual differences in stress reactivity. Physiol Behav 2003; 79: 359–71.
31. Stern JM, Offspring-induced nurturance: animal-human parallels. Dev Psychobiol 1997; 31: 19–37.
32. Weaver ICG, Cervoni N, D'Alessio AC et al. Epigenetic

lates catecholamine release in hypothalamus and prefrontal cortex in freely moving rats as assessed by microdialysis. J Neurochem 1993; 60: 602–12.

programming through maternal behavior. Nature (Neuroscience) 2004; 7: 847–54.

33. Caldji C, Tannenbaum B, Sharma S et al. Maternal care during infancy regulates the development of neural systems mediating the expression of behavioral fearfulness in adulthood in the rat. Proc Natl Acad Sci 1998; 95:5335–40.

34. Owens MJ, Vargas MA, Knight DL, Nemeroff CB. The effects of alprazoplam on corticotropin-releasing factor neurons in the rat brain: acute time course, chronic treatment and abrupt withdrawal. J Pharmacol Exp Ther 1991; 258: 349–56.

35. Francis DD, Caldji CC, Champagne F, Plotsky PM, Meaney MJ. The role of corticotropin-releasing factor–norepinephrine systems in mediating the effects of early experience on the development of behavioral and dndocrine responses to stress. Biol Psychiatry 1999; 46: 1153–66

36. Fries E, Moragues N, Caldji CC, Hellhammer HH, Meaney MJ. Preliminary evidence of altered sensitivity to benzodiazepines as a function of maternal care in the rat. Ann NY Acad Sci 2004; 1032: 3204.

37. Francis DD, Champagne F, Meaney MJ. Variations in maternal behaviour are associated with differences in oxytocin receptor levels in the rat. J Neuroendocrinol 2000; 12: 1145–8.

38. Francis DD, Diorio J, Liu D, Meaney MJ. Nongenomic transmission across generations in maternal behavior and stress responses in the rat. Science 1999; 286: 1155–8.

39. Maccari S, Piazza PV, Kabbaj M, Barbazanges A, Simon H, Le Moal M. Adoption reverses the long-term impairments in glucocorticoid feedback induced by prenatal stress. J Neurosci 1995; 15:110–6.

40. McCarty R, Lee JH. Maternal influences on adult blood pressure of SHRs: a single pup cross-fostering study. Physiol Behav 1996; 59: 71–5.

41. Mitchell JB, Iny LJ, Meaney MJ. The role of serotonin in the development and environmental regulation of hippocampal type II corticosteroid receptors. Dev Brain Res 1991; 55: 231–5.

42. Smythe JW, Rowe W, Meaney MJ. Neonatal handling alters serotonin turnover and serotonin type 2 receptor density in selected brain regions, Dev Brain Res 1994; 80: 183–9.

43. Mitchell JB, Rowe W, Boksa P, Meaney MJ. Serotonin regulates type II, corticosteroid receptor binding in cultured hippocampal cells. J Neurosci 1990; 10: 1745–52.

44. Mitchell JB, Betito K, Rowe W, Boksa P, Meaney MJ. Serotonergic regulation of type II corticosteroid receptor binding in cultured hippocampal cells: the role of serotonin-induced increases in cAMP levels. Neuroscience 1992; 48: 631–9.

45. Laplante P, Diorio J, Meaney MJ. Serotonin regulates hippocampal glucocorticoid receptor expression via a 5-HT7 receptor. Brain Res Dev Brain Res 2002; 139: 199–203.

46. Meaney MJ, Diorio J, Francis DD, et al. Environmental regulation of the development of glucocorticoid receptor systems in the rat forebrain: The role of serotonin. Ann NY Acad Sci 1994; 746: 260–75.

47. Meaney MJ, Diorio J, Francis DD et al. Postnatal handling increases the expression of cAMP-inducible transcription factors in the rat hippocampus: the effects of thyroid hormones and serotonin. J Neurosci 2000; 20: 3926–35.

48. Hellstrom I, Weaver ICG, Diorio J et al. Ex vivo characterization of maternal programming of stress responses through modulation of the epigenome. Soc Neurosci Abst 2004; 23: 662.11

49. Mohammed AH, Henricksson BG, Söderström S et al. Environmental influences on the central nervous system and their implications for the aging rat. Behav Brain Res 1993; 57: 183–91.

50. McCormick JA, Lyons V, Jacobson MD et al. 5′-heterogeneity of glucocorticoid receptor messenger RNA is tissue specific: differential regulation of variant transcripts by early-life events. Mol Endocrinol 2000; 14: 506–17.

51. Chen FH, Watson CS, Gametchu B. Multiple glucocorticoid receptor transcripts in membrane glucocorticoid receptor-enriched S-49 mouse lymphoma cells. J Cell Biochem 1999; 74: 418–29.

52. Strähle U, Schmidt A, Kelsey G et al. At least three promoters direct expression of the mouse glucocorticoid receptor gene. Proc Natl Acad Sci USA 1992; 89: 6731–5.

53. Crosby SD, Puetz JJ, Simburger KS, Fahrner TJ, Milbrandt J. The early response gene NGFI-C encodes a zinc finger transcriptional activator and is a member of the GCGGGGGCG (GSG) element-binding protein family. Mol Cell Biol 1991; 11: 3835–41.

54. Diorio J, Weaver S, Meaney MJ. Postnatal handling increases NGFI-A and AP-2 binding to a glucocorticoid receptor promoter. Soc Neurosci Abst 1997; 23: 1151.

55. Turner B. Chromatin structure and the regulation of gene expression, Blackwell Sci. (2001).

56. Roth SY, Denu JM, Allis CD. Histone acetyltransferases. Annu Rev Biochem 2001; 70: 81–120.

57. Bird AP. Methylation talk between histones and DNA. Science 2001; 294: 2113–15.

58. Bird A, Wolffe AP, Methylation-induced repression – belts, braces, and chromatin. Cell 1999; 99: 451–4.

59. Li E. Chromatin modification and epigenetic reprogramming in mammalian development. Nature Rev Genet 2003; 3: 662–73.

60. Razin A, Riggs AD. DNA methylation and gene function. Science 1980; 210: 604–10.

61. Wolffe AP, Jones PL, Wade PA. DNA demethylation. Proc Natl Acad Sci USA 1999; 96: 5894–6.

62. Razin A, Szyf M, DNA methylation patterns. Formation and function. Biochim Biophys Acta 1984; 782: 331–42.

63. Reik W, Dean W, Walter J. Epigenetic reprogramming in mammalian development. Science 2000; 293: 1089–93.

64. Szyf M. Towards a pharmacology of DNA methylation. Trends Pharmacol Sci 2001; 22: 350–4.

65. Ramchandani S, Bhattacharya SK, Cervoni N, Szyf M. DNA methylation is a reversible biological signal. Proc Natl Acad Sci USA 1999; 96; 6107–12.

66. Razin A, Cedar H. Distribution of 5-methylcytosine in chromatin. Proc Natl Acad Sci USA 1977; 74: 2725–8.

67. Kadonaga JT. Eukaryotic transcription: an interlaced network of transcription factors and chromatin-modifying machines. Cell 1998; 92: 307–13.

68. Hashimshony T, Zhang J, Keshet I, Bustin M, Cedar H. The role of DNA methylation in setting up chromatin structure during development. Nat Genet 2003; 34: 187–92.

69. Nan X, Ng HH, Johnson CA et al. Transcriptional repression by the methyl-CpG-binding protein MeCP2 involves a histone deacetylase complex. Nature, 393: 386–9.

70. Jones PL, Veenstra GJ, Wade PA et al. Methylated DNA and MeCP2 recruit histone deacetylase to repress transcription. Nat Genet 1998; 19: 187–91.

71. Cervoni N, Detich N, Seo SB, Chakravarti D, Szyf M. The oncoprotein Set/TAF-1beta, an inhibitor of histone acetyltransferase, inhibits active demethylation of DNA, integrating DNA methylation and transcriptional silencing. J Biol Chem 2002; 277: 25026–31.

72. Cervoni N, Szyf M. Demethylase is directed by histone acetylation. J Biol Chem 2001; 276: 40778–87.

73. Detich N, Bovenzi V, Szyf M, Valproate induces replication-independent active DNA demethylation. J Biol Chem 2003; 278: 27586–92.

74. Szyf M, Pakneshan P, Rabbani SA. DNA methylation and breast cancer. Biochem Pharmacol 2004; 68: 1187–97.

75. Fuks F, Hurd PJ, Wolf D et al. The methyl-CpG-binding protein MeCP2 links DNA methylation to histone methylation. J Biol Chem 2003; 278: 4035–40.

76. Razin A. CpG methylation, chromatin structure and gene silencing – a three-way connection. *EMBO J* 1998; 17: 4905–8.

77. Prendergast GC, Ziff EB, Methylation-sensitive sequence-specific DNA binding by the c-myc basic region. Science 1991; 251: 186–9.

78. Kudo, S. Methyl-CpG-binding protein mecp2 represses sp1-activated transcription of the human leukosialin gene when the promoter is methylated. Mol Cell Biol 1998; 18: 5492–9.

79. Frommer M, McDonald LE, Millar DS et al. A genomic sequencing protocol that yields a positive display of 5-methylcytosine residues in individual DNA strands. Proc Natl Acad Sci USA 1992; 89: 1827–31.

80. Sapienza C. Parental imprinting of genes. Sci Am 1990; 263: 52–60.

81. Milbrandt J. A nerve growth factor-induced gene encodes a possible transcriptional regulatory factor. Science 1987; 238: 797–9.

82. Hershko AY, Kafri T, Fainsod A, Razin A. Methylation of HoxA5 and HoxB5 and its relevance to expression during mouse development. Gene 2003; 302: 65–72.

83. Meaney MJ, Aitken DH, The effects of early postnatal handling on the development of hippocampal glucocorticoid receptors: Temporal parameters. Dev Brain Res 1985; 22: 301–4.

84. Weaver ICG, Diorio J, Hellstrom I, Szyf M, Meaney MJ. Intro programming of hippocampal glucocorticoid receptor expression through 5-HT-cAMP induced demethylation of a gluccorticoid receptor promoter. Submitted.

85. Bhattacharya SK, Ramchandani S, Cervoni N, Szyf M. A mammalian protein with specific demethylase activity for mCpG DNA. Nature 1999; 397: 579–83.

86. Bruniquel D, Schwartz RH. Selective, stable demethylation of the interleukin-2 gene enhances transcription by an active process. Nature Immunl 2003; 4: 235–40.

87. Hendrich B, Bird AP. Identification and characterization of a family of mammalian methyl-cpg binding proteins. Mol Cell Biol 1998; 18: 6538–47.

88. Cervoni N, Szyf M. Demethylase is directed by histone acetylation. J Biol Chem 2001; 276: 40778–87.

89. Detich N, Theberge J, Szyf M. Promoter-specific activation and demethylation by MBD2/demethylase. J Biol Chem 2002; 277: 35791–4.

90. Goel A, Saroj P, Mathupala P, Pedersen PL. Glucose metabolism in cancer. Evidence that demethylation events play a role in activating type II hexokinase gene expression. J Biol Chem 2003; 278: 15333–40.

91. Hattori M, Sakamoto H, Yamamoto T. DNA demethylase expression correlates with lung resistance protein expression in common epithelial ovarian cancers. J Int Med Res 2001; 29: 204–13.

92. Hattori M, Sakamoto H, Satoh K, Yamamoto T. DNA demethylase is expressed in ovarian cancers and the expression correlates with demethylation of CpG sites in the promoter region of c-erbB-2 and survivin genes. Cancer Lett 2001; 169: 155–64.

93. Fang JY, Cheng ZH, Chen YX et al. Expression of Dnmt1, demethylase, MeCP2 and methylation of tumor-related genes in human gastric cancer. World J Gastroenterol 2004; 10: 3394–8.

94. Marhold J, Zbylut M, Lankenau DH et al. Stage-specific chromosomal association of *Drosophila* dMBD2/3 during genome activation. Chromosoma 2002; 111: 13–21.

95. Mousseau TA, Fox CW, The adaptive significance of maternal effects. Trends Evol Ecol 1998; 13: 403–7.

96. Meaney MJ. The development of individual differences in behavioral and endocrine responses to stress. Annu Rev Neurosci 2001; 24: 1161–92.

Index

Note for users: Page references in **bold** refer to figures; those in *italic* refer to tables or boxed material